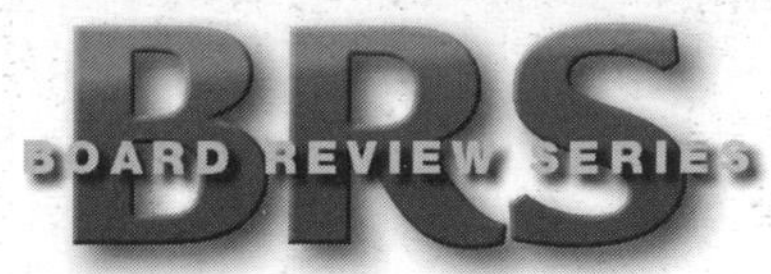

Gross Anatomy

EIGHTH EDITION

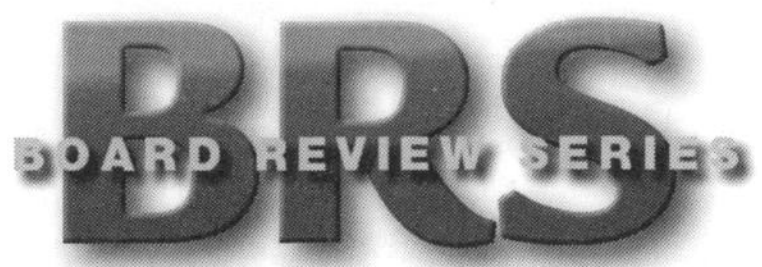

Gross Anatomy

EIGHTH EDITION

Kyung Won Chung, Ph.D.
David Ross Boyd Distinguished Professor Emeritus
Former Director, Medical Gross Anatomy
Department of Cell Biology, College of Medicine
University of Oklahoma Health Sciences Center
Oklahoma City, Oklahoma, USA

Harold M. Chung, M.D.
Associate Professor of Medicine
VCU Medical Center
Virginia Commonwealth University
Division of Hematology and Oncology
Bone Marrow Transplant Program
Director, Radioimmunotherapy Program
Richmond, Virginia, USA

Nancy L. Halliday, Ph.D.
Associate Professor
Codirector, Human Structure
Department of Cell Biology, College of Medicine
University of Oklahoma Health Sciences Center
Oklahoma City, Oklahoma, USA

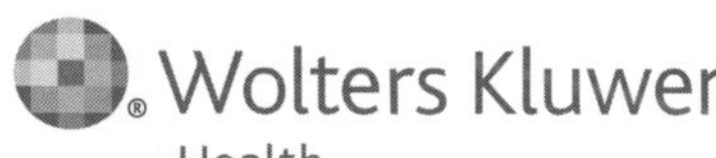

New Delhi • Philadelphia • Baltimore • New York
London • Buenos Aires • Hong Kong • Sydney • Tokyo

Eighth Edition

Two Commerce Square
2001 Market Street
Philadelphia, PA 19103

First Indian Reprint, 2016
Second Indian Reprint, 2017

Indian Reprint ISBN-13: 978-93-5129-595-2
Original ISBN-13: 978-1-4511-9307-7

Published by Wolters Kluwer (India) Pvt. Ltd., New Delhi

Printed and bound at Sanat Printers

To Young Hee, my wife, closest friend, and companion, for her love,
care, inspiration, and encouragement.
KWC

To Kathie, my wife, best friend, and soul partner, and to my daughters,
Kira, Liah, and Maia, for their love, support, and understanding.
HMC

To Frank, my husband and best friend, with love, respect,
and deep gratitude for his unwavering support and encouragement.
NLH

Preface

Anatomy is the science of studying and understanding the structure and organization of the body. The art of medicine requires a strong foundation in the basic medical sciences, and anatomy is a keystone in that foundation. This concise review of human anatomy is designed for medical, dental, graduate, physician associate, nursing, physical therapy, and other health science students. It is intended to help students prepare for the United States Medical Licensing Examination (USMLE), the National Board Dental Examination, as well as other board examinations for students in health-related professions. It presents the essentials of human anatomy in the form of condensed descriptions and simple illustrations. The text is concisely outlined with related board-type questions following each section. An attempt has been made to include all board-relevant information without introducing a vast amount of material or entangling students in a web of details. Even though this book is in summary form, its content presents key elements of the full-text version with abundant clinical information. However, it is not intended to be used as a primary textbook for a comprehensive study of difficult concepts and fundamentals.

CHANGE OF ORGANIZATION

The new eighth edition begins with a brief introduction to the skeletal, muscular, nervous, circulatory, and organ systems. The introductory chapter is followed by chapters on regional anatomy. These include the introduction, back, thorax, abdomen, perineum and pelvis, lower limb, upper limb, head and neck, and cranial and autonomic nerves of the head and neck. The cranial and autonomic nerves are separated from the head and neck chapter and are described more extensively with high-quality illustrations to facilitate thorough understanding of cranial and autonomic nerve functions and memory retention of information.

Once more, anatomy forms a foundation of clinical medicine and surgery and is a visual science of human structures. Thus, the success of learning and understanding largely depends on the quality of dissection and on clear, accurate illustrations. Many of the illustrations are simple schematic drawings, which are used to enhance the student's understanding of the descriptive text. A few of the illustrations are more complex, attempting to exhibit important anatomic relations. The considerable number of tables of muscles will prove particularly useful as a summary and review. In addition, the high-yield topics at the end of each chapter emphasize more important facts of anatomy and clinical medicine. These include numerous concise charts for the cranial nerves and their lesions, autonomic nerve functions, summary charts for muscle innervation and action, autonomic ganglia, and foramina of the skull and their contents in order to highlight pertinent aspects of the body system.

Test questions at the end of each chapter emphasize important information and lead to a better understanding of the material. These questions also serve as a self-evaluation to help the student uncover areas of weakness. Answers and explanations are provided after the questions.

FEATURES OF THE NEW EDITION

- **Illustrations and Extensive Medical Art**
  Illustrations play critical roles in assisting students to visualize anatomic structures, clarify difficult concepts, and help identify their functional and clinical characteristics. Some illustrations have been rearranged or redrawn, and many new figures and images have been incorporated. Furthermore, the addition of new illustrations reflects more artistic efforts, illuminates the beauty of the anatomical architecture of human tissues and organs, clarifies intricate concepts, enhances the quality and clarity of the images, and facilitates comprehension and quick recall of the text materials. Many new diagrams, line drawings, and angiograms are included in the text, aiding the process of learning and relating anatomic structures with their functional and clinical application.
- **Expanded and Updated Clinical Correlations**
  Clinical correlations emphasize the importance of anatomical knowledge by relating basic anatomy to actual medical practice. They are designed to challenge the student, enhance genuine understanding of anatomy, and encourage assimilation of information. The clinical correlates are set in boxes and placed at relevant locations in the text. Many clinical correlation boxes have been edited, updated, combined, or regrouped.
- **High-Yield Topics with End-of-Chapter Summaries**
  The high-yield topics with chapter summaries presented at the end of each chapter are one of the major feature changes of the new edition. These allow students to develop the anatomical knowledge base, problem-solving skills, critical thinking, and integration of essential anatomical and clinical problems and concepts. The high-yield topics help students learn and understand most efficiently, review and recall essential information quickly, reinforce key concepts, and highlight most likely tested materials in course examinations as well as the state and national board examinations.
- **Developmental Anatomy**
  The study of human embryology (normal development) and teratology (abnormal development) provides an important basis for the understanding of definitive human anatomy and is useful in guiding the students to apply the knowledge of human embryology to the clinical settings and problem-solving skills. Moreover, short summaries highlight the most important embryologic concepts in an effective, logical, and understandable way.
- **Review Test at the End of Each Chapter**
  The chapter review tests consist of questions and answers that reflect the guidelines set forth by the National Board of Medical Examiners and the current USMLE format. The questions reinforce the key information and test basic anatomic knowledge and the students' ability to interpret their observations and solve clinical problems. Therefore, clinically oriented questions and applications have been significantly increased because their fundamental utility is based on the relationship of anatomy to clinical medicine. More embryology questions are added and many test questions have been rewritten and updated. They are centered on a clinical situation that requires in-depth anatomic knowledge, problem-solving skills, and clinical applications. Expanded rationales for correct and incorrect answers are provided.

- **Comprehensive Examination**
  As before, the comprehensive examination is placed at the end of the book. It is useful in identifying specific knowledge deficits, filling the gaps in knowledge of clinical anatomy, and serving as an independent study, review resource, and self-assessment tool in preparation for the course final and state and national board examinations.

It is the authors' intention to invite feedback comments, constructive criticisms, and valuable suggestions from students and colleagues who choose this book as an aid to learning and teaching basic and clinical anatomy.

Kyung Won Chung
Harold M. Chung
Nancy L. Halliday

Acknowledgments

We express our sincere thanks to the many students, colleagues, and friends who have made valuable suggestions that have led to the improvement of the eighth edition. We are particularly grateful to John M. Chung, MD, for providing his invaluable criticism of the text and clinically oriented test questions as well as for his copy editing during the preparation phases of previous and current editions. Our grateful appreciation is also extended to Daniel O'Donoghue, PhD, for his encouragement, constructive criticism of the clinical notes, and helpful suggestions during the preparation of this new edition. Finally, we greatly appreciate and enjoy the privilege of working with the Wolters Kluwer staff, including Crystal Taylor, acquisitions editor; Dana Battaglia and Amy Weintraub, development editors; and Joy Fisher-Williams, marketing manager. We thank the staff for their constant guidance, enthusiasm, and unfailing support throughout the preparation, production, and completion of this new edition.

Contents

7. UPPER LIMB 273

8. HEAD AND NECK 337

chapter 1 Introduction

Studies of gross anatomy can be approached in several different ways, including systemic, regional, or clinical anatomy. **Systemic anatomy** is an approach to anatomic study organized by organ systems, such as the respiratory, digestive, or reproductive systems, which relates structure to function. **Regional anatomy** is an approach to anatomic study based on regions, and deals with structural relationships among the parts of the body, such as the thorax and abdomen, emphasizing the relationships among various systemic structures such as muscles, nerves, and blood vessels. Anatomy is best learned by emphasizing its connection to clinical medicine, and thus **clinical anatomy** emphasizes the practical application of anatomical knowledge to the solution of clinical problems and has real pertinence to the practice of medicine. In this introductory chapter, the systemic approach to the study of anatomy is used. In subsequent chapters, the clinical and regional approaches to the study of anatomy are used because many injuries and diseases involve specific body regions, and dissections and surgical procedures are performed region by region. In addition, clinical correlations are presented throughout the text.

SKELETAL SYSTEM

- Consists of the **axial skeleton** (bones of the head, vertebral column, ribs, and sternum) and the **appendicular skeleton** (bones of the extremities).

I. BONES

- Are calcified connective tissue consisting of cells (**osteocytes**) embedded in a matrix of ground substance and collagen fibers, have a superficial thin layer of **compact bone** around a central mass of **spongy bone**, and contain internal soft tissue, the **marrow**, where blood cells are formed.
- Serve as a **reservoir** for **calcium** and **phosphorus** and act as biomechanical **levers** on which muscles act to produce the movements permitted by joints.
- Are classified, according to shape, into long, short, flat, irregular, and sesamoid bones and, according to their developmental history, into endochondral and membranous bones.

A. Long Bones

- Include the humerus, radius, ulna, femur, tibia, fibula, metacarpals, and phalanges.
- Develop by replacement of hyaline cartilage plate (**endochondral ossification**).
- Have a shaft (**diaphysis**) and two ends (**epiphyses**). The **metaphysis** is a part of the diaphysis adjacent to the epiphyses.

1. Diaphysis

- Forms the **shaft** (central region) and is composed of a thick tube of **compact bone** that encloses the **marrow cavity**.

2. **Metaphysis**
   - Is a part of the diaphysis, the growth zone between the diaphysis and epiphysis during bone development.
3. **Epiphyses**
   - Are **expanded articular ends**, separated from the shaft by the epiphyseal plate during bone growth and composed of a **spongy bone** surrounded by a thin layer of **compact bone**.

B. Short Bones

- Include the carpal and tarsal bones and are approximately cuboid-shaped.
- Are composed of **spongy bone** and **marrow** surrounded by a thin outer layer of **compact bone**.

C. Flat Bones

- Include the ribs, sternum, scapulae, and bones in the vault of the skull.
- Consist of **two layers** of **compact bone** enclosing **spongy bone** and **marrow space** (**diploë**).
- Have articular surfaces that are covered with fibrocartilage and grow by the replacement of connective tissue.

D. Irregular Bones

- Include bones of mixed shapes such as bones of the skull, vertebrae, and coxa.
- Contain mostly **spongy bone** enveloped by a thin outer layer of **compact bone**.

E. Sesamoid Bones

- **Develop in** certain **tendons** and reduce friction on the tendon, thus protecting it from excessive wear.
- Are commonly found where tendons cross the ends of long bones in the limbs, as in the wrist and the knee (i.e., patella).

CLINICAL CORRELATES

Osteoblast synthesizes new bone and **osteoclast** functions in the resorption (break down bone matrix and release calcium and minerals) and remodeling of bone. Parathyroid hormone causes mobilization of calcium by promoting bone resorption, whereas calcitonin suppresses mobilization of calcium from bone. Osteoid is the organic matrix of bone prior to calcification.

Osteomalacia is a gradual softening of the bone due to failure of the bone to calcify because of lack of vitamin D or renal tubular dysfunction. **Osteopenia** is a decreased calcification of bone or a reduced bone mass due to an inadequate osteoid synthesis. **Osteoporosis** is an age-related disorder characterized by decreased bone mass and increased susceptibility to fractures of the hip, vertebra, and wrist. It occurs when bone resorption outpaces bone formation, since bone constantly undergoes cycles of resorption and formation (remodeling) to maintain the concentration of calcium and phosphate in the extracellular fluid. Signs of osteoporosis are vertebral compression, loss of body height, development of kyphosis, and hip fracture. **Osteopetrosis** is an abnormally dense bone, obliterating the marrow cavity, due to defective resorption of immature bone.

II. JOINTS

- Are places of union between two or more bones.
- Are innervated as follows: The nerve supplying a joint also supplies the muscles that move the joint and the skin covering the insertion of such muscles (**Hilton's law**).
- Are classified on the basis of their structural features into fibrous, cartilaginous, and synovial types.

A. Fibrous Joints (Synarthroses)

- Are joined by fibrous tissue, have **no joint cavities**, and permit little movement.

1. **Sutures**
   - Are connected by fibrous connective tissue and found between the flat bones of the skull.

2. **Syndesmoses**
   - Are connected by fibrous connective tissue.
   - Occur as the inferior tibiofibular and tympanostapedial syndesmoses.

B. Cartilaginous Joints

- Are united by **cartilage** and have **no joint cavity**.

1. **Primary Cartilaginous Joints (Synchondroses)**
   - Are united by **hyaline cartilage** and permit little to no movement but allow for growth in length during childhood and adolescence.
   - Include epiphyseal cartilage plates (the union between the epiphysis and the diaphysis of a growing bone) and sphenooccipital and manubriosternal synchondroses.
2. **Secondary Cartilaginous Joints (Symphyses)**
   - Are joined by **fibrocartilage** and are slightly movable joints.
   - Include the pubic symphysis and the intervertebral disks.

C. Synovial (Diarthrodial) Joints

- Permit a great degree of free movement and are classified according to the shape of the articulation and/or the type of movement.
- Are characterized by four features: joint cavity, articular (hyaline) cartilage, synovial membrane (which produces synovial fluid), and articular capsule.

1. **Plane (Gliding) Joints**
   - Are united by two flat articular surfaces and allow a simple **gliding** or sliding of one bone over the other.
   - Occur in the proximal tibiofibular, intertarsal, intercarpal, intermetacarpal, carpometacarpal, sternoclavicular, and acromioclavicular joints.
2. **Hinge (Ginglymus) Joints**
   - Resemble **door hinges** and allow only flexion and extension.
   - Occur in the elbow, ankle, and interphalangeal joints.
3. **Pivot (Trochoid) Joints**
   - Are formed by a central bony pivot turning within a bony ring and allow **only rotation** (movement around a single longitudinal axis).
   - Occur in the superior and inferior radioulnar joints and in the atlantoaxial joint.
4. **Condylar (Ellipsoidal) Joints**
   - Have two convex condyles articulating with two concave condyles. (The shape of the articulation is **ellipsoidal**.)
   - Allow flexion and extension and occur in the wrist (radiocarpal), metacarpophalangeal, knee (tibiofemoral), and atlantooccipital joints.
5. **Saddle (Sellar) Joints**
   - Resemble a **saddle** on a horse's back and allow flexion and extension, abduction and adduction, and circumduction but no axial rotation.
   - Occur in the carpometacarpal joint of the thumb and between the femur and patella.
6. **Ball-and-Socket (Spheroidal or Cotyloid) Joints**
   - Are formed by the reception of a globular (ball-like) head into a cup-shaped cavity and allow movement in many directions.
   - Allow flexion and extension, abduction and adduction, medial and lateral rotations, and circumduction, and occur in the shoulder and hip joints.

CLINICAL CORRELATES **Osteoarthritis** is a noninflammatory degenerative joint disease characterized by degeneration of the articular cartilage and osseous outgrowth at the margins. It results from wear and tear of the joints; commonly affects the hands, fingers, hips, knees, feet, and spine; and is accompanied by pain and stiffness. **Rheumatoid arthritis** is an inflammatory disease primarily of the joints. It is an autoimmune disease in which the immune system attacks the synovial membranes and articular structures, leading to deformities and disability. There is no cure for rheumatoid arthritis, and its most common symptoms are joint swelling, stiffness, and pain. **Gout** is a painful form of arthritis and is caused by too much uric acid in the blood. Uric acid crystals are deposited in and around the joints, causing inflammation and pain, heat, redness, stiffness, tenderness, and swelling of the joint tissues.

[...]LAR SYSTEM

I. MUSCLE

- Consists predominantly of **contractile cells**, produces the **movements** of various parts of the body by contraction, and occurs in three types:

A. Skeletal Muscle

- Is voluntary and striated; makes up approximately 40% of the total body mass; and functions to produce movement of the body, generate body heat, and maintain body posture.
- Has two attachments, an **origin** (which is usually the more fixed and proximal attachment) and an **insertion** (which is the more movable and distal attachment).
- Is enclosed by **epimysium**, a thin layer of connective tissue. Smaller bundles of muscle fibers are surrounded by **perimysium**. Each muscle fiber is enclosed by **endomysium**.

CLINICAL CORRELATES **Lou Gehrig disease** (amyotrophic lateral sclerosis) is a fatal neurologic disease that attacks the neurons responsible for controlling voluntary muscles. The muscles gradually weaken and atrophy; the brain is unable to control voluntary movement of the arms, legs, and body; and patients lose the ability to breath, swallow, and speak. The earliest symptoms may include cramping, twitching, and muscle weakness.

B. Cardiac Muscle

- Is involuntary and striated and forms the **myocardium**, the middle layer of the heart.
- Is innervated by the autonomic nervous system (ANS) but contracts spontaneously without any nerve supply.
- Includes specialized myocardial fibers that form the cardiac **conducting system**.

C. Smooth Muscle

- Is involuntary and nonstriated and generally arranged in two layers, **circular** and **longitudinal**, in the walls of many visceral organs.
- Is innervated by the ANS, regulating the size of the lumen of a tubular structure.
- Undergoes rhythmic contractions called **peristaltic waves** in the walls of the gastrointestinal (GI) tract, uterine tubes, ureters, and other organs.

II. STRUCTURES ASSOCIATED WITH MUSCLES

A. Tendons

- Are **fibrous bands** of dense connective tissue that **connect muscles to bones** or cartilage.
- Are supplied by sensory fibers extending from muscle nerves.

B. Ligaments

- Are **fibrous bands** that **connect bones to bones** or cartilage or are folds of peritoneum serving to support visceral structures.

C. Raphe

- Is the line of union of symmetrical structures by a fibrous or tendinous band such as the pterygomandibular, pharyngeal, and scrotal raphes.

D. Aponeuroses

- Are **flat fibrous sheets** or expanded broad tendons that attach to muscles and serve as the means of origin or insertion of a flat muscle.

E. Retinaculum

- Is a fibrous band that holds a structure in place in the region of joints.

F. Bursae

- Are fluid-filled **flattened sacs of synovial membrane** that facilitate movement by minimizing friction.

G. Synovial Tendon Sheaths

- Are synovial fluid-filled **tubular sacs** around **muscle tendons** that facilitate movement by reducing friction.

H. Fascia

- Is a **fibrous sheet** that envelops the body under the skin and invests the muscles and may limit the spread of pus and extravasated fluids such as urine and blood.

1. Superficial Fascia

- Is a loose connective tissue between the dermis and the deep (investing) fascia and has a **fatty superficial layer** (fat, cutaneous vessels, nerves, lymphatics, and glands) and a **membranous deep layer**.

2. Deep Fascia

- Is a sheet of fibrous tissue that **invests the muscles** and helps support them by serving as an elastic sheath or stocking.
- Provides origins or insertions for muscles, forms fibrous sheaths or retinacula for tendons, and forms potential pathways for infection or extravasation of fluids.

NERVOUS SYSTEM

I. NERVOUS SYSTEM

- Is divided anatomically into the central nervous system (CNS), consisting of the brain and spinal cord, and the peripheral nervous system (PNS), consisting of 12 pairs of cranial nerves and 31 pairs of spinal nerves, and their associated ganglia.
- Is divided functionally into the **somatic** nervous system, which controls primarily voluntary activities, and the **visceral (autonomic)** nervous system, which controls primarily involuntary activities.
- Is composed of **neurons** and **neuroglia** (nonneuronal cells such as astrocytes, oligodendrocytes, and microglia) and controls and integrates the body activity.

II. NEURONS

- Are the structural and functional units of the nervous system (neuron doctrine).
- Are specialized for the reception, integration, transformation, and transmission of information.

A. Components of Neurons

1. Cell bodies are located in the gray matter of the CNS, and their collections are called ganglia in the PNS and nuclei in the CNS.
2. Dendrites (dendron means "tree") are usually short and highly branched and carry impulses toward the cell body.
3. Axons are usually single and long, have fewer branches (collaterals), and carry impulses away from the cell body.

B. Classification of Neurons

1. Unipolar (Pseudounipolar) Neurons

- Have **one process**, which divides into a central branch that functions as an axon and a peripheral branch that serves as a dendrite.

called pseudounipolar because they were originally bipolar, but their two processes fuse ing development to form a single process that bifurcates at a distance from the cell body. ensory neurons of the PNS and found in spinal and cranial nerve ganglia.

2. Bipolar Neurons

- Have **two processes** (one dendrite and one axon), are sensory, and are found in the olfactory epithelium, the retina, and the inner ear.

3. Multipolar Neurons

- Have **several dendrites** and **one axon** and are most common in the CNS (e.g., motor cells in anterior and lateral horns of the spinal cord, autonomic ganglion cells).

C. Ganglion

- Is a collection of neuron cell bodies **outside the CNS**, and a **nucleus** is a collection of neuron cell bodies **within the CNS**.

D. Other Components of the Nervous System

1. Cells That Support Neurons

- Include **Schwann cells** and **satellite cells** in the PNS.
- Are called **neuroglia** in the CNS and are composed mainly of three types: **astrocytes; oligodendrocytes,** which play a role in myelin formation and transport of material to neurons; and **microglia**, which phagocytose waste products of nerve tissue.

2. Myelin

- Is the fatlike substance forming a sheath around certain nerve fibers.
- Is formed by **Schwann cells in the PNS** and **oligodendrocytes in the CNS**.

3. Synapses

- Are the **sites of functional contact** of a neuron with another neuron, an effector (muscle, gland) cell, or a sensory receptor cell.
- Are classified by the site of contact as axodendritic, axoaxonic, or axosomatic.
- Subserve the transmission of nerve impulses, commonly from the axon terminals (presynaptic elements) to the plasma membranes (postsynaptic elements) of the receiving cell.

III. CENTRAL NERVOUS SYSTEM

A. Brain

- Is enclosed within the cranium, or the brain case.
- Has a **cortex**, which is the **outer part** of the cerebral hemispheres, and is composed of **gray matter**. This matter consists largely of the **nerve cell bodies**, dendrites, and neuroglia.
- Has an interior part composed of **white matter**, which consists largely of **axons** forming tracts or pathways, and ventricles, which are filled with cerebrospinal fluid (CSF).

B. Spinal Cord

- Is **cylindrical**, occupies approximately the upper two-thirds of the vertebral canal, and is enveloped by the meninges.
- Has cervical and lumbar enlargements for the nerve supply of the upper and lower limbs.
- Has centrally located **gray matter**, in contrast to the cerebral hemispheres, and peripherally located **white matter**.
- Grows more slowly than the vertebral column during fetal development, and hence, its terminal end gradually shifts to a higher level.
- Has a conical end known as the **conus medullaris** and ends at the level of L2 (or between L1 and L2) in the adult and at the level of L3 in the newborn.

C. Meninges

- Consist of three layers of connective tissue membranes (**pia**, **arachnoid**, and **dura mater**) that surround and protect the brain and the spinal cord.
- Contain the **subarachnoid space**, which is the interval between the arachnoid and pia mater, filled with CSF.

D. Cerebrospinal Fluid

- Is produced by vascular choroid plexuses in the brain ventricles and found in the ventricle and subarachnoid space.

CLINICAL CORRELATES Multiple sclerosis (MS) is a nervous system disease that causes **destruction of myelin** in the spinal cord and brain, leading to sensory disorders and muscle weakness. Signs and symptoms include numbness or tingling, visual disturbances (swelling of the optic nerve), cognitive impairments, muscle weakness, difficulty with coordination and balance, slurred speech, bladder incontinence, fatigue, depression, and memory problems. MS may be caused by a virus, a gene defect, or an autoimmune disease, in which the immune system **attacks the myelin around axons in the CNS,** thereby disrupting the conduction of nerve signals along the axons. MS affects women more than men.

IV. PERIPHERAL NERVOUS SYSTEM

A. Cranial Nerves

- Consist of **12 pairs** and are connected to the brain rather than to the spinal cord.
- Have motor fibers with cell bodies located within the CNS and sensory fibers with cell bodies that form sensory ganglia located outside the CNS.
- Emerge from the ventral aspect of the brain (except for the trochlear nerve, cranial nerve IV).
- Contain all four functional components of the spinal nerves and three additional components (see Nervous System: IV. C; Nerves of the Head and Neck: Chapter 8).

B. Spinal Nerves (Figure 1.1)

- Consist of **31 pairs**: 8 cervical, 12 thoracic, 5 lumbar, 5 sacral, and 1 coccygeal.

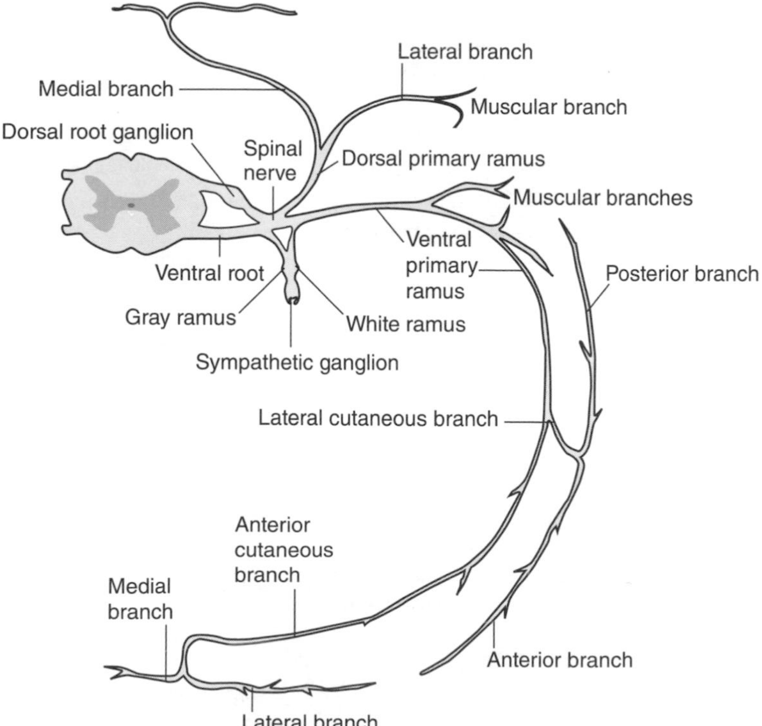

FIGURE 1.1. Typical spinal nerve (anterior = ventral; posterior = dorsal).

- Are formed from dorsal and ventral roots; each dorsal root has a ganglion that is within the intervertebral foramen.
- Are connected with the sympathetic chain ganglia by **rami communicantes.**
- Contain sensory fibers with cell bodies in the dorsal root ganglion (general somatic afferent [GSA] and general visceral afferent [GVA] fibers), motor fibers with cell bodies in the anterior horn of the spinal cord (general somatic efferent [GSE] fibers), and motor fibers with cell bodies in the lateral horn of the spinal cord (general visceral efferent [GVE] fibers) between T1 and L2.
- Are divided into the **ventral and dorsal primary rami**. The ventral primary rami enter into the formation of plexuses (i.e., cervical, brachial, and lumbosacral); the dorsal primary rami innervate the skin and deep muscles of the back.

C. Functional Components in Peripheral Nerves (Figures 1.2 and 1.3)

1. General Somatic Afferent Fibers

- Transmit pain, temperature, touch, and proprioception from the body to the CNS.

2. General Somatic Efferent Fibers

- Carry motor impulses to the skeletal muscles of the body.

3. General Visceral Afferent Fibers

- Convey sensory impulses from visceral organs to the CNS.

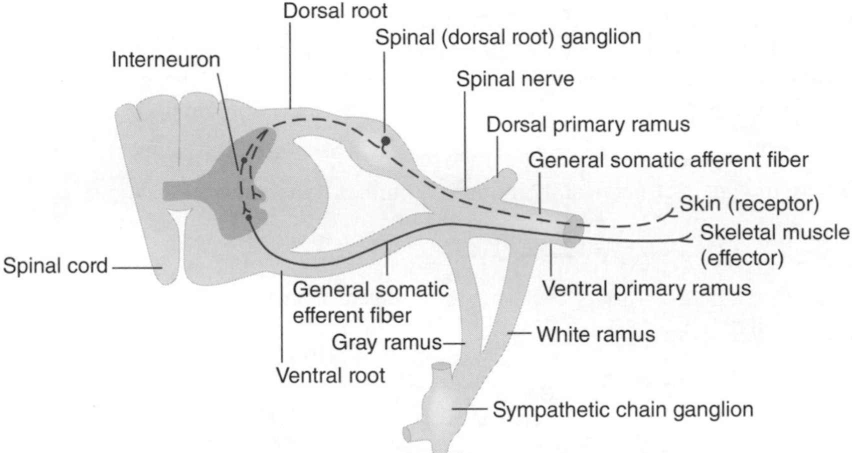

FIGURE 1.2. General somatic afferent and efferent nerves.

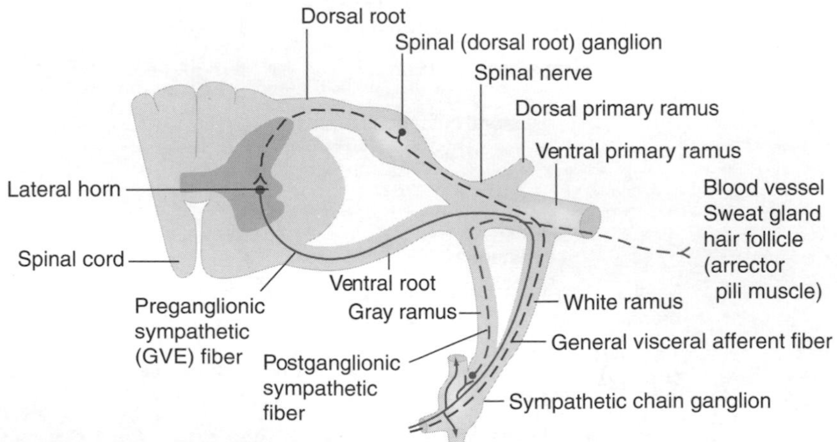

FIGURE 1.3. General visceral efferent (autonomic) and afferent nerves.

4. **General Visceral Efferent Fibers (Autonomic Nerves)**
   - Transmit motor impulses to smooth muscle, cardiac muscle, and glandular tissues.
5. **Special Somatic Afferent Fibers**
   - Convey special sensory impulses of vision, hearing, and equilibration to the CNS.
6. **Special Visceral Afferent Fibers**
   - Transmit smell and taste sensations to the CNS.
7. **Special Visceral Efferent Fibers**
   - Conduct motor impulses to the muscles of the head and neck.
   - Arise from branchiomeric structures such as muscles for mastication, muscles for facial expression, and muscles for elevation of the pharynx and movement of the larynx.

V. AUTONOMIC NERVOUS SYSTEM

- Is responsible for the motor innervation of smooth muscle, cardiac muscle, and glands of the body. It is divided into the **sympathetic** (thoracolumbar outflow), **parasympathetic** (craniosacral outflow), and **enteric divisions**.
- Is composed of two neurons, preganglionic and postganglionic, which are GVE neurons. It has **cholinergic** fibers (sympathetic preganglionic, parasympathetic pre- and postganglionic) and **adrenergic** fibers (sympathetic postganglionic) except those to sweat glands (cholinergic).
- **Preganglionic neurons** with cell bodies are located **in the CNS**, whereas **postganglionic neurons** with cell bodies are in ganglia **in the PNS**.

A. Sympathetic Nerve Fibers (See Figure 1.3)

- Have preganglionic nerve cell bodies that are located in the lateral horn of the thoracic and upper lumbar levels (L2 or L1–L3) of the spinal cord.
- Have **preganglionic fibers** that pass through ventral roots, spinal nerves, and white rami communicantes. These fibers enter adjacent sympathetic chain ganglia, where they synapse or travel up or down the chain to synapse in remote ganglia or run further through the splanchnic nerves to synapse in collateral ganglia, located along the major abdominal blood vessels.
- Have **postganglionic fibers** from the chain ganglia that return to spinal nerves by way of gray rami communicantes and supply the skin with secretory fibers to sweat glands, motor fibers to smooth muscles of the hair follicles (arrectores pilorum), and vasomotor fibers to the blood vessels.
- Function primarily in **emergencies** or catabolism (energy consumption), preparing individuals for **fight** or **flight**, and thus increase the heart rate, inhibit GI motility and secretion, and dilate pupils and bronchial lumen. They liberate norepinephrine (except sweat glands) and are classified as adrenergic.

B. Parasympathetic Nerve Fibers

- Comprise the preganglionic fibers that arise from the brain stem (cranial nerves III, VII, IX, and X) and sacral part of the spinal cord (second, third, and fourth sacral segments).
- Are, with few exceptions, characterized by **long preganglionic fibers** and **short postganglionic fibers**.
- Are distributed to the walls of the visceral organs and glands of the digestive system but not to the skin or to the periphery.
- Decrease the heart rate, increase GI peristalsis, and stimulate secretory activity.
- Function primarily in **homeostasis** or anabolism (energy conservation), tending to promote quiet and orderly processes of the body. They liberate acetylcholine and are classified as cholinergic.

C. Enteric Division

- Consists of enteric ganglia (parasympathetic postganglionic neuron cell bodies) and plexus of the GI tract, including the myenteric (Auerbach's) and submucosal (Meissner's) plexuses.
- Plays an important role in the control of GI motility and secretion.

Functions of Autonomic Nerves

Organs	Sympathetic Nerve	Parasympathetic Nerve
Eyes	Dilates pupil	Constricts pupil; contracts ciliary muscle to thicken lens
Lacrimal gland	Slightly reduces secretion	Promotes secretion
Salivary gland	Reduces secretion and more viscid	Increases secretion and watery
Sweat gland	Stimulates secretion	No effect
Blood vessels	Constricts	No effect
Heart	Increases rate and ventricular contraction; dilates coronary vessels	Decreases rate and ventricular contraction; constricts coronary vessels
Bronchi	Dilates lumen; reduces bronchial secretion	Constricts lumen; promotes secretion
GI tract	Inhibits motility and secretion; constricts sphincters	Stimulates motility and secretion; relaxes sphincters
Liver	Promotes glycogen breakdown	Promotes glycogen formation and bile secretion
Suprarenal medulla	Secretes epinephrine and norepinephrine	No effect
Kidney	Reduces urine formation by constriction of renal vessels	May cause vasodilation of renal vascular bed
Urinary bladder	Contracts sphincter vesicae	Relaxes sphincter vesicae; contracts detrusor muscle, causing urination
Genital organs	Causes vasoconstriction and ejaculation; contracts uterus	Causes vasodilation and erection; relaxes uterus

CIRCULATORY SYSTEM

I. VASCULAR SYSTEM

- Functions to transport vital materials such as **oxygen**, **nutrients**, and **waste products**, including carbon dioxide, hormones, defense elements, and cells involved in wound healing.
- Consists of the **heart** and **vessels** (arteries, capillaries, veins) that transport blood through all parts of the body.
- Includes the **lymphatic vessels**, a set of channels that begin in the tissue spaces and return excess tissue fluid to the bloodstream.

A. Circulatory Loops

1. Pulmonary Circulation

- Transports blood from the right ventricle through the pulmonary arteries to the lungs for the exchange of oxygen and carbon dioxide and returns it to the left atrium of the heart through the pulmonary veins.

2. Systemic Circulation

- Transports blood from the left ventricle through the aorta to all parts of the body and returns it to the right atrium through the superior and inferior venae cavae and the cardiac veins.

B. Heart

- Is a hollow, muscular, four-chambered organ that **pumps blood to** two separate circulatory loops, the **pulmonary circulation** and the **systemic circulation**.
- Is regulated in its pumping rate and strength by the ANS, which controls a **pacemaker** (i.e., sinoatrial node).
- Receives oxygenated blood from the right and left coronary arteries, which arise from the ascending aorta.

C. Blood Vessels

- Carry blood to the lungs, where carbon dioxide is exchanged for oxygen.
- Carry blood to the intestines, where nutritive materials in fluid form are absorbed, and to the endocrine glands, where hormones pass through the vessel walls and are distributed to target cells.
- Transport the waste products of tissue fluid to the kidneys, intestines, lungs, and skin, where they are excreted.
- Are of four types: arteries, veins, capillaries, and sinusoids.

1. Arteries

- Carry blood from the heart to the capillary beds and have thicker walls than do veins.
- Consist of three main types: **elastic** arteries, **muscular** arteries, and **arterioles**.

2. Capillaries

- Are composed of endothelium and its basement membrane and connect the arterioles to the venules.
- Are the **sites for the exchange** of carbon dioxide, oxygen, nutrients, and waste products between the tissues and the blood.
- Are absent in the cornea, epidermis, and hyaline cartilage and may be absent in some areas where the arterioles and venules have direct connections (**arteriovenous anastomoses** or **shunts**), which may occur in the skin of the nose, lips, fingers, and ears, where they conserve body heat.

CLINICAL CORRELATES

Aneurysm is a circumscribed dilation of the wall of an artery or the heart and is caused by a weakness of the arterial wall, an atherosclerosis (accumulation of fat, cholesterol, and calcium which form plaque in the arterial wall), or high blood pressure, giving a greater risk of rupture.

Atherosclerosis is a **narrowing** of the artery because of plaque formation by fat, cholesterol, and calcium deposits in the arterial walls. Narrowing and blockage of arteries in the brain cause **stroke**, and narrowed and blocked coronary arteries lead to **heart attacks** (myocardial infarctions).

Arteriosclerosis is a thickening and **hardening** of the arterial walls with resulting loss of elasticity. It may be caused by fibrosis and calcification of the arterial walls and develops with aging, high blood pressure, diabetes, and other conditions.

Varicose veins are enlarged and tortuous veins that develop most commonly in the superficial veins of the lower limb because of reduced elasticity and incompetent valves in the veins or thrombophlebitis of the deep veins.

3. Veins

- Return blood to the heart from the capillary beds and consist of the **pulmonary veins**, which return oxygenated blood to the heart from the lungs, and the **systemic veins**, which return deoxygenated blood to the heart from the rest of the body.
- Contain valves that prevent the reflux of blood and have **venae comitantes** that closely accompany muscular arteries in the limbs.

4. Sinusoids

- Are wider and more irregular than capillaries and substitute for capillaries in some organs, such as the liver, spleen, red bone marrow, adenohypophysis, suprarenal cortex, and parathyroid glands.
- Often contain phagocytic cells on their walls and form a part of the **reticuloendothelial system**, which is concerned chiefly with phagocytosis and antibody formation.

5. Portal System

- Is a system of vessels in which blood collected from one capillary network passes through a large vessel(s) and then a second capillary network before it returns to the systemic circulation.
- Consists of the **hepatic portal system** in which blood from the intestinal capillary bed passes through the hepatic portal vein and then hepatic capillaries (sinusoids) to the hepatic veins and the **hypophyseal portal system** in which blood from the hypothalamic capillaries passes through the hypophyseal portal veins and then the pituitary capillary sinusoids to the hypophyseal veins.

II. LYMPHATIC SYSTEM

- Provides an important **immune mechanism** for the body.
- Is involved in the **metastasis** of cancer cells and provides a route for transporting fat and large protein molecules absorbed from the intestine to the thoracic duct.

A. Lymphatic Vessels

- Serve as one-way drainage toward the heart and return lymph to the bloodstream through the **thoracic duct** (the largest lymphatic vessel) or the right lymphatic duct.
- Are not usually visible in dissections but are the major route by which cancer metastasizes.
- Function to **absorb large protein molecules** and transport them to the bloodstream because the molecules cannot pass through the walls of the blood capillaries back into the blood.
- Carry lymphocytes from lymphatic tissues to the bloodstream.
- Have valves, which are constricted at the sites of valves, showing a beaded appearance.
- Are absent in the brain, spinal cord, eyeballs, bone marrow, splenic pulp, hyaline cartilage, nails, and hair.

B. Lymphatic Capillaries

- Begin blindly in most tissues, collect tissue fluid, and join to form large collecting vessels that pass to regional lymph nodes.
- **Absorb lymph** from tissue spaces and transport it back to the venous system.
- Are called **lacteals** in the villi of the small intestine, where they absorb emulsified fat.

C. Lymph Nodes

- Are organized collections of lymphatic tissue permeated by lymph channels.
- Produce **lymphocytes** and **plasma cells** and **filter the lymph**.
- Trap **bacteria** drained from an infected area and contain reticuloendothelial cells and **phagocytic cells** (macrophages) that ingest these bacteria.
- Are hard and often palpable when there is a metastasis and are enlarged and tender during infection.

D. Lymph

- Is a clear, watery fluid that is collected from the intercellular spaces.
- Contains no cells until lymphocytes are added in its passage through the lymph nodes. Its constituents are similar to those of blood plasma (e.g., proteins, fats, lymphocytes).
- Often contains fat droplets (called **chyle**) when it comes from intestinal organs.
- Is filtered by passing through several lymph nodes before entering the venous system.

ORGAN SYSTEMS

I. DIGESTIVE SYSTEM

- Consists of three divisions including the **mouth**, the **pharynx**, and the **alimentary canal**, comprising the esophagus, the stomach, the small intestine, and the large intestine.
- Performs specific functions: essential food-processing activities. In the mouth, the food is moistened by saliva; is masticated and mixed by the mandible, teeth, and tongue; and is propelled by the pharynx and esophagus into the stomach, where it is mixed with the gastric juice and converted into chyme.
- Performs specific functions: in the **small intestine**, the food or chyme is **digested** by secretions from glands in the intestinal wall and from the liver, gallbladder, and pancreas; digested end products are **absorbed** into the blood and lymph capillaries in the intestinal wall.
- Performs specific functions: in the **large intestine**, **water** and **electrolytes** are **absorbed** and the waste products are transported to the rectum and anal canal, where they are eliminated as feces.

II. RESPIRATORY SYSTEM

- Consists of a **conducting portion** and a **respiratory portion**. Air is transported to the lungs through the conducting portion, which comprises the nose, nasal cavity and paranasal sinuses, pharynx, larynx, trachea, and bronchi. As the air passes through these organs, it is filtered, humidified, and warmed by their mucous membranes.
- Consists of a respiratory portion: the **lungs**, which contain the terminal air sacs, or **alveoli**, where **exchange occurs** between oxygen in the air and carbon dioxide in the blood with the aid of the diaphragm and thoracic cage.
- Is concerned with speech, which involves the intermittent release of exhaled air and the opening and closing of the glottis.

III. URINARY SYSTEM

- Comprises the **kidneys**, which remove wastes from the blood and produce the urine; the **ureters**, which carry urine from the kidney to the urinary bladder; the **bladder**, which stores urine; and the **urethra**, which drains urine from the bladder and conveys it out of the body.
- Contains the kidneys, which are important in maintaining the body water and electrolyte balance and the acid–base balance, in regulating the urine volume and composition and the blood volume and blood pressure, and in eliminating waste products from the blood.

IV. REPRODUCTIVE SYSTEM

A. Male Reproductive System

- Consists of (a) the **testes**, which produce **spermatozoa** and sex hormones; (b) a system of ducts, through which spermatozoa travel from the testis to reach the exterior; (c) various glands such as the seminal vesicles, prostate gland, and bulbourethral glands, which contribute secretions to the seminal fluid; and (d) the urethrae, which pass the ejaculate to an opening at the tip of the external genital organ, the penis.
- Has **ducts**: leading from each testis are the duct of the epididymis, the ductus deferens, and the ejaculatory duct, which opens into the urethra.
- Has **glands**: the prostate, the seminal vesicles, and the bulbourethral glands, all of which secrete into the urethra.

B. Female Reproductive System

- Consists of ovaries, uterine tubes, uterus, vagina, and external genital organs. The **ovaries** produce **oocytes** (ova or eggs) that are conveyed from the ovaries through the uterine tubes to the cavity of the uterus and also produce the steroid hormones. Each ovulated oocyte is released into the peritoneal cavity of the pelvis; one of the uterine tubes captures the oocyte by the fimbriae, where it begins its journey toward the uterus. The **uterine tubes** transmit spermatozoa in the opposite direction, and **fertilization** of an oocyte usually occurs within the expanded **ampulla** of a uterine tube. A fertilized oocyte becomes embedded in the wall of the uterus, where it develops and grows into a fetus, which passes through the uterus and vagina (together called the birth canal). The **vagina** provides a passage for delivery of an infant; it also receives the penis and semen during sexual intercourse.
- Includes female external genitalia: the **mons pubis**, which is a fatty eminence anterior to the symphysis pubis; the **labia majora**, which are two large folds of skin; the **labia minora**, which are two smaller skin folds, commence at the glans clitoris, lack hair, and contain no fat; the **vestibule**, which is an entrance of the vagina between the two labia minora and has the hymen at the vaginal orifice; and the **clitoris**, which is composed largely of erectile tissue, has crura, body, and glans (head), and is hooded by the prepuce of the clitoris.

V. ENDOCRINE SYSTEM

- Is a series of ductless or endocrine glands that secrete messenger molecules called **hormones** directly into the blood circulation and are carried to body cells.
- **Controls** and **integrates** the **functions** of other organ systems and plays a very important role in reproduction, growth, and metabolism, which are slower processes than the rapid processes of the nervous system.
- Comprises pure endocrine organs such as the pituitary, pineal, thyroid, parathyroid, and suprarenal glands; other endocrine cells are contained in the pancreas, thymus, gonads, hypothalamus, kidneys, liver, and stomach.
- Includes **tropic hormones**, which affect other organs and regulate the functional states of other endocrine glands and control a variety of physiologic responses.

VI. INTEGUMENTARY

- Consists of the skin (integument) and its appendages, including sweat glands, sebaceous glands, hair, and nails.
- Contains sense organs called **sensory receptors** associated with nerve endings for pain, temperature, touch, and pressure.

A. Skin

- Is the largest organ of the body and consists of the **epidermis**, a superficial layer of stratified epithelium that develops from ectoderm, and the **dermis**, a deeper layer of connective tissue that develops largely from mesoderm. The dermis contains downgrowths from the epidermis, such as hairs and glands, and the epidermis is an avascular keratinized layer of stratified squamous epithelium that is thickest on the palms and the soles. Just deep to the skin lies a fatty layer called the **hypodermis**.
- Not only is a protective layer and an extensive sensory organ but also is significant in body temperature regulation, production of vitamin D, and absorption.

B. Appendages of the Skin

- Have the **sweat glands** that develop as epidermal downgrowths, have the excretory functions of the body, and regulate body temperature; have the **sebaceous glands** that develop from the epidermis (as downgrowths from hair follicles into the dermis) and empty into hair follicles, and their oily sebum provides a lubricant to the hair and skin and protects the skin from drying; have **hairs** that develop as epidermal downgrowths, and their functions include protection, regulation of body temperature, and facilitation of evaporation of perspiration; and have **nails** that develop as epidermal thickenings and that protect the sensitive tips of the digits.

HIGH-YIELD TOPICS

- **Axial skeleton** includes the skull, vertebral column, ribs, and sternum.
- **Bones** serve as a **reservoir for calcium and phosphorus** and act as biomechanical levers on which muscles act to produce the movements.
- **Long bones** have a shaft **(diaphysis)** and two ends **(epiphyses)**. The **metaphysis** is a part of the diaphysis, the **growth zone** between the diaphysis and epiphysis during bone development.
- **Sesamoid bones** develop in certain tendons and reduce friction on the tendon.
- **Osteoblast** synthesizes new bone and **osteoclast** functions in the resorption and remodeling of bone.

- **Osteomalacia** is a gradual softening of the bone due to failure of the bone to calcify. **Osteopenia** is a decreased calcification of bone or a reduced bone mass.
- **Osteoporosis** is an age-related disorder characterized by decreased bone mass and increased susceptibility to factures. It occurs when bone resorption outpaces bone formation.
- **Osteopetrosis** is an abnormally dense bone, obliterating the marrow cavity, due to defective resorption of immature bone.
- The nerve supplying a joint also supplies the muscles that move the joint and the skin covering the insertion of such muscles **(Hilton's law).**
- **Osteoarthritis** is a noninflammatory degenerative joint disease characterized by degeneration of the articular cartilage and osseous outgrowth at the margins.
- **Rheumatoid arthritis** is an inflammatory disease of the joints. It is an autoimmune disease in which the immune system attacks the synovial membranes and articular structures, leading to deformities and disability.
- **Gout** is a painful form of arthritis and is caused by too much uric acid in the blood. Uric acid crystals are deposited in and around the joints, causing inflammation and pain, stiffness, and swelling of the joint tissues.
- **Lou Gehrig disease (amyotrophic lateral sclerosis)** is a fatal neurologic disease that attacks the neurons responsible for controlling voluntary muscles. The **muscles gradually weaken and atrophy;** the brain is unable to control voluntary movement of the body; and patients lose the ability to breath, swallow, and speak.
- **Nervous system** is divided into the central nervous system (**CNS**), consisting of the brain and spinal cord, and the peripheral nervous system (**PNS**), consisting of 12 pairs of cranial nerves and 31 pairs of spinal nerves, and their associated ganglia. It is divided functionally into the somatic and visceral (autonomic) nervous system.
- **Ganglion is a collection of neuron cell bodies outside the CNS,** and the **nucleus is a collection of neuron cell bodies within the CNS.**
- **Neurons** in cranial or spinal ganglia are **unipolar (pseudounipolar)** types.
- **Axons carry impulses away from the cell body,** whereas the **dendrites carry impulses toward the cell body.**
- **Myelin** is the fatlike substance forming a sheath around certain nerve fibers and is formed by **Schwann cells in the PNS** and **oligodendrocytes in the CNS.**
- Autonomic nervous system (**ANS**) is responsible for the motor innervation of smooth muscle, cardiac muscle, and glands, and is divided into the sympathetic, parasympathetic, and enteric divisions. Preganglionic neurons with cell bodies are in the CNS, and postganglionic neurons with cell bodies are in ganglia in the PNS. ANS consists of **cholinergic** fibers (sympathetic preganglionic, parasympathetic pre- and postganglionic) and **adrenergic** fibers (sympathetic postganglionic) except those to **sweat glands (cholinergic).**
- **Sympathetic nervous system** functions in **emergencies** or catabolism (energy consumption), preparing for fight or flight, whereas the parasympathetic nerve functions in homeostasis or anabolism (energy conservation), tending to promote quiet and orderly processes of the body.
- **C**erebrospinal fluid is produced by vascular choroid plexuses in the brain ventricles and found in the subarachnoid space.
- Multiple sclerosis (**MS**) is a nervous system disease that causes **destruction of myelin in the CNS** (spinal cord and brain), leading to sensory disorders and muscle weakness. Symptoms also include numbness, visual and cognitive impairments, loss of coordination and balance, slurred speech, bladder incontinence, fatigue, and depression.
- **Coronary arteries** arise from the ascending aorta and supply blood to the **heart.**
- **Portal venous system** consists of the **hepatic portal system** in which blood from the intestinal capillary bed passes through the hepatic portal vein and then hepatic capillaries (sinusoids) to the hepatic veins, and the **hypophyseal portal system** in which blood from the hypothalamic capillaries passes through the hypophyseal portal veins and then the pituitary capillary sinusoids to the hypophyseal veins.
- **Varicose veins** are dilated veins that develop in the superficial veins of the lower limb because of reduced elasticity and incompetent valves in the veins or thrombophlebitis of the deep veins.
- **Aneurysm** is a circumscribed dilation of the wall of an artery or the heart and caused by a **weakness of the arterial wall,** an atherosclerosis (accumulation of fat, cholesterol, and calcium which form plaque in the arterial wall), or high blood pressure, giving a greater risk of rupture.

- **Atherosclerosis** is a **narrowing** of the artery because of fatty **plaque** formation in the arterial wall. Narrowing and blockage of arteries in the brain cause **stroke,** and narrowed and blocked coronary arteries lead to **heart attacks. Arteriosclerosis** is a thickening and **hardening** of the arterial wall.
- **Lymphatic system** provides an important immune mechanism, is involved in the metastasis of cancer cells, and provides a route for transporting fat and large protein molecules.
- **Thoracic duct** begins in the abdomen at the cisterna chili, drains the lower limbs, pelvis, abdomen, left thorax, left upper limb, and left side of the head and neck, and empties into the junction of the left internal jugular and subclavian veins.
- **Right lymphatic duct** drains the right sides of the thorax, upper limb, head, and neck, and empties into the junction of the right internal jugular and subclavian veins.
- **Lymph nodes** are organized collections of lymphatic tissue and are an important part of the immune system. Lymph nodes are the main source of lymphocytes of the peripheral blood, play a role in antibody production, and as part of the reticuloendothelial system, serve as a defense mechanism by removing noxious agents, such as bacteria and toxins.

Review Test

Directions: Each of the numbered items or incomplete statements in this section is followed by answers or by completions of the statement. Select the **one-**lettered answer or completion that is **best** in each case.

1. A 22-year-old man presented to his family physician with a laceration of the fibrous sheets or bands that cover his body under the skin and invest the muscles. Which of the following structures would most likely be injured?

(A) Tendon
(B) Fascia
(C) Synovial tendon sheath
(D) Aponeurosis
(E) Ligament

2. On the basis of the examination at her doctor's office, a patient is told that her parasympathetic nerves are damaged. Which of the following muscles would most likely be affected?

(A) Muscles in the hair follicles
(B) Muscles in blood vessels
(C) Muscles that act at the elbow joint
(D) Muscles in the gastrointestinal (GI) tract
(E) Muscles enclosed by epimysium

3. A 46-year-old male patient with high blood pressure was examined in the emergency department, and his physician found a leakage of blood from the blood vessel that normally carries richly oxygenated blood. Which of the following vessels would most likely be damaged?

(A) Superior vena cava
(B) Pulmonary arteries
(C) Pulmonary veins
(D) Portal vein
(E) Coronary sinus

4. A 16-year-old patient received a stab wound, and axons of the general somatic efferent (GSE) neurons to the shoulder muscles were severed. The damaged axons:

(A) Would carry impulses toward the cell bodies
(B) Would carry impulses away from the cell bodies
(C) Would carry pain impulses
(D) Are several in numbers for multipolar neurons
(E) Are found primarily in the gray matter

5. A 16-year-old patient received a laceration of the posterior intercostal nerves by a penetrated knife blade. A pathologist obtained needle biopsy tissues and observed numerous degenerated cell bodies of the unipolar or pseudounipolar neurons. Which of the following structures would most likely provide the abnormal cell morphology?

(A) Ventral horn of the spinal cord
(B) Lateral horn of the spinal cord
(C) Dorsal horn of the spinal cord
(D) Dorsal root ganglion
(E) Sympathetic chain ganglion

6. A 19-year-old college student came to his doctor's office for a neurologic examination. His physician told him that normally synapses are absent in or on which of the following structures?

(A) Anterior horn of the spinal cord
(B) Dorsal root ganglia
(C) Sympathetic chain ganglia
(D) Dendrites
(E) Cell bodies

7. A 27-year-old woman involved in a car accident is brought into the emergency department. Her magnetic resonance imaging reveals that she has a laceration of the spinal cord at the L4 spinal cord level. Which of the following structures would you expect to be intact?

(A) Dorsal horn
(B) Lateral horn
(C) Ventral horn
(D) Gray matter
(E) White matter

8. A 33-year-old male patient complains of feeling severe pain when he tries to turn his neck. The physician realizes that the problem is in his pivot (trochoid) joint. Which of the following joints would most likely be examined?

(A) Atlantooccipital joint
(B) Atlantoaxial joint
(C) Carpometacarpal joint
(D) Proximal tibiofibular joint
(E) Intervertebral disks

9. A patient presents with a loss of sensation to the skin over the shoulder. Injury to which of the following nerve cells would most likely affect the conduction of sensory information to the central nervous system?

(A) Multipolar neurons
(B) Bipolar neurons
(C) Unipolar or pseudounipolar neurons
(D) Neurons in the ventral horn
(E) Neurons in sympathetic chain ganglia

10. A 7-year-old girl comes to the emergency department with severe diarrhea. Tests show that the diarrhea is due to decreased capacity of normal absorption in one of her organs. Which of the following organs is involved?

(A) Stomach
(B) Gallbladder
(C) Large intestine
(D) Liver
(E) Pancreas

11. A 16-year-old girl with urinary diseases comes to a local hospital. Her urologist's examination and laboratory test results reveal that she has difficulty in removing wastes from the blood and in producing urine. Which of the following organs may have abnormal functions?

(A) Ureter
(B) Spleen
(C) Urethra
(D) Bladder
(E) Kidney

12. A 53-year-old man with a known history of emphysema is examined in the emergency department. Laboratory findings along with examination indicate that the patient is unable to exchange oxygen in the air and carbon dioxide in the blood. This exchange occurs in which portion of the respiratory system?

(A) Bronchi
(B) Alveolar (air) sac
(C) Nasal cavity
(D) Larynx
(E) Trachea

13. A 26-year-old woman has an amenorrhea, followed by uterine bleeding, pelvic pain, and pelvic mass. Her obstetrician performed a thorough examination, and the patient was diagnosed as having an ectopic pregnancy. Which of the following organs is most likely to provide a normal site of fertilization?

(A) Fundus of the uterus
(B) Ampulla of the uterine tube
(C) Fimbriae
(D) Infundibulum of the uterine tube
(E) Body of the uterus

14. A 29-year-old woman with abdominal pain was admitted to a local hospital, and examination shows that a retroperitoneal infection is affecting a purely endocrine gland. Which of the following structures is infected?

(A) Ovary
(B) Suprarenal gland
(C) Pancreas
(D) Liver
(E) Stomach

15. A 36-year-old woman received a first-degree burn on her neck, arm, and forearm from a house fire. Which of the following skin structures or functions is most likely damaged or impaired?

(A) GSE nerves
(B) Parasympathetic general visceral efferent nerves
(C) Trophic hormone production
(D) Exocrine gland secretion
(E) Vitamin A production

16. A 9-year-old boy is diagnosed with multiple sclerosis (MS). Which of the following nervous structures would most likely be affected by this disease?

(A) Trigeminal ganglion
(B) Superior cervical ganglion
(C) Optic nerve
(D) Facial nerve
(E) Spinal accessory nerve

Answers and Explanations

1. **The answer is B.** The fascia is a fibrous sheet or band that covers the body under the skin and invests the muscles. Although fasciae are fibrous, tendons connect muscles to bones or cartilage, aponeuroses serve as the means of origin or insertion of a flat muscle, and ligaments connect bones to bones or cartilage. Synovial tendon sheaths are tubular sacs filled with synovial fluid that wrap around the tendons.

2. **The answer is D.** Smooth muscles in the gastrointestinal tract are innervated by both parasympathetic and sympathetic nerves. Smooth muscles in the wall of the blood vessels and arrector pili muscles in hair follicles are innervated only by sympathetic nerves. Muscles that act at the elbow joint and muscles enclosed by epimysium are skeletal muscles that are innervated by somatic motor (general somatic efferent [GSE]) nerves.

3. **The answer is C.** Pulmonary veins return oxygenated blood to the heart from the lungs. Pulmonary arteries carry deoxygenated blood from the heart to the lungs for oxygen renewal. The portal vein carries deoxygenated blood with nutrients from the intestine to the liver. The superior vena cava and coronary sinus carry deoxygenated blood to the right atrium.

4. **The answer is B.** The axons of the neurons carry impulses away from the cell bodies, and dendrites carry impulses to the cell bodies. The axons contain sensory or motor fibers. Multipolar neurons have several dendrites and one axon. The GSE neurons do not carry sensory impulses. The gray matter of the central nervous system consists largely of neuron cell bodies, dendrites, and neuroglia, whereas the white matter consists largely of axons and neuroglia.

5. **The answer is D.** Ventral, lateral, and dorsal horns and sympathetic chain ganglia contain multipolar neurons, whereas the dorsal root ganglion contains unipolar or pseudounipolar neurons. A laceration of the intercostal nerve injures GSE, postganglionic sympathetic general visceral efferent (GVE), general visceral afferent (GVA), and general somatic afferent (GSA) fibers, whose cell bodies are located in the anterior horn, sympathetic chain ganglia, and dorsal root ganglia.

6. **The answer is B.** Dorsal root ganglia consist of cell bodies of the unipolar or pseudounipolar neurons and have no synapses. Axosomatic and axodendritic synapses are the most common, but axoaxonal and dendrodendritic contacts are also found in many nerve tissues.

7. **The answer is B.** The lateral horns are found in the gray matter of the spinal cord between T1 and L2 and also between S2 and S4. Therefore, the lateral horns are absent at the L4 spinal cord level.

8. **The answer is B.** The atlantoaxial joint is the pivot or trochoid joint. The atlantooccipital joints are the condyloid (ellipsoidal) joints, the carpometacarpal joint of the thumb is the saddle (sellar) joint, and the proximal tibiofibular joint is the plane (gliding) joint. The intervertebral disk is the secondary cartilaginous (symphysis) joint.

9. **The answer is C.** Sensation from the skin is carried by GSA fibers, and their cells are unipolar or pseudounipolar types located in the dorsal root ganglia. Multipolar neurons and neurons in the ventral horn and in sympathetic chain ganglia are motor neurons. Bipolar neurons are sensory neurons, but they are not somatic sensory neurons.

10. **The answer is C.** The large intestine absorbs water, salts, and electrolytes. Hence, the patient's diarrhea stems from an absorption problem. The stomach mixes food with mucus and gastric juice, which contains hydrochloric acid and enzymes, and forms chyme. The gallbladder receives bile, concentrates it, and stores it. The liver produces bile, whereas the pancreas secretes pancreatic juice, which contains digestive enzymes and which releases hormones, such as insulin and glucagon.

11. The answer is E. The urinary system includes the kidneys, which remove wastes from the blood and produce the urine; the ureters, which carry urine; the urinary bladder, which stores urine; and the urethra, which conveys urine from the bladder to the exterior of the body. The spleen filters blood to remove particulate matter and cellular residue, stores red blood cells, and produces lymphocytes. Because the patient is not producing urine properly, the malfunctioning organs are the kidneys.

12. The answer is B. The respiratory portion of the lung contains the alveolar (air) sacs or alveoli, which are surrounded by networks of pulmonary capillaries. Oxygen and carbon dioxide exchange occurs across the thin walls of the alveoli and blood capillaries with the aid of the diaphragm and thoracic cage. The nasal cavity, larynx, trachea, and bronchi are air-conducting portions.

13. The answer is B. Fertilization occurs in the ampulla of the uterine tube, and a fertilized oocyte forms a blastocyst by day 7 after fertilization and becomes embedded or implanted in the wall of the uterus during the progestational (secretory) phase of the menstrual cycle. Fertilization is the process beginning with the penetration of the secondary oocyte by the sperm and completed by fusion of the male and female pronuclei.

14. The answer is B. The suprarenal gland is a retroperitoneal organ and is a purely endocrine gland. The pancreas is a retroperitoneal organ and contains endocrine cells, but it is not a purely endocrine gland. The liver and stomach contain endocrine cells, but they are not purely endocrine glands and also are surrounded by peritoneum. The ovary contains endocrine cells and is located in the pelvic cavity.

15. The answer is D. Skin has sweat glands and sebaceous glands, which are exocrine glands. Skin produces vitamin D, but it does not produce a trophic hormone and does not produce vitamin A. In addition, skin contains no GSE and parasympathetic GVE nerve fibers.

16. The answer is C. Multiple sclerosis affects only axons in the CNS (spinal cord and brain) that have myelin sheaths formed by oligodendrocytes. The optic nerve is considered to be part of the CNS, as it is derived from an outpouching of the diencephalon. All other nervous structures are in the PNS and have their myelin sheaths formed by Schwan cells.

chapter 2

Back

VERTEBRAL COLUMN

I. GENERAL CHARACTERISTICS (Figures 2.1 to 2.3)

- The vertebral column consists of 33 vertebrae (7 cervical, 12 thoracic, 5 lumbar, 5 fused sacral, and 4 fused coccygeal vertebrae). It protects the spinal cord, supports the weight of the head and the trunk, and allows the movement of the rib cage for respiration by articulating with the ribs.
- The **primary curvatures** are located in the thoracic and sacral regions and develop during embryonic and fetal periods, whereas the **secondary curvatures** are located in the cervical and lumbar regions and develop after birth and during infancy.

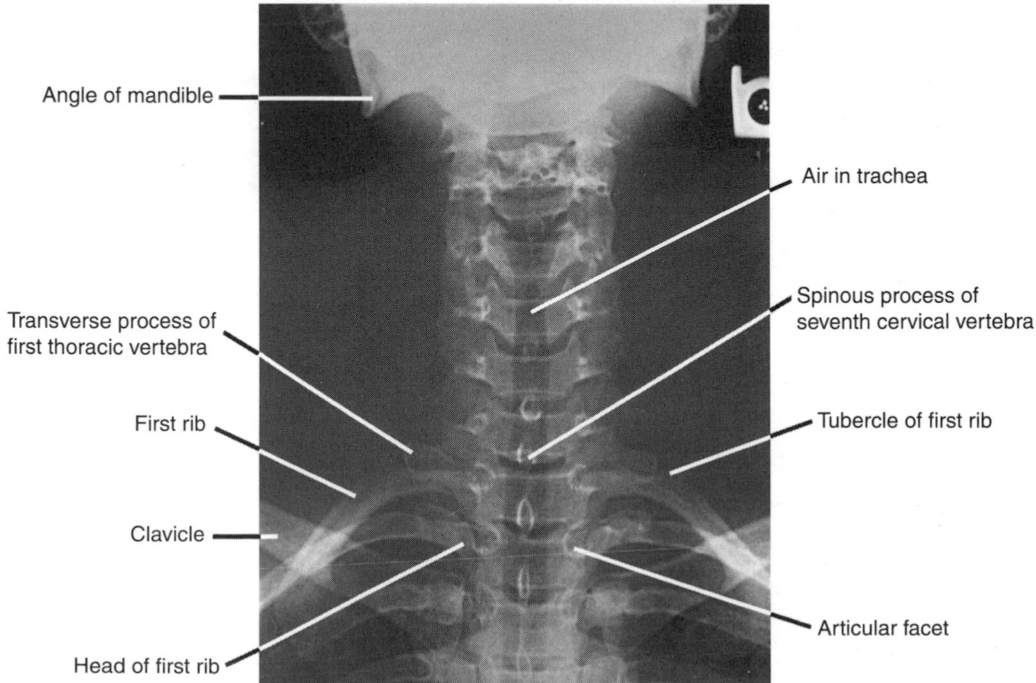

FIGURE 2.1. Anteroposterior radiograph of the cervical and upper thoracic vertebrae.

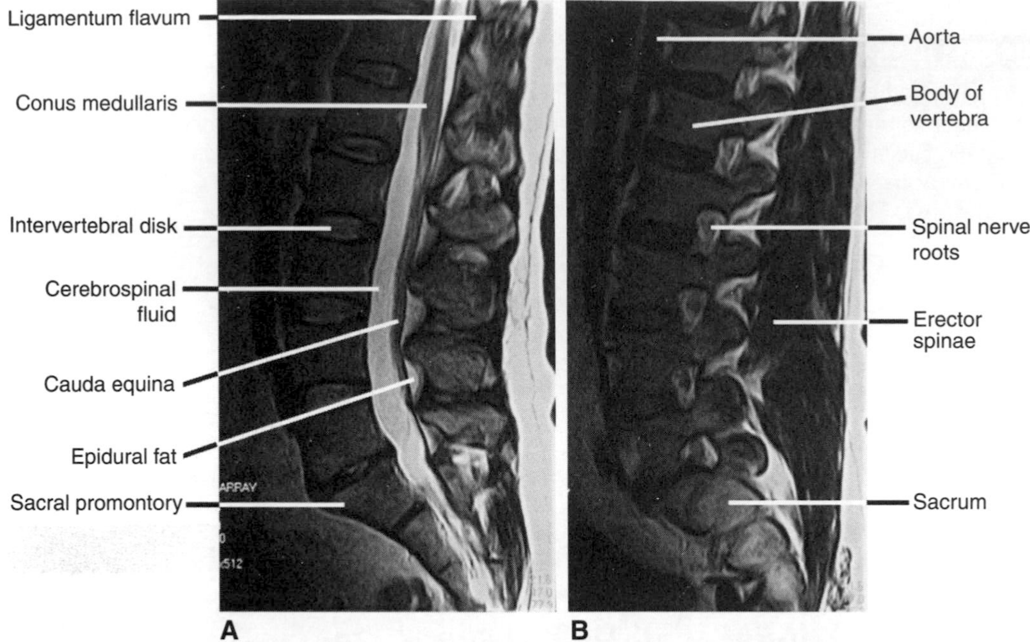

FIGURE 2.2. Sagittal magnetic resonance imaging (MRI) scans of the vertebral column. **A:** Midsagittal view. **B:** Parasagittal view.

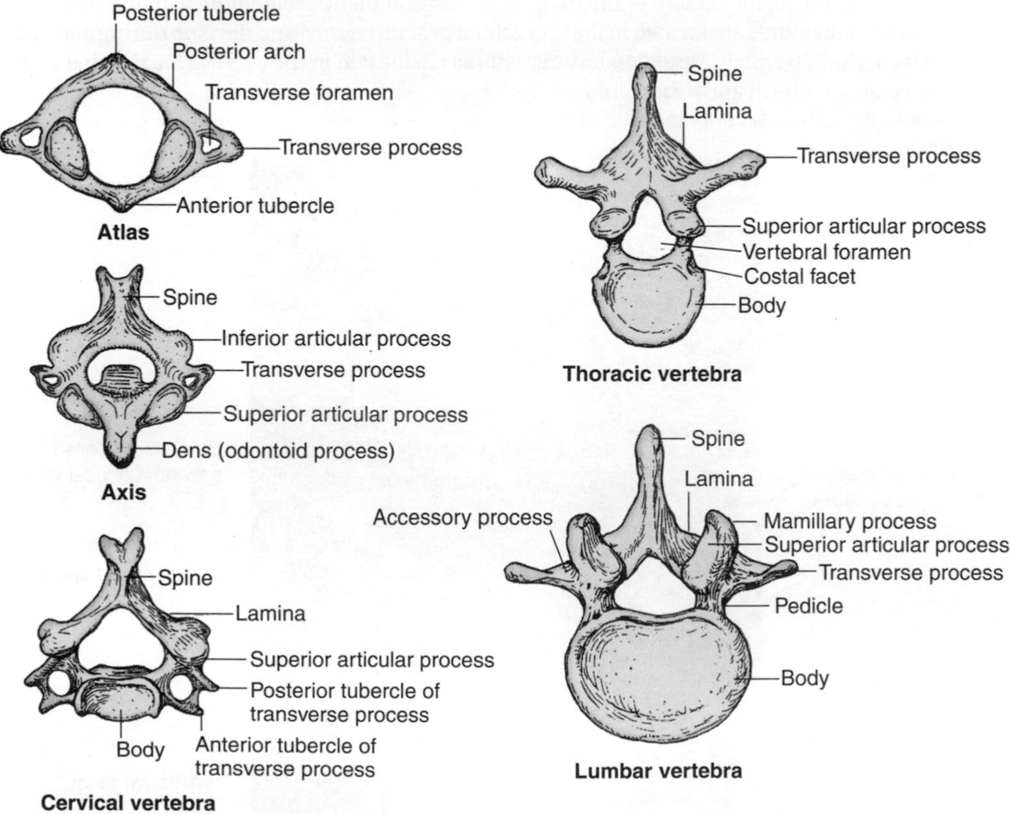

FIGURE 2.3. Typical cervical, thoracic, and lumbar vertebrae.

CLINICAL CORRELATES

Abnormal curvatures of the vertebral column include (a) **kyphosis** (hunchback or humpback), an abnormally **increased thoracic curvature** resulting from osteoporosis; (b) **lordosis** (swayback or saddle back), an abnormally **increased lumbar curvature** resulting from trunk muscular weakness or osteomalacia; and (c) **scoliosis**, a condition of **lateral deviation** resulting from unequal growth of the vertebral column, pathologic erosion of vertebral bodies, or asymmetric paralysis or weakness of vertebral muscles.

II. TYPICAL VERTEBRA (Figure 2.3)

- Consists of a **body** and a **vertebral arch** with several processes for muscular and articular attachments.

A. Body

- Is a short cylinder, **supports weight**, and is separated and also bound together by the **intervertebral disks**, forming the **cartilaginous joints**.
- Has **costal facets or processes of the thoracic vertebrae** anterior to the pedicles, which articulate with the heads of the corresponding and subjacent (just below) ribs.

CLINICAL CORRELATES

Spondylolisthesis is a forward displacement of one vertebra over another, usually of the fifth lumbar over the body of the sacrum, or of the fourth lumbar over the fifth; it is usually due to a developmental defect or traumatic fracture of the pedicle, lamina, or facets (pars interarticularis). It causes lower back pain, stiffness, muscle tightness, sciatica, or a shortened trunk.

Spondylosis (ankylosis or immobility of the vertebra) is a degenerative change due to osteoarthritis of the vertebral joints. It may cause pressure on nerve roots, producing pain and muscle weakness.

Spondylitis (inflammation of the vertebrae): Ankylosing spondylitis is a form of rheumatoid arthritis that affects the vertebral joints, especially the lower back. It produces pain, stiffness, swelling, and limited motion. The affected vertebrae fuse or grow together, resulting in a rigid spine (bamboo spine), poor posture, and deformities.

CLINICAL CORRELATES

Scheuermann disease (juvenile kyphosis) is epiphysial osteochondrosis (necrosis) of vertebral bodies commonly in the thoracic vertebrae in juveniles. Symptoms include intermittent back pain and tight hamstrings.

Pott disease (tuberculous spondylitis) is tuberculosis of the spine that results from softening and collapse of the vertebrae, often causing thoracic kyphosis. Common symptoms are paravertebral swelling or abscess (causing spinal cord compression), paraplegia, back pain, fever, cough, sweats, anorexia, and weight loss.

B. Vertebral (Neural) Arch

- Consists of paired **pedicles** laterally and paired **laminae** posteriorly.
- Forms the vertebral foramen with the vertebral body and protects the spinal cord and associated structures.

CLINICAL CORRELATES

Spina bifida is a developmental anomaly characterized by defective closure of the vertebral arch associated with maternal folic acid deficiency and is classified as follows (Figure 2.4): (a) **spina bifida occulta**—failure of the vertebral arch to fuse (bony defect only with a small tuft of hair over the affected area of skin), (b) **meningocele**—protrusion of the meninges through the unfused arch of the vertebra (spina bifida cystica), (c) **meningomyelocele**—protrusion of the spinal cord and the meninges, and (d) **myeloschisis (rachischisis)**—a cleft spinal cord due to failure of neural folds to close.

CLINICAL CORRELATES

Laminectomy is excision of the posterior arch of a vertebra by transecting the pedicles. It is often performed to relieve pressure on the spinal cord or nerve roots caused by a tumor or herniated disk.

A baby with spina bifida should be delivered by cesarean delivery, because passage of the baby through the narrow birth canal is likely to compress the meningocele and damage the spinal cord.

C. Processes Associated with the Vertebral Arch

1. Spinous Process

- Projects posteriorly from the junction of two laminae of the vertebral arch.
- Is bifid in the cervical region, spinelike in the thoracic region, and oblong in the lumbar region.

2. Transverse Processes

- Project laterally on each side from the junction of the pedicle and the lamina; articulate with the tubercles of ribs 1 to 10 in the thoracic region.
- Have transverse foramina in the cervical region.

3. Articular Processes (Facets)

- Are two superior and two inferior projections from the junction of the laminae and pedicles.
- Articulate with other articular processes of the arch above or below, forming **plane synovial joints.**

4. Mamillary Processes

- Are tubercles on the superior articular processes of the **lumbar vertebrae.**

5. Accessory Processes

- Project backward from the base of the transverse process and lateral and inferior to the mamillary process of a lumbar vertebra.

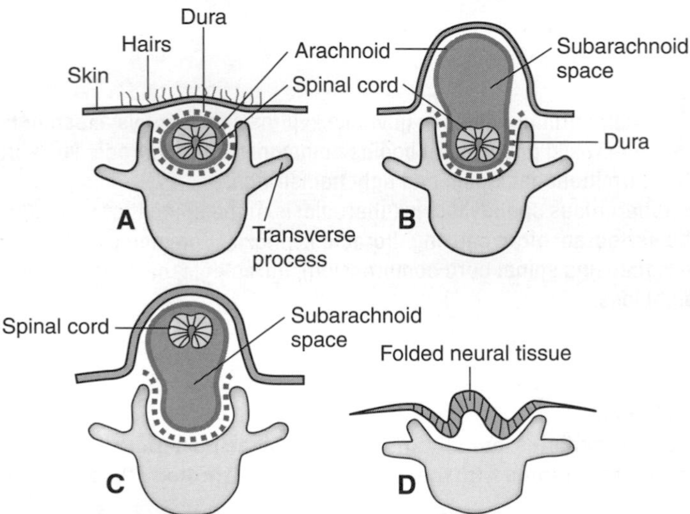

FIGURE 2.4. Various types of spina bifida. **A:** Spina bifida occulta. **B:** Meningocele. **C:** Meningomyelocele. **D:** Rachischisis. (Redrawn with permission from Langman J. *Medical embryology.* 4th ed. Baltimore, MD: Williams & Wilkins; 1981:331.)

D. Foramina Associated with the Vertebral Arch

1. Vertebral Foramina

- Are formed by the vertebral bodies and vertebral arches (pedicles and laminae).
- Collectively form the **vertebral canal** and transmit the **spinal cord** with its meningeal coverings, nerve roots, and associated vessels.

2. Intervertebral Foramina

- Are located between the inferior and superior surfaces of the pedicles of adjacent vertebrae.
- Transmit the **spinal nerves** and accompanying vessels as they exit the vertebral canal.

3. Transverse Foramina

- Are present in **transverse processes** of the cervical vertebrae.
- Transmit the vertebral artery (except for C7), **vertebral veins**, and **autonomic nerves**.

CLINICAL CORRELATES **Klippel–Feil syndrome** is a congenital defect manifested as a short, stiff neck resulting from reduction in the number of cervical vertebrae or extensive fusion of the cervical vertebrae, which causes low hairline and limited motion of the neck.

CLINICAL CORRELATES **Whiplash injury of the neck** is produced by a force that drives the trunk forward while the head lags behind, causing **the head** (with the upper part of the neck) **to hyperextend and the lower part of the neck to hyperflex rapidly**, as occurs in rear-end automobile collisions. This injury occurs frequently at the junction of vertebrae C4 and C5; thus, vertebrae C1 to C4 act as the lash, and vertebrae C5 to C7 act as the handle of the whip. It results in neck pain, stiff neck, and headache and can be treated by supporting the head and neck with a cervical collar that is higher in the back than in the front; the collar keeps the cervical vertebral column in a flexed position.

III. INTERVERTEBRAL DISKS (See Figures 2.2 and 2.5)

- Form the secondary cartilaginous joints between the bodies of two vertebrae from the axis to the sacrum **(there is no disk between the atlas and the axis)**.

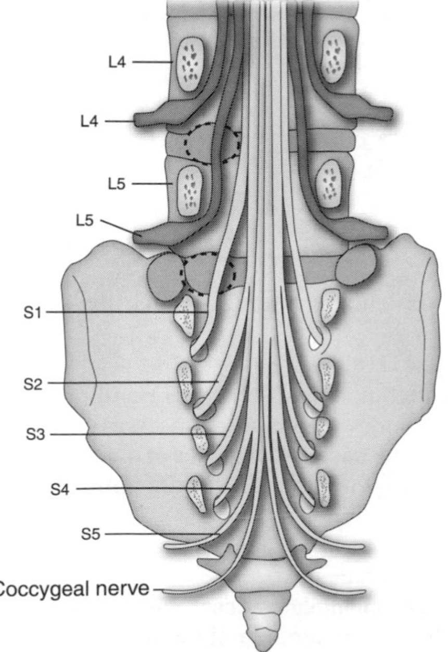

FIGURE 2.5. Note lower lumbar disk protrusion: Posterolateral protrusion at disk level L4 to L5 affects L5 spinal nerve, not L4 spinal nerve.

- Consist of a central mucoid substance **(nucleus pulposus)** with a surrounding fibrocartilaginous lamina **(annulus fibrosus).**
- Comprise one-fourth (25%) of the length of the vertebral column.
- Allow movements between the vertebrae and serve as a **shock absorber**.
- Are avascular except for their peripheries, which are supplied from adjacent blood vessels.

A. Nucleus Pulposus

- Is a remnant of the embryonic **notochord** and is situated in the central portion of the intervertebral disk.
- Consists of reticular and collagenous fibers embedded in **mucoid material.**
- May **herniate** or protrude through the annulus fibrosus, thereby impinging on the roots of the spinal nerve.
- Acts as a shock-absorbing mechanism by equalizing pressure.

B. Annulus Fibrosus

- Consists of concentric layers of fibrous tissue and fibrocartilage.
- **Binds the vertebral column together, retains the nucleus pulposus**, and permits a limited amount of movement.
- Acts as a shock absorber.

CLINICAL CORRELATES **A herniated (slipped) disk** is a **protrusion of the nucleus pulposus** through the annulus fibrosus of the intervertebral disk into the intervertebral foramen or into the vertebral canal, compressing the spinal nerve root. It commonly occurs posterolaterally where the annulus fibrosus is not reinforced by the posterior longitudinal ligament and frequently affects the lumbar region. A posterolateral herniation of the disk at the level L4 to L5, for example, would be likely to damage fifth lumbar nerve roots, not fourth lumbar nerve roots, due to a more oblique descending of the fourth and fifth lumbar nerve roots within the subarachnoid space (see Figure 2.5).

CLINICAL CORRELATES **Sciatica** is pain in the lower back and hip radiating into the buttock and into the lower limb and is most commonly caused by herniation of a lower lumbar intervertebral disk, compressing or irritating roots of the sciatic nerve. It causes muscular weakness, numbness, tingling, and pain along the path of the sciatic nerve.

IV. REGIONAL CHARACTERISTICS OF VERTEBRAE (See Figure 2.3)

A. First Cervical Vertebra (Atlas)

- **Supports the skull**, thus its name. According to Greek mythology, Atlas supported Earth on his shoulders.
- Is the widest of the cervical vertebrae.
- Has **no body** and **no spine** but consists of anterior and posterior arches, two **lateral masses** (which support the skull), and two transverse processes.
- Articulates superiorly with the **occipital condyles** of the skull to form the **atlantooccipital joints** and inferiorly with the **axis** to form the **atlantoaxial joints**.

B. Second Cervical Vertebra (Axis)

- Has **the smallest transverse process.**
- Is characterized by the **dens (odontoid process)**, which projects superiorly from the body of the axis and articulates with the **anterior arch of the atlas**, thus forming the pivot around which the atlas rotates. It is supported by the cruciform, apical, and alar ligaments and the tectorial membrane.

CLINICAL CORRELATES

Fracture of the atlas occurs by strong vertical forces as would result from a blow to the top of the head or striking the bottom of a shallow pool in a diving accident, causing **fracture of the lateral masses** and rupture of the transverse ligament. A burst fracture of the ring of the atlas, involving fracture of the anterior and posterior arches, is called **Jefferson fracture**.

Fracture of the axis occurs as a result of hyperextension of the head on the neck in such condition as an execution of a criminal by hanging.

Hangman fracture is a fracture of the pedicles of the axis (C2), which may occur as a result of judicial hanging or automobile accidents. In this fracture, the cruciform ligament is torn and the spinal cord is crushed, causing death.

C. **Third to Sixth Cervical Vertebrae**
- Are typical cervical vertebrae and have short bifid spinous processes and transverse processes with anterior and posterior tubercles and transverse foramina for the vertebral vessels.

D. **Seventh Cervical Vertebra (C7)**
- Is called the **vertebra prominens** because it has a long spinous process that is nearly horizontal, ends in a single tubercle (not bifid), and forms a visible protrusion.
- Provides an attachment site for the **ligamentum nuchae, supraspinous ligaments**, and numerous back muscles.

E. **Thoracic Vertebrae**
- Have costal facets; the superior costal facet on the body articulates with the head of the corresponding rib, whereas the inferior facet articulates with the subjacent rib (just below).
- Have a transverse process that articulates with the tubercle of the corresponding rib.
- Have the **typical thoracic vertebrae**, which are the second to the eighth thoracic vertebrae.

F. **Lumbar Vertebrae**
- Are distinguished by their large bodies, sturdy laminae, and absence of costal facets. The **fifth lumbar vertebra** has the **largest body** of the vertebrae.
- Are characterized by a strong, massive transverse process and have **mamillary and accessory processes.**

G. **Sacrum** (Figure 2.6; See Figure 2.2)
- Is a large, triangular, wedge-shaped bone composed of **five fused sacral vertebrae.**
- Has **four pairs of foramina** for the exit of the ventral and dorsal primary rami of the first four sacral nerves.
- Forms the posterior part of the pelvis and provides strength and **stability to the pelvis.**

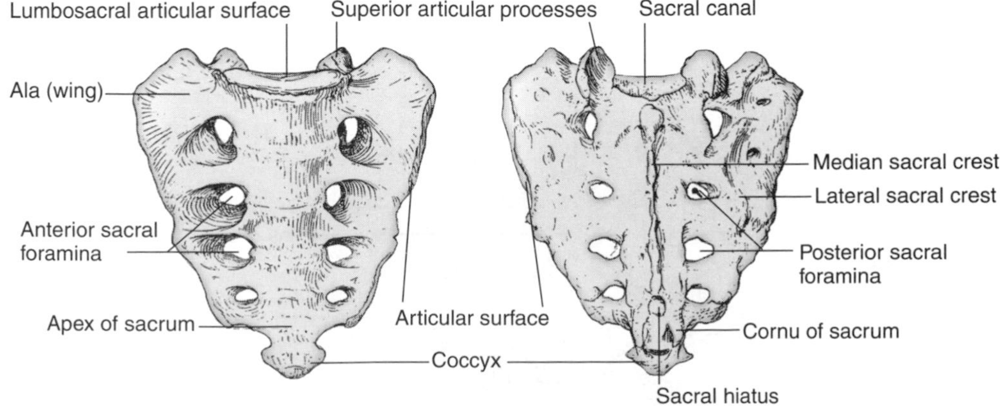

FIGURE 2.6. Sacrum.

- Is characterized by the following structures:
  1. **Promontory**
     - The prominent anterior edge of the first sacral vertebra (S1).
  2. **Ala**
     - The superior and lateral part of the sacrum, which is formed by the fused transverse processes and fused costal processes of the first sacral vertebra.
  3. **Median sacral crest**
     - Formed by the fused spinous processes.
  4. **Sacral hiatus**
     - Formed by the failure of the **laminae** of vertebra S5 to fuse. It is used for the administration of **caudal (extradural) anesthesia.**
  5. **Sacral cornu or horn**
     - Formed by the **pedicles** of the fifth sacral vertebra. It is an important landmark for locating the sacral hiatus.

H. Coccyx

- Is a wedge-shaped bone formed by the union of the four coccygeal vertebrae.
- Provides attachment for the coccygeus and levator ani muscles.

V. LIGAMENTS OF THE VERTEBRAL COLUMN (Figure 2.7)

A. Anterior Longitudinal Ligament

- Runs from the skull (occipital bone) to the sacrum on the anterior surface of the vertebral bodies and intervertebral disks.
- Is narrowest at the upper end but **widens as it descends**, maintaining the stability of the joints.

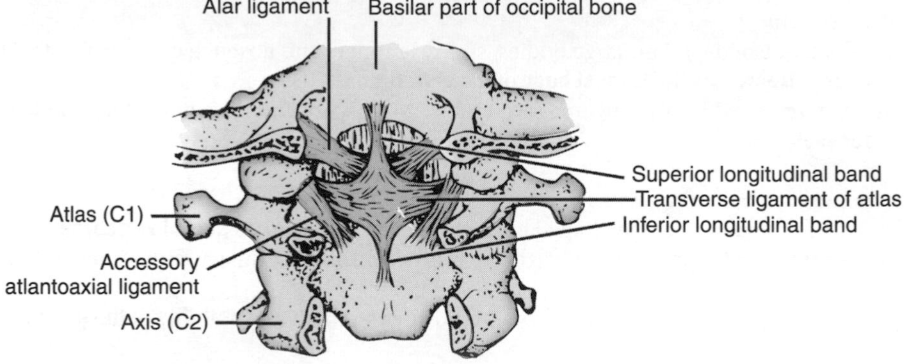

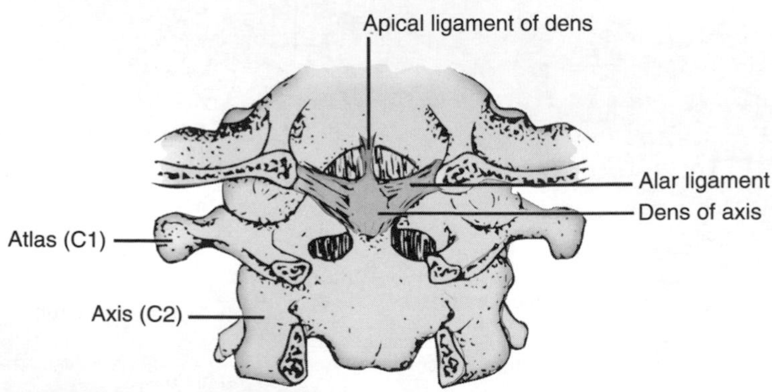

FIGURE 2.7. Ligaments of the atlas and the axis.

- **Limits extension** of the vertebral column, **supports the annulus fibrosus** anteriorly, and resists gravitational pull.

B. Posterior Longitudinal Ligament

- Interconnects the vertebral bodies and intervertebral disks posteriorly and **narrows as it descends**.
- **Supports** the posterior aspect of the **vertebral bodies** and the **annulus fibrosus**, but it runs anterior to the spinal cord within the vertebral canal.
- **Limits flexion** of the vertebral column and resists gravitational pull.

C. Ligamentum Flavum

- Connects the **laminae** of two adjacent vertebrae and functions to **maintain the upright posture**.
- Forms the posterior wall of the vertebral canal between the vertebrae and may be pierced during **lumbar (spinal) puncture**.

D. Ligamentum Nuchae (Back of Neck)

- Is a **triangular-shaped median fibrous septum** between the muscles on the two sides of the posterior aspect of the neck.
- Is formed by **thickened supraspinous ligaments** that extend from vertebra C7 to the external occipital protuberance and crest.
- Is also attached to the posterior tubercle of the atlas and to the spinous processes of the other cervical vertebrae.

E. Other Ligaments

- Include the interspinous (between two adjacent spinous processes), intertransverse (between two adjacent transverse processes), and supraspinous (between tips of two adjacent spinous processes) ligaments.

VI. VERTEBRAL VENOUS SYSTEM

- Is a valveless plexiform of veins, forming interconnecting channels.

A. Internal Vertebral Venous Plexus

- Lies in the **epidural space** between the wall of the vertebral canal and the dura mater and receives tributaries from the spinal cord and vertebrae, vertebral veins, basilar plexus, and occipital and sigmoid dural sinuses.
- Forms anterior and posterior ladderlike configurations by anastomosing longitudinal and transverse veins.
- Drains into segmental veins by the **intervertebral veins** that pass through the intervertebral and sacral foramina. The anterior veins receive the **basivertebral veins**, which lie within the vertebral bodies.
- Also communicates superiorly with the cranial dural sinuses, inferiorly with the pelvic vein, and in the thoracic and abdominal regions with both the azygos and caval systems.
- Is thought to be the **route of early metastasis of carcinoma** from the lung, breast, and prostate gland to bones and the central nervous system (CNS).

B. External Vertebral Venous Plexus

- Consists of the anterior part, which lies in front of the vertebral column, and the posterior part, which lies on the vertebral arch.
- Communicates with the internal venous plexus by way of the **intervertebral** and **basivertebral veins** and also with the vertebral, posterior intercostal, lumbar, and lateral sacral veins.

C. Vertebral Vein

- Arises from the **venous plexuses around the foramen magnum** and **in the suboccipital region**, passes with the vertebral artery through the transverse foramina of the upper six cervical vertebrae, and empties into the **brachiocephalic vein**.

SOFT TISSUES OF THE BACK

I. SUPERFICIAL TISSUES

A. Triangles and Fascia

1. Triangle of Auscultation (See Figure 2.8)

- Is bounded by the upper border of the **latissimus dorsi**, the lateral border of the **trapezius**, and the medial border of the **scapula**.
- Has a floor formed by the **rhomboid major**.
- Is the site where **breathing sounds** can be heard most clearly using a stethoscope invented by Laennec in 1816.

2. Lumbar Triangle (of Petit)

- Is formed by the iliac crest, latissimus dorsi, and posterior free border of the external oblique abdominal muscle; its floor is formed by the internal oblique abdominal muscle. It may be the site of an abdominal hernia.

3. Thoracolumbar (Lumbodorsal) Fascia

- Invests the deep muscles of the back, having an **anterior layer** that lies anterior to the erector spinae and attaches to the vertebral **transverse process**, and a **posterior layer** that lies posterior to the erector spinae and attaches to the **spinous processes**.
- Provides the origins for the latissimus dorsi and the internal oblique and transverse abdominis muscles.

B. Superficial or Extrinsic Muscles (Figure 2.8; Table 2.1)

C. Blood Vessels (See Figure 2.8)

1. Occipital Artery

- Arises from the external carotid artery, runs deep to the sternocleidomastoid muscle, and lies on the obliquus capitis superior and the semispinalis capitis.

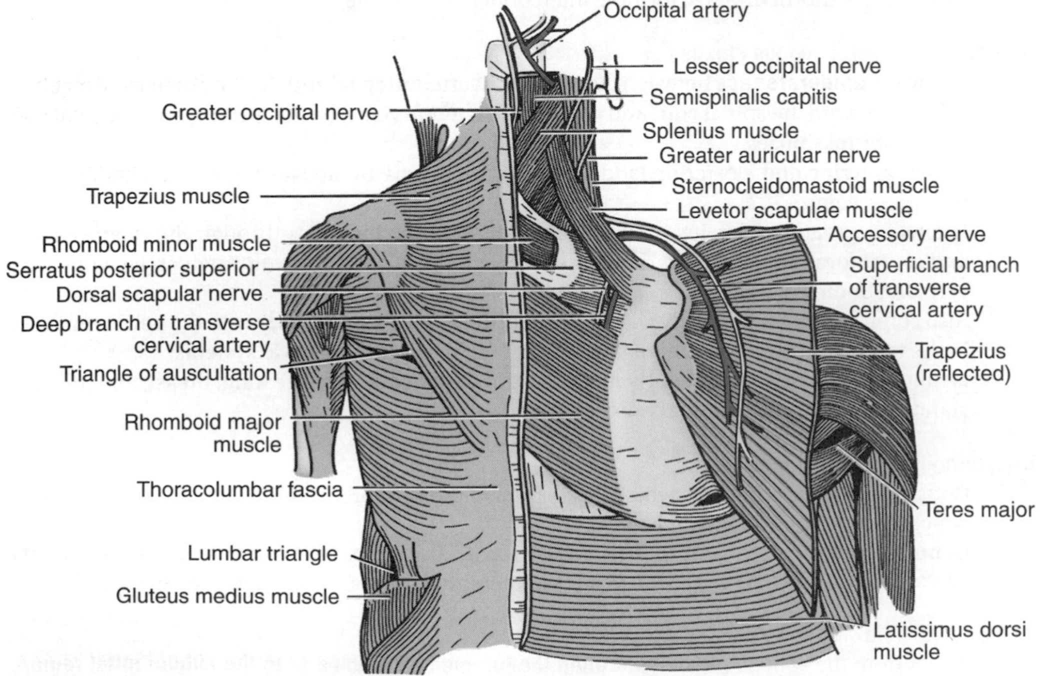

FIGURE 2.8. Superficial muscles of the back, with particular attention to the shoulder region.

table 2.1 Superficial Muscles of the Back

Muscle	Origin	Insertion	Nerve	Action
Trapezius	External occipital protuberance, superior nuchal line, ligamentum nuchae, and spines of C7–T12	Spine of scapula, acromion, and lateral third of clavicle	Spinal accessory nerve; C3–C4	Adducts, rotates, elevates, and depresses scapula
Levator scapulae	Transverse processes of C1–C4	Medial border of scapula	Dorsal scapular nerve (C5); C3–C4	Elevates scapula and rotates glenoid cavity
Rhomboid minor	Spines of C7–T1	Root of spine of scapula	Dorsal scapular nerve (C5)	Adducts scapula
Rhomboid major	Spines of T2–T5	Medial border of scapula	Dorsal scapular nerve (C5)	Adducts scapula
Latissimus dorsi	Spines of T7–T12, thoracodorsal fascia, iliac crest, and ribs 9–12	Floor of bicipital groove of humerus	Thoracodorsal nerve	Adducts, extends, and rotates arm medially; depresses scapula
Serratus posterior superior	Ligamentum nuchae, supraspinal ligament, and spines of C7–T3	Upper border of ribs 2–5	Intercostal nerve (T1–T4)	Elevates ribs
Serratus posterior inferior	Supraspinous ligament and spines of T11–L2	Lower border of ribs 9–12	Intercostal nerve (T9–T12)	Depresses ribs

- Pierces the trapezius, is accompanied by the **greater occipital nerve (C2)**, and supplies the scalp in the occipital region.
- Gives off the descending branch, which divides into the **superficial branch**, which anastomoses with the transverse cervical artery, and the **deep branch**, which anastomoses with the deep cervical artery from the costocervical trunk.

2. Transverse Cervical Artery

- Arises from the thyrocervical trunk of the subclavian artery and divides into the superficial and deep branches.
- Has a **superficial branch** (superficial cervical artery) that divides into an ascending branch that supplies the upper part of the trapezius and adjacent muscles and a descending branch that accompanies the **spinal accessory nerve** on the deep surface of the trapezius.
- Has a **deep branch** (dorsal scapular or descending scapular artery) that accompanies the **dorsal scapular nerve (C5)** deep to the levator scapulae and the rhomboids along the medial side of the scapula.

D. Nerves (See Figure 2.8)

1. Accessory Nerve

- Consists of a cranial portion that joins the vagus nerve and a spinal portion that runs deep to the sternocleidomastoid, lies on the levator scapulae, and passes deep to the trapezius.
- Supplies the sternocleidomastoid and trapezius muscles.

2. Dorsal Scapular Nerve (C5)

- Is derived from the **ventral primary ramus** of the fifth cervical spinal nerve, runs along with the deep branch of the transverse cervical artery, and supplies the rhomboid major and minor and levator scapulae muscles.

3. Greater Occipital Nerve (C2)

- Is derived as a medial branch of the **dorsal primary ramus**, the second cervical spinal nerve.
- Crosses obliquely between the obliquus inferior and the semispinalis capitis, pierces the semispinalis capitis and the trapezius, and supplies cutaneous innervation in the occipital region.

- May innervate the semispinalis capitis and communicates with the suboccipital and third occipital nerves.

4. **Third (Least) Occipital Nerve (C3)**
   - Is derived from the **dorsal primary ramus** of the third cervical spinal nerve.
   - Ascends across the suboccipital region, pierces the trapezius, and supplies cutaneous innervation in the occipital region.
5. **Lesser Occipital Nerve (C2)**
   - Is derived from the **ventral primary ramus** of the second cervical spinal nerve.
   - Is a cutaneous branch of the cervical plexus and ascends along the posterior border of the sternocleidomastoid to the scalp behind the auricle.

II. DEEP TISSUES

A. Deep or Intrinsic Muscles

1. **Muscles of the Superficial Layer: Spinotransverse Group**
   - Consist of the **splenius capitis** and the **splenius cervicis**.
   - Originate from the spinous processes and insert into the transverse processes (splenius cervicis) and on the mastoid process and the superior nuchal line (splenius capitis).
   - Are innervated by the dorsal primary rami of the middle and lower cervical spinal nerves.
   - **Extend, rotate**, and laterally **flex** the head and the neck.
2. **Muscles of the Intermediate Layer: Sacrospinalis Group**
   - Consist of the **erector spinae (sacrospinalis)**, which is divided into three columns: iliocostalis (lateral column), longissimus (intermediate column), and spinalis (medial column).
   - Originate from the sacrum, ilium, ribs, and spinous processes of lumbar and lower thoracic vertebrae.
   - Insert on the ribs **(iliocostalis)**; on the ribs, transverse processes, and mastoid process **(longissimus)**; and on the spinous processes **(spinalis)**.
   - Are innervated by the dorsal primary rami of the spinal nerves.
   - **Extend, rotate**, and laterally **flex** the vertebral column and head.
3. **Muscles of the Deep Layer: Transversospinalis Group**
   - Consist of the **semispinalis** (capitis, cervicis, and thoracis), the **multifidus**, and the **rotators**.
   - The **semispinalis** muscles originate from the transverse processes and insert into the skull (semispinalis capitis) and the spinous processes (semispinalis cervicis and thoracis).
   - The **rotators** run from the transverse processes to the spinous processes, two vertebrae above and one vertebra above (longus and brevis respectively).
   - The **multifidus** originates from the sacrum, ilium, and transverse processes and inserts on the spinous processes. It is best developed in the lumbar region.
   - Are innervated by the dorsal primary rami of the spinal nerves.
   - **Extend** and **rotate** the head, neck, and trunk.

B. Segmental Muscles

- Are innervated by the dorsal primary rami of the spinal nerves.
- Consist of the following.

1. **Interspinales**
   - Run between adjacent spinous processes and aid in extension of the vertebral column.
2. **Intertransversarii**
   - Run between adjacent transverse processes and aid in lateral flexion of the vertebral column.
3. **Levatores Costarum (Longus and Brevis)**
   - Extend from the transverse processes to ribs, elevate the ribs, and are innervated by the intercostal nerves.

III. SUBOCCIPITAL AREA (Figure 2.9)

A. Suboccipital Triangle

- Is bound medially by the rectus capitis posterior major muscle, laterally by the obliquus capitis superior muscle, and inferiorly by the obliquus capitis inferior muscle.
- Has a roof formed by the semispinalis capitis and longissimus capitis.
- Has a floor formed by the posterior arch of the atlas and posterior atlantooccipital membrane.
- Contains the vertebral artery and suboccipital nerve and vessels.

B. Suboccipital Muscles (Table 2.2)

C. Suboccipital Nerve

- Is derived from the dorsal ramus of C1 and emerges between the vertebral artery above and the posterior arch of the atlas below.
- Supplies the muscles of the suboccipital triangle and semispinalis capitis.
- Contains skeletal motor fibers and no cutaneous sensory fibers, but occasionally has a cutaneous branch.

D. Vertebral Artery

- Arises from the subclavian artery and ascends through the transverse foramina of the upper six cervical vertebrae.
- Winds behind the lateral mass of the atlas, runs in a groove on the superior surface of the posterior arch of the atlas, pierces the dura mater to enter the vertebral canal, and ascends into the cranial cavity through the foramen magnum.
- Gives off an anterior spinal and two posterior spinal arteries.

E. Vertebral Veins

- Are formed in the suboccipital triangle by union of tributaries from the venous plexus around the foramen magnum, the suboccipital venous plexus, the intervertebral veins, and the internal and external vertebral venous plexus.
- Do not emerge from the cranial cavity with the vertebral artery through the foramen magnum, but they enter the transverse foramen of the atlas and descend through the next five successive foramina, emptying into the brachiocephalic vein. The small accessory vertebral veins arise from the plexus, traverse the seventh cervical transverse foramina, and end in the brachiocephalic vein.

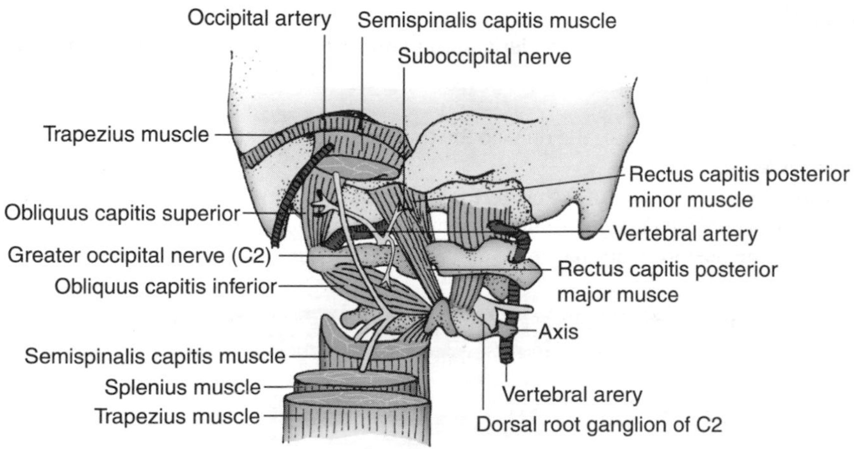

FIGURE 2.9. Suboccipital triangle.

table 2.2 Suboccipital Muscles of the Back

Muscle	Origin	Insertion	Nerve	Action
Rectus capitis posterior major	Spine of axis	Lateral portion of inferior nuchal line	Suboccipital	Extends, rotates, and flexes head laterally
Rectus capitis posterior minor	Posterior tubercle of atlas	Occipital bone below inferior nuchal line	Suboccipital	Extends and flexes head laterally
Obliquus capitis superior	Transverse process of atlas	Occipital bone above inferior nuchal line	Suboccipital	Extends, rotates, and flexes head laterally
Obliquus capitis inferior	Spine of axis	Transverse process of atlas	Suboccipital	Extends and rotates head laterally

F. Joints

1. Atlantooccipital Joint

- Is a **condylar synovial joint** that occurs between the superior articular facets of the atlas and the occipital condyles.
- Is involved primarily in flexion, extension, and lateral flexion of the head.

2. Atlantoaxial Joints

- Are **synovial joints** consisting of two lateral **plane joints**, which are between the articular facets of the atlas and the axis, and one median **pivot joint** between the dens of the axis and the anterior arch of the atlas.
- Are involved in **rotation of the atlas and head** as a unit on the axis.

CLINICAL CORRELATES **Atlantoaxial dislocation (subluxation)** occurs after rupture of the cruciform ligament caused by trauma or rheumatoid arthritis. It may result from a congenital absence of the dens, a fracture of the dens, or a direct trauma frequently caused by traffic accidents. This subluxation may injure the spinal cord and medulla, and its symptoms include pain in the cervical area and in the back of the neck or painful restriction of mobility.

G. Components of the Occipitoaxial Ligament (See Figure 2.7)

1. Cruciform Ligament

a. Transverse Ligament

- Runs between the lateral masses of the atlas, arching over the dens of the axis.

b. Longitudinal Ligament

- Extends from the dens of the axis to the anterior aspect of the foramen magnum and to the body of the axis.

2. Apical Ligament

- Extends from the apex of the dens to the anterior aspect of the foramen magnum (of the occipital bone).

3. Alar Ligament

- Extends from the apex of the dens to the tubercle on the medial side of the occipital condyle.

4. Tectorial Membrane

- Is an upward extension of the posterior longitudinal ligament from the body of the axis to the basilar part of the occipital bone anterior to the foramen magnum.
- Covers the posterior surface of the dens and the apical, alar, and cruciform ligaments.

SPINAL CORD AND ASSOCIATED STRUCTURES

I. SPINAL CORD (Figure 2.10; See Figure 2.2)

- Is cylindrical, occupies approximately the **upper two-thirds** of the **vertebral canal**, and is enveloped by the three **meninges**.

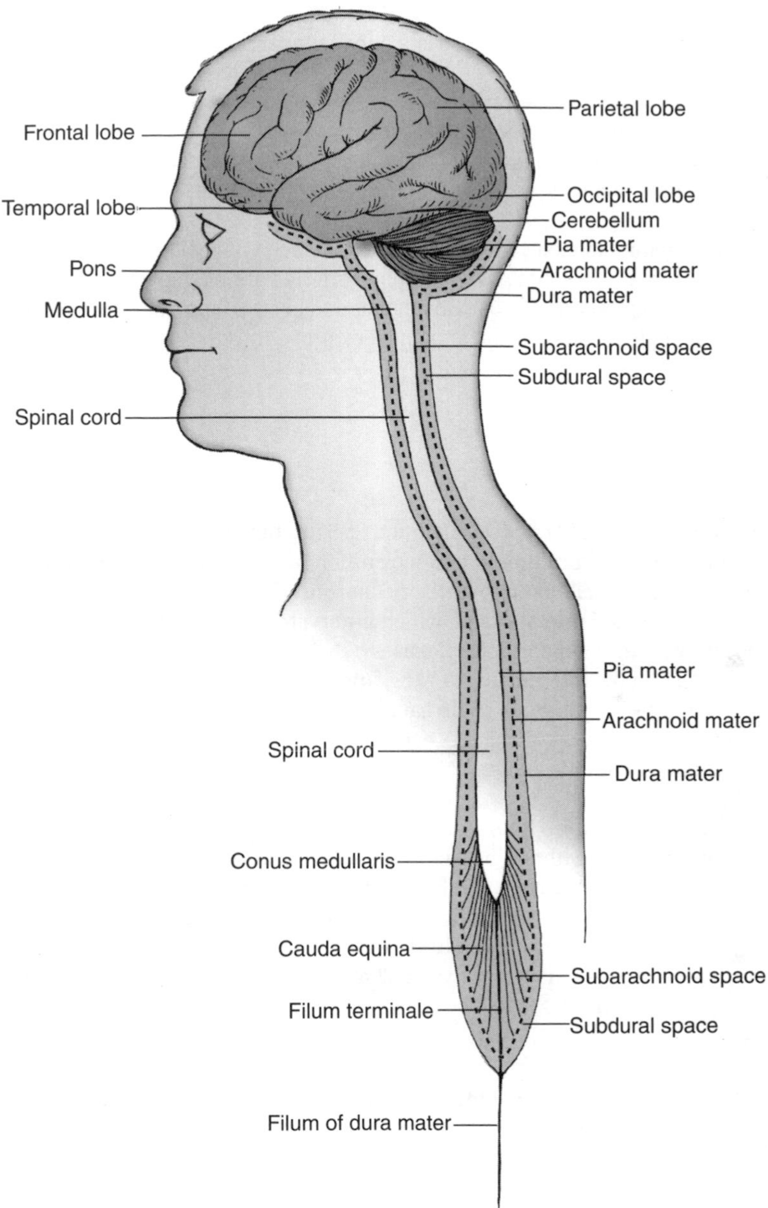

FIGURE 2.10. Meninges.

- Has cervical and lumbar enlargements for nerve supply of the upper and lower limbs, respectively.
- Contains **gray matter**, which is located in the interior (in contrast to the cerebral hemispheres); the spinal cord is surrounded by **white matter.**
- Has a conical end known as the **conus medullaris**, which terminates at the level of L2 vertebra or the intervertebral disk between L1 and L2 vertebrae.
- Grows much more slowly than the bony vertebral column during fetal development; thus, its end gradually shifts to a higher level and ends at the level of L2 vertebra in the adult and at the level of L3 vertebra in the newborn.
- Receives blood from the anterior spinal artery and two posterior spinal arteries and from branches of the vertebral, cervical, and posterior intercostal and lumbar arteries.

CLINICAL CORRELATES **Tethered cord syndrome** is a congenital anomaly resulting from defective closure of the neural tube. It is characterized by the abnormally low conus medullaris, which is tethered by a short thickened filum terminale, leading to such conditions as progressive neurologic defects in the legs and feet and scoliosis.

Arnold–Chiari (or Chiari) deformity is a congenital cerebellomedullary malformation in which the cerebellum and medulla oblongata protrude down into the vertebral canal through the foramen magnum.

Spinal cord ischemia can easily occur because the blood supply to the spinal cord is surprisingly meager. The anterior and posterior spinal arteries are of small and variable diameter, and the reinforcing segmental arteries vary in number and in size. Ischemia may be caused by aortic disease and surgery, regional anesthesia, or pain block procedures.

II. SPINAL NERVES

- Consist of **31 pairs** of nerves (8 cervical, 12 thoracic, 5 lumbar, 5 sacral, 1 coccygeal).
- Are formed within an intervertebral foramen by union of the ventral root and the dorsal root with ganglion, which contains cell bodies of sensory neurons.
- Are divided into the **dorsal primary rami**, which innervate the skin and deep muscles of the back; the **ventral primary rami**, which form the plexuses (C1–C4, cervical; C5–T1, brachial; L1–L4, lumbar; and L4–S4, sacral); and the **intercostal** (T1–T11) and **subcostal** (T12) **nerves**.
- Are connected with the sympathetic chain ganglia by **rami communicantes**.
- Are mixed nerves, containing all of the **general functional components** (i.e., general somatic afferent [GSA], general somatic efferent [GSE], general visceral afferent [GVA], and general visceral efferent [GVE]).
- Contain **sensory (GSA and GVA) fibers** with cell bodies in the dorsal root ganglion.
- Contain **motor (GSE) fibers** with cell bodies in the anterior horn of the spinal cord.
- Contain **preganglionic sympathetic (GVE) fibers** with cell bodies in the intermediolateral cell column in the lateral horn of the spinal cord (segments between T1 and L2).
- Contain **preganglionic parasympathetic (GVE) fibers** with cell bodies in the intermediolateral cell column of the spinal cord segments between S2 and S4. These GVE fibers leave the sacral nerves via the pelvic splanchnic nerves.

CLINICAL CORRELATES **Shingles (herpes zoster)** is an infectious disease caused by the **varicella zoster virus** that remains latent in the dorsal root ganglia of spinal nerves and the sensory ganglia of cranial nerves. It results from activation of the virus, which travels down the sensory nerve to produce severe neuralgic pain, an eruption of groups of vesicles, or a rash in the dermatome of the nerve. Herpes zoster is frequently associated with spina bifida and results in such conditions as a short neck and obstructive hydrocephalus.

Chicken pox (varicella) is caused by the **varicella zoster virus**, which later resides latent in the cranial (i.e., trigeminal) or dorsal root ganglia. It is marked by vesicular eruption of the skin and mucous membranes. It is contagious, and a patient may have a runny or stuffy nose, sneezing, cough, itchy rash, fever, and abdominal pain.

III. MENINGES (See Figures 2.2 and 2.10)

A. Pia Mater

- Is the innermost meningeal layer; it is closely applied to the spinal cord and thus cannot be dissected from it. It also enmeshes blood vessels on the surfaces of the spinal cord.
- Has lateral extensions **(denticulate ligaments)** between dorsal and ventral roots of spinal nerves and an inferior extension known as the **filum terminale**.

CLINICAL CORRELATES **Meningitis** is inflammation of the meninges caused by viral or bacterial infection. Viral meningitis is milder and occurs more often than bacterial meningitis. Bacterial meningitis (purulent meningitis) is an extremely serious illness and may result in brain damage or death, even if treated. Meningitis is also caused by fungi, chemical irritation or drug allergies, and tumors. Its symptoms include fever, headache, stiff neck, brain swelling, shock, convulsions, nausea, and vomiting. Antibiotics are effective for treating bacterial meningitis but are ineffective for treating viral meningitis.

B. Arachnoid Mater

- Is a filmy, transparent, spidery layer connected to the pia mater by weblike trabeculations.
- Forms the **subarachnoid space**, the space between the arachnoid layer and the pia mater that is filled with **cerebrospinal fluid (CSF)** and that extends to the second sacral vertebral level. The enlarged subarachnoid space between vertebrae L1 and S2 is called the **lumbar cistern.**

C. Dura Mater

- Is the tough, fibrous, outermost layer of the meninges.
- The **subdural space** is a potential space between the arachnoid and the dura. It extends inferiorly to the second sacral vertebral level and contains only sufficient fluid to moisten the surfaces of two membranes.
- The **epidural space** is external to it and contains the internal vertebral venous plexus and epidural fat.

CLINICAL CORRELATES **Caudal (epidural) anesthesia** is used to **block the spinal nerves in the epidural space** by injection of local anesthetic agents via the sacral hiatus located between the sacral cornua. It is used for surgery on the rectum, anus, genitals, or urinary tract and for culdoscopy. Obstetricians use this method of nerve block to relieve the pains during labor and childbirth, and its advantage is that the anesthetic does not affect the infant.

Saddle block is the introduction of anesthesia into the dural sac in the region corresponding with the areas of the buttocks, perineum, and medial aspects of the thighs that impinge on the saddle in riding.

Lumbar puncture (spinal tap) is the tapping of the subarachnoid space in the lumbar region (lumbar cistern), usually between the laminae of vertebrae L3 and L4 or vertebrae L4 and L5 during maximally flexing the vertebral column. It allows measurement of CSF pressure and withdrawal of a sample of the fluid for microbial or chemical analysis and also allows introduction of anesthesia, drugs, or radiopaque material into the subarachnoid space.

IV. STRUCTURES ASSOCIATED WITH THE SPINAL CORD

A. Cauda Equina ("Horse's Tail")

- Is formed by a great lash of dorsal and ventral roots of the lumbar and sacral spinal nerves that surround the **filum terminale**.
- Is located within the subarachnoid space (lumbar cistern) below the level of the conus medullaris.
- Is free to float in the CSF within the lumbar cistern and therefore is not damaged during a spinal tap.

B. Denticulate Ligaments

- Are lateral extensions of the spinal **pia mater**, consisting of **21 pairs** of toothpick-like processes.
- Extend laterally from the pia through the arachnoid to the dura mater between the dorsal and ventral roots of the spinal nerves.
- Help **hold the spinal cord** in position within the subarachnoid space.

C. Filum Terminale (Internum)

- Is a prolongation of the **pia mater** from the tip (conus medullaris) of the spinal cord at the level of L2.

- Lies in the midst of the cauda equina and ends at the level of S2 by attaching to the apex of the dural sac.
- Blends with the dura at the apex of the dural sac, and then the dura continues downward as the **filum terminale externum** (filum of the dura mater of the coccygeal ligament), which is attached to the dorsum of the coccyx.

D. Cerebrospinal Fluid

- Is contained in the subarachnoid space between the arachnoid and pia mater.
- Is formed by **vascular choroid plexuses** in the ventricles of the brain.
- Circulates through the ventricles, enters the subarachnoid space, and eventually filters into the venous system through arachnoid villi, projecting into the dural venous sinuses, particularly the superior sagittal sinus.

V. DERMATOME, MYOTOME, AND SCLEROTOME

A. Dermatome (See Figure 2.11)

- Is an area of skin innervated by sensory fibers derived from a particular spinal nerve or segment of the spinal cord. Knowledge of the segmental innervation is useful clinically to produce a region of anesthesia or to determine which nerve has been damaged.

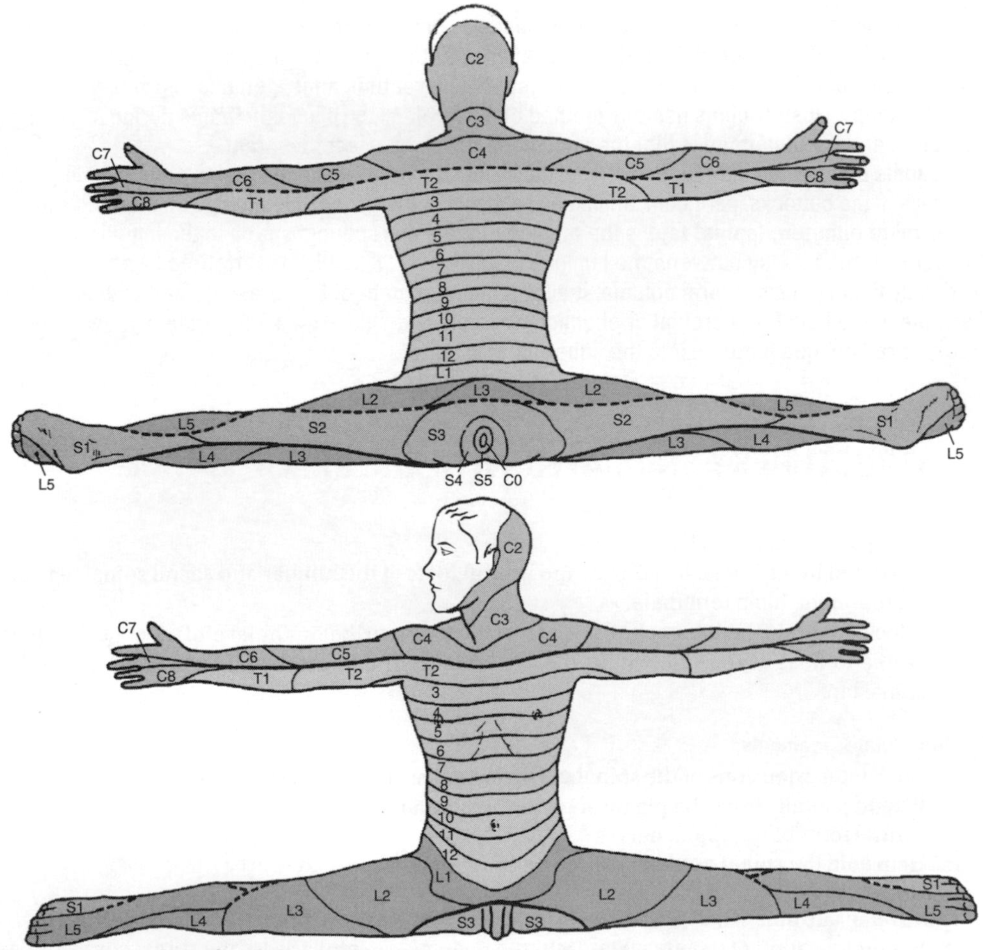

FIGURE 2.11. Schematic demarcation of dermatomes shown as distinct segments.

B. Myotome

- Is a group of muscles innervated by motor fibers derived from a single spinal nerve segment.

C. Sclerotome

- Is the area of a bone innervated from a single spinal segment.

VI. DEVELOPMENT OF BACK STRUCTURES

A. Development of Vertebral Column

- The embryonic mesoderm differentiates into the paraxial mesoderm, intermediate mesoderm, and lateral mesoderm.
- The paraxial mesoderm divides into **somites**, and each somite differentiates into the **sclerotome** (a ventromedial part) and the **dermatomyotome** (a dorsolateral part), which further differentiates into the **myotome** and the **dermatome**.
- Mesenchymal cells from the sclerotome form condensations around the neural tube and the notochord.
- The caudal half of one sclerotome fuses with the cranial half of the next sclerotome to form a **vertebral body**.
- The notochord degenerates in the vertebral body, but it forms the nucleus **pulposus** in the intervertebral disks.
- The **annulus fibrosus** of the intervertebral disk is derived from mesenchymal cells of sclerotome situated between adjacent vertebral bodies.

B. Development of Spinal Cord and Meninges (See Figure 2.10)

1. Neural Tube Formation (Neurulation)

- The **notochord** induces the overlying ectoderm to differentiate into neuroectoderm to form the neural plate.
- The **neural plate** (neuroectoderm) folds to form the neural tube. As the neural plate folds, some cells differentiate into neural crest cells.
- The **neural tube** initially remains open at cranial and caudal neuropores.
- The brain develops from cranial swellings of neural tube after closure of cranial neuropore.
- The spinal cord develops from caudal neural tube on closure of caudal neuropore.
- Neuroblasts form all neurons within the brain and spinal cord, including preganglionic sympathetic and parasympathetic neurons.

2. Neural Crest Cells

- Develop from the junction of the neural tube and surface ectoderm.
- Give rise to dorsal root ganglia, autonomic ganglia, and adrenal medulla.

3. Meninges

- The **dura mater** arises from the mesoderm that surrounds the neural tube.
- The **pia mater** and the arachnoid membrane arise from neural crest cells.

C. Development of Back Muscles

- Differentiating somites give rise to segmental myotomes, and each myotome splits into dorsal **epimere** (dorsal part of a myotome) and ventral **hypomere** (ventrolateral part of a myotome).
- The epimere gives rise to deep back (epaxial) muscles that are innervated by dorsal primary rami of spinal nerves.
- The hypomere gives rise to body-wall (hypaxial) muscles that are innervated by ventral primary rami of spinal nerves. The prevertebral and postvertebral muscles develop from the segmental myotomes.
- Limb muscles that arise from the hypomere migrate into limb buds and are innervated by ventral primary rami of spinal nerves.
- Superficial muscles of the back are muscles of the upper limb that develop from limb bud mesoderm and migrate into the back and are innervated by ventral primary rami of spinal nerves.

HIGH-YIELD TOPICS

- **Vertebral column** consists of 33 vertebrae, including the 7 cervical, 12 thoracic, 5 lumbar, 5 fused sacral, and 4 fused coccyx or 26 vertebrae (if the sacrum and coccyx are considered as a fused 1 bone each).
- **Atlas** is the C1 vertebra, supports the skull and helps make nodding movements possible. The **axis** has a dens that helps the head to rotate.
- **Alar ligament** prevents excessive rotation of the head. The **ligamentum nuchae** is the extension of the supraspinous ligament in the cervical region. The **ligamentum flavum** connects adjacent laminae.
- **Intervertebral disks** consist of a central **nucleus pulposus** with a surrounding **annulus fibrosus** and serve as shock absorbers. The nucleus pulposus arises from the embryonic notochord and may **herniate** through the ruptured annulus fibrosus, thereby impinging on the roots of the spinal nerve. Most herniated disk occurs at L4 to L5.
- **Primary curvatures** are located in the thoracic and sacral regions and develop during embryonic and fetal periods, whereas the **secondary curvatures** are located in the cervical and lumbar regions.
- **Spina bifida** is a defective closure of the vertebral arch associated with maternal folic acid deficiency and includes (a) **spina bifida occulta**—a failure of the vertebral arch to fuse (bony defect only with a small tuft of hair over the affected area of skin), (b) **meningocele**—a protrusion of the meninges through the unfused arch of the vertebra (spina bifida cystica), (c) **meningomyelocele**—a protrusion of the spinal cord and the meninges, and (d) **myeloschisis (rachischisis)**—a cleft spinal cord due to failure of neural folds to close.
- **Lumbar spondylosis** (ankylosis) is a degenerative joint disease affecting the lumbar vertebrae and intervertebral disks, causing pain, muscle weakness, and stiffness, sometimes with sciatic radiation resulting from nerve root pressure by associated protruding disks or osteophytes.
- **Klippel–Feil syndrome** is a congenital defect manifested as a short, stiff neck resulting from reduction in the number of cervical vertebrae or extensive fusion of the cervical vertebrae.
- **Arnold–Chiari (or Chiari) deformity** is a congenital cerebellomedullary malformation in which the cerebellum and medulla oblongata protrude down into the vertebral canal through the foramen magnum.
- **Atlantooccipital joint** is a condylar synovial joint and involved in flexion, extension, and lateral flexion of the head. The **atlantoaxial joints** consist of two lateral plane joints and one median pivot joint (between the anterior arch of the atlas and the dens of the axis), and are involved in rotation of the atlas and head as a one unit on the axis.
- **Atlantoaxial dislocation (subluxation)** occurs after rupture of the cruciform ligament caused by trauma or rheumatoid arthritis. It may result from a congenital absence of the dens, a fracture of the dens, or a direct trauma frequently caused by traffic accidents.
- **Compression fracture** is produced by collapse of the vertebral bodies resulting from trauma, results in kyphosis or scoliosis, and may cause spinal nerve compression.
- **Whiplash injury of the neck** is produced by a force that drives the trunk forward while the head lags behind, causing **the head** (with the upper part of the neck) **to hyperextend** and **the lower part of the neck to hyperflex rapidly**, as occurs in rear-end automobile collisions.
- **Herniated (slipped) disk** is a **protrusion of the nucleus pulposus** through the annulus fibrosus of the intervertebral disk into the intervertebral foramen or into the vertebral canal, compressing the spinal nerve root. It commonly occurs posterolaterally.
- **Sciatica** is pain in the lower back and hip, radiating into the buttock and into the lower limb and is most commonly caused by herniation of a lower lumbar intervertebral disk, compressing or irritating roots of the sciatic nerve. It causes muscular weakness, numbness, tingling, and pain along the path of the sciatic nerve.
- **Hangman fracture** is a fracture of the pedicles of the axis (C2), which may occur as a result of judicial hanging or automobile accidents. In this fracture, the cruciform ligament is torn and the spinal cord is crushed, causing death.
- **Spinal cord** occupies approximately the upper two-thirds of the vertebral canal, is enveloped by three meninges, and has cervical and lumbar enlargements for nerve supply of the upper and

lower limbs, respectively. It has a conical end known as the **conus medullaris**, which terminates at the level of L2 vertebra.

- **Denticulate ligaments** are 21 pairs of lateral extensions of the pia mater; the **filum terminale** internus is an inferior extension of the pia mater; **CSF** is formed by vascular choroid plexuses in the ventricles of the brain and is contained in the subarachnoid space; and the **cauda equina** (horse's tail) is formed by dorsal and ventral roots of the lumbar and sacral spinal nerves.
- **Tethered cord syndrome** is a congenital anomaly resulting from defective closure of the neural tube. It is characterized by the abnormally low conus medullaris, which is tethered by a short thickened filum terminale, leading to such conditions as progressive neurologic defects in the legs and feet and scoliosis.
- **Spinal nerves** consist of 31 pairs of nerves (8 cervical, 12 thoracic, 5 lumbar, 5 sacral, and 1 coccygeal). The **cervical spinal nerves** exit above the correspondingly numbered vertebrae except the eighth cervical nerves, which emerge below the seventh cervical vertebra; the remaining spinal nerves exit below the correspondingly numbered vertebrae.
- **Shingles (herpes zoster)** is caused by the **varicella zoster virus** that remains latent in the dorsal root ganglia of spinal nerves and the sensory ganglia of cranial nerves. It results from activation of the virus, which travels down the sensory nerve to produce severe neuralgic pain, an eruption of groups of vesicles, or a rash in the dermatome of the nerve.
- **Caudal (epidural) anesthesia** is used to **block the spinal nerves in the epidural space** by injection of local anesthetic agents via the sacral hiatus located between the sacral cornua.
- **Saddle block** is the introduction of anesthesia into the dural sac in the region corresponding with the areas of the buttocks, perineum, and medial aspects of the thighs that impinge on the saddle in riding.
- **Lumbar puncture (spinal tap)** is the tapping of the subarachnoid space in the lumbar region (lumbar cistern), usually between the laminae of vertebrae L3 and L4 or vertebrae L4 and L5. It allows measurement of CSF pressure and withdrawal of a fluid sample for microbial or chemical analysis and also allows introduction of anesthesia, drugs, or radiopaque material into the subarachnoid space.
- **Meninges** consist of a pia mater (innermost layer), arachnoid mater (transparent spidery layer), and dura mater (tough fibrous outermost layer). The **subarachnoid space** between the pia and arachnoid maters contains CSF, the **subdural space** between the arachnoid and dura maters contains moistening fluid, and the **epidural space** external to the dura mater contains the internal vertebral venous plexus.
- **Meningitis** is inflammation of the meninges caused by viral or bacterial infection. Bacterial meningitis (purulent meningitis) is an extremely serious illness and may result in brain damage or death, even if treated. Meningitis is also caused by fungi, chemical irritation or drug allergies, and tumors.
- **Vertebral artery** arises from the subclavian artery and ascends through the transverse foramina of the upper six cervical vertebrae.
- **Vertebral veins** are formed in the suboccipital triangle by tributaries from the venous plexus around the foramen magnum and the suboccipital venous plexus and descend through the transverse foramina.
- **Internal vertebral venous plexus** lies in the epidural space and communicates superiorly with the cranial dural sinuses and inferiorly with the pelvic veins and with both the azygos and caval systems in the thoracic and abdominal regions. This venous plexus is the route of early metastasis of carcinoma from the lung, breast, and prostate gland or uterus to bones and the CNS.
- **External vertebral venous plexus** lies in front of the vertebral column and on the vertebral arch and communicates with the internal vertebral venous plexus.
- **Superficial muscles** of the back are involved in moving the shoulder and arm and are innervated by ventral primary rami of the spinal nerves.
- **Intermediate muscles** are muscles of respiration.
- **Deep muscles** of the back are responsible for extension of the spine and head and are innervated by dorsal primary rami of the spinal nerves.
- **Triangle of auscultation** is bounded by the latissimus dorsi, trapezius, and scapula (medial border) and is the site where breathing sounds can be heard most clearly. The **lumbar triangle** is formed

by the iliac crest, latissimus dorsi, and external oblique abdominal muscles. It may be the site of an abdominal hernia.

- **Suboccipital triangle** is bounded by the rectus capitis posterior major, obliquus capitis superior, and obliquus capitis inferior muscles. The suboccipital muscles are innervated by the suboccipital nerve (dorsal primary ramus of C1).
- **Accessory nerve** consists of a cranial portion that joins the vagus nerve and a spinal portion that supplies the sternocleidomastoid and trapezius muscles.
- **Dorsal scapular nerve** (C5) supplies the rhomboid major and minor and levator scapulae muscles.
- **Suboccipital nerve** (C1) supplies the muscles of the suboccipital region. **The greater occipital nerve (C2)** is derived from the dorsal primary ramus and communicates with the suboccipital and third occipital nerves and may supply the semispinalis capitis.

Review Test

Directions: Each of the numbered items or incomplete statements in this section is followed by answers or by completions of the statement. Select the **one**-lettered answer or completion that is **best** in each case.

1. During an outbreak of meningitis at a local college, a 20-year-old student presents to a hospital emergency department complaining of headache, fever, chills, and stiff neck. On examination, it appears that he may have meningitis and needs a lumbar puncture or a spinal tap. Cerebrospinal fluid (CSF) is normally withdrawn from which of the following spaces?

(A) Epidural space
(B) Subdural space
(C) Space between the spinal cord and the pia mater
(D) Subarachnoid space
(E) Space between the arachnoid and dura maters

2. A 23-year-old jockey falls from her horse and complains of headache, backache, and weakness. Radiologic examination would reveal blood in which of the following spaces if the internal vertebral venous plexus was ruptured?

(A) Space deep to the pia mater
(B) Space between the arachnoid and dura maters
(C) Subdural space
(D) Epidural space
(E) Subarachnoid space

3. A 42-year-old woman with metastatic breast cancer is known to have tumors in the intervertebral foramina between the fourth and fifth cervical vertebrae and between the fourth and fifth thoracic vertebrae. Which of the following spinal nerves may be damaged?

(A) Fourth cervical and fourth thoracic nerves
(B) Fifth cervical and fifth thoracic nerves
(C) Fourth cervical and fifth thoracic nerves
(D) Fifth cervical and fourth thoracic nerves
(E) Third cervical and fourth thoracic nerves

4. A 39-year-old woman with headaches presents to her primary care physician with a possible herniated disk. Her magnetic resonance imaging (MRI) scan reveals that the posterolateral protrusion of the intervertebral disk between L4 and L5 vertebrae would most likely affect nerve roots of which of the following spinal nerves?

(A) Third lumbar nerve
(B) Fourth lumbar nerve
(C) Fifth lumbar nerve
(D) First sacral nerve
(E) Second sacral nerve

5. A 57-year-old woman comes into her physician's office complaining of fever, nausea, vomiting, and the worst headache of her life. Tests and physical examination suggest hydrocephalus (widening ventricles) resulting from a decrease in the absorption of cerebrospinal fluid (CSF). A decrease of flow in the CSF through which of the following structures would be responsible for these findings?

(A) Choroid plexus
(B) Vertebral venous plexus
(C) Arachnoid villi
(D) Internal jugular vein
(E) Subarachnoid trabeculae

6. After a 26-year-old man's car was broadsided by a large truck, he is brought to the emergency department with multiple fractures of the transverse processes of the cervical and upper thoracic vertebrae. Which of the following muscles might be affected?

(A) Trapezius
(B) Levator scapulae
(C) Rhomboid major
(D) Serratus posterior superior
(E) Rectus capitis posterior major

7. A 27-year-old mountain climber falls from a steep rock wall and is brought to the emergency department. His physical examination and computed tomography (CT) scan reveal dislocation fracture of the upper thoracic vertebrae. The fractured body of the T4 vertebra articulates with which of the following parts of the ribs?

(A) Head of the third rib
(B) Neck of the fourth rib
(C) Tubercle of the fourth rib
(D) Head of the fifth rib
(E) Tubercle of the fifth rib

8. A young toddler presents to her pediatrician with rather new onset of bowel and bladder dysfunction and loss of the lower limb function. Her mother had not taken enough folic acid (to the point of a deficiency) during her pregnancy. On examination, the child has protrusion of the spinal cord and meninges and is diagnosed with which of the following conditions?

(A) Spina bifida occulta
(B) Meningocele
(C) Meningomyelocele
(D) Myeloschisis
(E) Syringomyelocele

9. A 34-year-old woman crashes into a tree during a skiing lesson and is brought to a hospital with multiple injuries that impinge the dorsal primary rami of several spinal nerves. Such lesions could affect which of the following muscles?

(A) Rhomboid major
(B) Levator scapulae
(C) Serratus posterior superior
(D) Iliocostalis
(E) Latissimus dorsi

10. During a domestic dispute, a 16-year-old boy receives a deep stab wound around the superior angle of the scapula near the medial border, which injures both the dorsal scapular and spinal accessory nerves. Such an injury could result in paralysis or weakness of which of the following muscles?

(A) Trapezius and serratus posterior superior
(B) Rhomboid major and trapezius
(C) Rhomboid minor and latissimus dorsi
(D) Splenius cervicis and sternocleidomastoid
(E) Levator scapulae and erector spinae

11. An elderly man at a nursing home is known to have degenerative brain disease. When cerebrospinal fluid (CSF) is withdrawn by lumbar puncture for further examination, which of the following structures is most likely penetrated by the needle?

(A) Pia mater
(B) Filum terminale externum
(C) Posterior longitudinal ligament
(D) Ligamentum flavum
(E) Annulus fibrosus

12. A 27-year-old stuntman is thrown out of his vehicle prematurely when the car used for a particular scene speeds out of control. His spinal cord is crushed at the level of the fourth lumbar spinal segment. Which of the following structures would most likely be spared from destruction?

(A) Dorsal horn
(B) Ventral horn
(C) Lateral horn
(D) Gray matter
(E) Pia mater

13. A 24-year-old woman comes to a hospital to deliver her baby. Her obstetrician uses a caudal anesthesia during labor and childbirth to block the spinal nerves in the epidural space. Local anesthetic agents are most likely injected via which of the following openings?

(A) Intervertebral foramen
(B) Sacral hiatus
(C) Vertebral canal
(D) Dorsal sacral foramen
(E) Ventral sacral foramen

14. In a freak hunting accident, a 17-year-old boy was shot with an arrow that penetrated into his suboccipital triangle, injuring the suboccipital nerve between the vertebral artery and the posterior arch of the atlas. Which of the following muscles would be unaffected by such a lesion?

(A) Rectus capitis posterior major
(B) Semispinalis capitis
(C) Splenius capitis
(D) Obliquus capitis superior
(E) Obliquus capitis inferior

15. A 26-year-old heavyweight boxer was punched on his mandible, resulting in a slight subluxation (dislocation) of the atlantoaxial joint. The consequence of the injury was decreased range of motion at that joint. What movement would be most affected?

(A) Extension
(B) Flexion
(C) Abduction
(D) Adduction
(E) Rotation

16. A crush injury of the vertebral column can cause the spinal cord to swell. Which structure would be trapped between the dura and the vertebral body by the swelling spinal cord?

(A) Anterior longitudinal ligament
(B) Alar ligament
(C) Posterior longitudinal ligament
(D) Cruciform ligament
(E) Ligamentum nuchae

17. A 44-year-old woman comes to her physician and complains of headache and backache. On examination, she is found to have fluid accumulated in the spinal epidural space because of damage to blood vessels or meninges. Which of the following structures is most likely ruptured?

(A) Vertebral artery
(B) Vertebral vein
(C) External vertebral venous plexus
(D) Internal vertebral venous plexus
(E) Lumbar cistern

18. A 69-year-old man has an abnormally increased curvature of the thoracic vertebral column. Which of the following conditions is the most likely diagnosis?

(A) Lordosis
(B) Spina bifida occulta
(C) Meningocele
(D) Meningomyelocele
(E) Kyphosis

19. During a snowstorm, a 52-year-old man is brought to the emergency department after a multiple car accident. Which of the following conditions is produced by a force that drives the trunk forward while the head lags behind in a rear-end automobile collision?

(A) Scoliosis
(B) Hangman fracture
(C) Meningomyelocele
(D) Whiplash injury
(E) Herniated disk

20. A 37-year-old man is brought to the emergency department with a crushed second cervical vertebra (axis) that he suffered after a stack of pallets fell on him at work. Which of the following structures would be intact after the accident?

(A) Alar ligament
(B) Apical ligament
(C) Semispinalis cervicis muscle
(D) Rectus capitis posterior minor
(E) Obliquus capitis inferior

21. A middle-aged coal miner injures his back after an accidental explosion. His magnetic resonance imaging (MRI) scan reveals that his spinal cord has shifted to the right because the lateral extensions of the pia mater were torn. Function of which of the following structures is most likely impaired?

(A) Filum terminale internum
(B) Coccygeal ligament
(C) Denticulate ligament
(D) Choroid plexus
(E) Tectorial membrane

22. A 25-year-old man with congenital abnormalities at birth has a lesion of the dorsal scapular nerve, making him unable to adduct his scapula. Which of the following muscles is most likely paralyzed?

(A) Semispinalis capitis
(B) Rhomboid major
(C) Multifidus
(D) Rotator longus
(E) Iliocostalis

23. After an automobile accident, a back muscle that forms the boundaries of the triangle of auscultation and the lumbar triangle receives no blood. Which of the following muscles might be ischemic?

(A) Levator scapulae
(B) Rhomboid minor
(C) Latissimus dorsi
(D) Trapezius
(E) Splenius capitis

24. A 38-year-old woman with a long history of shoulder pain is admitted to a hospital for surgery. Which of the following muscles becomes ischemic soon after ligation of the superficial or ascending branch of the transverse cervical artery?

(A) Latissimus dorsi
(B) Multifidus
(C) Trapezius
(D) Rhomboid major
(E) Longissimus capitis

25. A 25-year-old soldier suffers a gunshot wound on the lower part of his back and is unable to move his legs. A neurologic examination and magnetic resonance imaging (MRI) scan reveal injury of the cauda equina. Which of the following is most likely damaged?

(A) Dorsal primary rami
(B) Ventral primary rami
(C) Dorsal roots of the thoracic spinal nerves
(D) Ventral roots of the sacral spinal nerves
(E) Lumbar spinal nerves

Questions 26 to 30: Choose the appropriate lettered structure in this magnetic resonance imaging (MRI) scan of the back (see Figure below).

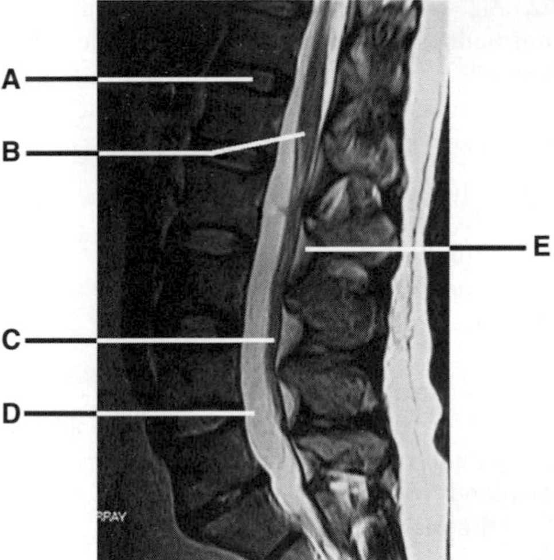

26. When the internal vertebral venous plexus is ruptured, venous blood may spread into which tissue and space?

27. Dorsal and ventral roots of the lower lumbar and sacral nerves are lacerated. Which structure is most likely damaged?

28. The spinal cord is crushed at the level of the upper part of the first lumbar vertebra. Which structure is most likely damaged?

29. Which structure may herniate through the annulus fibrosus, thereby impinging on the roots of the spinal nerve?

30. Cerebrospinal fluid (CSF) is produced by vascular choroid plexuses in the ventricles of the brain and accumulated in which space?

Answers and Explanations

1. **The Answer is D.** Cerebrospinal fluid (CSF) is found in the subarachnoid space, which is a wide interval between the arachnoid layer and the pia mater. The epidural space contains the internal vertebral venous plexus and epidural fat. The subdural space between the arachnoid and the dura contains a little fluid to moisten the meningeal surface. The pia mater closely covers the spinal cord and enmeshes blood vessels on the surfaces of the spinal cord. Thus, the space between the spinal cord and the pia is a potential space.

2. **The Answer is D.** The space between the vertebral canal and the dura mater is the epidural space, which contains the internal vertebral venous plexus. The spinal cord and blood vessels lie deep to the pia mater. The space between the arachnoid and dura maters is the subdural space, which contains a film of fluid. The subarachnoid space contains cerebrospinal fluid (CSF).

3. **The Answer is D.** All cervical spinal nerves exit through the intervertebral foramina above the corresponding vertebrae, except the eighth cervical nerves, which run inferior to the seventh cervical vertebra. All other spinal nerves exit the intervertebral foramina below the corresponding vertebrae. Therefore, the fifth cervical nerve passes between the fourth and fifth cervical vertebrae, and the fourth thoracic nerve runs between the fourth and fifth thoracic vertebrae.

4. **The Answer is C.** A posterolateral herniation of the intervertebral disk at disk level L4 to L5 affects the fifth lumbar nerve root but rarely affects the fourth lumbar nerve root because of a progressive descending obliquity of the fourth and fifth lumbar nerve roots. The first seven cervical nerves exit above the corresponding vertebra, and the eighth cervical nerve exits below the seventh cervical vertebra because there are eight cervical nerves but only seven cervical vertebrae. The rest of the spinal nerves exit below their corresponding vertebrae.

5. **The Answer is C.** Cerebrospinal fluid (CSF) is absorbed into the venous system primarily through the arachnoid villi projecting into the cranial dural venous sinuses, particularly the superior sagittal sinus. CSF is produced by the choroid plexuses of the ventricles of the brain and is circulated in the subarachnoid space, in which subarachnoid trabeculae are also found. The vertebral venous plexus and internal jugular vein are not involved in the absorption of CSF.

6. **The Answer is B.** The levator scapulae arise from the transverse processes of the upper cervical vertebrae and inserts on the medial border of the scapula. The other muscles are attached to the spinous processes of the vertebrae.

7. **The Answer is D.** The body of vertebra T4 articulates with the heads of the fourth and fifth ribs. The body of the T3 vertebra articulates with the head of the third and fourth ribs. The neck of a rib does not articulate with any part of the vertebra. The transverse process of the vertebra articulates with the tubercle of the corresponding rib. Therefore, the transverse process of vertebra T4 articulates with the tubercle of the fourth rib.

8. **The Answer is C.** Meningomyelocele is protrusion of the meninges and spinal cord through the unfused arch of the vertebra. A sufficient amount of folic acid during pregnancy is shown to prevent these kinds of neural tube defects. Spina bifida occulta is failure of the vertebral arch to fuse (only bony defect). Meningocele is protrusion of the meninges through the defective vertebral arch. Syringomyelocele is protrusion of the meninges and a pathologic tubular cavity in the spinal cord or brain.

9. **The Answer is D.** The dorsal primary rami of the spinal nerves innervate the deep muscles of the back, including the iliocostalis. The other muscles are the superficial muscles of the back, which are innervated by the ventral primary rami of the spinal nerves.

10. **The Answer is B.** The dorsal scapular nerve innervates the levator scapulae and rhomboid muscles, whereas the accessory nerve innervates the trapezius and sternocleidomastoid muscles. The serratus posterior superior is innervated by ventral primary rami of the spinal nerves, whereas the splenius cervicis and erector spinae are innervated by dorsal primary rami of the spinal nerves.

11. **The Answer is D.** The cerebrospinal fluid (CSF) is located in the subarachnoid space, between the arachnoid layer and the pia mater. In a lumbar puncture, the needle penetrates the skin, fascia, ligamentum flavum, epidural space, dura mater, subdural space, and arachnoid mater. The pia mater forms the internal boundary of the subarachnoid space; thus, it cannot be penetrated by needle. The posterior longitudinal ligament lies anterior to the spinal cord; thus, it is not penetrated by the needle. The filum terminale externum is the downward prolongation of the spinal dura mater from the second sacral vertebra to the dorsum of the coccyx. The annulus fibrosus consists of concentric layers of fibrous tissue and fibrocartilage surrounding and retaining the nucleus pulposus of the intervertebral disk, which lies anterior to the spinal cord.

12. **The Answer is C.** The lateral horns, which contain sympathetic preganglionic neuron cell bodies, are present between the first thoracic and second lumbar spinal cord levels (T1–L2). The lateral horns of the second, third, and fourth sacral spinal cord levels (S2–S4) contain parasympathetic preganglionic neuron cell bodies. The entire spinal cord is surrounded by the pia mater and has the dorsal horn, ventral horn, and gray matter. Note that the fourth lumbar spinal cord level is not the same as the fourth vertebral level.

13. **The Answer is B.** Caudal (epidural) anesthesia is used to block the spinal nerves in the epidural space by injecting local anesthetic agents via the sacral hiatus located between the sacral cornua. An intervertebral foramen transmits the dorsal and ventral primary rami of the spinal nerves. The vertebral canal accommodates the spinal cord. Dorsal and ventral sacral foramina transmit the dorsal and ventral primary rami of the sacral nerves.

14. **The Answer is C.** The splenius capitis is innervated by dorsal primary rami of the middle and lower cervical nerves. The suboccipital nerve (dorsal primary ramus of C1) supplies the muscles of the suboccipital area, including the rectus capitis posterior major, obliquus capitis superior and inferior, and the semispinalis capitis.

15. **The Answer is E.** The atlantoaxial joints are synovial joints that consist of two plane joints and one pivot joint and are involved primarily in rotation of the head. Other movements do not occur at this joint.

16. **The Answer is C.** The posterior longitudinal ligament interconnects the vertebral bodies and intervertebral disks posteriorly and runs anterior to the spinal cord within the vertebral canal. The ligamentum nuchae is formed by supraspinous ligaments that extend from the seventh cervical vertebra to the external occipital protuberance and crest. The anterior longitudinal ligament runs anterior to the vertebral bodies. The alar and cruciform ligaments also lie anterior to the spinal cord.

17. **The Answer is D.** The internal vertebral venous plexus is located in the spinal epidural space. The vertebral artery and vein occupy the transverse foramina of the upper six cervical vertebrae. The external vertebral venous plexus consists of the anterior part, which lies in front of the vertebral column, and the posterior part, which lies on the vertebral arch. The lumbar cistern is the enlargement of the subarachnoid space between the inferior end of the spinal cord and the inferior end of the subarachnoid space.

18. **The Answer is E.** Kyphosis (hunchback or humpback) is an abnormally increased thoracic curvature, usually resulting from osteoporosis. Lordosis is an abnormal accentuation of the lumbar curvature. Spina bifida occulta is failure of the vertebral arch to fuse (only bony defect). Meningocele is a protrusion of the meninges through the unfused arch of the vertebra, whereas meningomyelocele is a protrusion of the spinal cord and the meninges.

19. **The Answer is D.** Whiplash injury of the neck is produced by a force that drives the trunk forward while the head lags behind. Scoliosis is a lateral deviation resulting from unequal growth of the spinal column. Hangman fracture is a fracture of the neural arch through the pedicle of the axis that may occur as a result of hanging or motor vehicle accidents. Meningomyelocele is

a protrusion of the spinal cord and its meninges. A herniated disk compresses the spinal nerve roots when the nucleus pulposus is protruded through the annulus fibrosus.

20. **The Answer is D.** The rectus capitis posterior minor arises from the posterior tubercle of the atlas and inserts on the occipital bone below the inferior nuchal line. The alar ligament extends from the apex of the dens to the medial side of the occipital bone. The apical ligament extends from the dens of the axis to the anterior aspect of the foramen magnum of the occipital bone. The semispinalis cervicis arises from the transverse processes and inserts on the spinous processes. The obliquus capitis inferior originates from the spine of the axis and inserts on the transverse process of the atlas.

21. **The Answer is C.** The denticulate ligament is a lateral extension of the pia mater. The filum terminale (internum) is an inferior extension of the pia mater from the tip of the conus medullaris. The coccygeal ligament, which is also called the filum terminale externum or the filum of the dura, extends from the tip of the dural sac to the coccyx. The vascular choroid plexuses produce the cerebrospinal fluid (CSF) in the ventricles of the brain. The tectorial membrane is an upward extension of the posterior longitudinal ligaments from the body of the axis to the basilar part of the occipital bone.

22. **The Answer is B.** The rhomboid major is a superficial muscle of the back; is innervated by the dorsal scapular nerve, which arises from the ventral primary ramus of the fifth cervical nerve; and adducts the scapula. The semispinalis capitis, multifidus, rotator longus, and iliocostalis muscles are deep muscles of the back, are innervated by dorsal primary rami of the spinal nerves, and have no attachment to the scapula.

23. **The Answer is C.** The latissimus dorsi forms boundaries of the auscultation and lumbar triangles and receives blood from the thoracodorsal artery. The levator scapulae, rhomboid minor, and splenius capitis muscles do not form boundaries of these two triangles. The trapezius muscle forms a boundary of the auscultation triangle but not the lumbar triangle. The levator scapulae, rhomboid minor, and trapezius muscles receive blood from the transverse cervical artery. The splenius capitis muscle receives blood from the occipital and transverse cervical arteries.

24. **The Answer is C.** The trapezius receives blood from the superficial branch of the transverse cervical artery. The latissimus dorsi receives blood from the thoracodorsal artery. The rhomboid major receives blood from the deep or descending branch of the transverse cervical artery. The multifidus and longissimus capitis receive blood from the segmental arteries.

25. **The Answer is D.** The cauda equina is the collection of dorsal and ventral roots of the lower lumbar and sacral spinal nerves below the spinal cord. Dorsal and ventral primary rami and dorsal roots of the thoracic spinal nerves and lumbar spinal nerves do not participate in the formation of the cauda equina.

26. **The Answer is E.** Epidural fat is shown in the magnetic resonance imaging (MRI) scan. In addition, the internal vertebral venous plexus lies in the epidural space; thus, venous blood from the plexus may spread into epidural fat.

27. **The Answer is C.** The cauda equina is formed by a great lash of the dorsal and ventral roots of the lumbar and sacral nerves.

28. **The Answer is B.** The conus medullaris is a conical end of the spinal cord and terminates at the level of the L2 vertebra or the intervertebral disk between L1 and L2 vertebrae. A spinal cord injury at the level of the upper part of the first lumbar vertebra damages the conus medullaris.

29. **The Answer is A.** The intervertebral disk lies between the bodies of two vertebrae and consists of a central mucoid substance, the nucleus pulposus, and a surrounding fibrous tissue and fibrocartilage, the annulus fibrosus. The nucleus pulposus may herniate through the annulus fibrosus, thereby impinging on the roots of the spinal nerves.

30. **The Answer is D.** The cerebrospinal fluid (CSF) is found in the lumbar cistern, which is a subarachnoid space in the lumbar area. CSF is produced by vascular choroid plexuses in the ventricles of the brain, circulated in the subarachnoid space, and filtered into the venous system through the arachnoid villi and arachnoid granulations.

chapter 3

Thorax

THORACIC WALL

I. SKELETON OF THE THORAX (See Figure 3.1)

A. Sternum

- Is a flat bone and consists of the manubrium, the body, and the xiphoid process.
- Is relatively **shorter** and **thinner** in the female, and its body is more than twice as long as the manubrium in the male but is usually less in the female.

1. Manubrium

- Has a superior margin, the jugular notch, which can be readily palpated at the root of the neck.
- Has a clavicular notch on each side for articulation with the clavicle.
- Also articulates with the cartilage of the first rib, the upper half of the second rib, and the body of the sternum at the manubriosternal joint, or sternal angle.

2. Sternal Angle (Angle of Louis)

- Is the junction between the manubrium and the body of the sternum.
- Is located at the level where
  - **(a) The second ribs articulate with the sternum.**
  - **(b) The aortic arch begins and ends.**
  - **(c) The trachea bifurcates into the right and left bronchi at the carina.**
  - **(d) The inferior border of the superior mediastinum is demarcated.**
  - **(e) A transverse plane can pass through the intervertebral disk between T4 and T5.**

3. Body of the Sternum

- Articulates with the second to seventh costal cartilages.
- Also articulates with the xiphoid process at the **xiphisternal joint**, which is at level with the ninth thoracic vertebra.

4. Xiphoid Process

- Is a flat, cartilaginous process at birth that ossifies slowly from the central core and unites with the body of the sternum after middle age.
- Lies at the level of T10 vertebra, and the xiphisternal joint lies at the level of the T9 vertebral body, which marks the lower limit of the thoracic cavity in front, the upper surface of the liver, diaphragm, and lower border of the heart.
- Can be palpated in the epigastrium and is attached via its pointed caudal end to the **linea alba**.

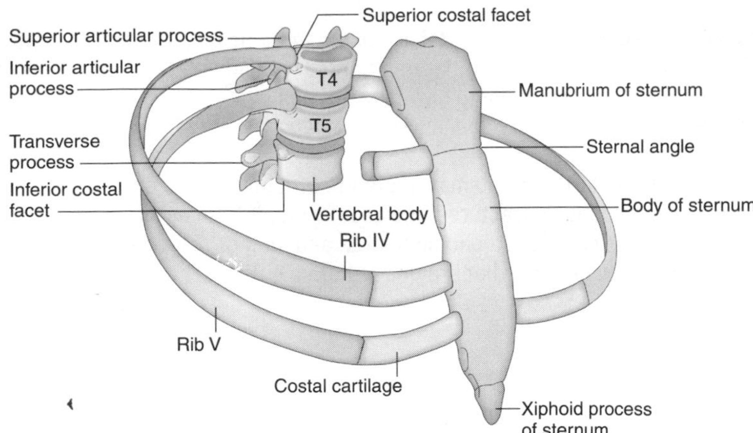

FIGURE 3.1. Articulations of the ribs with the vertebrae and the sternum.

CLINICAL CORRELATES The **sternum** is a common site for bone marrow biopsy because it possesses hematopoietic marrow throughout life and because of its breadth and subcutaneous position. It may be split in the median plane (median sternotomy) to allow the surgeon to gain easy access to the lungs, heart, and great vessels.

B. Ribs

- Consist of 12 pairs of bones that form the main part of the **thoracic cage**, extending from the vertebrae to or toward the sternum.
- **Increase** the anteroposterior and transverse **diameters** of the thorax by their movements.

1. Structure

- **Typical ribs** are ribs 3 through 9, each of which has a head, neck, tubercle, and body (shaft).
- The **head** articulates with the corresponding vertebral bodies and intervertebral disks and supraadjacent vertebral bodies.
- The **body** (shaft) is thin and flat and turns sharply anteriorly at the **angle** and has a **costal groove** that follows the inferior and internal surface of a rib and lodges the intercostal vessels and nerves.
- The tubercle articulates with the transverse processes of the corresponding vertebrae, with the exception of ribs 11 and 12.

2. Classification

(a) True Ribs

- Are the first seven ribs **(ribs 1–7)**, which are attached to the sternum by their costal cartilages.

(b) False Ribs

- Are the lower five ribs **(ribs 8–12)**; ribs 8 to 10 are connected to the costal cartilages immediately above, and thus, the 7th to 10th costal cartilages form the anterior **costal arch** or costal margin.

(c) Floating Ribs

- Are the last two ribs **(ribs 11 and 12)**, which are connected only to the vertebrae.

CLINICAL CORRELATES **Thoracic outlet syndrome** is the compression of neurovascular structures in the thoracic outlet (a space between the clavicle and the first rib), causing a combination of pain, numbness, tingling, or weakness and fatigue in the upper limb caused by pressure on the brachial plexus (lower trunk or C8 and T1 nerve roots) by a **cervical rib** (mesenchymal or cartilaginous elongation of the transverse process of the seventh cervical vertebra). A cervical rib may also compress the subclavian artery in the thoracic outlet, resulting in ischemic muscle pain in the upper limb. Compression on the neurovascular bundle occurs as a result of cervical ribs or **abnormal insertions** of the anterior and middle scalene muscles.

CLINICAL CORRELATES **Flail chest** is a loss of stability of the thoracic cage that occurs when a segment of the anterior or lateral thoracic wall moves freely because of **multiple rib fractures**, allowing the loose segment to move inward on inspiration and outward on expiration. Flail chest is an extremely painful injury and impairs ventilation, thereby affecting oxygenation of the blood and causing respiratory failure.

Rib fractures: Fracture of the first rib may injure the brachial plexus and subclavian vessels. The middle ribs are most commonly fractured and usually result from direct blows or crushing injuries. The broken ends of ribs may cause pneumothorax and lung or spleen injury. Lower rib fractures may tear the diaphragm, resulting in a diaphragmatic hernia.

3. First Rib

- Is the **broadest** and **shortest** of the true ribs.
- Has a single articular facet on its head, which articulates with the first thoracic vertebra.
- Has a **scalene tubercle** for the insertion of the anterior scalene muscle and **two grooves** for the subclavian artery and vein.

4. Second Rib

- Has two articular facets on its head, which articulate with the bodies of the first and second thoracic vertebrae.
- Is about twice as long as the first rib.

5. Tenth Rib

- Has a single articular facet on its head, which articulates with the 10th thoracic vertebra.

6. Eleventh and Twelfth Ribs

- Have a single articular facet on their heads.
- Have no neck or tubercle.

II. ARTICULATIONS OF THE THORAX (See Figure 3.1)

A. Sternoclavicular Joint

- Is a saddle-type synovial joint with two separate synovial cavities and provides the only bony attachment between the appendicular and axial skeletons.

B. Sternocostal (Sternochondral) Joints

- Are the articulation of the sternum with the first seven cartilages. The sternum (manubrium) forms synchondrosis with the first costal cartilage, whereas the second to seventh costal cartilages form synovial plane joints with the sternum.

C. Costochondral Joints

- Are synchondroses in which the ribs articulate with their respective costal cartilages.

D. Manubriosternal Joint

- Is symphysis (secondary cartilaginous joint) between manubrium and body of the sternum.

E. Xiphisternal Joint

- Is synchondrosis articulation between xiphoid process and body of the sternum.

F. Costovertebral Joints

- Are synovial plane joints of heads of ribs with corresponding and supraadjacent vertebral bodies.

G. Costotransverse Joint

- Is synovial plane joint of tubercle of rib with transverse process of corresponding vertebra.

H. Interchondral Joints

- Are synovial plane joints between 6th and 10th costal cartilages of ribs.

III. BREASTS AND MAMMARY GLANDS (See Figure 7.10, Chapter 7)

IV. MUSCLES OF THE THORACIC WALL (Table 3.1)

V. NERVES AND BLOOD VESSELS OF THE THORACIC WALL

A. Intercostal Nerves

- Are the **anterior primary rami** of the first 11 thoracic spinal nerves. The anterior primary ramus of the 12th thoracic spinal nerve is the **subcostal nerve**, which runs beneath the 12th rib.
- Run between the internal and innermost layers of muscles, with the intercostal veins and arteries above (**v**eins, **a**rteries, **n**erves [**VAN**]).
- Are lodged in the **costal grooves** on the inferior surface of the ribs.
- Give rise to lateral and anterior cutaneous branches and muscular branches.

B. Internal Thoracic Artery

- Usually arises from the **first part of the subclavian artery** and descends directly behind the first six costal cartilages, just lateral to the sternum.
- Gives rise to two anterior intercostal arteries in each of the upper six intercostal spaces and terminates at the sixth intercostal space by dividing into the musculophrenic and superior epigastric arteries.

1. Pericardiophrenic Artery

- Accompanies the phrenic nerve between the pleura and the pericardium to the diaphragm.
- Supplies the pleura, pericardium, and diaphragm (upper surface).

2. Anterior Intercostal Arteries

- Are **12 small arteries**, 2 in each of the upper 6 intercostal spaces that run laterally, one each at the upper and lower borders of each space. The upper artery in each intercostal space anastomoses with the **posterior intercostal artery**, and the lower one joins the **collateral branch** of the posterior intercostal artery.
- Provide muscular branches to the intercostal, serratus anterior, and pectoral muscles.

3. Anterior Perforating Branches

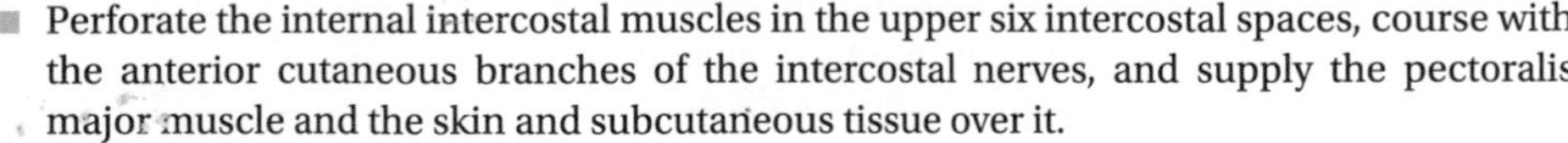

- Perforate the internal intercostal muscles in the upper six intercostal spaces, course with the anterior cutaneous branches of the intercostal nerves, and supply the pectoralis major muscle and the skin and subcutaneous tissue over it.
- Provide the **medial mammary branches** (second, third, and fourth branches).

table 3.1 Muscles of the Thoracic Wall

Muscle	Origin	Insertion	Nerve	Action
External intercostals	Lower border of ribs	Upper border of rib below	Intercostal	Elevate ribs in inspiration
Internal intercostals	Lower border of ribs	Upper border of rib below	Intercostal	Depress ribs (costal part); elevate ribs (interchondral part)
Innermost intercostals	Lower border of ribs	Upper border of rib below	Intercostal	Elevate ribs
Transversus thoracis	Posterior surface of lower sternum and xiphoid	Inner surface of costal cartilages 2–6	Intercostal	Depresses ribs
Subcostalis	Inner surface of lower ribs near their angles	Upper borders of ribs 2 or 3 below	Intercostal	Elevates ribs
Levator costarum	Transverse processes of T7–T11	Subjacent ribs between tubercle and angle	Dorsal primary rami of C8–T11	Elevates ribs

4. Musculophrenic Artery

- Follows the costal arch on the inner surface of the costal cartilages.
- Gives rise to two anterior arteries in the seventh, eighth, and ninth spaces; perforates the diaphragm; and ends in the 10th intercostal space, where it anastomoses with the **deep circumflex iliac artery**.
- Supplies the pericardium, diaphragm, and muscles of the abdominal wall.

5. Superior Epigastric Artery

- Descends on the deep surface of the rectus abdominis muscle within the rectus sheath; supplies this muscle and anastomoses with the **inferior epigastric artery**.
- Supplies the diaphragm, peritoneum, and anterior abdominal wall.

C. Internal Thoracic Vein

- Is formed by the confluence of the superior epigastric and musculophrenic veins, ascends on the medial side of the artery, receives the upper six anterior intercostal and pericardiacophrenic veins, and ends in the brachiocephalic vein.

D. Thoracoepigastric Vein

- Is a venous connection between the lateral thoracic vein and the superficial epigastric vein.

VI. LYMPHATIC DRAINAGE OF THE THORAX

A. Sternal or Parasternal (Internal Thoracic) Nodes

- Are placed along the **internal thoracic artery**.
- Receive lymph from the medial portion of the breast, intercostal spaces, diaphragm, and supraumbilical region of the abdominal wall.
- Drain into the junction of the internal jugular and subclavian veins.

B. Intercostal Nodes

- Lie near the heads of the ribs.
- Receive lymph from the intercostal spaces and the pleura.
- Drain into the **cisterna chyli** or the **thoracic duct**.

C. Phrenic Nodes

- Lie on the thoracic surface of the diaphragm.
- Receive lymph from the pericardium, diaphragm, and liver.
- Drain into the sternal and posterior mediastinal nodes.

VII. THYMUS

- Is a bilobed structure, lying in the neck anterior to the trachea and the anterior part of the superior mediastinum, attains its greatest relative size in the neonate, playing a key role in the development of the immune system in early life but continues to grow until puberty, and then undergoes a gradual involution, in which the thymic tissue is replaced by fat.
- Precursors of both B cells and T cells are produced in the bone marrow. T-lymphocyte precursors migrate to the thymus, where they develop into T lymphocytes. After the thymus undergoes involution, T lymphocytes (thymocytes) migrate out of the thymus to the peripheral lymphoid organs such as spleen, tonsils, and lymph nodes, where they further differentiate into mature immunologically competent cells, which are responsible for cell-mediated immune reactions. (However, B-lymphocyte precursors remain in the bone marrow to develop into B lymphocytes, which migrate to the peripheral lymphoid organs, where they become mature immunocompetent

B cells, which are responsible for the humeral immune response. Also, B cells differentiate into plasma cells that synthesize antibodies [immunoglobulins].)

- Arises from the third pharyngeal pouches, is supplied by the inferior thyroid and internal thoracic artery, and produces a hormone, thymosin, which promotes T-lymphocyte differentiation and maturation.

VIII. DIAPHRAGM AND ITS OPENINGS (See Figure 4.17, Chapter 4)

MEDIASTINUM, PLEURA, AND ORGANS OF RESPIRATION

I. MEDIASTINUM (See Figure 3.2)

- Is an **interpleural space** (area between the pleural cavities) in the thorax and is bounded laterally by the pleural cavities, anteriorly by the sternum and the transversus thoracis muscles, and posteriorly by the vertebral column (does not contain the lungs).
- Consists of the superior mediastinum above the pericardium and the three lower divisions: anterior, middle, and posterior.

A. Superior Mediastinum

- Is bounded superiorly by the oblique plane of the first rib and inferiorly by the imaginary line running from the sternal angle to the intervertebral disk between the fourth and fifth thoracic vertebrae.
- Contains the superior vena cava (SVC), brachiocephalic veins, **arch of the aorta**, thoracic duct, **trachea**, esophagus, vagus nerve, left recurrent laryngeal nerve, and phrenic nerve.
- Also contains the thymus, which is a lymphoid organ; is the site at which immature lymphocytes develop into T lymphocytes; and secretes thymic hormones, which cause T lymphocytes to gain immunocompetence. It begins involution after puberty.

B. Anterior Mediastinum

- Lies anterior to the pericardium and posterior to the sternum and the transverse thoracic muscles.
- Contains the remnants of the thymus gland, lymph nodes, fat, and connective tissue.

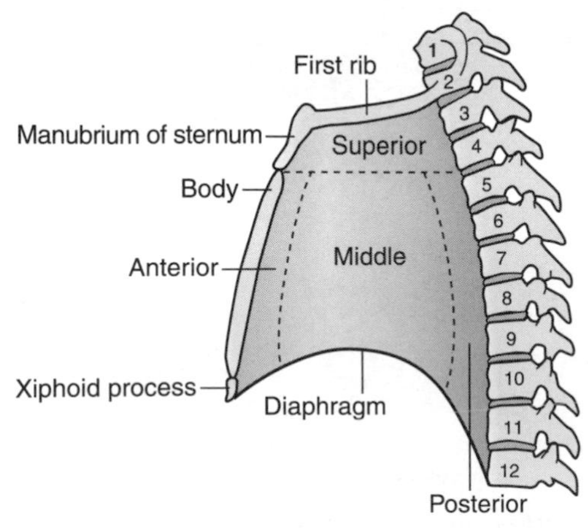

FIGURE 3.2. Mediastinum.

C. Middle Mediastinum

- Lies between the right and left pleural cavities.
- Contains the heart, pericardium, phrenic nerves, roots of the great vessels (aorta, pulmonary arteries and veins, and vena cavae), **arch of the azygos vein**, and main bronchi.

D. Posterior Mediastinum (See Structures in the Posterior Mediastinum)

- Lies posterior to the pericardium between the mediastinal pleurae.
- Contains the esophagus, thoracic aorta, azygos and hemiazygos veins, thoracic duct, vagus nerves, sympathetic trunk, and splanchnic nerves.

II. TRACHEA AND BRONCHI (See Figure 3.3)

A. Trachea

- Begins at the inferior border of the **cricoid cartilage** (C6) as a continuation of the larynx and ends by bifurcating into the right and left main stem bronchi at the level of the **sternal angle** (disk between T4 and T5).
- Is approximately 12 cm in length and has **16 to 20 incomplete hyaline cartilaginous rings** that open posteriorly toward the esophagus and prevent the trachea from collapsing.

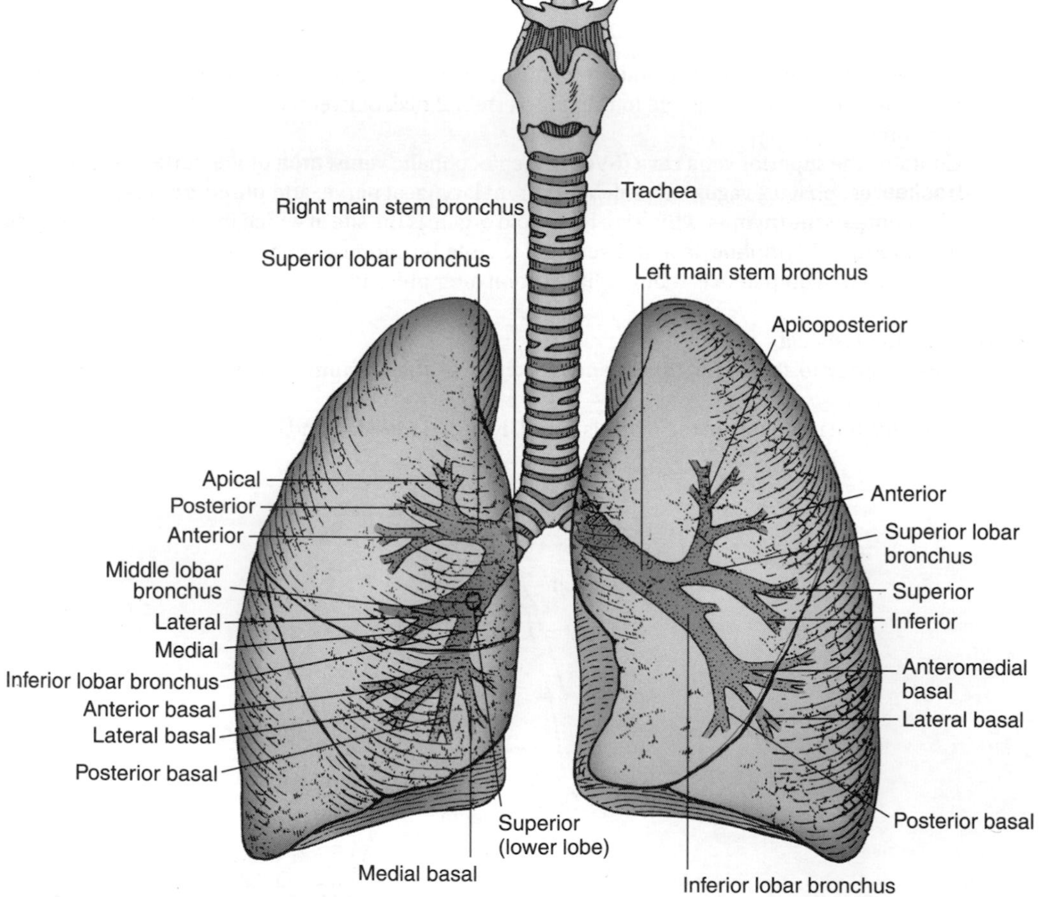

FIGURE 3.3. Anterior view of the trachea, bronchi, and lungs.

- May be compressed by an aortic arch aneurysm, a goiter, or thyroid tumors, causing dyspnea.
- Has the **carina**, a downward and backward projection of the last tracheal cartilage, which lies at the level of the sternal angle and forms a keel-like ridge separating the openings of the right and left main bronchi.
- **Carina** may be distorted, widened posteriorly, and immobile in the presence of a bronchogenic carcinoma. The mucous membrane over the carina is one of the most sensitive areas of the tracheobronchial tree and is associated with the cough reflex.

B. Right Main (Primary) Bronchus

- Is **shorter, wider**, and **more vertical** than the left main bronchus; therefore, more foreign bodies that enter through the trachea are lodged in this bronchus or inferior lobar bronchus.
- Runs under **the arch of the azygos vein** and divides into 3 lobar or secondary **(superior, middle,** and **inferior) bronchi** and finally into 10 segmental bronchi. The right superior lobar (secondary) bronchus is known as the **eparterial** (above the artery) **bronchus** because it passes above the level of the pulmonary artery. All others are the **hyparterial bronchi**.

C. Left Main (Primary) Bronchus

- Runs inferolaterally **inferior to the arch of the aorta**, crosses anterior to the esophagus and thoracic aorta, and divides into **2 lobar or secondary bronchi**, the upper and lower, and finally into 8 to 10 segmental bronchi.
- Is also **crossed superiorly by the arch of the aorta** over its proximal part **and by the left pulmonary artery** over its distal part.
- Dilates its lumen by sympathetic nerves and constricts by parasympathetic stimulation.

CLINICAL CORRELATES

Chronic obstructive pulmonary disease (COPD) is a group of lung diseases associated with chronic obstruction of airflow through the airways and lungs. It consists of **chronic bronchitis** and **emphysema**, which are the most common forms and is caused primarily by cigarette smoking. Symptoms of COPD include chronic cough, difficulty in breathing, chronic sputum production, and wheezing. It is treated with bronchodilators and glucocorticoids.

Chronic bronchitis is an **inflammation of the airways**, which results in **excessive mucus production** that plugs up the airways, causing a cough and breathing difficulty.

Emphysema is an accumulation of **air in the terminal bronchioles and alveolar sacs** (air is trapped in the lungs) **due to destruction of the alveolar walls**, reducing the surface area available for the exchange of oxygen and carbon dioxide and thereby reducing oxygen absorption. **Barrel chest** is a chest resembling the shape of a barrel, with increased anteroposterior diameter that occurs as a result of long-term overinflation of the lungs, sometimes seen in cases of emphysema or asthma.

CLINICAL CORRELATES

Asthma is a **chronic inflammation of the bronchi** that causes **swelling** and **narrowing** (constriction) of the airways. It causes an **airway obstruction** and is characterized by dyspnea (difficulty in breathing), cough, and wheezing because of spasmodic contraction of smooth muscles in the bronchioles.

Bronchiectasis is a **chronic dilation of bronchi and bronchioles** resulting from destruction of bronchial elastic and muscular elements, which may cause **collapse of the bronchioles**. It may be caused by pulmonary infections (e.g., pneumonia, tuberculosis [TB]) or by a bronchial obstruction with heavy sputum production. Signs and symptoms include a chronic cough with expectoration of large volumes of sputum. COPD may include asthma and bronchiectasis.

III. PLEURAE AND PLEURAL CAVITIES (See Figures 3.4 to 3.5)

A. Pleura

- Is a thin serous membrane that consists of a parietal pleura and a visceral pleura.

1. Parietal Pleura

- Lines the inner surface of the thoracic wall and the mediastinum and has costal, diaphragmatic, mediastinal, and cervical parts. The cervical pleura **(cupula)** is the dome of the pleura, projecting into the neck above the neck of the first rib. It is reinforced by **Sibson fascia** (suprapleural membrane), which is a thickened portion of the **endothoracic fascia**, and is attached to the first rib and the transverse process of the seventh cervical vertebra.
- Is separated from the thoracic wall by the endothoracic fascia, which is an extrapleural fascial sheet lining the thoracic wall.
- Is innervated by the **intercostal nerves** (costal pleura and the peripheral portion of the diaphragmatic pleura) and the **phrenic nerves** (central portion of the diaphragmatic pleura and the mediastinal pleura). The parietal pleura is **very sensitive to pain**.
- Is supplied by branches of the internal thoracic, superior phrenic, posterior intercostal, and superior intercostal arteries. However, the visceral pleura is supplied by the bronchial arteries. The veins from the parietal pleura joins systemic veins.
- Forms the **pulmonary ligament**, a two-layered vertical fold of mediastinal pleura, which extends along the mediastinal surface of each lung from the **hilus** to the **base** (diaphragmatic surface) and ends in a free falciform border. It supports the lungs in the **pleural sac** by retaining the lower parts of the lungs in position.

2. Visceral Pleura (Pulmonary Pleura)

- Intimately invests the lungs and dips into all of the fissures.
- Is supplied by bronchial arteries, but its venous blood is drained by pulmonary veins.
- Is insensitive to pain but is sensitive to stretch and contains vasomotor fibers and sensory endings of vagal origin, which may be involved in respiratory reflexes.

CLINICAL CORRELATES

Pleurisy (pleuritis) is an **inflammation of the pleura** with exudation (escape of fluid from blood vessels) into its cavity, causing the pleural surfaces to be roughened. This roughening produces friction, and a **pleural rub** can be heard with the stethoscope on respiration. The exudate forms dense adhesions between the visceral and parietal pleurae, forming pleural adhesions. Symptoms are a chill followed by fever and dry cough. Treatments consist of relieving pain with analgesics, as necessary, and lidocaine for intercostal nerve block.

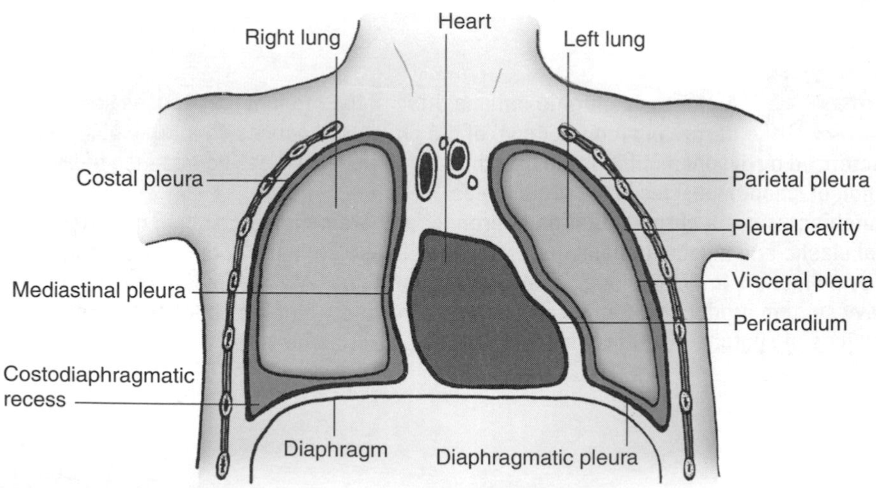

FIGURE 3.4. Frontal section of the thorax.

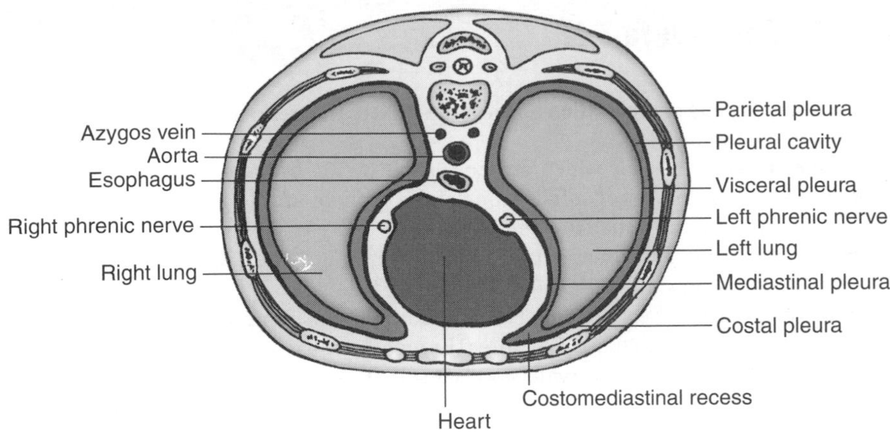

FIGURE 3.5. Horizontal section through the thorax.

B. Pleural Cavity

- Is a **potential space** between the parietal and visceral pleurae.
- Represents a closed sac with no communication between right and left parts.
- Contains a film of fluid that lubricates the surface of the pleurae and facilitates the movement of the lungs.

1. Costodiaphragmatic Recesses

- Are the **pleural recesses** formed by the reflection of the costal and diaphragmatic pleurae.
- Can accumulate fluid when in the erect position.
- Allow the lungs to be pulled down and expanded during inspiration.

2. Costomediastinal Recesses

- Are part of the pleural cavity where the costal and mediastinal pleurae meet.

CLINICAL CORRELATES

Pneumothorax is an accumulation of **air** in the pleural cavity, and thus, the **lung collapses** because the negative pressure necessary to keep the lung expanded has been eliminated. It results from an injury to the thoracic wall or the lung. **Tension pneumothorax** is a life-threatening pneumothorax in which air enters during inspiration and is trapped during expiration; therefore, the resultant increased pressure displaces the mediastinum to the opposite side, with consequent cardiopulmonary impairment. Major **symptoms** of pneumothorax are chest pain and dyspnea (shortness of breath). It can be **treated** by draining the pleural air collection by simple aspiration using an intravenous catheter or chest tube thoracostomy.

CLINICAL CORRELATES

Pleural effusion is an abnormal accumulation of excess fluid in the pleural space. There are two types of pleural effusion: the transudate (clear watery fluid) and the exudate (cloudy viscous fluid). A **transudate** is caused by congestive heart failure or, less commonly, liver or kidney disease, whereas an **exudate** is caused by inflammation, pneumonia, lung cancer, TB, asbestosis, or pulmonary embolism. Symptoms include shortness of breath, chest pain, and cough. It can be treated by removing fluid by thoracentesis.

CLINICAL CORRELATES

Thoracentesis (pleuracentesis or pleural tap) is a surgical puncture of the thoracic wall into the pleural cavity for aspiration of fluid. An accumulation of fluid in the pleural cavity has a clinical name such as a **hydrothorax** (water), a **hemothorax** (blood), a **chylothorax** (lymph), and a **pyothorax** (pus). It is performed at or posterior to the **midaxillary line**, one or two intercostal spaces below the fluid level but not below the ninth intercostal space. The ideal site is seventh, eighth, or ninth intercostal space, as this site avoids possible accidental puncture of the lung, liver, spleen, and diaphragm. A needle should be inserted immediately above the superior margin of a rib to avoid injury to the intercostal neurovascular bundle.

IV. LUNGS (See Figure 3.3)

- Are the **essential organs of respiration** and are attached to the heart and trachea by their roots and the pulmonary ligaments.
- Contain nonrespiratory tissues, which are nourished by the **bronchial arteries** and drained by the **bronchial veins** for the larger subdivisions of the bronchi and by the **pulmonary veins** for the smaller subdivisions of the bronchial tree.
- Have **bases** that rest on the convex surface of the diaphragm, descend during inspiration, and ascend during expiration.
- Receive parasympathetic fibers that innervate the smooth muscle and glands of the bronchial tree and probably are excitatory to these structures (bronchoconstrictor and secretomotor).
- Receive sympathetic fibers that innervate blood vessels, smooth muscle, and glands of the bronchial tree and probably are inhibitory to these structures (bronchodilator and vasoconstrictor).
- Have some sensory endings of vagal origin, which are stimulated by the stretching of the lung during inspiration and are concerned in the reflex control of respiration.

A. Right Lung

- Has an apex that projects into the neck and a concave base that sits on the diaphragm.
- Is **larger** and **heavier** than the left lung, but is **shorter** and **wider** because of the higher right dome of the diaphragm and the inclination of the heart to the left.
- Is divided into upper, middle, and lower lobes by the **oblique** and **horizontal** (accessory) **fissures**, but usually receives a single bronchial artery. The **oblique fissure** usually begins at the head of the fifth rib and follows roughly the line of the **sixth rib**. The **horizontal fissure** runs from the oblique fissure in the midaxillary line at the sixth rib level and extends forward to the fourth costal cartilage level.
- Has 3 lobar (secondary) bronchi and 10 segmental (tertiary) bronchi.
- Has grooves for various structures (e.g., SVC, arch of azygos vein, esophagus).

B. Left Lung

- Is divided into upper and lower lobes by an **oblique fissure** that follows the line of the sixth rib, is usually more vertical in the left lung than in the right lung, and usually receives two bronchial arteries.
- Contains the **lingula**, a tongue-shaped portion of the upper lobe that corresponds to the middle lobe of the right lung.
- Contains a **cardiac impression**, a **cardiac notch** (a deep indentation of the anterior border of the **superior lobe** of the left lung), and **grooves** for various structures (e.g., aortic arch, descending aorta, left subclavian artery).
- Has 2 lobar (secondary) bronchi and 8 to 10 segmental bronchi.

CLINICAL CORRELATES

Pneumonia (pneumonitis) is an inflammation of the lungs, which is of bacterial and viral origin. Symptoms are usually cough, fever, sputum production, chest pain, and dyspnea. It can be treated by administering antibiotics for initial therapy.

TB is an infectious lung disease caused by the bacterium ***Mycobacterium tuberculosis*** and is characterized by the formation of tubercles that can undergo caseous necrosis. Its symptoms are cough, fever, sweats, tiredness, and emaciation. TB is spread by coughing and mainly enters the body in inhaled air and can be treated with very effective drugs.

CLINICAL CORRELATES

Pancoast or superior pulmonary sulcus tumor is a malignant neoplasm of the lung apex and causes **Pancoast syndrome**, which comprises (a) **lower trunk brachial plexopathy** (which causes severe pain radiating toward the shoulder and along the medial aspect of the arm and atrophy of the muscles of the forearm and hand) and (b) **lesions of cervical**

sympathetic chain ganglia with **Horner syndrome** (ptosis, enophthalmos, miosis, anhidrosis, and vasodilation).

Superior pulmonary sulcus is a deep vertical groove in the posterior wall of the thoracic cavity on either side of the vertebral column formed by the posterior curvature of the ribs, lodging the posterior bulky portion of the lung.

CLINICAL CORRELATES **Pulmonary edema** involves fluid accumulation and swelling in the lungs caused by lung toxins (causing altered capillary permeability), mitral stenosis, or left ventricular failure that results in increased pressure in the pulmonary veins. As pressure in the pulmonary veins rises, **fluid** is pushed **into the alveoli** and becomes a barrier to normal oxygen exchange, resulting in shortness of breath. Signs and symptoms include rapid breathing, increased heart rate, heart murmurs, shortness of breath, difficulty breathing, cough, and excessive sweating. Treatments include supplemental oxygen, bed rest, and mechanical ventilation.

CLINICAL CORRELATES **Asbestosis** is caused by inhalation of asbestos fibers, and accumulated particles and fibers in the lungs can cause irritation and inflammation, leading to a breathing disorder, cough, chest pains, and a high risk of lung cancer. **Mesothelioma** is a rare form of cancer that is caused by previous exposure to asbestos and is found in the mesothelium primarily in the pleura. Its symptoms include shortness of breath due to pleural effusion, chest wall pain, cough, fatigue, and weight loss.

C. Bronchopulmonary Segment

- Is the anatomic, functional, and surgical unit (subdivision) of the lungs.
- Consists of a segmental (tertiary or lobular) bronchus, a segmental branch of the pulmonary artery, and a segment of the lung tissue, surrounded by a delicate connective tissue septum (intersegmental septum). It is drained by the intersegmental part of the pulmonary vein.
- Refers to the portion of the **lung supplied by each segmental bronchus and segmental artery**. The **pulmonary veins** are said to be **intersegmental**.
- Is clinically important because the intersegmental pulmonary veins form surgical landmarks; thus, a surgeon can remove a bronchopulmonary segment without seriously disrupting the surrounding lung tissue and major blood vessels.

CLINICAL CORRELATES **Atelectasis** is the **collapse** of a **lung** by blockage of the air passages or by very shallow breathing because of anesthesia or prolonged bed rest. It is caused by mucus secretions that plug the airway, foreign bodies in the airway, and tumors that compress or obstruct the airway. Signs and symptoms are breathing difficulty, chest pain, and cough.

CLINICAL CORRELATES **Lung cancer** has two types, small cell and non–small cell carcinomas, based on histology of the cell type of origin. **Small cell carcinoma** accounts for 20% and grow aggressively, while **non–small cell carcinoma** (80%) is divided further into squamous cell carcinoma, adenocarcinoma, and bronchoalveolar large cell carcinoma. Its symptoms include chronic cough, coughing up blood, shortness of breath, chest pain, and weight loss.

D. Conducting Portion (Airway)

- Includes the nasal cavity, nasopharynx, larynx, trachea, bronchi, bronchioles (possess no cartilage), and terminal bronchioles, whereas the **respiratory portion** includes the respiratory bronchioles, alveolar ducts, atria, and alveolar sacs. Oxygen and carbon dioxide exchange takes place across the wall (blood–air barrier) of lung alveoli and pulmonary capillaries.

V. RESPIRATION

- Is the vital exchange of oxygen and carbon dioxide that occurs in the lungs. The air–blood barrier consists of alveolar type I cells, basal lamina, and capillary endothelial cells. The alveolar type II cells secrete surfactant.

A. Inspiration

- Occurs when the ribs and sternum (or thoracic cage) are elevated by the following **muscles**: the **diaphragm**; external, internal (interchondral part), and innermost intercostal; sternocleidomastoid; levator costarum; serratus anterior; scalenus; pectoralis major and minor; and serratus posterior superior muscles.
- Involves the following processes:

1. Contraction of the Diaphragm

- Pulls the dome inferiorly into the abdomen, thereby **increasing the vertical diameter** of the thorax.

2. Enlargement of the Pleural Cavities and Lungs

- **Reduces** the intrapulmonary **pressure** (creates a **negative pressure**), thus allowing air to rush into the lungs passively because of atmospheric pressure.

3. Forced Inspiration

- Involves contraction of the **intercostal muscles and elevation of the ribs** (superolateral movement), with the sternum moving anteriorly like a **bucket handle**. (When the handle is raised, the convexity moves laterally.)
- Results in **increased transverse and anteroposterior diameters** of the thoracic cavity. The abdominal volume is decreased with an increased abdominal pressure.

B. Expiration

- Involves the following muscles: the **muscles of the anterior abdominal wall, internal intercostal** (costal part) **muscles**, and serratus posterior inferior muscles.
- Involves the following processes:

1. Overall Process

- Involves relaxation of the diaphragm, the internal intercostal muscles (costal part), and other muscles; decrease in thoracic volume; and increase in the intrathoracic pressure. The **abdominal pressure is decreased**, and the **ribs are depressed**.

2. Elastic Recoil of the Lungs

- Produces a **subatmospheric pressure** in the pleural cavities. Thus, much of the air is expelled. (**Quiet expiration** is a passive process caused by the elastic recoil of the lungs, whereas **quiet inspiration** results from contraction of the **diaphragm**.)

3. Forced Expiration

- Requires contraction of the anterior abdominal muscles and the internal intercostals (costal part).

VI. LYMPHATIC VESSELS OF THE LUNG (See Figure 3.6)

- Drain the bronchial tree, pulmonary vessels, and connective tissue septa.
- Run along the bronchiole and bronchi toward the hilus, where they drain to the pulmonary (intrapulmonary) and then **bronchopulmonary** nodes, which in turn drain to the inferior (carinal) and superior **tracheobronchial** nodes, the **tracheal** (paratracheal) nodes, **bronchomediastinal** nodes and trunks, and eventually to the **thoracic duct** on the left and right lymphatic duct on the right.
- Are not present in the walls of the pulmonary alveoli.

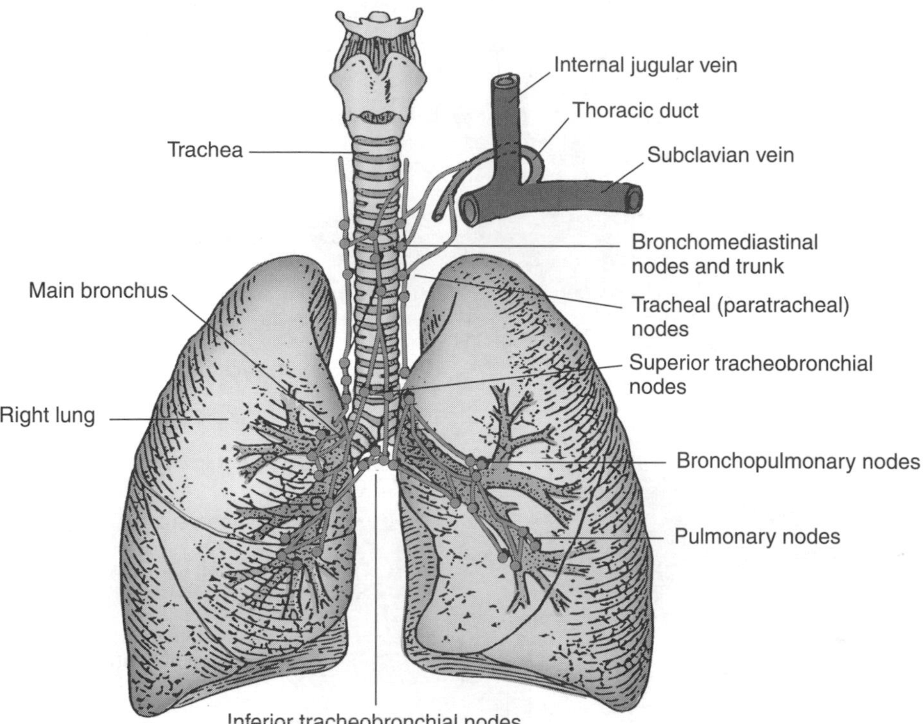

FIGURE 3.6. The trachea, bronchi, and lungs, plus associated lymph nodes.

VII. BLOOD VESSELS OF THE LUNG (See Figure 3.7)

A. Pulmonary Trunk

- Extends upward from the **conus arteriosus** of the right ventricle of the heart and carries poorly oxygenated blood to the lungs for oxygenation.
- Passes superiorly and posteriorly from the front of the ascending aorta to its left side for approximately 5 cm and bifurcates into the right and left pulmonary arteries within the concavity of the aortic arch at the level of the sternal angle.
- Has much lower blood pressure than that in the aorta and is contained within the fibrous pericardium.

1. Left Pulmonary Artery

- Carries deoxygenated blood to the left lung, is shorter and narrower than the right pulmonary artery, and **arches over the left primary bronchus**.
- Is connected to the arch of the aorta by the **ligamentum arteriosum**, the fibrous remains of the ductus arteriosus.

2. Right Pulmonary Artery

- Runs horizontally toward the hilus of the right lung **under the arch of the aorta** behind the ascending aorta and SVC and anterior to the right bronchus.

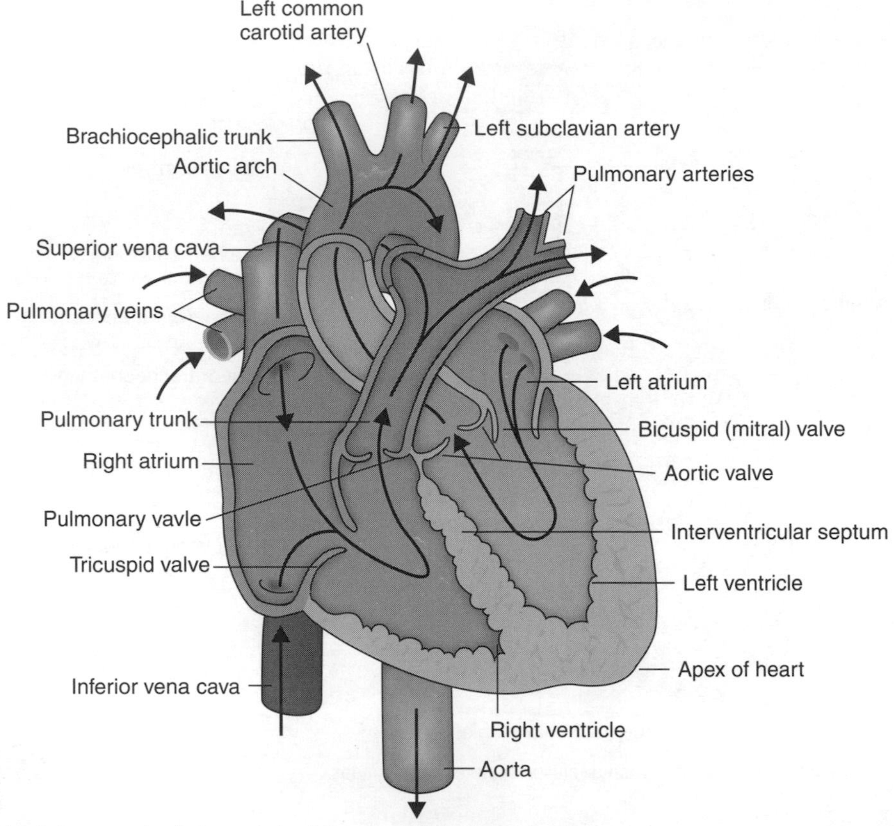

FIGURE 3.7. Pulmonary circulation and circulation through the heart chambers.

CLINICAL CORRELATES

Pulmonary embolism (pulmonary thromboembolism) is an obstruction of the pulmonary artery or one of its branches by an embolus (air, blood clot, fat, tumor cells, or other foreign material), which arises in the deep veins of the lower limbs or in the pelvic veins or occurs following an operation or after a fracture of a long bone with fatty marrow. Symptoms may be sudden onset of dyspnea, anxiety, and substernal chest pain. Treatments include heparin therapy and surgical therapy such as **pulmonary embolectomy**, which is surgical removal of massive pulmonary emboli.

B. Pulmonary Veins

- Are **intersegmental** in drainage (do not accompany the bronchi or the segmental artery within the parenchyma of the lungs).
- Leave the lung as five pulmonary veins, one from each lobe of the lungs. However, the right upper and middle veins usually join so that only four veins enter the **left atrium**.
- Carry oxygenated blood from the respiratory part (alveoli) of the lung and deoxygenated blood from the visceral pleura and from a part of the bronchioles to the left atrium of the heart. (Gas exchange occurs between the walls of alveoli and pulmonary capillaries, and the newly oxygenated blood enters venules and then pulmonary veins.)

C. Bronchial Arteries

- Arise from the **thoracic aorta**; usually there is one artery for the right lung and two for the left lung.
- Supply oxygenated blood to the **nonrespiratory conducting tissues of the lungs** and the visceral pleura. Anastomoses occur between the capillaries of the bronchial and pulmonary systems.

D. Bronchial Veins

- Receive blood from the bronchi and empty into the **azygos vein** on the right and into the **accessory hemiazygos vein** or the superior intercostal vein on the left.
- May receive twigs (small vessels) from the tracheobronchial lymph nodes.

VIII. NERVE SUPPLY TO THE LUNG

A. Pulmonary Plexus

- Receives afferent and efferent (parasympathetic preganglionic) fibers from the vagus nerve, joined by branches (sympathetic postganglionic fibers) from the sympathetic trunk and cardiac plexus.
- Is divided into the **anterior pulmonary plexus**, which lies in front of the root of the lung, and the **posterior pulmonary plexus**, which lies behind the root of the lung.
- Has branches that accompany the blood vessels and bronchi into the lung.
- Has **sympathetic** nerve fibers that **dilate the lumina** of the bronchi and constrict the pulmonary vessels, whereas **parasympathetic** fibers **constrict the lumina**, dilate the pulmonary vessels, and **increase glandular secretion**.

B. Phrenic Nerve

- Arises from the third through fifth cervical nerves (C3–C5) and lies in front of the anterior scalene muscle.
- Enters the thorax by passing deep to the subclavian vein and superficial to the subclavian arteries.
- Runs anterior to the root of the lung, whereas the vagus nerve runs posterior to the root of the lung.
- Is accompanied by the pericardiophrenic vessels of the internal thoracic vessels and descends between the mediastinal pleura and the pericardium.
- Innervates the fibrous pericardium, the mediastinal and diaphragmatic pleurae, and the diaphragm for motor and its central tendon for sensory functions.

CLINICAL CORRELATES

Lesion of the phrenic nerve may or may not produce complete paralysis of the corresponding half of the diaphragm because the **accessory phrenic nerve**, derived from the fifth cervical nerve as a branch of the nerve to the subclavius, usually joins the phrenic nerve in the root of the neck or in the upper part of the thorax.

Hiccup is an **involuntary spasmodic sharp contraction of the diaphragm**, accompanied by the approximation of the vocal folds and closure of the glottis of the larynx. It may occur as a result of the stimulation of nerve endings in the digestive tract or the diaphragm. When chronic, it can be stopped by **sectioning** or **crushing the phrenic nerve**.

IX. DEVELOPMENT OF THE RESPIRATORY SYSTEM

A. Development of the Trachea and Bronchi

- Primordium for the lower respiratory system appears as a **laryngotracheal groove** in the floor of the pharyngeal foregut. The groove evaginates to form the laryngotracheal (respiratory) diverticulum.
- **Laryngotracheal (respiratory) diverticulum** forms from the laryngotracheal groove in the ventral wall of the foregut, and soon after, the diverticulum is separated from the foregut proper by the formation of a tracheoesophageal septum.
- **Tracheoesophageal septum** divides the foregut into a ventral portion, the **laryngotracheal tube** (primordium of the larynx, trachea, bronchi, and lungs), and a dorsal portion (primordium of the oropharynx and esophagus).

- **Lung buds** develop at the distal end of the laryngotracheal diverticulum and divide into two bronchial buds, which branch into the primary, secondary, and tertiary bronchi. The tertiary bronchi continue to divide to form respiratory bronchioles.

B. Derivations or Sources

- Epithelium and glands in the trachea and bronchi are derived from the endoderm, whereas smooth muscles, connective tissue, and cartilage of the trachea and bronchi are derived from visceral (splanchnic) mesoderm.
- Visceral pleura is derived from visceral mesoderm covering the outside of the bronchi, whereas the parietal pleura is derived from somatic mesoderm covering the inside of the body wall.

C. Development of Lungs

- The lungs undergo four stages of development.

1. Glandular Period (Prenatal Weeks 5 to 17)

- The conducting (airway) system through the **terminal bronchioles** develops. Respiration is not possible.

2. Canalicular Period (Prenatal Weeks 13 to 25)

- Luminal diameter of the conducting system increases, and **respiratory bronchioles**, alveolar ducts, and terminal sacs begin to appear. Premature fetuses born before week 20 rarely survive.

3. Terminal Sac Period (Prenatal Weeks 24 to Birth)

- More **terminal sacs** form, and alveolar type I cells and **surfactant**-producing alveolar type II cells develop. Respiration is possible, and premature infants can survive with intensive care.

4. Alveolar Period (Late Fetal Stage to 8 Years)

- Respiratory bronchioles, terminal sacs, **alveolar ducts**, and **alveoli** increase in number.

PERICARDIUM AND HEART

I. PERICARDIUM

- Is a fibroserous sac that encloses the heart and the roots of the great vessels and occupies the **middle mediastinum.**
- Is composed of the fibrous pericardium and serous pericardium.
- Receives blood from the pericardiophrenic, bronchial, and esophageal arteries.
- Is innervated by vasomotor and sensory fibers from the phrenic and vagus nerves and the sympathetic trunks.

A. Fibrous Pericardium

- Is a strong, dense, fibrous layer that blends with the adventitia of the roots of the great vessels and the central tendon of the diaphragm.

B. Serous Pericardium

- Consists of the **parietal layer**, which lines the inner surface of the fibrous pericardium, and the **visceral layer**, which forms the outer layer (epicardium) of the heart wall and the roots of the great vessels.

CLINICAL CORRELATES

Pericarditis is an **inflammation of the pericardium**, which may result in cardiac tamponade, pericardial effusion, and precordial and epigastric pain. It also causes the **pericardial murmur** or **pericardial friction rub** (the surfaces of the pericardium become rough, and the resulting friction sounds like the rustle of silk, which can be heard on auscultation). It has symptoms of dysphagia, dyspnea and cough, inspiratory chest pain, and paradoxic pulse.

C. Pericardial Cavity

- Is a **potential space** between the visceral layer of the serous pericardium (epicardium) and the parietal layer of the serous pericardium lining the inner surfaces of the fibrous pericardium.

D. Pericardial Sinuses

1. Transverse Sinus

- Is a subdivision of the **pericardial sac**, lying posterior to the ascending aorta and pulmonary trunk, anterior to the SVC, and superior to the left atrium and the pulmonary veins.
- Is of great importance to the cardiac surgeon because while performing surgery on the aorta or pulmonary artery, a surgeon can pass a finger and make a ligature through the sinus between the arteries and veins, thus stopping the blood circulation with the ligature.

2. Oblique Sinus

- Is a subdivision of the **pericardial sac** behind the heart, surrounded by the reflection of the serous pericardium around the right and left pulmonary veins and the inferior vena cava (IVC).

CLINICAL CORRELATES

Cardiac tamponade is an **acute compression of the heart** caused by a rapid **accumulation of fluid** or blood in the pericardial cavity from wounds to the heart or **pericardial effusion** (passage of fluid from the pericardial capillaries into the pericardial sac). Tamponade can be treated by pericardiocentesis. It causes **compression of venous return** to the heart, resulting in decreased diastolic capacity (ventricular filling), **reduced cardiac output** with an increased heart rate, increased venous pressure with jugular vein distention, hepatic enlargement, and peripheral edema.

Pericardial effusion is an **accumulation of fluid** in the pericardial space resulting from inflammation caused by acute pericarditis, and the accumulated fluid compresses the heart, inhibiting cardiac filling. It has signs of an enlarged heart, a water bottle appearance of the cardiac silhouette, faint heart sounds, and vanished apex beat. It can be treated by pericardiocentesis.

Pericardiocentesis is a **surgical puncture of the pericardial cavity** for the aspiration of fluid, which is necessary to relieve the pressure of accumulated fluid in the heart. A needle is inserted into the pericardial cavity through the fifth intercostal space left to the sternum. Because of the cardiac notch, the needle misses the pleura and lungs, but it penetrates the pericardium.

II. HEART (Figures 3.8 to 3.10)

A. General Characteristics

- The **apex of the heart** is the blunt rounded extremity of the heart formed by the left ventricle and lies in the left fifth intercostal space slightly medial to the midclavicular (or nipple) line, approximately 9 cm from the midline. This location is useful clinically for determining the left border of the heart and for **auscultating the mitral valve**.
- Its posterior aspect, called the **base**, is formed primarily by the left atrium and only partly by the posterior right atrium.
- Its **right (acute) border** is formed by the SVC, right atrium, and IVC, and its **left (obtuse) border** is formed by the left ventricle. (In radiology, the left border consists of the aortic arch, pulmonary trunk, left auricle, and left ventricle.)
- The heart wall consists of three layers: inner **endocardium**, middle **myocardium**, and outer **epicardium**.
- The **sulcus terminalis**, a groove on the external surface of the right atrium, marks the junction of the primitive sinus venosus with the atrium in the embryo and corresponds to a ridge on the internal heart surface, the **crista terminalis**.
- The **coronary sulcus**, a groove on the external surface of the heart, marks the division between the atria and the ventricles. The **crux** is the point at which the interventricular and interatrial sulci cross the coronary sulcus.

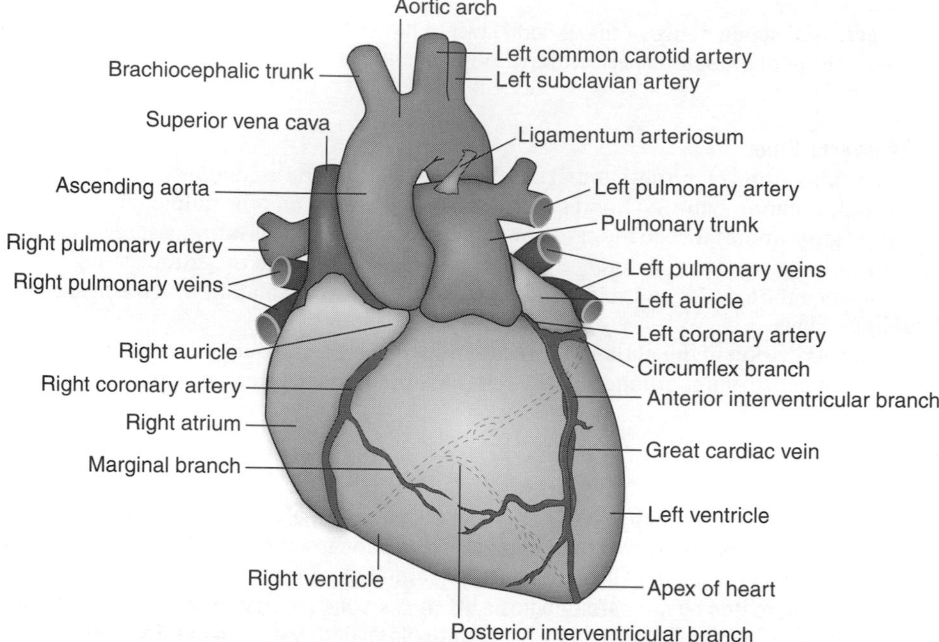

FIGURE 3.8. Anterior view of the heart with coronary arteries.

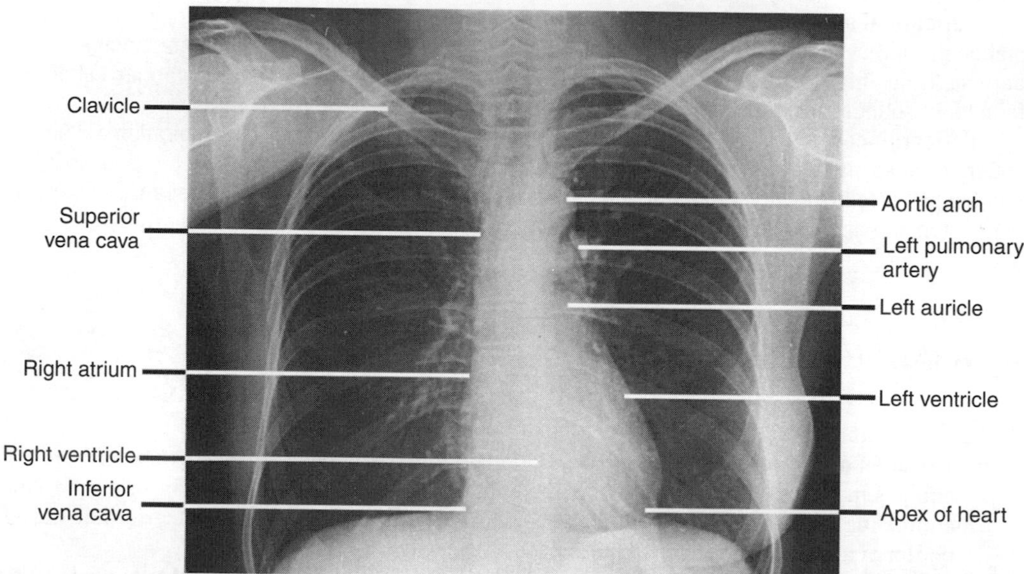

FIGURE 3.9. Posterior–anterior radiograph of the thorax showing the heart and great vessels.

- The **cardiovascular silhouette**, or cardiac shadow, is the contour of the heart and great vessels seen on **posterior–anterior chest radiographs**. Its **right border** is formed by the SVC, the right atrium, and the IVC. Its **left border** is formed by the aortic arch (which produces the **aortic knob**), the pulmonary trunk, the left auricle, and the left ventricle. Its **inferior border** is formed by the right ventricle, and the **left atrium** shows **no border**.

B. Internal Anatomy of the Heart (See Figures 3.9 to 3.11)

1. Right Atrium

- Has an anteriorly situated rough-walled **atrium proper** and the auricle lined with pectinate muscles and a posteriorly situated smooth-walled **sinus venarum**, into which the two venae cavae open.

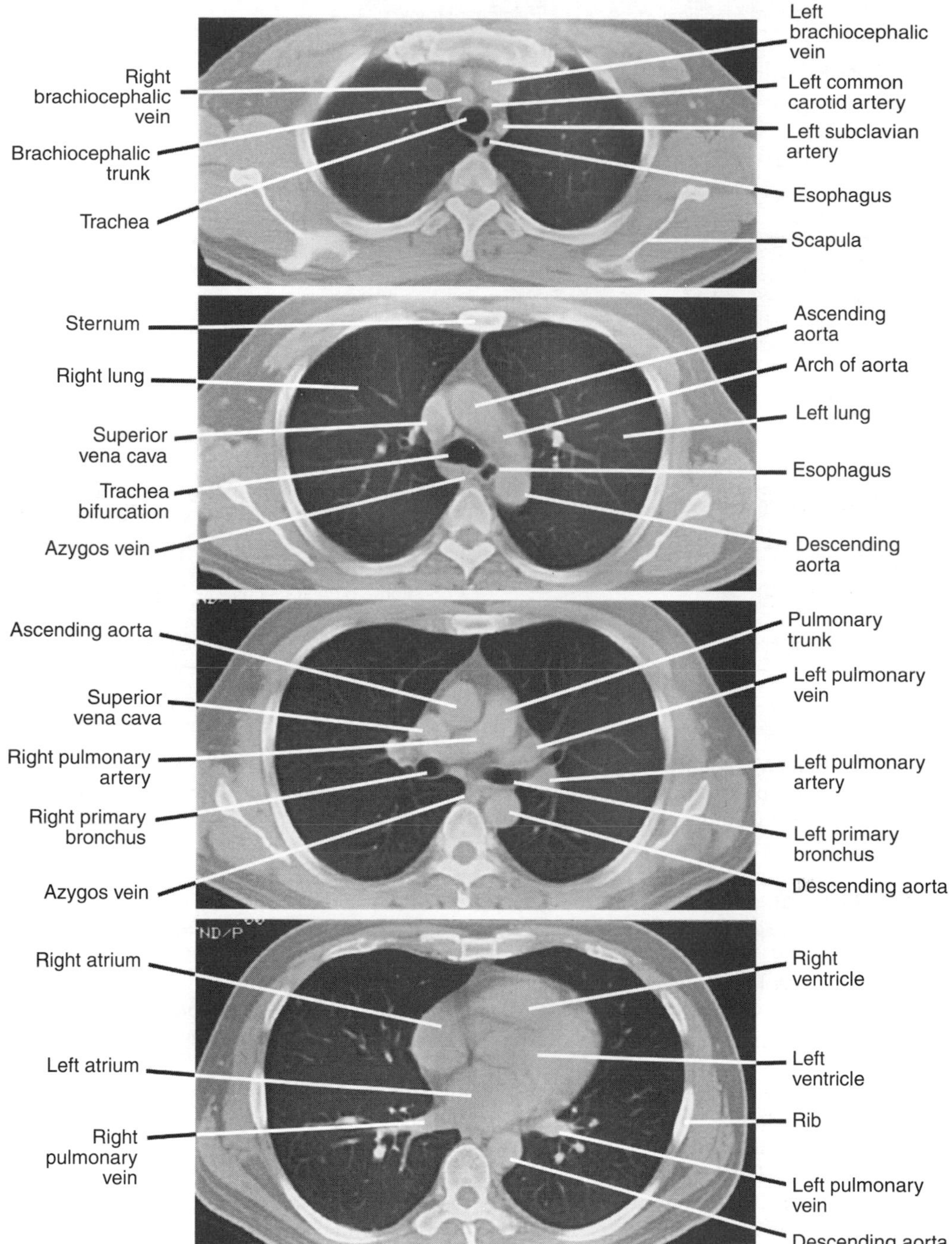

FIGURE 3.10. Contrast-enhanced computed tomography scan of the thorax at a setting that demonstrates soft tissues.

- Is larger than the left atrium but has a thinner wall, and its sinus venarum between two venae cavae is separated from the atrium proper by the crista terminalis.
- Has a **right atrial pressure** that is normally slightly lower than the left atrial pressure.
- Contains the valve (Eustachian) of the IVC and the valve (Thebesian) of the coronary sinus.

(a) Right Auricle

- Is the conical muscular pouch of the upper anterior portion of the right atrium, which covers the first part of the right coronary artery.

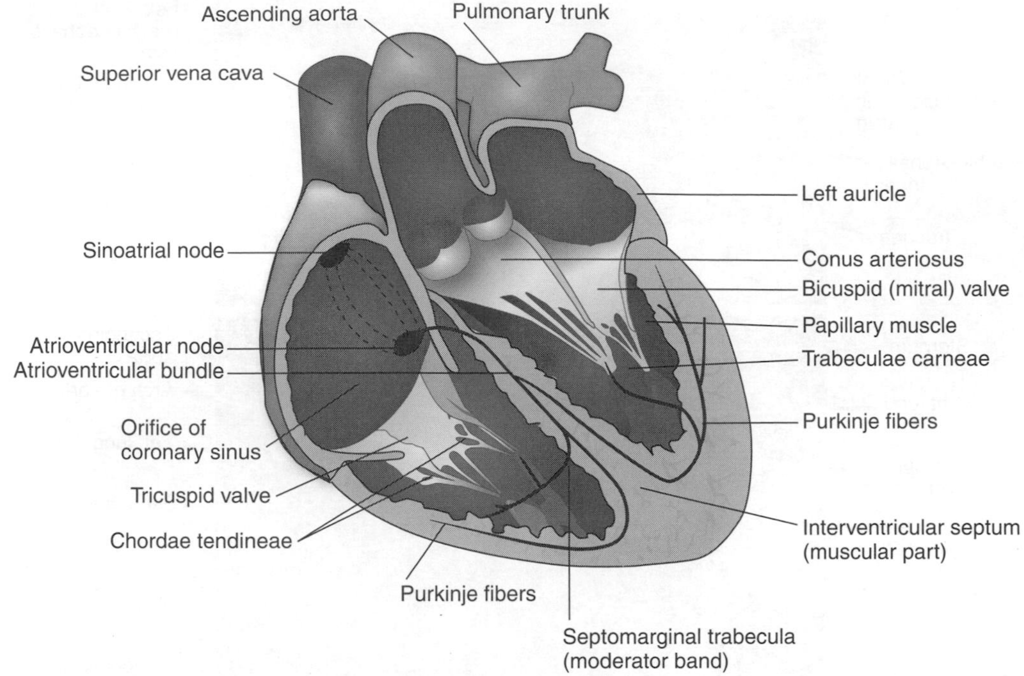

FIGURE 3.11. Internal anatomy and conducting system of the heart.

(b) Sinus Venarum (Sinus Venarum Cavarum)

- Is a posteriorly situated, smooth-walled area that is separated from the more muscular atrium proper by the **crista terminalis.**
- Develops from the embryonic **sinus venosus** and receives the SVC, IVC, coronary sinus, and anterior cardiac veins.

(c) Pectinate Muscles

- Are **prominent ridges of atrial myocardium** located in the interior of both auricles and the right atrium.

(d) Crista Terminalis

- Is a **vertical muscular ridge** running anteriorly along the **right atrial wall** from the opening of the SVC to the opening of the IVC, providing the **origin of the pectinate muscles.**
- Represents the junction between the **primitive sinus venarum** (a smooth-walled region) and the right atrium proper and is indicated externally by the **sulcus terminalis.**

(e) Venae Cordis Minimae

- Are the smallest cardiac veins, which begin in the substance of the heart (endocardium and innermost layer of the myocardium) and end chiefly in the atria at the **foramina venarum minimarum cordis.**

(f) Fossa Ovalis

- Is an oval-shaped depression in the interatrial septum and represents the site of the **foramen ovale**, through which blood runs from the right atrium to the left atrium before birth. The upper rounded margin of the fossa is called the **limbus fossa ovale.**

2. Left Atrium

- Is **smaller** and has **thicker walls** than the right atrium, but its walls are smooth, except for a few pectinate muscles in the auricle.
- Is the **most posterior** of the four chambers lying posterior to the right atrium but anterior to the esophagus and shows no structural borders on a posteroanterior radiograph.
- Receives oxygenated blood through four pulmonary veins.

3. **Right Ventricle**
   - Makes up the major portion of the anterior (sternocostal) surface of the heart.
   - Contains the following structures:

   (a) **Trabeculae Carneae Cordis**
   - Are anastomosing muscular ridges of myocardium in the ventricles.

   (b) **Papillary Muscles**
   - Are cone-shaped muscles enveloped by endocardium.
   - Extend from the anterior and posterior ventricular walls and the septum, and their apices are attached to the **chordae tendineae.**
   - Contract to tighten the chordae tendineae, **preventing** the cusps of the **tricuspid valve from being everted** into the atrium by the pressure developed by the pumping action of the heart. This **prevents regurgitation of ventricular blood** into the right atrium.

   (c) **Chordae Tendineae**
   - Extend from one papillary muscle to more than one cusp of the tricuspid valve.
   - **Prevent eversion of the valve cusps** into the atrium during ventricular contractions.

   (d) **Conus Arteriosus (Infundibulum)**
   - Is the upper smooth-walled portion of the right ventricle, which leads to the pulmonary trunk.

   (e) **Septomarginal Trabecula (Moderator Band)**
   - Is an isolated band of trabeculae carneae that forms a bridge between the **intraventricular (IV) septum** and the base of the anterior papillary muscle of the anterior wall of the right ventricle.
   - Is called the moderator band for its ability to **prevent overdistention** of the ventricle and carries the right limb (Purkinje fibers) of the **atrioventricular (AV) bundle** from the septum to the sternocostal wall of the ventricle.

   (f) **IV Septum**
   - Is the place of origin of the septal papillary muscle.
   - Is mostly muscular but has a small membranous upper part, which is a common site of ventricular septal defects (VSDs).

4. **Left Ventricle**
   - Lies at the back of the heart, and its apex is directed downward, forward, and toward the left.
   - Is divided into the left **ventricle proper** and the **aortic vestibule**, which is the upper anterior part of the left ventricle and leads into the aorta.
   - Contains two **papillary muscles** (anterior and posterior) with their **chordae tendineae** and a meshwork of muscular ridges, the **trabeculae carneae cordis**.
   - Performs **harder work**, has a **thicker** (two to three times as thick) wall, and is longer, narrower, and more conical-shaped than the right ventricle.

CLINICAL CORRELATES

Myocardial infarction is a **necrosis** of the myocardium because of local **ischemia** resulting from vasospasm or obstruction of the blood supply, most commonly by a thrombus or embolus in the coronary arteries. Symptoms are severe chest pain or pressure for a prolonged period (more than 30 minutes), congestive heart failure, and murmur of mitral regurgitation. It can be treated with nitroglycerin (prevents coronary spasm and reduces myocardial oxygen demand), morphine (relieves pain and anxiety), lidocaine (reduces ventricular arrhythmias), or atropine (restores conduction and increases heart rate).

Angina pectoris is characterized by attacks of **chest pain originating** in the heart and felt beneath the sternum, in many cases radiating to the left shoulder and down the arm. It is caused by an **insufficient supply of oxygen to the heart muscle** because of coronary artery disease or exertion (e.g., exercise, excitement) or emotion (e.g., stress, anger, frustration). Symptoms and treatment are similar to those of myocardial infarction.

Prinzmetal angina is a variant form of angina pectoris caused by transient coronary artery spasm. The vasospasm typically occurs at rest, and in many cases, the coronary arteries are normal. Electrocardiogram exhibits the ST segment elevation rather than depression during an attack, and the prolonged vasospasm may lead to myocardial infarction and sudden death. Nitroglycerin, nifedipine, amlodipine besylate, and calcium channel blockers can prevent artery spasm. Smoking is the most significant risk factor for the spasm.

C. **Heart Valves** (See Figure 3.12)

1. **Pulmonary Valve**
   - Lies behind the medial end of the left third costal cartilage and adjoining part of the sternum.
   - Is most audible over the **left second intercostal space** just lateral to the sternum.
   - Is opened by ventricular systole and **shut slightly after closure of the aortic valve**.
2. **Aortic Valve**
   - Lies behind the left half of the sternum opposite the third intercostal space.
   - Is **closed during ventricular diastole; its closure** at the beginning of ventricular diastole causes the **second ("dub") heart sound.**
   - Is most audible over the **right second intercostal space** just lateral to the sternum.
3. **Tricuspid (Right AV) Valve**
   - Lies between the right atrium and ventricle, behind the right half of the sternum opposite the fourth intercostal space, and is covered by endocardium.
   - Is most audible over the **right** (or left for some people) **lower part of the body of the sternum**.
   - Has anterior, posterior, and septal cusps, which are attached by the chordae tendineae to three papillary muscles that keep the valve closed against the pressure developed by the pumping action of the heart.
   - Is **closed during the ventricular systole** (contraction); **its closure** contributes to the **first ("lub") heart sound.**
4. **Bicuspid (Left AV) Valve**
   - Is called the **mitral valve** because it is shaped like a bishop's miter.
   - Lies between the left atrium and ventricle, behind the left half of the sternum at the fourth costal cartilage, and has two cusps: a larger anterior and a smaller posterior.
   - Is **closed slightly before the tricuspid valve** by the ventricular contraction (systole); **its closure** at the onset of ventricular systole causes the **first ("lub") heart sound**.
   - Is most audible over the apical region of the heart in the **left fifth intercostal space at the midclavicular line.**

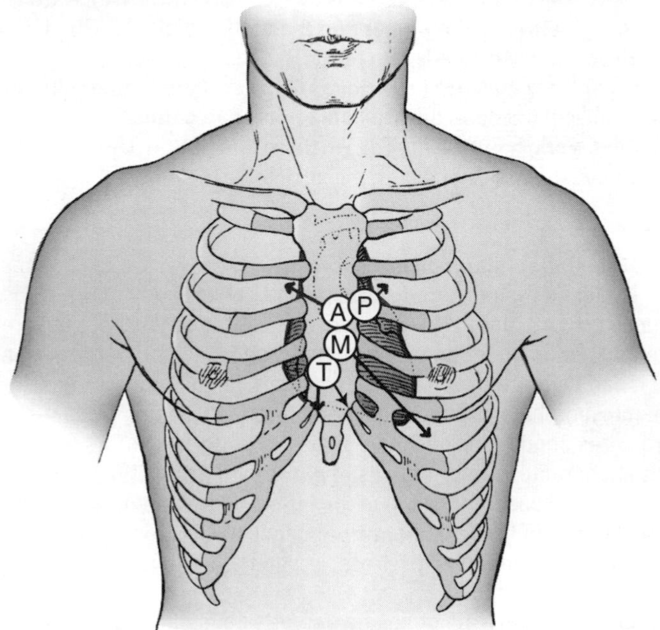

FIGURE 3.12. Positions of the valves of the heart and heart sounds. *A*, aortic valve; *M*, mitral valve; *P*, pulmonary valve; *T*, tricuspid valve. *Arrows* indicate positions of the heart sounds.

CLINICAL CORRELATES **Mitral valve prolapse** is a condition in which the valve everts into the left atrium and thus fails to close properly when the left ventricle contracts. It may produce chest pain, shortness of breath, palpitations, and cardiac arrhythmia. In most cases, no treatment is needed.

Endocarditis is an infection of the endocardium of the heart, most commonly involving the heart valves and is caused by a cluster of bacteria on the valves. The valves do not receive any blood supply, and white blood cells cannot enter, and thus they have no defense mechanisms. Symptoms include fatigue, weakness, fever, night sweats, anorexia, heart murmur, and shortness of breath. Risk factors include a damaged abnormal heart valve, mitral valve prolapse, and certain congenital heart defects. **Cardiac murmur** is a characteristic sound generated by turbulence of blood flow through an orifice of the heart.

D. **Heart Sounds**

1. **First ("Lub") Sound**
   - Is caused by the closure of the tricuspid and mitral valves at the onset of ventricular systole.
2. **Second ("Dub") Sound**
   - Is caused by the closure of the aortic and pulmonary valves (and vibration of walls of the heart and major vessels) at the onset of ventricular diastole.

E. **Conducting System of the Heart** (See Figure 3.11)

- Is composed of modified, specialized cardiac muscle cells that lie immediately beneath the endocardium and carry impulses throughout the cardiac muscle, signaling the heart chambers to contract in the proper sequence.

1. **Sinoatrial Node**
   - Is a small mass of specialized cardiac muscle fibers that lies in the myocardium at the **upper end of the crista terminalis** near the opening of the SVC in the right atrium.
   - Is known as the **pacemaker** of the heart and initiates the heartbeat, which can be altered by autonomic nervous stimulation (sympathetic stimulation speeds it up, and vagal stimulation slows it down). Impulses spread in a wave along the cardiac muscle fibers of the atria and also travel along an internodal pathway to the AV node.
   - Is supplied by the **sinus node artery**, which is a branch of the **right coronary artery**.
2. **AV Node**
   - Lies in the septal wall of the right atrium, superior and medial to the opening of the coronary sinus in the right atrium, receives the impulse from the sinoatrial (SA) node and passes it to the AV bundle.
   - Is supplied by the AV nodal artery, which usually arises from the **right coronary artery** opposite the origin of the posterior interventricular artery.
   - Is innervated by autonomic nerve fibers, although the cardiac muscle fibers lack motor endings.
3. **AV Bundle (Bundle of His)**
   - Begins at the **AV node** and runs along the membranous part of the interventricular septum.
   - Splits into right and left branches, which descend into the muscular part of the interventricular septum, and breaks up into terminal conducting fibers **(Purkinje fibers)** to spread out into the ventricular walls.

CLINICAL CORRELATES **Damage to the conducting system** causes a **heart block**, which interferes with the ability of the ventricles to receive the atrial impulses. A delay or disruption of the electrical signals produces an irregular and slower heartbeat, reducing the heart's efficiency in maintaining adequate circulation. Heart block requires a pacemaker to be implanted. **Atrial or ventricular fibrillation** is a cardiac arrhythmia resulting from rapid irregular uncoordinated contractions of the atrial or ventricular muscle due to fast repetitive excitation of myocardial fibers, causing palpitations, shortness of breath, angina, fatigue, congestive heart failure, and sudden cardiac death.

F. Coronary Arteries (See Figure 3.8)

- Arise from the ascending aorta and are filled with blood during the ventricular diastole.
- Have maximal blood flow during diastole and minimal blood flow during systole because of compression of the arterial branches in the myocardium during systole.

1. Right Coronary Artery

- Arises from the anterior (right) aortic sinus of the ascending aorta, runs between the root of the pulmonary trunk and the right auricle, and then descends in the right coronary sulcus, and generally supplies the right atrium and ventricle.
- Gives rise to the following:

(a) SA Nodal Artery

- Passes between the right atrium and the root of the ascending aorta, encircles the base of the SVC, and supplies the SA node and the right atrium.

(b) Marginal Artery

- Runs along the inferior border toward the apex and supplies the inferior margin of the right ventricle.

(c) Posterior IV (Posterior Descending) Artery

- Is a larger terminal branch and supplies a part of the IV septum and left ventricle and the AV node.

(d) AV Nodal Artery

- Arises opposite the origin of its posterior IV artery and supplies the AV node.

CLINICAL CORRELATES

Coronary atherosclerosis is characterized by the presence of **sclerotic plaques** containing cholesterol and lipoid material that impair myocardial blood flow, leading to ischemia and **myocardial infarction.**

Coronary angioplasty is an angiographic reconstruction (radiographic view of vessels after the injection of a radiopaque material) of a blood vessel made by enlarging a narrowed coronary arterial lumen. It is performed by peripheral introduction of a balloon-tip catheter and **dilation of the lumen on withdrawal of the inflated catheter tip**. A metal stent is often placed during angioplasty.

CLINICAL CORRELATES

Coronary bypass involves a connection of a section of vessel, usually the saphenous vein, or of the internal thoracic artery or other conduit between the aorta and a coronary artery distal to an obstruction in the coronary artery, shunting blood from the aorta to the coronary arteries. Alternatively, the internal thoracic artery is connected to the coronary artery distal to the obstructive lesion.

2. Left Coronary Artery

- Arises from the left aortic sinus of the ascending aorta, just above the **aortic semilunar valve.**
- Is shorter than the right coronary artery and usually is distributed to more of the myocardium.
- Gives rise to the following:

(a) Anterior IV (Left Anterior Descending) Artery

- Generally supplies anterior aspects of the right and left ventricles and is the chief source of blood to the IV septum and the apex.

(b) Circumflex Artery

- Runs in the coronary sulcus, gives off the left marginal artery, supplies the left atrium and left ventricle, and anastomoses with the terminal branch of the right coronary artery.

G. Cardiac Veins and Coronary Sinus (See Figure 3.13)

1. Coronary Sinus

- Is the **largest vein draining the heart** and lies in the **coronary sulcus**, which separates the atria from the ventricles.

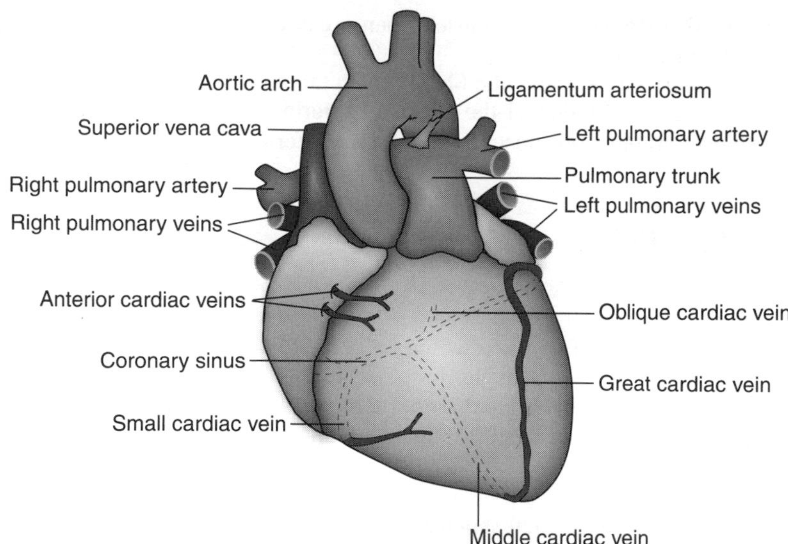

FIGURE 3.13. Anterior view of the heart.

- Opens into the right atrium between the opening of the IVC and the AV opening.
- Has a one-cusp valve at the right margin of its aperture.
- Receives the great, middle, and small cardiac veins; the oblique vein of the left atrium; and the posterior vein of the left ventricle.

2. **Great Cardiac Vein**
   - Begins at the apex of the heart and ascends along with the IV branch of the left coronary artery.
   - Turns to the left to lie in the coronary sulcus and continues as the **coronary sinus**.
3. **Middle Cardiac Vein**
   - Begins at the apex of the heart and ascends in the **posterior IV groove**, accompanying the posterior IV branch of the right coronary artery.
   - Drains into the right end of the coronary sinus.
4. **Small Cardiac Vein**
   - Runs along the right margin of the heart in company with the marginal artery and then posteriorly in the coronary sulcus to end in the right end of the coronary sinus.
5. **Oblique Vein of the Left Atrium**
   - Descends to empty into the coronary sinus, near its left end.
6. **Anterior Cardiac Vein**
   - Drains the anterior right ventricle, crosses the coronary groove, and ends directly in the right atrium.
7. **Smallest Cardiac Veins (Venae Cordis Minimae)**
   - Begin in the wall of the heart and empty directly into its chambers.

H. Lymphatic Vessels of the Heart

- Receive lymph from the myocardium and epicardium.
- Follow the right coronary artery to empty into the **anterior mediastinal nodes** and follow the left coronary artery to empty into a tracheobronchial node.

I. Cardiac Plexus

- Receives the superior, middle, and inferior cervical and thoracic cardiac nerves from the sympathetic trunks and vagus nerves.
- Is divisible into the **superficial cardiac plexus**, which lies beneath the arch of the aorta in front of the pulmonary artery, and the **deep cardiac plexus**, which lies posterior to the arch of the aorta in front of the bifurcation of the trachea.
- Richly innervates the conducting system of the heart: the right sympathetic and parasympathetic branches terminate chiefly in the region of the **SA node**, and the left branches end chiefly in the

region of the **AV node**. The cardiac muscle fibers are devoid of motor endings and are activated by the conducting system.

- Supplies the heart with **sympathetic fibers**, which **increase the heart rate** and the force of the heartbeat and cause **dilation of the coronary arteries**, and **parasympathetic fibers**, which **decrease the heart rate** and constrict the coronary arteries.

III. GREAT VESSELS

A. Ascending Aorta

- Takes its origin from the left ventricle within the pericardial sac and ascends behind the sternum to end at the level of the sternal angle.
- Lies in the **middle mediastinum**, has three aortic sinuses located immediately above the cusps of the aortic valve, and gives off the right and left coronary artery.

B. Arch of the Aorta

- Is found within the **superior mediastinum**, begins as a continuation of the ascending aorta, and **arches over the right pulmonary artery** and the **left main bronchus**.
- Forms a prominence that is visible on the radiograph as the **aortic knob**.
- Gives rise to the brachiocephalic, left common carotid, and left subclavian arteries.

CLINICAL CORRELATES **Aneurysm of the aortic arch** is a sac formed by dilation of the aortic arch that compresses the left recurrent laryngeal nerve, leading to coughing, hoarseness, and paralysis of the ipsilateral vocal cord. It may cause **dysphagia** (difficulty in swallowing), resulting from pressure on the esophagus, and **dyspnea** (difficulty in breathing), resulting from pressure on the trachea, root of the lung, or phrenic nerve.

CLINICAL CORRELATES **Marfan syndrome** is an inheritable disorder of connective tissue that affects the skeleton (causing long limbs), eyes (dislocated lens), lungs (pneumothorax), and heart and blood vessels (aortic root dilation, aortic aneurysm, aortic regurgitation, and mitral valve prolapse). It may be treated with β-blocker medications that reduce aortic root dilation.

C. Superior Vena Cava

- Is formed by the union of the right and left brachiocephalic veins and returns blood from all structures superior to the diaphragm, except the lungs and heart.
- Descends on the right side of the ascending aorta, receives the **azygos vein**, and enters the right atrium. Its upper half is in the **superior mediastinum**, and its lower half is in the **middle mediastinum**.

D. Pulmonary Trunk

- Arises from the conus arteriosus of the right ventricle, passes obliquely upward and backward across the origin and on the left side of the ascending aorta within the fibrous pericardium, and bifurcates into the right and left pulmonary arteries in the concavity of the aortic arch.

IV. DEVELOPMENT OF THE HEART (See Figure 3.14)

- Begins to form angiogenic cell clusters formed in the **splanchnic mesoderm**.
- Involves fusion of two endocardial tubes into a single **primitive heart tube**.

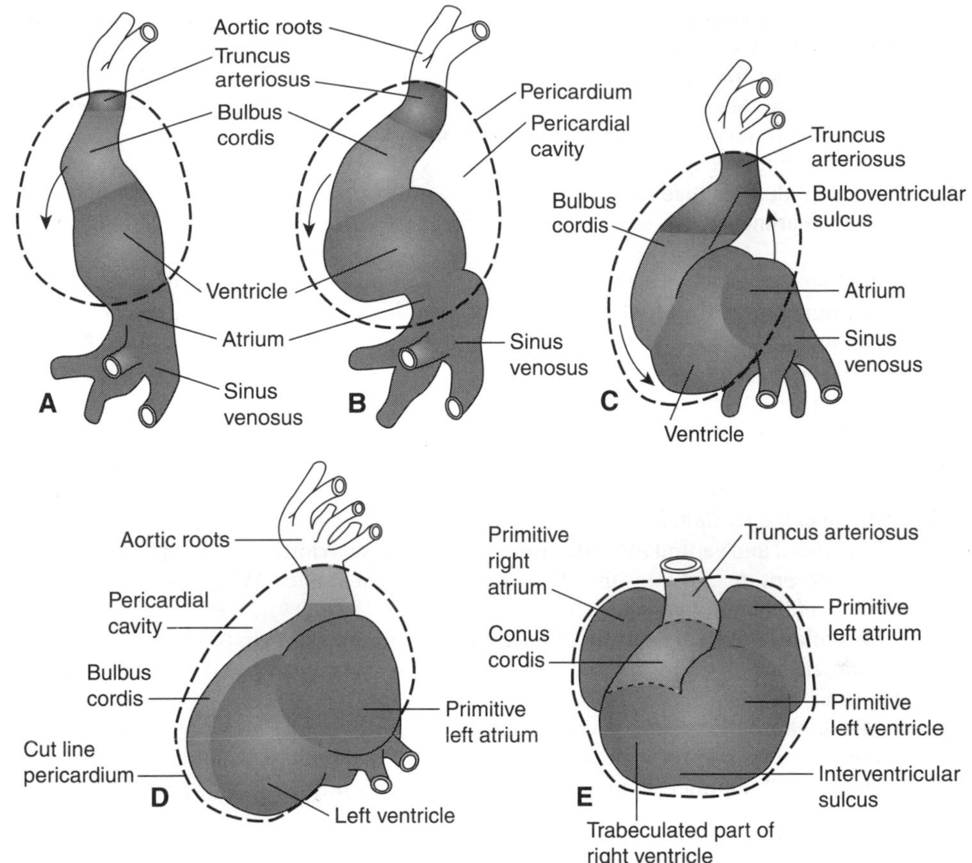

FIGURE 3.14. Formation of the cardiac loop and heart. **A–C:** Cardiac loop. **D** and **E:** Heart.
(Reprinted with permission from Langman J. *Medical embryology.* 4th ed. Baltimore, MD: Williams & Wilkins; 1981:162.)

A. Primitive Heart Tube

- It is formed by fusion of two endocardial heart tubes of mesodermal origin in the cardiogenic region.
- It develops into the endocardium, and the splanchnic mesoderm surrounding the tube develops into the myocardium and epicardium.
- It forms five dilations, including the truncus arteriosus, bulbus cordis, primitive ventricle, primitive atrium, and sinus venosus.
- It undergoes a folding into a U-shape, bringing the arterial and venous ends of the heart together and moving the ventricle caudally and the atrium cranially.

B. Fate of Five Dilations of the Primitive Heart Tube

- **Truncus arteriosus** (ventral aorta) forms aorta and pulmonary trunk by formation of the aorticopulmonary (AP) septum.
- **Bulbus cordis** forms conus cordis or conus arteriosus (smooth part of right ventricle) and aortic vestibule (smooth part of left ventricle at the root of the aorta).
- **Primitive ventricle** forms trabeculated part of right and left ventricles.
- **Primitive atrium** forms trabeculated part of right and left atrium.
- **Sinus venosus** forms **sinus venarum** (smooth part of right atrium), coronary sinus, and oblique vein of left atrium.

C. Division of the Heart Into Four Chambers

- Heart divides into its four chambers by formation of its septum and valves.

- Four main septa involved in dividing the heart include the AP septum, the atrial septum, the AV septum, and the IV septum.

1. **Partition of the Truncus Arteriosus and Bulbus Cordis**
   - The **truncal ridges** and the **bulbar ridges** derived from neural crest mesenchyme grow in a spiral fashion and fuse to form the **AP septum.**
   - The **AP septum** divides the truncus arteriosus into the aorta and pulmonary trunk.
2. **Partition of the Primitive Atrium**
   - **Septum primum** grows toward the AV endocardial cushions from the roof of the primitive atrium.
   - **Septum secundum** forms to the right of the septum primum and fuses with the septum primum to form the **atrial septum**, which separates the right and left atria.
   - **Foramen primum** forms between the free edge of the septum primum and the **AV septum**, allowing a passage between the right and left atria. The foramen is closed by growth of the septum primum.
   - **Foramen secundum** forms in the center of the septum primum.
   - **Foramen ovale** is an oval opening in the septum secundum that provides a communication between the atria. See Fetal Circulation: VII. A.1.
3. **Partition of the AV Canal**
   - The dorsal and ventral AV endocardial cushions fuse to form the AV septum.
   - The AV septum partitions the AV canal into the right and left AV canals.
4. **Partition of the Primitive Ventricle**
   - **Muscular IV septum** develops as outgrowth of muscular wall in the floor of the primitive ventricle and grows toward the AV septum but stops to create the IV foramen, leaving the septum incomplete.
   - **Membranous IV septum** forms by fusion of the bulbar ridges with the endocardial cushion, the AP septum, and the muscular part of the IV septum. The membranous IV septum closes the IV foramen, completing partition of the ventricles.

CLINICAL CORRELATES

Tetralogy of Fallot occurs when the **AP septum** fails to align properly with the AV septum, resulting in (1) **pulmonary stenosis** (obstruction to right ventricular outflow), (2) **VSD**, (3) **overriding aorta** (dextraposition of aorta), and (4) **right ventricular hypertrophy**. It is characterized by right-to-left shunting of blood and **cyanosis. Overriding aorta** (dextraposition of aorta) is that the aorta (its outlet) lies over both ventricles (instead of over the left ventricle), directly above the VSD, causing the aorta to arise from both ventricles.

Transposition of the great vessels occurs when the AP septum fails to develop in a spiral fashion, causing the aorta to arise from the right ventricle and the pulmonary trunk to arise from the left ventricle. It results in right-to-left shunting of blood and **cyanosis**. Thus, the transposition must be accompanied by a VSD or a patent ductus arteriosus for the infant to survive.

CLINICAL CORRELATES

Atrial septal defect (ASD) is a congenital defect in the septum between the atria due to **failure of the foramen primum or secundum to close** normally, resulting in a **patent foramen ovale**. This congenital heart defect shunts blood from the left atrium to the right atrium and causes hypertrophy of the right atrium, right ventricle, and pulmonary trunk, and thus mixing of oxygenated and deoxygenated blood, producing cyanosis. Symptoms of the defect are dyspnea (difficulty breathing), shortness of breath, and palpitations, and its signs include abnormal heart sounds, murmur, and heart failure. It can be treated by surgical closure of the defect and a new procedure without surgery, which introduces a catheter through the femoral vein and advances it into the heart where the closure device is placed across the ASD and the defect is closed. A **blood clot**, which usually forms in the deep veins of the thigh or the leg, travels to the right atrium, the left atrium through the ASD, the left ventricle, the systemic circulation, and eventually to the brain, causing a **stroke**.

CLINICAL CORRELATES

VSD occurs commonly in the membranous part of the IV septum because of the failure of the membranous IV septum to develop, resulting in left-to-right shunting of blood through the IV foramen, which increases blood flow to the lungs and causes pulmonary hypertension. Symptoms of the defect are shortness of breath, fast heart rate and breathing, sweating, and paleness, and its signs include a loud, continuous murmur and congestive heart failure. It may be treated with medications such as digitalis (digoxin) and diuretics.

V. DEVELOPMENT OF THE ARTERIAL SYSTEM

A. Formation

- The arterial system develops from the aortic arches and branches of the dorsal aorta.

B. Aortic Arch Derivatives

- Aortic arch 1 has no derivative because it disappears soon after development.
- Aortic arch 2 has no derivative because it persists only during the early development.
- Aortic arch 3 forms the common carotid arteries and the proximal part of the internal carotid arteries.
- Aortic arch 4 forms the **aortic arch** on the left and the **brachiocephalic** artery and the proximal **subclavian** artery on the right.
- Aortic arch 5 has no derivative.
- Aortic arch 6 forms the proximal pulmonary arteries and ductus arteriosus.

C. Dorsal Aorta

1. Posterolateral Branches

- Form the intercostal, lumbar, vertebral, cervical, internal thoracic, and epigastric arteries and arteries to upper and lower limbs.

2. Lateral Branches

- Form the renal, suprarenal, and gonadal arteries.

3. Ventral Branches

- Vitelline arteries form the celiac (foregut), superior mesenteric (midgut), and inferior mesenteric (hindgut) arteries.
- Umbilical arteries form a part of the internal iliac and superior vesical arteries.

VI. DEVELOPMENT OF THE VENOUS SYSTEM

- The venous system develops from the vitelline, umbilical, and cardinal veins, which drain into the sinus venosus.

A. Vitelline Veins

- Return poorly oxygenated blood from the yolk sac.
- Right vein forms the hepatic veins and sinusoids, ductus venosus, hepatic portal, superior mesenteric, inferior mesenteric, and splenic veins and part of the IVC.
- Left vein forms the hepatic veins and sinusoids and ductus venosus.

B. Umbilical Veins

- Carry well-oxygenated blood from the placenta.
- Right vein degenerates during early development.
- Left vein forms the ligamentum teres hepatis.

C. Cardinal Veins

- Return poorly oxygenated blood from the body of the embryo.
- Anterior cardinal vein forms the internal jugular veins and SVC.
- Posterior cardinal vein forms a part of the IVC and common iliac veins.
- Subcardinal vein forms a part of the IVC, renal veins, and gonadal veins.
- Supracardinal vein forms a part of the IVC, intercostal, azygos, and hemiazygos veins.

VII. FETAL CIRCULATION (See Figure 3.15)

A. The Fetus

- Has blood that is oxygenated in the placenta rather than in the lungs.
- Has three shunts that partially bypass the lungs and liver.

1. Foramen Ovale

- Is an opening in the septum secundum.
- Usually closes functionally at birth, but with anatomic closure occurring later.
- Shunts blood from the right atrium to the left atrium, partially bypassing the lungs (pulmonary circulation).

2. Ductus Arteriosus

- Is derived from the sixth aortic arch and connects the bifurcation of the pulmonary trunk with the aorta.
- Closes functionally soon after birth, with anatomic closure requiring several weeks.
- Becomes the ligamentum arteriosum, which connects the left pulmonary artery (at its origin from the pulmonary trunk) to the concavity of the arch of the aorta.
- Shunts blood from the pulmonary trunk to the aorta, partially bypassing the lungs (pulmonary circulation).

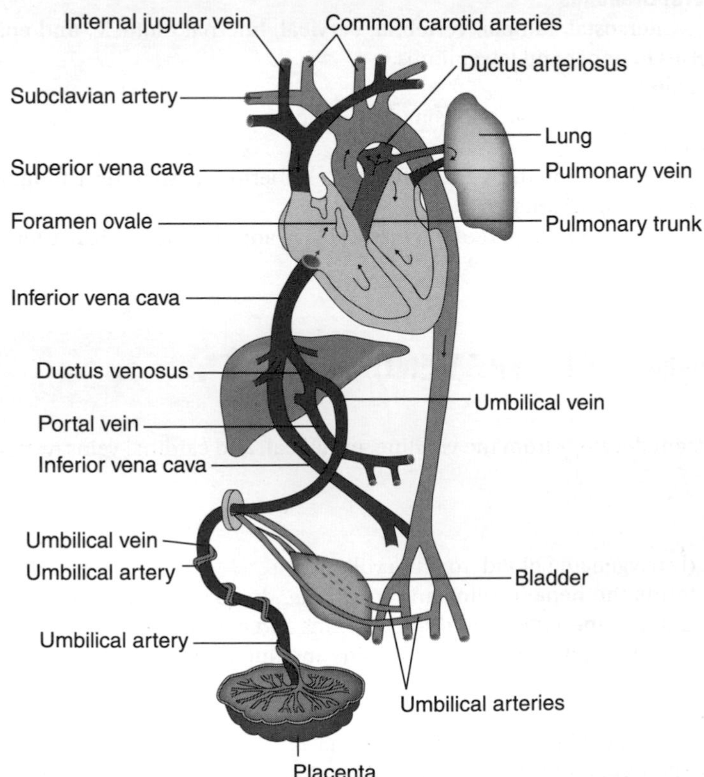

FIGURE 3.15. Fetal circulation.

CLINICAL CORRELATES **Patent ductus arteriosus** results from failure of the ductus arteriosus to close after birth, and it is common in premature infants. The **ductus arteriosus** takes origin from the left sixth arch.

3. Ductus Venosus

- Shunts oxygenated blood from the umbilical vein (returning from the placenta) to the IVC, partially bypassing the liver (portal circulation).
- Joins the left branch of the portal vein to the IVC and is obliterated to become the ligamentum venosum after birth.

B. Umbilical Arteries

- Carry blood to the placenta for reoxygenation before birth.
- Become medial umbilical ligaments after birth, after their distal parts have atrophied.

C. Umbilical Veins

- Carry highly oxygenated blood from the placenta to the fetus.
- Consists of the right vein, which is obliterated during the embryonic period, and the left vein, which is obliterated to form the ligamentum teres hepatis after birth.

STRUCTURES IN THE POSTERIOR MEDIASTINUM

I. ESOPHAGUS

- Is a muscular tube (approximately 10 in. long) that extends from the pharynx to the stomach, descending behind the trachea.
- Has **three constrictions**: (1) upper or pharyngoesophageal constriction at the **beginning of the esophagus** at the level of the cricoid cartilage (C6) is caused by the **cricopharyngeus** muscle; (2) middle or thoracic constriction where it is crossed by the **aortic arch** and then **left main bronchus** and; (3) inferior or diaphragmatic constriction at the **esophageal hiatus** of the diaphragm (T10). The left atrium also presses against the anterior surface of the esophagus.
- Has a physiologic sphincter, which is the circular layer of smooth muscle at the gastroesophageal junction. This is called the **inferior esophageal sphincter** by clinicians.
- Receives blood from the **inferior thyroid** artery in the neck and branches of the **aorta** (bronchial and esophageal arteries) and from the **left gastric** and **left inferior phrenic** arteries in the thorax.

CLINICAL CORRELATES **Achalasia of esophagus** is a condition of **impaired esophageal contractions** because of failure of relaxation of the **inferior esophageal sphincter**, resulting from degeneration of myenteric (Auerbach) plexus in the esophagus. It causes an obstruction to the passage of food in the terminal esophagus and exhibits symptoms of dysphagia for solids and liquids, weight loss, chest pain, nocturnal cough, and recurrent bronchitis or pneumonia.

Systemic sclerosis (scleroderma) is a systemic collagen vascular disease and has clinical features of dysphagia for solids and liquids, severe heartburn, and **esophageal stricture**.

II. BLOOD VESSELS AND LYMPHATIC VESSELS (See Figures 3.16 to 3.17)

A. Thoracic Aorta

- Begins at the level of the fourth thoracic vertebra.
- Descends on the left side of the vertebral column and then approaches the median plane to end in front of the vertebral column by passing through the **aortic hiatus** of the diaphragm.
- Gives rise to nine pairs of **posterior intercostal arteries** and one pair of **subcostal arteries.** The first two intercostal arteries arise from the highest intercostal arteries of the costocervical trunk. The posterior intercostal artery gives rise to a collateral branch, which runs along the upper border of the rib below the space.
- Also gives rise to pericardial, bronchial (one right and two left), esophageal, mediastinal, and superior phrenic branches.

CLINICAL CORRELATES

Coarctation of the aorta (Figure 3.16) occurs when the aorta is abnormally constricted just inferior to the ductus arteriosus, in which case an adequate collateral circulation develops before birth. It causes (a) a characteristic rib notching and a high risk of cerebral hemorrhage; (b) tortuous and enlarged blood vessels, especially the internal thoracic, intercostal, epigastric, and scapular arteries; (c) an elevated blood pressure in the radial artery and decreased pressure in the femoral artery; and (d) the femoral pulse to occur after the radial pulse (normally, the femoral pulse occurs slightly before the radial pulse). It leads to the development of the important **collateral circulation** over the thorax, which occurs between the (a) **anterior intercostal** branches of the internal thoracic artery and the **posterior intercostal** arteries; (b) **superior epigastric** branch of the **internal thoracic** artery and the inferior epigastric artery; (c) superior intercostal branch of the costocervical trunk and the **third posterior intercostal** artery; and (d) **posterior intercostal** arteries and the **descending** scapular (or dorsal scapular) artery, which anastomoses with the suprascapular and circumflex scapular arteries around the scapula.

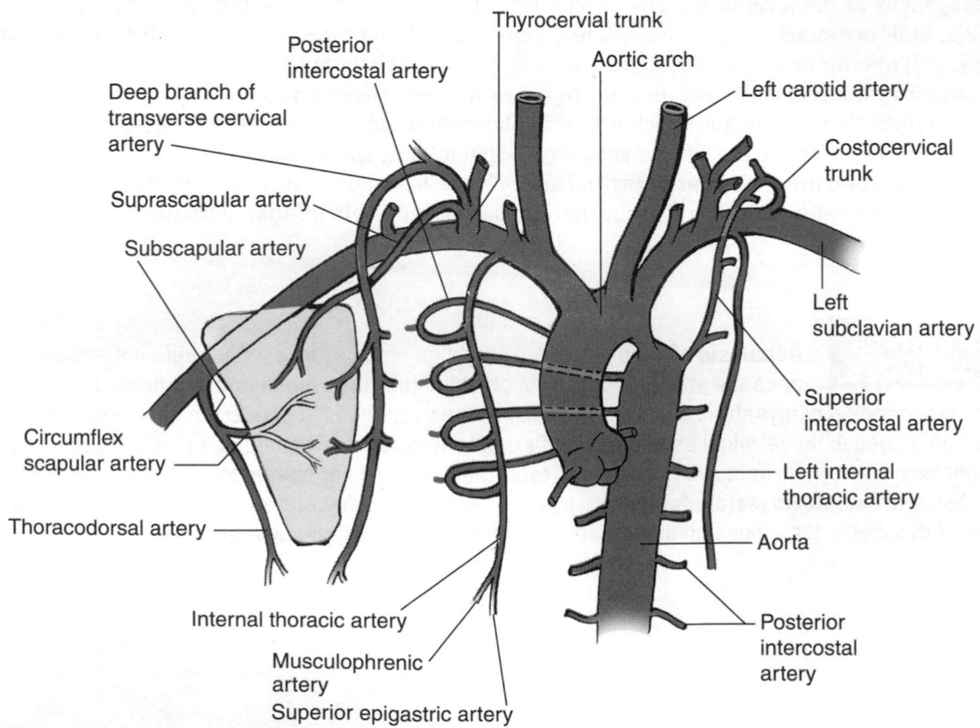

FIGURE 3.16. Coarctation of the aorta.

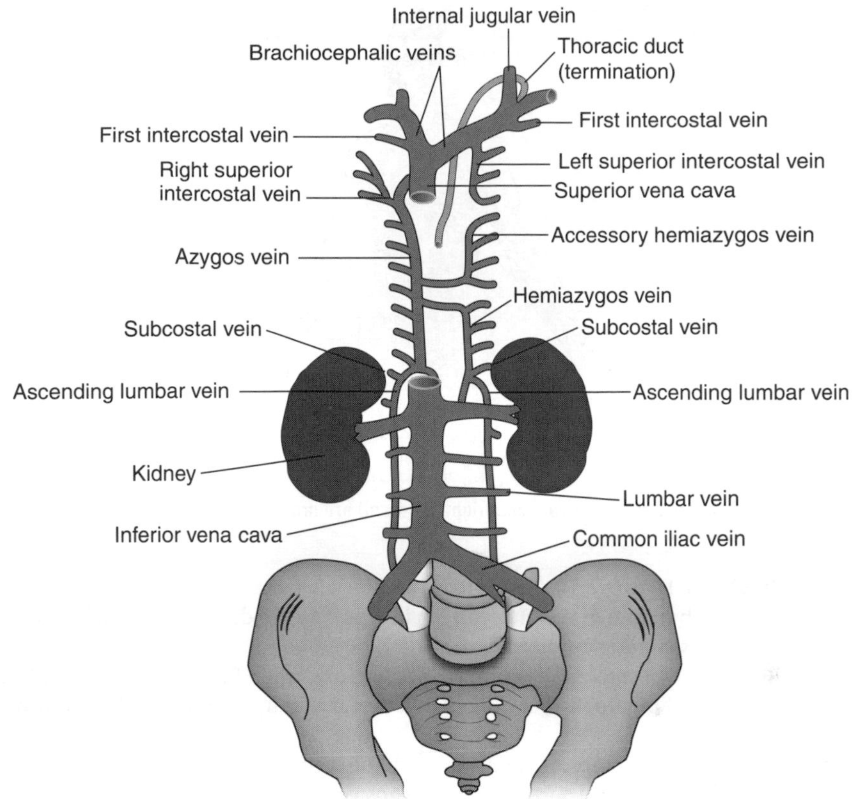

FIGURE 3.17. Azygos venous system.

B. Azygos Venous System (See Figure 3.17)

1. Azygos (Unpaired) Vein

- Is formed by the union of the right ascending lumbar and right subcostal veins. Its lower end is connected to the IVC.
- Enters the thorax through the aortic opening of the diaphragm.
- Receives the right intercostal veins, the **right superior intercostal vein**, and the hemiazygos and accessory hemiazygos veins.
- **Arches over the root of the right lung and empties into the SVC**, of which it is the first tributary.

2. Hemiazygos Vein

- Is formed by the union of the left subcostal and ascending lumbar veins. Its lower end is connected to the left renal vein.
- Ascends on the left side of the vertebral bodies behind the thoracic aorta, receiving the 9th, 10th, and 11th posterior intercostal veins.

3. Accessory Hemiazygos Vein

- Begins at the fourth or fifth intercostal space; descends, receiving the fourth or fifth to eighth intercostal veins; turns to the right; passes behind the aorta; and terminates in the azygos vein.

4. Superior Intercostal Vein

- Is formed by a union of the second, third, and fourth posterior intercostal veins and drains into the azygos vein on the right and the brachiocephalic vein on the left.

5. Posterior Intercostal Veins

- The first intercostal vein on each side drains into the corresponding brachiocephalic vein.
- The second, third, and often the fourth intercostal veins join to form the **superior intercostal vein**.
- The rest of the veins drain into the azygos vein on the right and into the hemiazygos or accessory hemiazygos veins on the left.

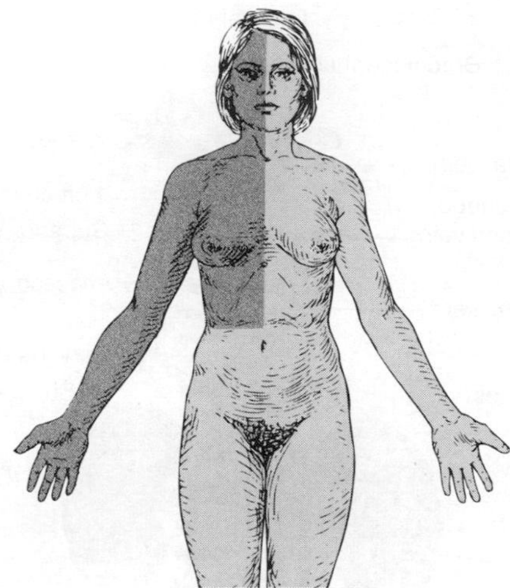

FIGURE 3.18. All areas except the *shaded* area (upper right quadrant) are drained by the thoracic duct.

C. Lymphatics

1. Thoracic Duct (See Figures 3.10, 3.17, and 3.18)

- Begins in the abdomen at the **cisterna chyli**, which is the dilated junction of the intestinal, lumbar, and descending intercostal trunks.
- Is usually beaded because of its numerous valves and often forms double or triple ducts.
- Drains the lower limbs, pelvis, abdomen, left thorax, left upper limb, and left side of the head and neck.
- Passes through the aortic opening of the diaphragm and ascends through the posterior mediastinum between the aorta and the azygos vein.
- Arches laterally over the apex of the left pleura and between the left carotid sheath in front and the vertebral artery behind, runs behind the left internal jugular vein, and then usually empties into the junction of the left internal jugular and subclavian veins.

2. Right Lymphatic Duct

- Drains the right sides of the thorax, upper limb, head, and neck.
- Empties into the junction of the right internal jugular and subclavian veins.

III. AUTONOMIC NERVOUS SYSTEM IN THE THORAX (Figure 3.19)

- Is composed of motor, or efferent, nerves through which **cardiac muscle**, **smooth muscle**, and **glands** are innervated.
- Involves two neurons: **preganglionic** and **postganglionic**. It may include **general visceral afferent (GVA) fibers** because they run along with **general visceral efferent (GVE) fibers**.
- Consists of sympathetic (or thoracolumbar outflow) and parasympathetic (or craniosacral outflow) systems.
- Consists of **cholinergic** fibers (sympathetic preganglionic, parasympathetic preganglionic, and postganglionic), which use acetylcholine as the neurotransmitter and **adrenergic** fibers (sympathetic postganglionic), which use norepinephrine as the neurotransmitter (except those to sweat glands [cholinergic]).

A. Sympathetic Nervous System

- Is a **catabolic (energy-consuming)** system that enables the body to cope with crises or emergencies, and thus often is referred to as the **fight-or-flight** division.
- Contains preganglionic cell bodies that are located in the lateral horn or intermediolateral cell column of the spinal cord segments between T1 and L2.

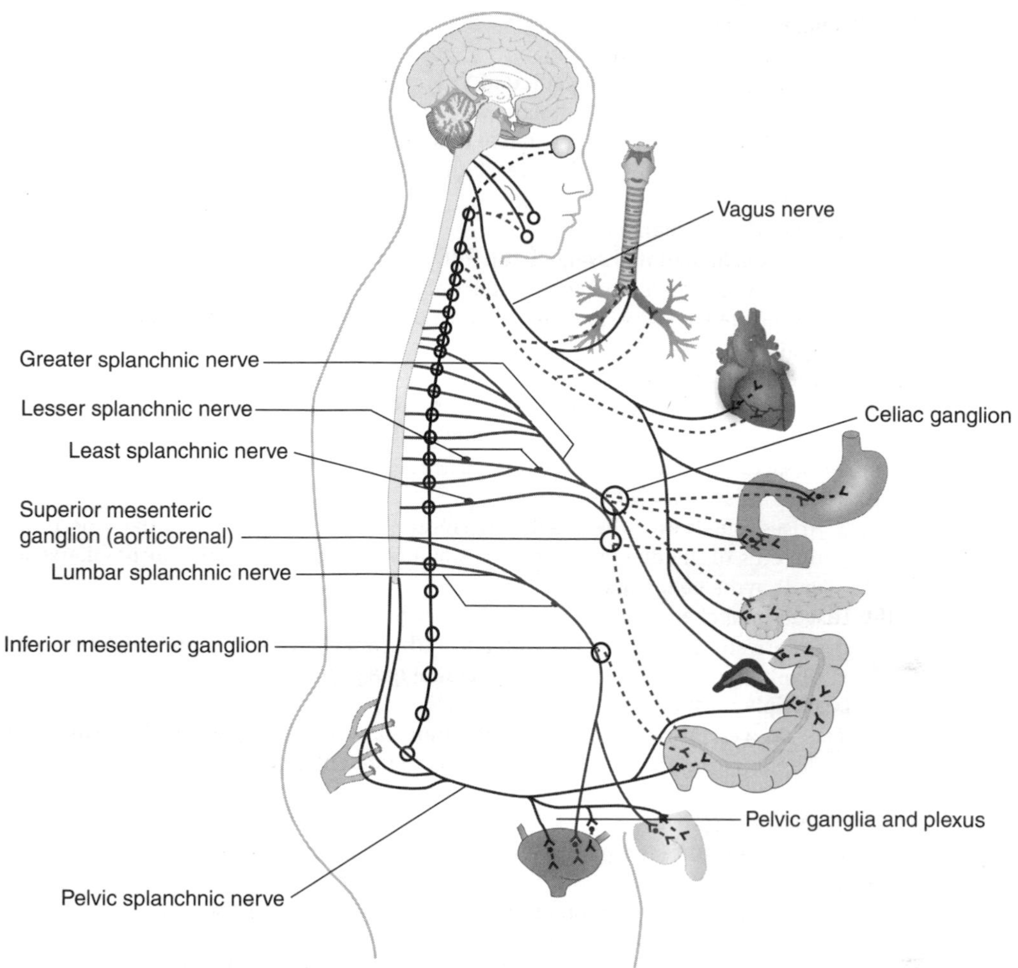

FIGURE 3.19. Autonomic nervous system.

- Has preganglionic fibers that pass through the white rami communicantes and enter the sympathetic chain ganglion, where they synapse.
- Has postganglionic fibers that join each spinal nerve by way of the gray rami communicantes and supply the blood vessels, hair follicles (arrector pili muscles), and sweat glands.
- Increases the **heart rate** and dilates the **bronchial lumen** and the **coronary arteries**.

1. Sympathetic Trunk

- Is composed primarily of ascending and descending preganglionic sympathetic fibers and visceral afferent fibers and contains the cell bodies of the postganglionic sympathetic (GVE) fibers.
- Descends in front of the neck of the ribs and the posterior intercostal vessels.
- Contains the **cervicothoracic (or stellate) ganglion**, which is formed by fusion of the inferior cervical ganglion with the first thoracic ganglion.
- Enters the abdomen through the crus of the diaphragm or behind the medial lumbocostal arch.
- Gives rise to cardiac, pulmonary, mediastinal, and splanchnic branches.
- Is connected to the thoracic spinal nerves by gray and white rami communicantes.

CLINICAL CORRELATES

Stellate block is an injection of local anesthetic near the stellate ganglion by placing the tip of the needle near the neck of the first rib. It produces a temporary interruption of sympathetic function such as in a patient with excess vasoconstriction in the upper limb.

2. **Rami Communicantes**

(a) **White Rami Communicantes**

- Contain **preganglionic sympathetic GVE** (myelinated) fibers with **cell bodies** located in the **lateral horn** (intermediolateral cell column) of the spinal cord and **GVA** fibers with **cell bodies** located in the **dorsal root ganglia**.
- Are connected to the spinal nerves, limited to the spinal cord segments between T1 and L2.

(b) **Gray Rami Communicantes**

- Contain **postganglionic sympathetic GVE** (unmyelinated) fibers that supply the blood vessels, sweat glands, and arrector pili muscles of hair follicles.
- Are connected to every spinal nerve and contain fibers with **cell bodies** located in the **sympathetic trunk.**

3. **Thoracic Splanchnic Nerves**

- Contain **sympathetic preganglionic GVE** fibers with cell bodies located in the lateral horn (intermediolateral cell column) of the spinal cord and **GVA** fibers with cell bodies located in the dorsal root ganglia.

(a) **Greater Splanchnic Nerve**

- Arises usually from the fifth through ninth thoracic sympathetic ganglia, perforates the crus of the diaphragm or occasionally passes through the aortic hiatus, and ends in the **celiac ganglion**.

(b) **Lesser Splanchnic Nerve**

- Is derived usually from the 10th and 11th thoracic ganglia, pierces the crus of the diaphragm, and ends in the **aorticorenal ganglion**.

(c) **Least Splanchnic Nerve**

- Is derived usually from the 12th thoracic ganglion, pierces the crus of the diaphragm, and ends in the ganglia of the **renal plexus**.

B. Parasympathetic Nervous System

- Is a homeostatic or **anabolic (energy-conserving)** system, promoting quiet and orderly processes of the body.
- Is not as widely distributed over the entire body as sympathetic fibers; the body wall and extremities have no parasympathetic nerve supply.
- Has preganglionic fibers running in cranial nerves (CNs) III, VII, and IX that pass to cranial autonomic ganglia (i.e., the ciliary, submandibular, pterygopalatine, and otic ganglia), where they synapse with postganglionic neurons.
- Has preganglionic fibers in CN X and in **pelvic splanchnic nerves** (originating from S2 to S4) that pass to terminal ganglia, where they synapse.
- Has parasympathetic fibers in the **vagus nerve** (CN X) that supply all of the thoracic and abdominal viscera, except the descending and sigmoid colons and other pelvic viscera. These structures are innervated by the pelvic splanchnic nerves (S2–S4). The vagus nerve contains the parasympathetic preganglionic fibers with cell bodies located in the medulla oblongata and the GVA fibers with cell bodies located in the inferior (nodose) ganglion.
- **Decreases the heart rate**, **constricts bronchial lumen**, and causes **vasoconstriction** of the coronary arteries.

1. **Right Vagus Nerve**

- Gives rise to the **right recurrent laryngeal nerve**, which hooks around the right subclavian artery and ascends into the neck between the trachea and the esophagus.
- Crosses anterior to the right subclavian artery, runs posterior to the SVC, and descends at the right surface of the trachea and then posterior to the right main bronchus.
- Contributes to the cardiac, pulmonary, and esophageal plexuses.
- Forms the posterior vagal trunk (or gastric nerves) at the lower part of the esophagus and enters the abdomen through the esophageal hiatus.

2. **Left Vagus Nerve**

- Enters the thorax between the left common carotid and subclavian arteries and behind the left brachiocephalic vein and descends on the arch of the aorta.

- Gives rise to the **left recurrent laryngeal nerve**, which hooks around the arch of the aorta to the left of the ligamentum arteriosum. It ascends through the superior mediastinum and the neck in a groove between the trachea and esophagus.
- Gives off the thoracic cardiac branches, breaks up into the pulmonary plexuses, continues into the esophageal plexus, and then forms the anterior vagal trunk.

CLINICAL CORRELATES

Injury to the recurrent laryngeal nerve may be caused by a bronchogenic or esophageal carcinoma, enlargement of mediastinal lymph nodes, an aneurysm of the aortic arch, or thyroid and parathyroid surgeries, causing respiratory obstruction, hoarseness, and an inability to speak because of paralysis of the vocal cord.

Vagotomy is transection of the vagus nerves at the lower portion of the esophagus in an attempt to reduce gastric secretion in the treatment of peptic ulcer.

C. Organ-Specific Effects of Autonomic Activity

- Sympathetic stimulation increases heart rate, dilates coronary arteries, and thus increases blood flow through the vessels, supplying more oxygen and nutrients to the myocardium. Sympathetic nerve also produces bronchodilation and vasoconstriction of pulmonary vessels.
- Parasympathetic stimulation slows the heart rate, constricts the coronary arteries, produces bronchoconstriction (motor to smooth muscle) and vasodilation of the pulmonary vessels, and increases glandular secretion of the bronchial tree (secretomotor).

HIGH-YIELD TOPICS

- The **sternum** can be used for bone marrow biopsy because of its accessible location and it possesses hematopoietic marrow throughout life.
- The **sternal angle** (of Louis) is the junction between the manubrium and body of the sternum located at the level where (1) the second ribs articulate with the sternum, (2) the aortic arch begins and ends, (3) the trachea bifurcates into the right and left primary bronchi, and (4) it marks the plane of separation between the superior and inferior mediastinum.
- The **true ribs** are the first seven ribs (ribs 1–7), **the false ribs** are the lower five ribs (ribs 8–12), and the **floating ribs** are the last two ribs (ribs 11 and 12).
- **Flail chest** occurs when a segment of the anterior or lateral thoracic wall moves freely because of **multiple rib fractures**, allowing the loose segment to move inward on inspiration and outward on expiration.
- **Muscles of inspiration** include the diaphragm, external, internal (interchondral part), and innermost intercostal muscles, sternocleidomastoid, levator costarum, serratus anterior, serratus posterior superior, scalenus, and pectoral muscles.
- **Muscles of expiration** include anterior abdominal, internal intercostal (costal part), and serratus posterior inferior muscles. Quiet inspiration results from contraction of the diaphragm, whereas quiet expiration is a passive process caused by the elastic recoil of the lungs.
- The **trachea** begins at the inferior border of the cricoid cartilage (C6) and has 16 to 20 incomplete hyaline cartilaginous rings that prevent the trachea from collapsing and that open posteriorly toward the esophagus. It bifurcates into right and left primary bronchi at the level of the sternal angle.
- The **carina**, the last tracheal cartilage, separates the openings of the right and left primary bronchi. The **right primary bronchus** is shorter, wider, and more vertical than the left and divides into the superior (eparterial), middle, and inferior secondary (lobar) bronchi. The **left primary bronchus** divides into the superior and inferior lobar bronchi.
- The **bronchopulmonary segment** is the anatomical, functional, and surgical unit of the lungs and consists of a segmental (tertiary or lobular) bronchus, a segmental branch of the pulmonary artery,

and a segment of lung tissue, surrounded by a delicate connective tissue (intersegmental) septum. The pulmonary veins are intersegmental.

- **Bronchopulmonary (hilum) nodes** drain into tracheobronchial nodes, then to paratracheal nodes, and eventually to the thoracic duct.
- **Lung buds** arises from the laryngotracheal diverticulum in the embryonic foregut region.
- **Lungs** are the essential organs of respiration. The **right lung** is divided into the upper, middle, and lower lobes by the oblique and horizontal fissures. The **left lung** is divided into the upper and lower lobes by an oblique fissure and contains the lingula and the cardiac notch.
- **Most abscesses** occur in the right lung, because the right main bronchus is wider, shorter, and more vertical than the left, and thus aspirated infective agents gain easier access to the right lung.
- The **cupula** is the dome of cervical parietal pleura over the apex of the lung. It lies above the first rib and is vulnerable to trauma at the root of the neck.
- **Pancoast tumor** (superior pulmonary sulcus tumor) is a malignant neoplasm of the lung apex which may cause a lower trunk brachial plexopathy and a **lesion of cervical sympathetic chain** ganglia with **Horner syndrome** (ptosis, enophthalmos, miosis, anhidrosis, and vasodilation).
- **Chronic obstructive pulmonary disease (COPD)** is an obstruction of airflow through the airways and lungs and includes **chronic bronchitis** and **emphysema.** Shortness of breath in COPD occur when the walls of airways and air sacs get inflamed, destroyed, lose elasticity, and hypersecrete mucus.
- **Chronic bronchitis** is an **inflammation of the airways**, which results in **excessive mucus production** that plugs up the airways, causing a cough and dyspnea (difficulty in breathing).
- **Emphysema** is an accumulation of **trapped air in the alveolar sacs,** resulting in **destruction of the alveolar walls,** reducing the surface area for gas exchange.
- **Asthma** is an **airway obstruction** and is characterized by dyspnea, cough, and wheezing with **spasmodic contraction of smooth muscles** in the bronchi and bronchioles, narrowing the airways.
- **Barrel chest** is a chest resembling the shape of a barrel because the lungs are overinflated and the thoracic cage becomes enlarged, as seen in cases of emphysema or asthma.
- **Bronchiectasis** is a **chronic dilation of bronchi and bronchioles,** resulting from destruction of bronchial elastic and muscular elements, which may cause **collapse of the bronchioles**. It may be caused by pulmonary infections or by a bronchial obstruction with heavy sputum production.
- **Pleurisy (pleuritis)** is **inflammation of the pleura** with exudation (escape of fluid from blood vessels) into its cavity, causing the pleural surfaces to be roughened, producing friction.
- **Pneumothorax** is an accumulation of **air** in the pleural cavity because of an injury to the thoracic wall or the lung, causing no negative pressure in the chest and thus the lung collapses. **Tension pneumothorax** is a life-threatening pneumothorax in which air enters during inspiration and is trapped during expiration; therefore, the resultant increased pressure displaces the mediastinum to the opposite side, with consequent cardiopulmonary impairment.
- **Pleural effusion** is an abnormal accumulation of excess fluid in the pleural space, having two types; the **transudate** (clear watery fluid) and the **exudate** (cloudy viscous fluid).
- **Thoracentesis (pleuracentesis or pleural tap)** is a surgical procedure to collect pleural effusion for analysis. A needle or tube is inserted through thoracic wall into the pleural cavity posterior to the midaxillary line one or two intercostal spaces below the fluid level but not below the ninth intercostal space. Fluid in the pleural cavity includes **hydrothorax** (water), **hemothorax** (blood), **chylothorax** (lymph), and **pyothorax** (pus).
- **Pneumonia (pneumonitis)** is an infection in the lungs, which is of bacterial, viral, or mycoplasmal origin.
- **Tuberculosis (TB)** is an infectious lung disease caused by the bacterium ***Mycobacterium tuberculosis*** and is characterized by the formation of tubercles that can undergo necrosis.
- **Cystic fibrosis** (**CF**) is an inherited multisystem disease that has widespread dysfunction of the exocrine glands and pulmonary and gastrointestinal tracts. CF affects the respiratory system by causing an excess production of viscous mucus, obstructing the respiratory airway.
- **Pulmonary edema** involves fluid accumulation in the lungs caused by lung toxins. As pressure in the pulmonary veins rises, **fluid** is pushed **into the alveoli** and becomes a barrier to normal oxygen exchange, resulting in shortness of breath, increased heart rate, and cough.
- **Atelectasis** is the **collapse of a lung** by blockage of the air passages, pressure on the outside of the lung, or shallow breathing. It is caused by mucus secretions that plug the airway, foreign bodies in the airway, and tumors that compress or obstruct the airway.

- **Lung cancer** has two types, small cell and non-small cell carcinomas. **Small cell carcinoma** accounts for 20% and grow aggressively, while **non–small cell carcinoma** (80%) is further divided into **squamous cell carcinoma** (most common type), adenocarcinoma, and bronchoalveolar large cell carcinoma.
- **Pulmonary embolism** is an obstruction of the pulmonary artery or one of its branches by an embolus (air, blood clot, fat, tumor cells, or other foreign material). Its most common origin is deep leg veins (especially those in the calf).
- **Phrenic nerve** supplies somatic motor fibers to the diaphragm. The **central part** of diaphragm receives sensory fibers from the phrenic nerve, whereas the **peripheral part** receives sensory fibers from the intercostal nerves.
- **Phrenic nerve lesion** may not produce complete paralysis of the corresponding half of the diaphragm because the accessory phrenic nerve usually joins the phrenic nerve in the root of the neck.
- **Pain** from an infection of the pericardium (pericarditis) is carried in the **phrenic nerve.**
- **Pericarditis** is an **inflammation of the pericardium,** and the typical sign is **pericardial murmur or pericardial friction rub. Pericarditis** may result in **pericardial effusion** and **cardiac tamponade.**
- **Pericardial effusion** is an **accumulation of fluid** in the pericardial space, resulting from inflammation caused by acute pericarditis. The accumulated fluid compresses the heart, inhibiting cardiac filling. A radiograph will reveal an enlarged cardiac silhouette with a water bottle appearance.
- **Cardiac tamponade** is an **acute compression of the heart** caused by a rapid **accumulation of fluid** or blood in the pericardial cavity and can be treated by pericardiocentesis.
- **Pericardiocentesis** is a **surgical puncture of the pericardial cavity** for the aspiration of fluid. A needle is inserted into the pericardial cavity through the fifth intercostal space left of the sternum.
- The **crista terminalis** is a vertical muscular ridge running anteriorly along the right atrial wall from the opening of the SVC to the opening of the IVC, providing the origin of the pectinate muscles. It presents the junction between the primitive sinus venosus and the right atrium proper and is indicated externally by the sulcus terminalis.
- The **left atrium** is smaller with thicker walls than the right atrium and is the most posterior of the four chambers. The left ventricle forms the heart's apex, performs harder work, has a thicker wall, and is more conical-shaped than the right ventricle.
- The **papillary muscles** contract to tighten the **chordae tendineae**, preventing eversion of the AV valve cusps into the atrium, thus preventing regurgitation of ventricular blood into the atrium.
- The **septomarginal trabecula** (moderator band) is an isolated band of trabeculae carneae that forms a bridge between the interventricular septum and the base of the anterior papillary muscle of the right ventricle. It carries the right limb (Purkinje fibers) of the AV bundle.
- **Atrial septal defect (ASD)** is a congenital defect in the interatrial septum due to failure of the foramen primum or secundum to close normally, resulting in a **patent foramen ovale**. This defect shunts blood from the left atrium to the right atrium, thus mixing oxygenated and deoxygenated blood. A large ASD can cause hypertrophy of the right chambers and pulmonary trunk.
- **Ventricular septal defect (VSD)** occurs usually in the membranous part of the interventricular septum and is the most common congenital heart defect. The defect results in left-to-right shunting of blood through the IV foramen, increases blood flow to the lung, and causes pulmonary hypertension.
- The **first** ("lub") **sound** is caused by closure of the tricuspid and mitral valves at the onset of ventricular systole. The **second** ("dub") **sound** is caused by closure of the aortic and pulmonary valves and vibration of walls of the heart and major vessels at the onset of ventricular diastole.
- For **cardiac auscultation**, the stethoscope should be placed over the mitral valve area, in the left fifth intercostal space over the apex of the heart to hear the first heart sound ("lub").
- The **tricuspid** (right AV) valve is **most audible** over the right or left lower part of the body of the sternum, whereas the **bicuspid** or **mitral** (left AV) valve is most audible over the apical region of the heart in the left fifth intercostal space at the midclavicular line. The **pulmonary valve** is most audible over the left second intercostal space just lateral to the sternum, whereas the **aortic valve** is most audible over the right second intercostal space just lateral to the sternum.
- **Mitral valve stenosis** is a narrowing of the orifice of the mitral valve. This impedes the flow of blood from the left atrium to the left ventricle, causing an enlargement of the left atrium and pulmonary edema due to increased left atrial pressure.
- **Mitral valve prolapse** is a condition in which the valve everts into the left atrium when the left ventricle contacts and may produce chest pain, shortness of breath, and cardiac arrhythmia.

- **The SA node (pacemaker)** initiates the heartbeat. Impulse travels from the **SA node** to the AV node to the **AV bundle** (of His) that divides to right and left bundle branches, then to subendocardial Purkinje fibers, and the ventricular musculature. SA node is supplied by SA nodal branch of the right coronary artery.
- **Myocardial infarction** (MI) is **necrosis of the myocardium** due to local **ischemia.** Causes of ischemia include vasospasm or obstruction of the blood supply, most commonly by a thrombus or embolus in the coronary arteries. Major causes of MI include coronary atherosclerosis and thrombosis, and the left anterior descending is the most common site (40%–50%). MI symptoms range from none (silent MI) to severe chest pain or pressure for a prolonged period.
- **Angina pectoris** is characterized by **chest pain originating** in the heart and felt beneath the sternum, in many cases radiating to the left shoulder and down the arm. It is caused by an **insufficient supply of oxygen** to the heart muscle. It can be treated with nitroglycerin.
- **Endocarditis** is an infection of the endocardium of the heart, most commonly involving the heart valves and is caused by a cluster of bacteria on the valves. The valves have reduced defense mechanisms because they do not receive dedicated blood supply, thus immune cells cannot enter. Valve infections can cause cardiac murmur, which is a characteristic sound generated by turbulence of blood flow through an orifice of the heart.
- **Damage to the conducting system** interferes with the spread of electrical signals through the heart (heart block). A delay or disruption of the electrical signals produces an irregular and slower heartbeat, reducing the heart's efficiency in maintaining adequate circulation. Severe heart block requires implantation of a pacemaker.
- **Atrial or ventricular fibrillation** is a cardiac arrhythmia resulting from rapid irregular uncoordinated contractions of the atrial or ventricular muscle. Fibrillation causes palpitations, shortness of breath, angina, fatigue, congestive heart failure, and sudden cardiac death.
- **Coronary atherosclerosis** is characterized by presence of sclerotic plagues containing cholesterol and lipid material that impairs myocardial blood flow, leading to ischemia and myocardial infarction.
- **Coronary angioplasty** is an angiographic reconstruction of a blood vessel made by enlarging a narrowed coronary arterial lumen. It is performed by peripheral introduction of a balloon-tip catheter and dilation of the arterial lumen on withdrawal of the inflated catheter tip.
- **Coronary bypass** is connection of a healthy section of vessel (usually the saphenous vein or internal thoracic artery) between the aorta and a coronary artery distal to an obstruction. Alternatively, the internal thoracic artery is connected to the coronary artery distal to the obstructive lesion. Bypass creates a new pathway for blood flow to the heart muscle.
- **Aortic aneurysm** is a local dilation of the aorta that can lead to dissection or rupture. If located in the aortic arch, compression of the left recurrent laryngeal nerve may occur, leading to coughing, hoarseness, and paralysis of the ipsilateral vocal cord. Pressure on the esophagus may cause **dysphagia** (difficulty in swallowing), while **dyspnea** (difficulty in breathing) results from pressure on the trachea, root of the lung, or phrenic nerve.
- **Marfan syndrome** is an inheritable disorder of connective tissue. It most often affects the heart and blood vessels (aortic root dilation, aortic aneurysm, aortic regurgitation, and mitral valve prolapse), the skeleton (long limbs), eye (dislocated lens), and lungs (spontaneous pneumothorax).
- The **coronary arteries** arise from the ascending aorta. Systolic compression of the arterial branches in the myocardium reduces coronary blood flow. Therefore, maximal blood flow occurs during diastole.
- The **right coronary artery** has the SA nodal, marginal, posterior IV, and AV nodal branches. The left coronary artery is shorter than the right one and divides into the anterior IV and circumflex arteries.
- All **cardiac veins**, including the great, middle, small, and oblique cardiac veins, drain into the coronary sinus except the anterior cardiac vein, which drains into the right atrium.
- **Tetralogy of Fallot** includes (1) **pulmonary stenosis** (narrowing of right ventricular outflow), (2) large **overriding aorta** (drains both ventricles), (3) **VSD**, and (4) **right ventricular hypertrophy**. It is characterized by right-to-left shunting of blood and **cyanosis**.
- **Overriding aorta** (dextraposition of aorta) is that the aorta (its outlet) lies over both ventricles (instead of just the left ventricle), directly above the VSD, causing the aorta to arise from both ventricles.

- **Transposition of the great vessels** occurs when the AP septum fails to develop in a spiral fashion, causing the aorta to arise from the right ventricle and the pulmonary trunk to arise from the left ventricle.
- **Patent ductus arteriosus** results from failure of the ductus arteriosus to close after birth, and is common in premature infants. The **ductus arteriosus** takes origin from the left sixth aortic arch.
- The **fourth aortic arches** contribute to the right **subclavian artery** on the right side and the **aortic arch** on the left.
- The **mediastinum** is an **interpleural space** and consists of the superior mediastinum and inferior mediastinum. The inferior mediastinum further divides into the anterior, middle, and posterior mediastina.
- The **middle mediastinum** contains the heart. The **posterior mediastinum** contains the esophagus, thoracic aorta, azygos and hemiazygos veins, thoracic duct, vagus nerves, and sympathetic splanchnic nerves.
- **Achalasia** is a condition of **impaired esophageal contractions** resulting from degeneration of myenteric (Auerbach) plexus in the esophagus. The lower esophageal sphincter fails to relax during swallowing.
- **Systemic sclerosis (scleroderma)** is a systemic collagen vascular disease and has clinical features of dysphagia for solids and liquids, severe heartburn, and **esophageal stricture**.
- **Coarctation of the aorta** occurs when the aorta is abnormally constricted just inferior to the ductus arteriosus, in which case an adequate collateral circulation develops before birth. Clinical signs include hypertension and/or heart failure. It causes (a) a characteristic rib notching and a high risk of cerebral hemorrhage; (b) tortuous and enlarged blood vessels, especially the internal thoracic, intercostal, epigastric, and scapular arteries; (c) an elevated blood pressure in the radial artery and decreased pressure in the femoral artery; and (d) the femoral pulse to occur after the radial pulse (normally the femoral pulse occurs slightly before the radial pulse).
- **Stellate block** is an injection of local anesthetic near the stellate ganglion by placing the tip of the needle near the neck of the first rib. It produces a temporary interruption of sympathetic function such as in a patient with excess vasoconstriction in the upper limb.
- **Injury to the recurrent laryngeal nerve** may be caused by a bronchogenic or esophageal carcinoma, enlargement of mediastinal lymph nodes, an aneurysm of the aortic arch, or thyroid and parathyroid surgeries, causing respiratory obstruction, hoarseness, or an inability to speak because of paralysis of the vocal cord.
- **Vagotomy** is transection of the vagus nerves at the lower portion of the esophagus in an attempt to reduce gastric secretion in the treatment of peptic ulcer.
- The **azygos vein** is formed by the union of the right ascending lumbar and right subcostal veins. Its lower end is connected to the IVC. It **arches over the root of the right lung** and empties into the SVC.
- The **hemiazygos vein** is formed by the union of the left subcostal and ascending lumbar vein, receives the 9th, 10th, and 11th posterior intercostal veins, and enters the azygos vein. Its lower end is connected to the left renal vein. The **accessory hemiazygos vein** receives the fifth to eighth posterior intercostal veins and terminates in the azygos vein.
- The **superior intercostal vein** is formed by the second, third, and fourth intercostal veins and drains into the azygos vein on the right and the brachiocephalic vein on the left.
- The **thoracic duct** begins in the abdomen at the **cisterna chyli**, which is the dilated junction of the intestinal, lumbar, and descending intercostal **trunks**. It drains all parts of the body except the right head, neck, upper limb, and thorax, which are drained by the right lymphatic duct. It passes through the aortic opening of the diaphragm, ascends between the aorta and the azygos vein, and empties into the junction of the left internal jugular and subclavian veins.
- The **greater splanchnic nerve** arises from the fifth through ninth thoracic sympathetic ganglia and ends in the celiac ganglion. The **lesser splanchnic nerve** arises from the 10th and 11th thoracic sympathetic ganglia and ends in the aorticorenal ganglion. The **least splanchnic nerve** arises from the 12th thoracic sympathetic ganglia and ends in the renal plexus. All of these splanchnic nerves contain preganglionic sympathetic GVE fibers with cell bodies located in the lateral horn (intermediolateral cell column) of the spinal cord and GVA fibers with cell bodies located in the dorsal root ganglia.

- **White rami communicantes** contain preganglionic sympathetic GVE fibers with cell bodies located in the lateral horn of the spinal cord and GVA fibers with cell bodies located in the dorsal root ganglia. They are connected to the spinal nerves and limited to spinal cord segments between T1 and L2.
- **Gray rami communicantes** contain postganglionic sympathetic GVE fibers with cell bodies located in the sympathetic chain ganglia. They are connected to every spinal nerve and supply the blood vessels, sweat glands, and arrector pili muscles of hair follicles.
- Autonomic nerve functions in the thorax:

Functions of Autonomic Nerves

	Sympathetic Nerve	Parasympathetic Nerve
Heart	Increases rate and ventricular contraction; dilates coronary vessels	Decreases rate and ventricular contraction; constricts coronary vessels
Bronchi	Dilates lumen; reduces bronchial secretion	Constricts lumen; promotes secretion
Esophagus	Vasoconstriction	Peristalsis

Review Test

Directions: Each of the numbered items or incomplete statements in this section is followed by answers or by completions of the statement. Select the **one**-lettered answer or completion that is **best** in each case.

1. A 32-year-old patient who weighs 275 lb comes to the doctor's office. On the surface of the chest, the physician is able to locate the apex of the heart:

(A) At the level of the sternal angle
(B) In the left fourth intercostal space
(C) In the left fifth intercostal space
(D) In the right fifth intercostal space
(E) At the level of the xiphoid process of the sternum

2. A 43-year-old female patient has been lying down on the hospital bed for more than 4 months. Her normal, quiet expiration is achieved by contraction of which of the following structures?

(A) Elastic tissue in the lungs and thoracic wall
(B) Serratus posterior superior muscles
(C) Pectoralis minor muscles
(D) Serratus anterior muscles
(E) Diaphragm

3. A 23-year-old man received a gunshot wound, and his greater splanchnic nerve was destroyed. Which of the following nerve fibers would be injured?

(A) General somatic afferent (GSA) and preganglionic sympathetic fibers
(B) General visceral afferent (GVA) and postganglionic sympathetic fibers
(C) GVA and preganglionic sympathetic fibers
(D) General somatic efferent (GSE) and postganglionic sympathetic fibers
(E) GVA and GSE fibers

4. A 17-year-old boy was involved in a gang fight, and a stab wound severed the white rami communicantes at the level of his sixth thoracic vertebra. This injury would result in degeneration of nerve cell bodies in which of the following structures?

(A) Dorsal root ganglion and anterior horn of the spinal cord
(B) Sympathetic chain ganglion and dorsal root ganglion
(C) Sympathetic chain ganglion and posterior horn of the spinal cord
(D) Dorsal root ganglion and lateral horn of the spinal cord
(E) Anterior and lateral horns of the spinal cord

5. A 27-year-old cardiac patient with an irregular heartbeat visits her doctor's office for examination. Where should the physician place the stethoscope to listen to the sound of the mitral valve?

(A) Over the medial end of the second left intercostal space
(B) Over the medial end of the second right intercostal space
(C) In the left fourth intercostal space at the midclavicular line
(D) In the left fifth intercostal space at the midclavicular line
(E) Over the right half of the lower end of the body of the sternum

6. A 19-year-old man came to the emergency department, and his angiogram exhibited that he was bleeding from the vein that is accompanied by the posterior interventricular artery. Which of the following veins is most likely to be ruptured?

(A) Great cardiac vein
(B) Middle cardiac vein
(C) Anterior cardiac vein
(D) Small cardiac vein
(E) Oblique veins of the left atrium

7. A 37-year-old patient with palpitation was examined by her physician, and one of the diagnostic records included a posterior–anterior chest radiograph. Which of the following comprises the largest portion of the sternocostal surface of the heart seen on the radiograph?

(A) Left atrium
(B) Right atrium
(C) Left ventricle
(D) Right ventricle
(E) Base of the heart

8. A 5-year-old girl is brought to the emergency department because of difficulty breathing (dyspnea), palpitations, and shortness of breath. Doppler study of the heart reveals an atrial septal defect (ASD). This malformation usually results from incomplete closure of which of the following embryonic structures?

(A) Ductus arteriosus
(B) Ductus venosus
(C) Sinus venarum
(D) Foramen ovale
(E) Truncus arteriosus

9. A 54-year-old patient is implanted with an artificial cardiac pacemaker. Which of the following conductive tissues of the heart had a defective function that required the pacemaker?

(A) Atrioventricular (AV) bundle
(B) AV node
(C) Sinoatrial (SA) node
(D) Purkinje fiber
(E) Moderator band

10. A thoracic surgeon removed the right middle lobar (secondary) bronchus along with lung tissue from a 57-year-old heavy smoker with lung cancer. Which of the following bronchopulmonary segments must contain cancerous tissues?

(A) Medial and lateral
(B) Anterior and posterior
(C) Anterior basal and medial basal
(D) Anterior basal and posterior basal
(E) Lateral basal and posterior basal

11. The bronchogram of a 45-year-old female smoker shows the presence of a tumor in the eparterial bronchus. Which airway is most likely blocked?

(A) Left superior bronchus
(B) Left inferior bronchus
(C) Right superior bronchus
(D) Right middle bronchus
(E) Right inferior bronchus

12. An 83-year-old man with a typical coronary circulation has been suffering from an embolism of the circumflex branch of the left coronary artery. This condition would result in ischemia of which of the following areas of the heart?

(A) Anterior part of the left ventricle
(B) Anterior interventricular region
(C) Posterior interventricular region
(D) Posterior part of the left ventricle
(E) Anterior part of the right ventricle

13. A 44-year-old man with a stab wound was brought to the emergency department, and a physician found that the patient was suffering from a laceration of his right phrenic nerve. Which of the following conditions has likely occurred?

(A) Injury to only GSE fibers
(B) Difficulty in expiration
(C) Loss of sensation in the fibrous pericardium and mediastinal pleura
(D) Normal function of the diaphragm
(E) Loss of sensation in the costal part of the diaphragm

14. An 8-year-old boy with ASD presents to a pediatrician. This congenital heart defect shunts blood from the left atrium to the right atrium and causes hypertrophy of the right atrium, right ventricle, and pulmonary trunk. Which of the following veins opens into the hypertrophied atrium?

(A) Middle cardiac vein
(B) Small cardiac vein
(C) Oblique cardiac vein
(D) Anterior cardiac vein
(E) Right pulmonary vein

15. A 37-year-old patient with severe chest pain, shortness of breath, and congestive heart failure was admitted to a local hospital. His coronary angiograms reveal a thrombosis in the circumflex branch of the left coronary artery. Which of the following conditions could result from the blockage of blood flow in the circumflex branch?

(A) Tricuspid valve insufficiency
(B) Mitral valve insufficiency
(C) Ischemia of AV node
(D) Paralysis of pectinate muscle
(E) Necrosis of septomarginal trabecula

16. A 75-year-old patient has been suffering from lung cancer located near the cardiac notch, a deep indentation on the lung. Which of the following lobes is most likely to be excised?

(A) Superior lobe of the right lung
(B) Middle lobe of the right lung
(C) Inferior lobe of the right lung
(D) Superior lobe of the left lung
(E) Inferior lobe of the left lung

17. A thoracentesis is performed to aspirate an abnormal accumulation of fluid in a 37-year-old patient with pleural effusion. A needle should be inserted at the midaxillary line between which of the following two ribs so as to avoid puncturing the lung?

(A) Ribs 1 and 3
(B) Ribs 3 and 5
(C) Ribs 5 and 7
(D) Ribs 7 and 9
(E) Ribs 9 and 11

18. A newborn baby is readmitted to the hospital with hypoxia and upon testing is found to have pulmonary stenosis, dextraposition of the aorta, interventricular septal defect, and hypertrophy of the right ventricle. Which of the following is best described by these symptoms?

(A) ASD
(B) Patent ductus arteriosus
(C) Tetralogy of Fallot
(D) Aortic stenosis
(E) Coarctation of the aorta

19. A 33-year-old patient is suffering from a sudden occlusion at the origin of the descending (thoracic) aorta. This condition would most likely decrease blood flow in which of the following intercostal arteries?

(A) Upper six anterior
(B) All of the posterior
(C) Upper two posterior
(D) Lower anterior
(E) Lower six posterior

20. A 56-year-old patient recently suffered a myocardial infarction in the area of the apex of the heart. The occlusion by atherosclerosis is in which of the following arteries?

(A) Marginal artery
(B) Right coronary artery at its origin
(C) Anterior interventricular artery
(D) Posterior interventricular artery
(E) Circumflex branch of the left coronary artery

21. A 75-year-old woman was admitted to a local hospital, and bronchograms and radiographs revealed a lung carcinoma in her left lung. Which of the following structures or characteristics does the cancerous lung contain?

(A) Horizontal fissure
(B) Groove for superior vena cava (SVC)
(C) Middle lobe
(D) Lingula
(E) Larger capacity than the right

22. An 18-year-old girl is thrust into the steering wheel while driving and experiences difficulty in expiration. Which of the following muscles is most likely damaged?

(A) Levator costarum
(B) Innermost intercostal muscle
(C) External intercostal muscle
(D) Diaphragm
(E) Muscles of the abdominal wall

23. A 78-year-old patient presents with an advanced cancer in the posterior mediastinum. The surgeons are in a dilemma as to how to manage the condition. Which of the following structures is most likely damaged?

(A) Brachiocephalic veins
(B) Trachea
(C) Arch of the azygos vein
(D) Arch of the aorta
(E) Hemiazygos vein

24. A 46-year-old patient comes to his doctor's office and complains of chest pain and headache. His computed tomography (CT) scan reveals a tumor located just superior to the root of the right lung. Blood flow in which of the following veins is most likely blocked by this tumor?

(A) Hemiazygos vein
(B) Arch of the azygos vein
(C) Right subclavian vein
(D) Right brachiocephalic vein
(E) Accessory hemiazygos vein

25. A 21-year-old patient with a stab wound reveals a laceration of the right vagus nerve proximal to the origin of the recurrent laryngeal nerve. Which of the following conditions would most likely result from this lesion?

(A) Contraction of bronchial muscle
(B) Stimulation of bronchial gland secretion
(C) Dilation of the bronchial lumen
(D) Decrease in cardiac rate
(E) Constriction of coronary artery

26. A neonate appears severely cyanotic and breathing rapidly. Cardiac echocardiogram reveals that the aorta lies to the right of the pulmonary trunk. Which of the following is most likely occurred during development?

(A) AP septum failed to develop in a spiral fashion
(B) Excessive resorption of septum primum
(C) Pulmonary valve atresia
(D) Persistent truncus arteriosus
(E) Coarctation of the aorta

27. A 12-year-old boy was admitted to a local hospital with a known history of heart problems. His left ventricular hypertrophy could result from which of the following conditions?

(A) A constricted pulmonary trunk
(B) An abnormally small left AV opening
(C) Improper closing of the pulmonary valves
(D) An abnormally large right AV opening
(E) Stenosis of the aorta

28. A 31-year-old man was involved in a severe automobile accident and suffered laceration of the left primary bronchus. The damaged primary bronchus:

(A) Has a larger diameter than the right primary bronchus
(B) Often receives more foreign bodies than the right primary bronchus
(C) Gives rise to the eparterial bronchus
(D) Is longer than the right primary bronchus
(E) Runs under the arch of the azygos vein

29. A 62-year-old woman who is a heavy smoker has an advanced lung cancer that spread into her right third posterior intercostal space posterior to the midaxillary line. If cancer cells are carried in the venous drainage, they would travel first to which of the following veins?

(A) SVC
(B) Right superior intercostal vein
(C) Right brachiocephalic vein
(D) Azygos vein
(E) Hemiazygos vein

30. A radiologist examines posterior–anterior chest radiographs of a 27-year-old victim of a car accident. Which of the following structures forms the right border of the cardiovascular silhouette?

(A) Arch of the aorta
(B) Pulmonary trunk
(C) SVC
(D) Ascending aorta
(E) Left ventricle

31. A 37-year-old man is brought to the emergency department complaining of severe chest pain. His angiogram reveals thromboses of both brachiocephalic veins just before entering the superior vena cava. This condition would most likely cause a dilation of which of the following veins?

(A) Azygos
(B) Hemiazygos
(C) Right superior intercostal
(D) Left superior intercostal
(E) Internal thoracic

32. A cardiologist is on clinical rounds with her medical students. She asks them, "During the cardiac cycle, which of the following events occurs?"

(A) AV valves close during diastole
(B) Aortic valve closes during systole
(C) Pulmonary valve opens during diastole
(D) Blood flow in coronary arteries is maximal during diastole
(E) Aortic valve closes at the same time as AV valve

33. Coronary angiographs of a 44-year-old male patient reveal an occlusion of the circumflex branch of the left coronary artery. This patient has been suffering from myocardial infarction in which of the following areas?

(A) Right and left ventricles
(B) Right and left atria
(C) Interventricular septum
(D) Apex of the heart
(E) Left atrium and ventricle

34. A patient has a small but solid tumor in the mediastinum, which is confined at the level of the sternal angle. Which of the following structures would most likely be found at this level?

(A) Bifurcation of the trachea
(B) Beginning of the ascending aorta
(C) Middle of the aortic arch
(D) Articulation of the third rib with the sternum
(E) Superior border of the superior mediastinum

35. A 37-year-old house painter fell from a ladder and fractured his left third rib and the structures with which it articulated. Which of the following structures would most likely be damaged?

(A) Manubrium of the sternum
(B) Body of the second thoracic vertebra
(C) Spinous process of the third thoracic vertebra
(D) Body of the fourth thoracic vertebra
(E) Transverse process of the second thoracic vertebra

36. A 45-year-old woman presents with a tumor confined to the posterior mediastinum. This could result in compression of which of the following structures?

(A) Trachea
(B) Descending aorta
(C) Arch of the aorta
(D) Arch of the azygos vein
(E) Phrenic nerve

37. A 62-year-old patient with pericardial effusion comes to a local hospital for aspiration of pericardial fluid by pericardiocentesis. The needle is inserted into the pericardial cavity through which of the following intercostal spaces adjacent to the sternum?

(A) Right fourth intercostal space
(B) Left fourth intercostal space
(C) Right fifth intercostal space
(D) Left fifth intercostal space
(E) Right sixth intercostal space

38. The attending faculty in the coronary intensive care unit demonstrates to his students a normal heart examination. The first heart sound is produced by near-simultaneous closure of which of the following valves?

(A) Aortic and tricuspid
(B) Aortic and pulmonary
(C) Tricuspid and mitral
(D) Mitral and pulmonary
(E) Tricuspid and pulmonary

39. A 27-year-old patient with Marfan syndrome has an aneurysm of the aortic arch. This may compress which of the following structures?

(A) Right vagus nerve
(B) Left phrenic nerve
(C) Right sympathetic trunk
(D) Left recurrent laryngeal nerve
(E) Left greater splanchnic nerve

40. A 47-year-old man with a known atrial fibrillation returns to see his cardiologist for follow-up of his cardiac health. The right atrium is important in this case because it:

(A) Receives blood from the oblique cardiac vein
(B) Is associated with the apex of the heart
(C) Contains the SA node
(D) Receives the right pulmonary vein
(E) Is hypertrophied by pulmonary stenosis

41. A 57-year-old patient has a heart murmur resulting from the inability to maintain constant tension on the cusps of the AV valve. Which of the following structures is most likely damaged?

(A) Crista terminalis
(B) Septomarginal trabecula
(C) Chordae tendineae
(D) Pectinate muscle
(E) Anulus fibrosus

42. A mother with diabetes gives birth to a baby who is diagnosed as having dextroposition of the aorta and the pulmonary trunk with cyanosis and shortness of breath. Which of the following structures is required to remain patent until surgical correction of the deformity?

(A) Umbilical arteries
(B) Umbilical vein
(C) Ductus arteriosus
(D) Ductus venosus
(E) Sinus venosus

43. During early development of the respiratory system, the laryngotracheal tube maintains communication with the primitive foregut. Which of the following embryonic structures is most likely responsible for partitioning these two embryonic structures?

(A) Tracheoesophageal folds
(B) Tracheoesophageal fistula
(C) Tracheoesophageal septum
(D) Laryngotracheal diverticulum
(E) Laryngotracheal septum

44. A 32-year-old patient has a tension pneumothorax that can be treated with needle aspiration. To avoid an injury of the intercostal neurovascular bundle, the needle may be inserted in which of the following locations?

(A) Above the upper border of the ribs
(B) Deep to the upper border of the ribs
(C) Beneath the lower border of the ribs
(D) Between the external and internal intercostals
(E) Through the transversus thoracis muscle

45. A 9-month-old girl was admitted to the children's hospital with tachypnea (fast breathing) and shortness of breath. Physical examination further exhibits tachycardia (fast heart rate), a bounding peripheral pulse, and her angiographs reveal a patent ductus arteriosus. Which of the following embryonic arterial structures is most likely responsible for the origin of the patent ductus arteriosus?

(A) Right fourth arch
(B) Left fifth arch
(C) Right fifth arch
(D) Left sixth arch
(E) Right sixth arch

46. A 7-day-old baby is diagnosed as having congenital neonatal emphysema, which is caused by collapsed bronchi because of failure of bronchial cartilage development. Bronchial cartilages are derived from which of the following derivations?

(A) Ectoderm
(B) Mesoderm
(C) Endoderm
(D) Proctodeum
(E) Neuroectoderm

Questions 47 to 52: Choose the appropriate lettered site or structure in this CT scan (see Figure below) of the thorax from a 42-year-old man who complains of chest pain and breathing problems. His electrocardiogram shows left ventricular hypertrophy.

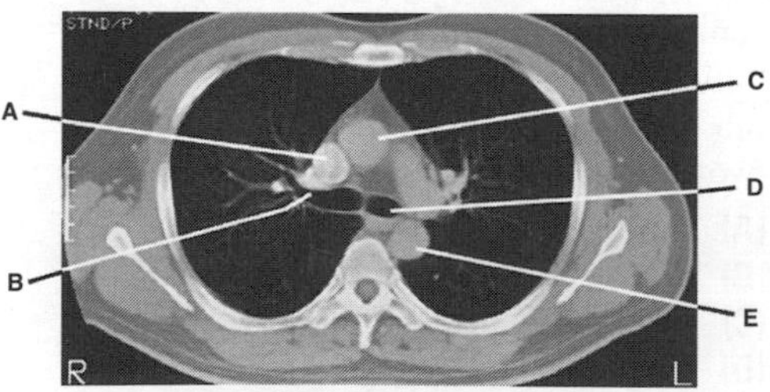

47. Stenosis of which structure may produce left ventricular hypertrophy?

48. Which structure is most likely to be removed by a pulmonary surgeon in a surgical resection of a lobe (lobectomy) to remove lung cancer in the apex of the right lung?

49. Which structure branches into the bronchial arteries?

50. Into which structure does the azygos vein drain venous blood?

51. The left coronary artery arises from which structure?

52. Which structure is crossed superiorly by the aortic arch and left pulmonary artery?

Questions 53 to 58: Choose the appropriate lettered site or structure in this CT scan (see Figure below) of the thorax. Which structure in this CT scan:

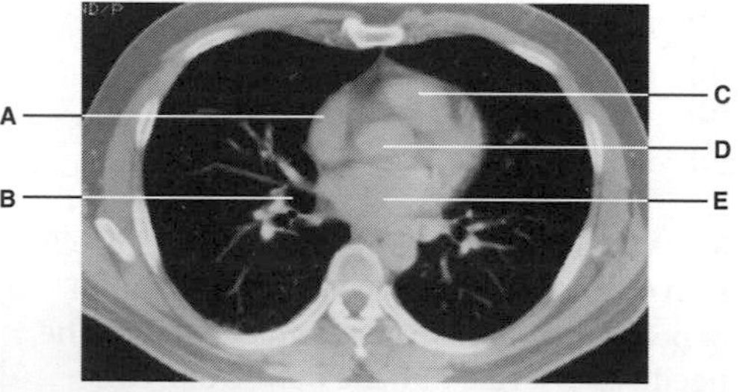

53. Can be removed in a surgical resection of a lobe to remove lung cancer on the diaphragmatic surface?

54. Becomes hypertrophied as result of the pulmonary stenosis?

55. Receives oxygenated blood via pulmonary veins?

56. Lies on the right side of the aortic arch and ascending aorta?

57. Contains the septomarginal trabecula?

58. Takes its origin from the left ventricle and ends at the sternal angle?

Answers and Explanations

1. **The answer is C.** On the surface of the chest, the apex of the heart can be located in the left fifth intercostal space slightly medial to the midclavicular (or nipple) line. The sternal angle is located at the level where the second ribs articulate with the sternum. The xiphoid process lies at the level of T10 vertebra.

2. **The answer is A.** Normal, quiet expiration is achieved by contraction of extensible tissue in the lungs and the thoracic wall. The serratus posterior superior muscles, diaphragm, pectoralis major, and serratus anterior are muscles of inspiration.

3. **The answer is C.** The greater splanchnic nerves contain general visceral afferent (GVA) and preganglionic sympathetic general visceral efferent (GVE) fibers.

4. **The answer is D.** The white rami communicantes contain preganglionic sympathetic GVE fibers and GVA fibers, whose cell bodies are located in the lateral horn of the spinal cord and the dorsal root ganglia. The sympathetic chain ganglion contains cell bodies of the postganglionic sympathetic nerve fibers. The anterior horn of the spinal cord contains cell bodies of the GSE fibers. The dorsal root ganglion contains cell bodies of GSA and GVA fibers.

5. **The answer is D.** The mitral valve (left atrioventricular [AV] valve) produces the apical beat (thrust) of the heart, which is most audible over the left fifth intercostal space at the midclavicular line. The pulmonary valve is most audible over the medial end of the second left intercostal space, the aortic valve is most audible over the medial end of the second right intercostal space, and the right AV valve is most audible over the right half of the lower end of the body of the sternum.

6. **The answer is B.** The middle cardiac vein ascends in the posterior interventricular groove, accompanied by the posterior interventricular branch of the right coronary artery. The great cardiac vein is accompanied by the anterior interventricular artery, the anterior cardiac vein drains directly into the right atrium, and the small cardiac vein is accompanied by the marginal artery.

7. **The answer is D.** The right ventricle forms a large part of the sternocostal surface of the heart. The left atrium occupies almost the entire posterior surface of the right atrium. The right atrium occupies the right aspect of the heart. The left ventricle lies at the back of the heart and bulges roundly to the left. The base of the heart is formed by the atria, which lie mainly behind the ventricles.

8. **The answer is D.** An atrial septal defect (ASD) is a congenital defect in the interatrial septum. During partitioning of the two atria, the opening in the foramen secundum (the foramen ovale) usually closes at birth. If this foramen ovale is not closed completely, this would result in an ASD, shunting blood from the left atrium to the right atrium.

9. **The answer is C.** The sinoatrial (SA) node initiates the impulse of contraction and is known as the pacemaker of the heart. Impulses from the SA node travel through the atrial myocardium to the AV node and then race through the AV bundle (bundle of His), which divides into the right and left bundle branches. The bundle breaks up into terminal conducting fibers (Purkinje fibers) to spread out into the ventricular walls. The moderate band carries the right limb of the AV bundle from the septum to the sternocostal wall of the ventricle.

10. **The answer is A.** The right middle lobar (secondary) bronchus leads to the medial and lateral bronchopulmonary segments. The right superior lobar bronchus divides into the superior, posterior, and anterior segmental (tertiary) bronchi. The right inferior lobar bronchus has the anterior, lateral, posterior, and anterior segmental bronchi.

11. **The answer is C.** The eparterial bronchus is the right superior lobar (secondary) bronchus; all of the other bronchi are hyparterial bronchi.

12. **The answer is D.** The circumflex branch of the left coronary artery supplies the posterior portion of the left ventricle. The anterior interventricular artery supplies the anterior aspects of the right and left ventricles and the anterior interventricular septum.

13. **The answer is C.** The phrenic nerve supplies the pericardium and mediastinal and diaphragmatic (central part) pleura and the diaphragm, an important muscle of inspiration. It contains general somatic efferent (GSE), general somatic afferent (GSA), and GVE (postganglionic sympathetic) fibers. The costal part of the diaphragm receives GSA fibers from the intercostal nerves.

14. **The answer is D.** The anterior cardiac vein drains into the right atrium. The middle, small, and oblique cardiac veins drain into the coronary sinus. The right and left pulmonary veins drain into the left atrium.

15. **The answer is B.** The circumflex branch of the left coronary artery supplies the left ventricle, and thus its blockage of blood flow results in necrosis of myocardium in the left ventricle, producing mitral valve insufficiency. The tricuspid valve, AV node, pectinate muscles, and septomarginal trabecula are present in the right atrium and ventricle.

16. **The answer is D.** The cardiac notch is a deep indentation of the anterior border of the superior lobe of the left lung. Therefore, the right lung is not involved.

17. **The answer is D.** A thoracentesis is performed for aspiration of fluid in the pleural cavity at or posterior to the midaxillary line, one or two intercostal spaces below the fluid level but not below the ninth intercostal space and, therefore, between ribs 7 and 9. Other intercostals spaces are not preferred.

18. **The answer is C.** Tetralogy of Fallot is a combination of congenital cardiac defects consisting of (a) pulmonary stenosis, (b) dextraposition of the aorta (so that it overrides the ventricular septum and receives blood from the right ventricle), (c) ventricular septal defect (VSD), and (d) right ventricular hypertrophy. ASD is a congenital defect in the atrial septum, resulting from a patent foramen ovale. Patent ductus arteriosus shunts blood from the pulmonary trunk to the aorta, bypassing the lungs. Aortic stenosis is an abnormal narrowing of the aortic valve orifice, impeding the blood flow. Coarctation of the aorta is a congenital constriction of the aorta, commonly occurs just distal to the left subclavian artery, causing upper limb hypertension and diminished blood flow to the lower limbs and abdominal viscera.

19. **The answer is E.** The first two posterior intercostal arteries are branches of the highest (superior) intercostal artery of the costocervical trunk; the remaining nine branches are from the thoracic aorta. The internal thoracic artery gives off the upper six anterior intercostal arteries and is divided into the superior epigastric and musculophrenic arteries, which gives off anterior intercostal arteries in the 7th, 8th, and 9th intercostal spaces and ends in the 10th intercostal space where it anastomoses with the deep circumflex iliac artery.

20. **The answer is C.** The apex of the heart typically receives blood from the anterior interventricular branch of the left coronary artery. The marginal artery supplies the right inferior margin of the right ventricle, the right coronary artery at its origin supplies the right atrium and ventricle, and the posterior interventricular artery and a circumflex branch of the left coronary artery supply the left ventricle.

21. **The answer is D.** The lingula is the tongue-shaped portion of the upper lobe of the left lung. The right lung has a groove for the horizontal fissure, superior vena cava (SVC), and middle lobe and has a larger capacity than the left lung.

22. **The answer is E.** The abdominal muscles are the major muscles of expiration, whereas the other distractors are muscles of inspiration.

23. **The answer is E.** The hemiazygos vein is located in the posterior mediastinum. The brachiocephalic veins, trachea, and arch of the aorta are located in the superior mediastinum, whereas the arch of the azygos vein is found in the middle mediastinum.

24. **The answer is B.** The azygos vein arches over the root of the right lung and empties into the SVC. Other veins do not pass over the root of the right lung.

25. **The answer is C.** The parasympathetic nerve fibers in the vagus nerve constrict the bronchial lumen, contract bronchial smooth muscle, stimulate bronchial gland secretion, decrease heart rate, and constrict the coronary artery. The vagus nerve also carries afferent fibers of pain, cough reflex, and stretch of the lung (during inspiration).

26. **The answer is A.** Failure of the aorticopulmonary septum results in transposition of the great vessels, exhibiting that the aorta is to the right of the pulmonary trunk. Cyanosis is common in transposition of the great vessels. Excessive resorption of septum primum results in a secundum type of ASD. Pulmonary valve atresia may result in cyanosis, but it will not cause the aorta to be to the right of the pulmonary trunk. A persistent truncus arteriosus is caused by lack of development of the aorticopulmonary septum resulting in a single outflow track. Coarctation of the aorta is a severe narrowing of the aorta.

27. **The answer is E.** Stenosis of the aorta can cause left ventricular hypertrophy. Right ventricular hypertrophy may occur as a result of pulmonary stenosis, pulmonary and tricuspid valve defects, or mitral valve stenosis.

28. **The answer is D.** The right primary bronchus is shorter than the left one and has a larger diameter. More foreign bodies enter it via the trachea because it is more vertical than the left primary bronchus. The right primary bronchus runs under the arch of the azygos vein and gives rise to the eparterial bronchus.

29. **The answer is B.** The superior intercostal vein is formed by the union of the second, third, and fourth posterior intercostal veins and drains into the azygos vein on the right and the brachiocephalic vein on the left. The azygos vein drains into the SVC. The hemiazygos vein usually drains into the azygos vein.

30. **The answer is C.** A cardiovascular silhouette or cardiac shadow is the contour of the heart and great vessels seen on posterior–anterior chest radiographs. Its right border is formed by the SVC, right atrium, and inferior vena cava; its left border is formed by the aortic arch (aortic knob), pulmonary trunk, left auricle, and left ventricle. The ascending aorta becomes the arch of the aorta and is found in the middle of the heart.

31. **The answer is D.** The left superior intercostal vein is formed by the second, third, and fourth posterior intercostal veins and drains into the left brachiocephalic vein. The right superior intercostal vein drains into the azygos vein, which in turn drains into the SVC. The hemiazygos vein drains into the azygos vein, whereas the internal thoracic vein empties into the brachiocephalic vein.

32. **The answer is D.** During diastole, the AV valves open, and the aortic and pulmonary valves close; whereas during systole, the AV valves close, and the aortic and pulmonary valves open.

33. **The answer is E.** The left atrium and ventricle receive blood from the circumflex branch of the left coronary artery. The interventricular septum and the apex of the heart are supplied by the anterior interventricular branch of the left coronary artery. The right ventricle receives blood from the anterior interventricular artery and the marginal branch of the right coronary artery. The right atrium receives blood from the right coronary artery.

34. **The answer is A.** The sternal angle is the junction of the manubrium and the body of the sternum. It is located at the level where the second rib articulates with the sternum, the trachea bifurcates into the right and left bronchi, and the aortic arch begins and ends. It marks the end of the ascending aorta and the beginning of the descending aorta, and it forms the inferior border of the superior mediastinum.

35. **The answer is B.** The third rib articulates with the body of the sternum, bodies of the second and third thoracic vertebrae, and transverse process of the third thoracic vertebra.

36. **The answer is B.** The descending aorta is found in the posterior mediastinum. The superior mediastinum contains the trachea and arch of the aorta, and the middle mediastinum contains

the ascending aorta, arch of the azygos vein, and main bronchi. The phrenic nerve runs in the middle mediastinum.

37. **The answer is D.** To aspirate pericardial fluid, the needle should be inserted into the pericardial cavity through the fifth intercostals space just left to the sternum. Because of the cardiac notch, the needle misses the pleura and lungs, but it penetrates the pericardium. Lung tissues lie beneath the fourth and sixth intercostal spaces.

38. **The answer is C.** The first heart sound ("lub") is produced by the closure of the tricuspid and mitral valves, whereas the second heart sound ("dub") is produced by the closure of the aortic and pulmonary valves.

39. **The answer is D.** The left recurrent laryngeal nerve loops around the arch of the aorta near the ligamentum arteriosum, whereas the right recurrent laryngeal nerve hooks around the right subclavian artery. All other nerves are not closely associated with the aortic arch.

40. **The answer is C.** The SA and AV nodes are in the wall of the right atrium and are not associated with the apex of the heart. The oblique cardiac vein drains into the coronary sinus, and the pulmonary veins empty into the left atrium. The right ventricle is hypertrophied by the pulmonary stenosis.

41. **The answer is C.** The chordae tendineae are tendinous strands that extend from the papillary muscles to the cusps of the valve. The papillary muscles and chordae tendineae prevent the cusps from being everted into the atrium during ventricular contraction.

42. **The answer is C.** A patent ductus arteriosus shunts blood from the pulmonary trunk to the aorta, partially bypassing the lungs, and thus allowing mixed blood to reach the body tissues and causing cyanosis. Dextroposition or transposition of the great arteries must be accompanied by a VSD or a patent ductus arteriosus for the infant to survive. The transposition causes oxygenated blood to pass from the left ventricle into the pulmonary trunk and then into the lungs, but deoxygenated blood travels from the right ventricle into the aorta and then into the systemic circulation.

43. **The answer is C.** The tracheoesophageal septum is formed by the fusion of the tracheoesophageal folds in the midline. This septum divides the foregut into a ventral portion, the laryngotracheal tube (primordium of the larynx, trachea, bronchi, and lungs), and a dorsal portion (primordium of the oropharynx and esophagus).

44. **The answer is A.** The intercostal veins, arteries, and nerves run in the costal groove beneath the inferior border of the ribs between the internal and innermost layers of muscles. The transversus thoracis muscles are situated in the internal surface of the lower anterior thoracic wall.

45. **The answer is D.** The left sixth aortic arch is responsible for the development of both the ductus arteriosus and the pulmonary arteries. The ductus arteriosus closes functionally in an infant soon after birth, with anatomic closure requiring several weeks.

46. **The answer is B.** Bronchial cartilages, smooth muscles, and connective tissue are derived from the mesoderm. The bronchial epithelium and glands are derived from the endoderm.

47. **The answer is C.** Stenosis of the ascending aorta results in left ventricular hypertrophy.

48. **The answer is B.** During surgical treatment for cancer in the apex of the right lung by a lobectomy, the right superior secondary (eparterial) bronchus should be removed.

49. **The answer is E.** The right and left bronchial arteries arise from the descending (thoracic) aorta.

50. **The answer is A.** The azygos vein drains venous blood into the SVC.

51. **The answer is C.** The right and left coronary arteries arise from the ascending aorta.

52. **The answer is D.** The left primary bronchus is crossed superiorly by the arch of the aorta and the pulmonary artery.

53. **The answer is B.** The right inferior lobar bronchus may be removed in a surgical resection of the inferior lobe of the right lung that is in contact with the diaphragm.

54. **The answer is C.** Pulmonary stenosis results in right ventricular hypertrophy.

55. **The answer is E.** The left atrium receives oxygenated blood from the lung by way of the pulmonary veins.

56. **The answer is A.** The SVC lies on the right side of the ascending aorta and the arch of the aorta.

57. **The answer is C.** The right ventricle contains the septomarginal trabecula.

58. **The answer is D.** The ascending aorta takes its origin from the left ventricle and ends at the level of the sternal angle by becoming the arch of the aorta.

chapter **4** Abdomen

ANTERIOR ABDOMINAL WALL

I. ABDOMEN (Figure 4.1)

- Is divided topographically by two transverse and two longitudinal planes into nine regions: right and left **hypochondriac, epigastric**, right and left **lumbar**, **umbilical**, right and left **inguinal (iliac)**, and **hypogastric (pubic)**.
- Is also divided by vertical and horizontal planes through the umbilicus into four quadrants: right and left upper quadrants and right and left lower quadrants. The **umbilicus** lies at the level of the intervertebral disk between the third and fourth lumbar vertebrae. Its region is innervated by the 10th thoracic nerve.

CLINICAL CORRELATES **Umbilical hernia** may occur due to failure of the midgut to return to the abdomen early in fetal life, and it occurs as a protrusion of intestines through a defect at the umbilicus. The hernia is covered by peritoneum, subcutaneous tissue, and skin; is not usually treated surgically, but closes spontaneously by 3 years of age. **Omphalocele** is a persistence of the herniation of abdominal contents, which remain outside the abdominal cavity and are covered only by the amniotic membrane; thus, immediate surgical repair is required. **Gastroschisis** is a protrusion of the abdominal viscera through a defect in the abdominal wall without involving the umbilical cord on the right side of the umbilicus.

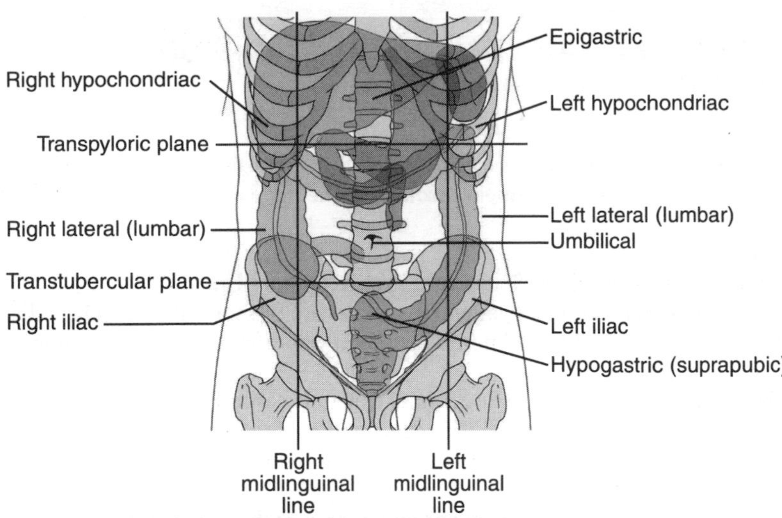

FIGURE 4.1. Planes of subdivision of the abdomen.

II. MUSCLES OF THE ANTERIOR ABDOMINAL WALL (Table 4.1)

table 4.1 Muscles of the Anterior Abdominal Wall

Muscle	Origin	Insertion	Nerve	Action
External oblique	External surface of lower eight ribs (5–12)	Anterior half of iliac crest; anterior superior iliac spine; pubic tubercle; linea alba	Intercostal (T7–T11); subcostal (T12)	Compresses abdomen; flexes trunk; active in forced expiration
Internal oblique	Lateral two-thirds of inguinal ligament; iliac crest; thoracolumbar fascia	Lower four costal cartilages; linea alba; pubic crest; pectineal line	Intercostal (T7–T11); subcostal (T12); iliohypogastric and ilioinguinal (L1)	Compresses abdomen; flexes trunk; active in forced expiration
Transverse	Lateral one-third of inguinal ligament; iliac crest; thoracolumbar fascia; lower six costal cartilages	Linea alba; pubic crest; pectineal line	Intercostal (T7–T12); subcostal (T12); iliohypogastric and ilioinguinal (L1)	Compresses abdomen; depresses ribs
Rectus abdominis	Pubic crest and pubic symphysis	Xiphoid process and costal cartilages fifth to seventh	Intercostal (T7–T11); subcostal (T12)	Depresses ribs; flexes trunk
Pyramidal	Pubic body	Linea alba	Subcostal (T12)	Tenses linea alba
Cremaster	Middle of inguinal ligament; lower margin of internal oblique muscle	Pubic tubercle and crest	Genitofemoral	Retracts testis

III. FASCIAE AND LIGAMENTS OF THE ANTERIOR ABDOMINAL WALL

- Are organized into superficial (tela subcutanea) and deep fasciae. The superficial fascia has two layers: the superficial fatty layer (**Camper fascia**) and the deep membranous layer (**Scarpa fascia**).

A. Superficial Fascia

1. Superficial (Fatty) Layer of the Superficial Fascia (Camper Fascia)

- Continues over the inguinal ligament to merge with the superficial fascia of the thigh.
- Continues over the pubis and perineum as the superficial layer of the superficial perineal fascia.

2. Deep (Membranous) Layer of the Superficial Fascia (Scarpa Fascia)

- Is attached to the **fascia lata** just below the inguinal ligament.
- Continues over the pubis and perineum as the membranous layer (**Colles fascia**) of the superficial perineal fascia.
- Continues over the penis as the **superficial fascia of the penis** and over the scrotum as the **tunica dartos**, which contains smooth muscle.
- May contain extravasated urine between this fascia and the deep fascia of the abdomen, resulting from rupture of the spongy urethra.

B. Deep Fascia

- Covers the muscles and continues over the spermatic cord at the superficial inguinal ring as the **external spermatic fascia**.
- Continues over the penis as the deep fascia of the penis (Buck fascia) and over the pubis and perineum as the deep perineal fascia.

C. Linea Alba

- Is a **tendinous median raphe** between the two rectus abdominis muscles, formed by the fusion of the aponeuroses of the external oblique, internal oblique, and transverse abdominal muscles.
- Extends from the xiphoid process to the pubic symphysis and, in pregnancy, it becomes a pigmented vertical line (**linea nigra**), probably due to hormone stimulation to produce more melanin.

CLINICAL CORRELATES **Epigastric hernia** is a protrusion of extraperitoneal fat or a small piece of greater omentum through a defect in the linea alba above the umbilicus and may contain a small portion of intestine, which may become trapped within the hernia, leading to incarcerated and/or strangulated. Its symptoms include nausea, vomiting, and discomfort because of nerves and tissue being irritated or stretched.

D. Linea Semilunaris

- Is a **curved line** along the lateral border of the rectus abdominis.

E. Linea Semicircularis (Arcuate Line)

- Is a **crescent-shaped line** marking the inferior limit of the posterior layer of the rectus sheath just below the level of the iliac crest.

F. Lacunar Ligament (Gimbernat Ligament)

- Represents the medial triangular expansion of the inguinal ligament to the pectineal line of the pubis.
- Forms the medial border of the femoral ring and the floor of the inguinal canal.

G. Pectineal (Cooper) Ligament

- Is a strong fibrous band that extends laterally from the lacunar ligament along the pectineal line of the pubis.

H. Inguinal Ligament (Poupart Ligament)

- Is the folded lower border of the aponeurosis of the external oblique muscle, extending between the anterior superior iliac spine and the pubic tubercle.
- Forms the floor (inferior wall) of the inguinal canal.

I. Iliopectineal Arcus or Ligament

- Is a **fascial partition** that separates the muscular (lateral) and vascular (medial) lacunae deep to the inguinal ligament.
  1. The **muscular lacuna** transmits the iliopsoas muscle.
  2. The **vascular lacuna** transmits the femoral sheath and its contents, including the femoral vessels, a femoral branch of the genitofemoral nerve, and the femoral canal.

J. Reflected Inguinal Ligament

- Is formed by fibers derived from the medial portion of the inguinal ligament and lacunar ligament and runs upward over the conjoint tendon to end at the **linea alba**.

K. Falx Inguinalis (Conjoint Tendon)

- Is formed by the aponeuroses of the internal oblique and transverse muscles of the abdomen and is inserted into the pubic tubercle and crest.
- Strengthens the posterior wall of the medial half of the **inguinal canal**.

L. Rectus Sheath (Figure 4.2)

- Is formed by fusion of the aponeuroses of the external oblique, internal oblique, and transverse muscles of the abdomen.
- Encloses the rectus abdominis and sometimes the pyramidal muscle.
- Also contains the superior and inferior epigastric vessels and the ventral primary rami of thoracic nerves 7 to 12.
  1. **Anterior Layer of the Rectus Sheath**
     - **(a) Above the arcuate line**: aponeuroses of the external and internal oblique muscles.
     - **(b) Below the arcuate line**: aponeuroses of the external oblique, internal oblique, and transverse muscles.

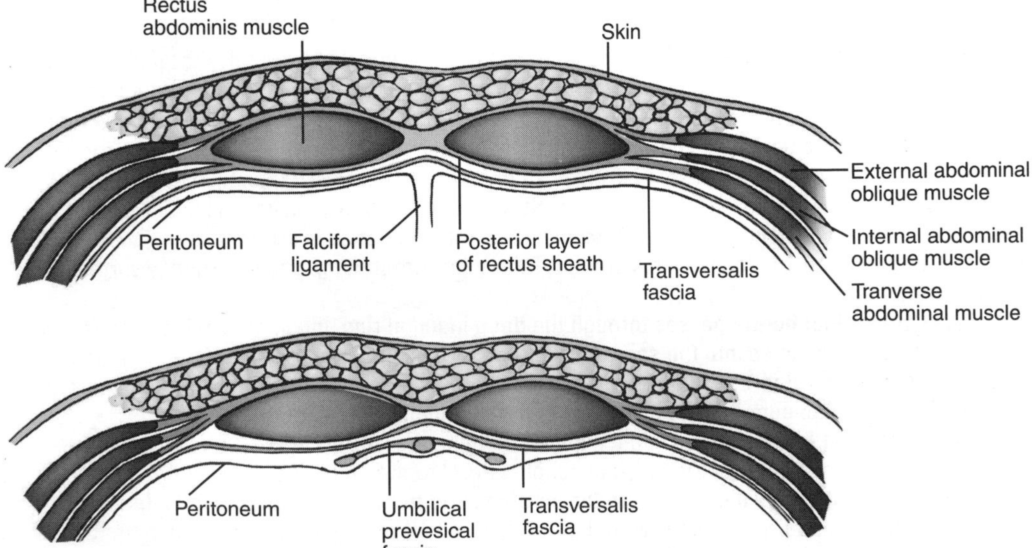

FIGURE 4.2. Arrangement of the rectus sheath above the umbilicus (**top**) and below the arcuate line (**bottom**).

2. **Posterior Layer of the Rectus Sheath**
   (a) **Above the arcuate line**: aponeuroses of the internal oblique and transverse muscles.
   (b) **Below the arcuate line**: rectus abdominis is in contact with the transversalis fascia.

IV. INGUINAL REGION

A. Inguinal (Hesselbach) Triangle

- Is bounded medially by the linea semilunaris (lateral edge of the rectus abdominis), laterally by the inferior epigastric vessels, and inferiorly by the inguinal ligament.
- Is an area of potential weakness and hence is a common site of a **direct inguinal hernia**.

B. Inguinal Rings

1. Superficial Inguinal Ring

- Is a **triangular opening** in the aponeurosis of the external oblique muscle that lies just lateral to the pubic tubercle.

2. Deep Inguinal Ring

- Lies in the transversalis fascia, just lateral to the inferior epigastric vessels.

C. Inguinal Canal

- Begins at the deep inguinal ring and terminates at the superficial ring.
- Transmits the spermatic cord or the round ligament of the uterus and the genital branch of the genitofemoral nerve, both of which also run through the **deep inguinal ring** and the **inguinal canal**. An indirect inguinal hernia (if present) also passes through this canal. Although the ilioinguinal nerve runs through part of the inguinal canal and the superficial inguinal ring, it does not pass through the deep inguinal ring.
  1. **Anterior wall**: aponeuroses of the external oblique and internal oblique muscles.
  2. **Posterior wall**: aponeurosis of the transverse abdominal muscle and transversalis fascia.
  3. **Superior wall (roof)**: arching fibers of the internal oblique and transverse muscles.
  4. **Inferior wall (floor)**: inguinal and lacunar ligaments.

CLINICAL CORRELATES

Inguinal hernia arises when a portion of intestine protrudes through a weak spot in the inguinal canal or in the inguinal triangle. **Inguinal hernia** occurs superior to the inguinal ligament and lateral to the pubic tubercle, and occurs more in males than in females. **Reducible hernia** is a hernia in which the contents of the hernial sac can be returned to their normal position. **Incarcerated hernia** is an irreducible hernia in which the contents of the hernial sac are entrapped or stuck in the groin. **Strangulated hernia** is an irreducible hernia in which the intestine becomes tightly trapped or twisted; thus, the circulation is arrested, and gangrene (death of tissue) occurs unless relief is prompt. This is life-threatening, and emergency surgical repair is required.

Indirect inguinal hernia passes through the deep inguinal ring, inguinal canal, and superficial inguinal ring and descends into the scrotum. Indirect hernias lie lateral to the inferior epigastric vessels, are **congenital** (present at birth), derived from persistence of the processus vaginalis, and covered by the peritoneum and the coverings of the spermatic cord (Figure 4.3).

Direct inguinal hernia occurs in the inguinal triangle directly through the abdominal wall muscles (posterior wall of the inguinal canal), lateral to the edge of the conjoint tendon (falx inguinalis), and rarely descends into the scrotum. The hernia lies medial to the inferior epigastric vessels and protrudes forward (but rarely through) the superficial inguinal ring. It is **acquired** (develops after birth) and has a sac formed by peritoneum and occasionally transversalis fascia.

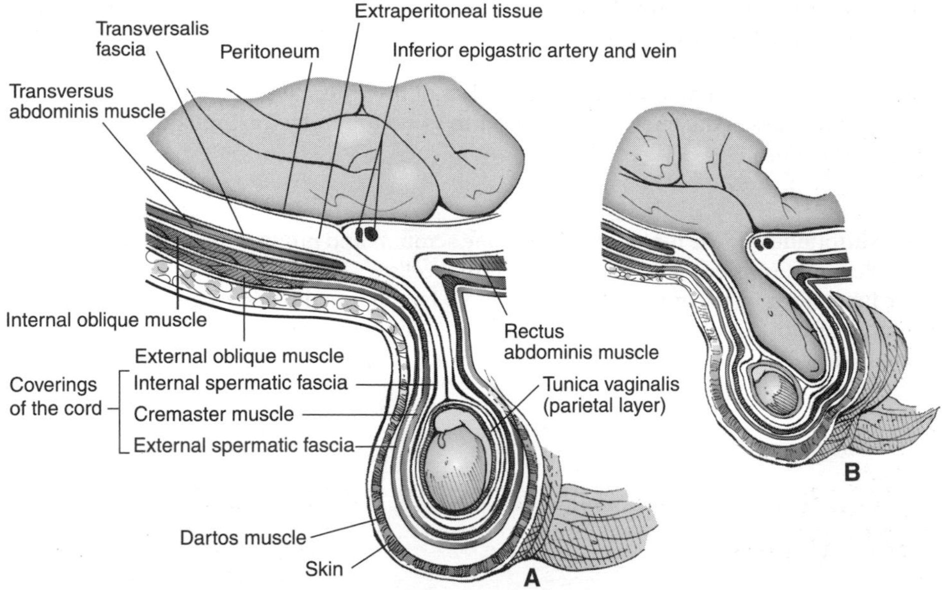

FIGURE 4.3. A: Coverings of spermatic cord and testis. **B:** Inguinal hernia.

V. SPERMATIC CORD, SCROTUM, AND TESTIS

A. Spermatic Cord (Figure 4.3)

- Is composed of the **ductus deferens**; **testicular**, cremasteric, and deferential arteries; pampiniform plexus of **testicular veins; genital branch of the genitofemoral** and cremasteric nerves and the testicular sympathetic plexus; and lymph vessels. These are all interconnected by loose connective tissue.
- Has several fasciae:
  1. **External spermatic fascia**, derived from the aponeurosis of the external oblique muscle.
  2. **Cremasteric fascia** (cremaster muscle and fascia), originating in the internal oblique muscle.
  3. **Internal spermatic fascia**, derived from the transversalis fascia.

B. Fetal Structures

1. Processus Vaginalis Testis

- Is a **peritoneal diverticulum** in the fetus that evaginates into a developing scrotum and forms the visceral and parietal layers of the **tunica vaginalis testis.**
- Normally closes before birth or shortly thereafter and loses its connection with the peritoneal cavity.
- May result in a **congenital indirect inguinal hernia** if it persists.
- May cause **fluid accumulation** (hydrocele processus vaginalis) if it is occluded.

2. Tunica Vaginalis

- Is a **double serous membrane**, a peritoneal sac that covers the front and sides of the **testis** and **epididymis.**
- Is derived from the abdominal peritoneum and forms the **innermost layer of the scrotum.**

3. Gubernaculum Testis

- Is the **fetal ligament** that connects the bottom of the fetal testis to the developing scrotum.
- Appears to be important in **testicular descent** (pulls the testis down as it migrates).
- Is homologous to the ovarian ligament and the round ligament of the uterus.

C. Scrotum

- Consists of a thin pigmented skin and **dartos** fascia, a layer of smooth muscle fibers; when contracted, it wrinkles to regulate the temperature.

- Is innervated by genital branch of the genitofemoral, anterior scrotal branch of the ilioinguinal, posterior scrotal branch of the perineal, and perineal branch of the posterior femoral cutaneous nerves.
- Receives blood from anterior scrotal branches of the external pudendal artery and posterior scrotal branches of the internal pudendal artery and drains lymph initially into the superficial inguinal nodes.

D. Testes

- Are surrounded by the tunica vaginalis in the scrotum and produce sperm in the seminiferous tubules and testosterone by interstitial (Leydig) cells.
- Are innervated by the autonomic nerves, drain lymph into the deep inguinal nodes and to the lumbar and preaortic nodes, receive blood from the testicular arteries arising from the aorta, and drain venous blood by testicular veins, which empty into the inferior **vena cava (IVC)** on the right and the renal vein on the left.

VI. INNER SURFACE OF THE ANTERIOR ABDOMINAL WALL (Figure 4.4)

A. Supravesical Fossa

- Is a depression on the anterior abdominal wall between the median and medial umbilical folds of the peritoneum.

B. Medial Inguinal Fossa

- Is a depression on the anterior abdominal wall between the medial and lateral umbilical folds of the peritoneum. It lies lateral to the supravesical fossa.
- Is the fossa where most **direct inguinal hernias occur.**

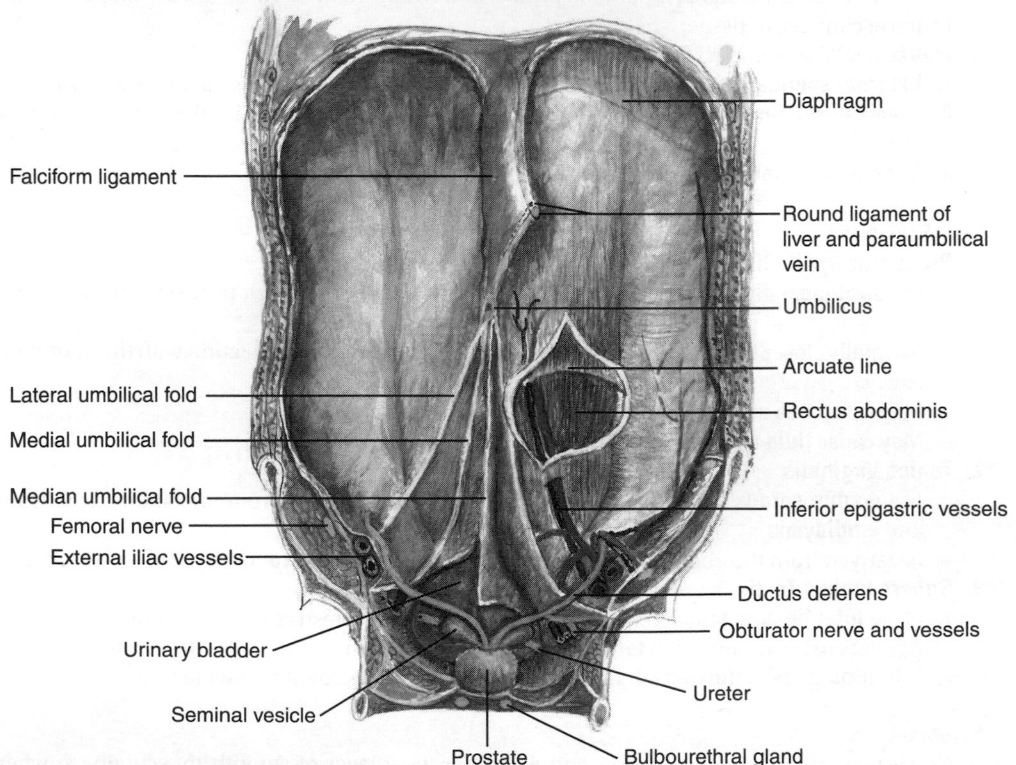

FIGURE 4.4. Umbilical folds over the anterior abdominal wall.

C. Lateral Inguinal Fossa

- Is a depression on the anterior abdominal wall, lateral to the lateral umbilical fold of the peritoneum.

D. Umbilical Folds or Ligaments

1. Median Umbilical Ligament or Fold

- Is a fibrous cord, the remnant of the obliterated **urachus**, which forms a **median umbilical fold** of the peritoneum.
- Lies between the transversalis fascia and the peritoneum and extends from the apex of the bladder to the umbilicus.

2. Medial Umbilical Ligament or Fold

- Is a fibrous cord, the remnant of the **obliterated umbilical artery**, which forms a medial umbilical fold and extends from the side of the bladder to the umbilicus.

3. Lateral Umbilical Fold

- Is a fold of the peritoneum that covers inferior epigastric vessels and extends from the medial side of the deep inguinal ring to the arcuate line.

E. Transversalis Fascia

- Is the lining fascia of the entire abdominopelvic cavity between the parietal peritoneum and the inner surface of the abdominal muscles.
- Continues with the diaphragmatic, psoas, iliac, pelvic, and quadratus lumborum fasciae.
- Forms the **deep inguinal ring** and gives rise to the femoral sheath and the internal spermatic fascia.
- Is directly in contact with the rectus abdominis below the arcuate line.

VII. NERVES OF THE ANTERIOR ABDOMINAL WALL

A. Subcostal Nerve

- Is the ventral ramus of the 12th thoracic nerve and innervates the muscles of the anterior abdominal wall.
- Has a **lateral cutaneous branch** that innervates the skin of the side of the hip.

B. Iliohypogastric Nerve

- Arises from the **first lumbar nerve** and innervates the internal oblique and transverse muscles of the abdomen.
- Divides into a **lateral cutaneous branch** to supply the skin of the lateral side of the buttocks and an **anterior cutaneous branch** to supply the skin above the pubis.

C. Ilioinguinal Nerve

- Arises from the **first lumbar nerve**, pierces the internal oblique muscle near the deep inguinal ring, and accompanies the spermatic cord through the inguinal canal and then through the superficial inguinal ring.
- Innervates the internal oblique and transverse muscles.
- Gives rise to a **femoral branch**, which innervates the upper and medial parts of the anterior thigh, and the **anterior scrotal nerve**, which innervates the skin of the root of the penis (or the skin of the mons pubis) and the anterior part of the scrotum (or the labium majus).

CLINICAL CORRELATES

Cremasteric reflex is a **drawing up of the testis** by contraction of the cremaster muscle when the skin on the upper medial side of the thigh is stroked. The efferent limb of the reflex arc is the **genital branch of the genitofemoral nerve**; the afferent limb is a **femoral branch of the genitofemoral nerve** and also of the ilioinguinal nerve.

VIII. LYMPHATIC DRAINAGE OF THE ANTERIOR ABDOMINAL WALL

A. Lymphatics in the Region above the Umbilicus

- Drain into the axillary lymph nodes.

B. Lymphatics in the Region below the Umbilicus

- Drain into the superficial inguinal nodes.

C. Superficial Inguinal Lymph Nodes

- Receive lymph from the lower abdominal wall, buttocks, penis, scrotum, labium majus, and the lower parts of the vagina and anal canal. Their efferent vessels primarily enter the external iliac nodes and, ultimately, the lumbar (aortic) nodes.

IX. BLOOD VESSELS OF THE ANTERIOR ABDOMINAL WALL

A. Superior Epigastric Artery

- Arises from the **internal thoracic artery**, enters the rectus sheath, and descends on the posterior surface of the rectus abdominis.
- Anastomoses with the inferior epigastric artery within the rectus abdominis.

B. Inferior Epigastric Artery

- Arises from the **external iliac artery** above the inguinal ligament, enters the rectus sheath, and ascends between the rectus abdominis and the posterior layer of the rectus sheath.
- Anastomoses with the superior epigastric artery, providing collateral circulation between the subclavian and external iliac arteries.
- Gives rise to the **cremasteric artery**, which accompanies the spermatic cord.

C. Deep Circumflex Iliac Artery

- Arises from the **external iliac artery** and runs laterally along the inguinal ligament and the iliac crest between the transverse and internal oblique muscles.
- Forms an ascending branch that anastomoses with the **musculophrenic artery**.

D. Superficial Epigastric Arteries

- Arise from the **femoral artery** and run superiorly toward the umbilicus over the inguinal ligament.
- Anastomose with branches of the inferior epigastric artery.

E. Superficial Circumflex Iliac Artery

- Arises from the **femoral artery** and runs laterally upward, parallel to the inguinal ligament.
- Anastomoses with the deep circumflex iliac and lateral femoral circumflex arteries.

F. Superficial (External) Pudendal Arteries

- Arise from the femoral artery, pierce the cribriform fascia, and run medially to supply the skin above the pubis.

G. Thoracoepigastric Veins

- Are longitudinal venous connections between the lateral thoracic vein and the superficial epigastric vein.
- Provide a collateral route for venous return if a caval or portal obstruction occurs.

PERITONEUM AND PERITONEAL CAVITY

I. PERITONEUM

- Is a **serous membrane** lined by mesothelial cells.
- Consists of the **parietal peritoneum** and the **visceral peritoneum**.

A. Parietal Peritoneum
- Lines the abdominal and pelvic walls and the inferior surface of the diaphragm.
- Is innervated by **somatic nerves** such as the phrenic, lower intercostal, subcostal, iliohypogastric, and ilioinguinal nerves.

B. Visceral Peritoneum
- Covers the viscera, is innervated by visceral nerves, and is insensitive to pain.

II. PERITONEAL REFLECTIONS (Figure 4.5)

- Support the viscera and provide pathways for associated neurovascular structures.

A. Omentum
- Is a fold of peritoneum extending from the stomach to adjacent abdominal organs.

1. Lesser Omentum
- Is a **double layer of peritoneum** extending from the porta hepatis of the liver to the lesser curvature of the stomach and the beginning of the duodenum.

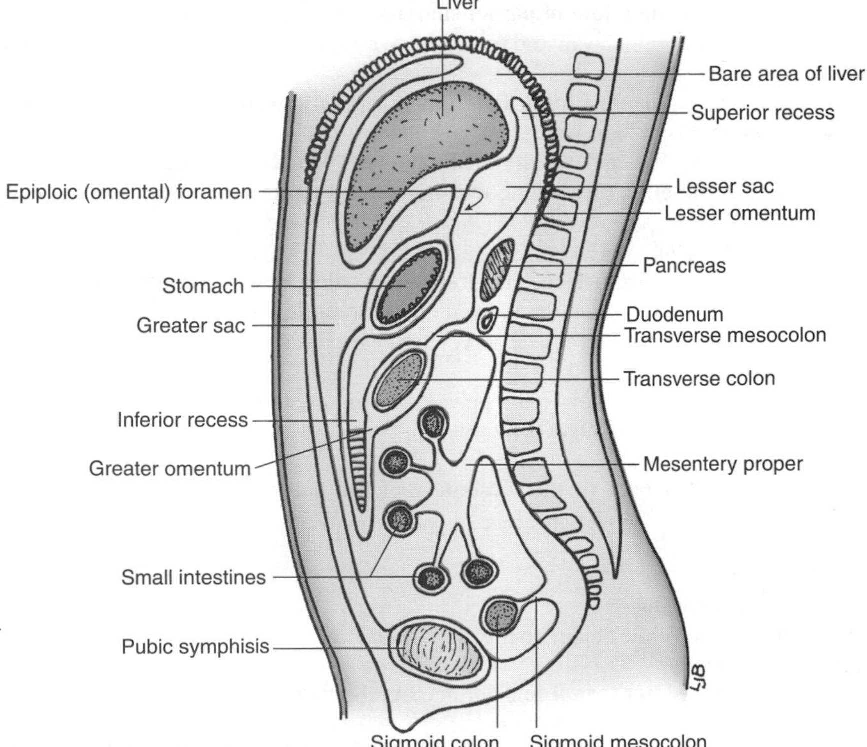

FIGURE 4.5. Sagittal section of the abdomen.

- Consists of the **hepatogastric and hepatoduodenal ligaments** and forms the anterior wall of the lesser sac of the peritoneal cavity.
- Transmits the left and right gastric vessels, which run between its two layers along the lesser curvature.
- Has a right free margin that contains the **proper hepatic artery**, **bile duct**, and **portal vein**.

2. Greater Omentum

- Is derived from the embryonic dorsal mesentery.
- Hangs down like an apron from the greater curvature of the stomach, covering the transverse colon and other abdominal viscera.
- Transmits the right and left gastroepiploic vessels along the greater curvature.
- Plugs the neck of a hernial sac, preventing the entrance of coils of the small intestine.
- Adheres to areas of inflammation and wraps itself around the inflamed organs, thus preventing serious diffuse **peritonitis**. Peritonitis is an inflammation of the peritoneum, characterized by an accumulation of peritoneal fluid that contains fibrin and leukocytes (pus).
- Consists of the gastrolienal, lienorenal, gastrophrenic, and gastrocolic ligaments.

(a) Gastrolienal (Gastrosplenic) Ligament

- Extends from the left portion of the greater curvature of the stomach to the hilus of the spleen and contains the **short gastric** and **left gastroepiploic** vessels.

(b) Lienorenal (Splenorenal) Ligament

- Runs from the hilus of the spleen to the left kidney and contains the **splenic** vessels and the **tail** of the pancreas.

(c) Gastrophrenic Ligament

- Runs from the upper part of the greater curvature of the stomach to the diaphragm.

(d) Gastrocolic Ligament

- Runs from the greater curvature of the stomach to the transverse colon.

B. Mesenteries

1. Mesentery of the Small Intestine (Mesentery Proper)

- Is a fan-shaped **double fold of peritoneum** that suspends the jejunum and the ileum from the posterior abdominal wall and transmits nerves and blood vessels to and from the small intestine.
- Forms a root that extends from the duodenojejunal flexure to the right iliac fossa and is approximately 15 cm (6 in.) long.
- Has a free border that encloses the **small intestine**, which is approximately 6 m (20 ft) long.
- Contains the superior mesenteric and intestinal (jejunal and ileal) vessels, nerves, and lymphatics.

2. Transverse Mesocolon

- Connects the posterior surface of the **transverse colon** to the posterior abdominal wall.
- Fuses with the greater omentum to form the **gastrocolic ligament**.
- Contains the middle colic vessels, nerves, and lymphatics.

3. Sigmoid Mesocolon

- Connects the sigmoid colon to the pelvic wall and contains the sigmoid vessels. Its line of attachment may form an inverted V.

4. Mesoappendix

- Connects the **appendix** to the mesentery of the ileum and contains the appendicular vessels.

C. Other Peritoneal Ligaments

1. Phrenicocolic Ligament

- Runs from the left colic flexure to the diaphragm.

2. Falciform Ligament

- Is a **sickle-shaped peritoneal fold** connecting the **liver** to the diaphragm and the anterior abdominal wall.
- Contains the **ligamentum teres hepatis** and the **paraumbilical vein**, which connects the left branch of the portal vein with the subcutaneous veins in the region of the **umbilicus**.

3. Ligamentum Teres Hepatis (Round Ligament of the Liver)

- Lies in the free margin of the falciform ligament and ascends from the umbilicus to the inferior (visceral) surface of the liver, lying in the fissure that forms the left boundary of the quadrate lobe of the liver.
- Is formed after birth from the remnant of the **left umbilical vein**, which carries oxygenated blood from the placenta to the left branch of the portal vein in the fetus. (The right umbilical vein is obliterated during the embryonic period.)

4. Coronary Ligament

- Is a peritoneal reflection from the diaphragmatic surface of the liver onto the diaphragm and encloses a triangular area of the right lobe, the **bare area of the liver**.
- Has right and left extensions that form the **right and left triangular ligaments**.

5. Ligamentum Venosum

- Is the fibrous remnant of the **ductus venosus**.
- Lies in the fissure on the inferior surface of the liver, forming the left boundary of the **caudate lobe of the liver**.

D. Peritoneal Folds

1. Umbilical Folds

- Are five folds of peritoneum below the umbilicus, including the median, medial, and lateral umbilical folds.

2. Rectouterine Fold

- Extends from the cervix of the uterus, along the side of the rectum, to the posterior pelvic wall, forming the rectouterine pouch (of Douglas).

3. Ileocecal Fold

- Extends from the terminal ileum to the cecum.

III. PERITONEAL CAVITY (See Figure 4.5)

- Is a **potential space** between the parietal and visceral peritoneum and contains a film of fluid that lubricates the surface of the peritoneum and facilitates free movements of the viscera.
- Is a completely closed sac in the male but is open in the female through the uterine tubes, uterus, and vagina. It is divided into the lesser and greater sacs.

CLINICAL CORRELATES

Peritonitis is inflammation and/or infection of the peritoneum. Common causes include leakage of fecal material from a burst appendix, a penetrating wound to the abdomen, perforating ulcer that leaks stomach contents into the peritoneal cavity (lesser sac), or poor sterile technique during abdominal surgery. Peritonitis can be treated by rinsing the peritoneum with large amounts of sterile saline solution and giving antibiotics.

Paracentesis (abdominal tap) is a procedure in which a needle is inserted 1 to 2 in. through the abdominal wall into the peritoneal cavity to obtain a sample or drain fluid while the patient is sitting upright. The entry site is midline at approximately 2 cm below the umbilicus or lateral to McBurney's point, avoiding the inferior epigastric vessels.

A. Lesser Sac (Omental Bursa)

- Is an irregular space that lies behind the liver, lesser omentum, stomach, and upper anterior part of the greater omentum.
- Is a closed sac, except for its communication with the greater sac through the **epiploic (omental) foramen**.
- Presents three recesses: (a) **superior recess**, which lies behind the stomach, lesser omentum, and left lobe of the liver; (b) **inferior recess**, which lies behind the stomach, extending into the layers of the greater omentum; and (c) **splenic recess**, which extends to the left at the hilus of the spleen.

B. Greater Sac

- Extends across the entire breadth of the abdomen and from the diaphragm to the pelvic floor and presents numerous recesses.

1. **Subphrenic (Suprahepatic) Recess**
   - Is a peritoneal pocket between the diaphragm and the anterior and superior part of the liver and is separated into right and left recesses by the **falciform ligament**.
2. **Subhepatic Recess or Hepatorenal Recess (Morrison Pouch)**
   - Is a deep peritoneal pocket between the liver anteriorly and the kidney and suprarenal gland posteriorly and communicates with the lesser sac via the epiploic foramen and the right paracolic gutter, thus the pelvic cavity.
3. **Paracolic Recesses (Gutters)**
   - Lie lateral to both the ascending colon (right paracolic gutter) and the descending colon (left paracolic gutter).

C. Epiploic or Omental (Winslow) Foramen

- Is a natural opening between the lesser and greater sacs.
- Is bounded superiorly by peritoneum on the **caudate lobe** of the liver, inferiorly by peritoneum on the **first part of the duodenum**, anteriorly by the **free edge of the lesser omentum**, and posteriorly by peritoneum covering the **IVC**.

GASTROINTESTINAL (GI) VISCERA

I. ESOPHAGUS (ABDOMINAL PORTION)

- Is a muscular tube (approximately 10 in. or 25 cm long) that extends from the pharynx to the stomach, but the short abdominal part (1/2 in. long) extends from the diaphragm to the cardiac orifice of the stomach, entering the abdomen through an opening in the right crus of the diaphragm.
- Has a **physiologic esophageal sphincter**, which is the circular layer of smooth muscle at the terminal portion of the esophagus. The tonic contraction of this sphincter prevents the stomach contents from regurgitating into the esophagus. It is also known that, at the gastroesophageal junction, the diaphragmatic musculature forming the esophageal hiatus functions as a physiologic esophageal sphincter.

CLINICAL CORRELATES

Gastroesophageal reflux disease (GERD) is caused by a lower esophageal sphincter dysfunction (relaxation or weakness) and/or hiatal hernia, causing reflux of stomach contents. This reflux disease has symptoms of heartburn or acid indigestion, painful swallowing, burping, and feeling of fullness in the chest. It can be treated surgically by moving the herniated area of stomach back into the abdominal cavity and then tightening the esophageal hiatus.

Hiatal or esophageal hernia is a herniation of part of the stomach through the esophageal hiatus into the thoracic cavity. The hernia is caused by an abnormally large esophageal hiatus in the diaphragm, a relaxed and weakened lower esophageal sphincter, increased pressure in the abdomen resulting from coughing, vomiting, straining, constipation, or pregnancy. It may cause gastroesophageal reflux, strangulation of the esophagus or stomach, or vomiting in an infant after feeding and usually does not require treatment, but it may need surgery to reduce its size or to prevent strangulation.

II. STOMACH (Figures 4.6, 4.7, and 4.8)

- Rests, in the supine position, on the **stomach bed**, which is formed by the pancreas, spleen, left kidney, left suprarenal gland, transverse colon and its mesocolon, and diaphragm.
- Is covered entirely by peritoneum and is located in the left hypochondriac and epigastric regions of the abdomen.

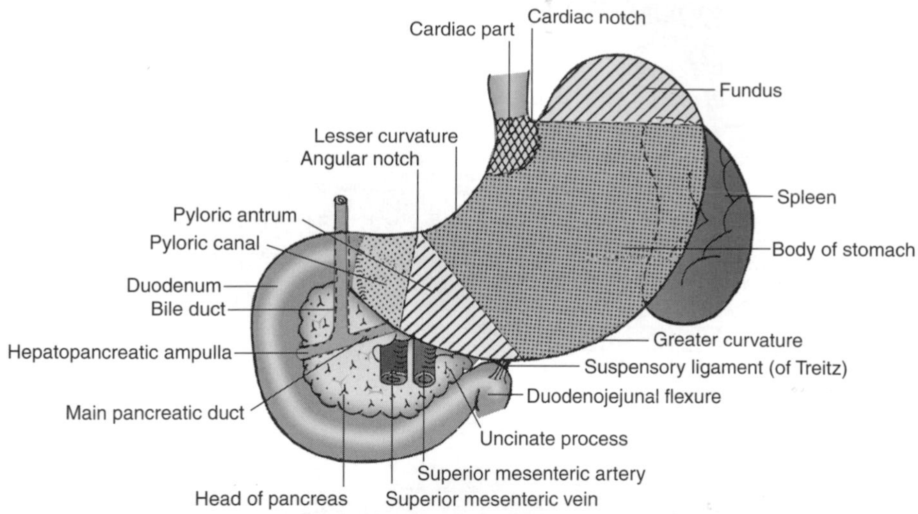

FIGURE 4.6. Stomach and duodenum.

- Has **greater and lesser curvatures**, anterior and posterior walls, cardiac and pyloric openings, and cardiac and angular notches.
- Is divided into four regions: **cardia**, **fundus**, **body**, and **pylorus**. The fundus lies inferior to the apex of the heart at the level of the fifth rib. The pylorus is divided into the **pyloric antrum** and **pyloric canal**. The pyloric orifice is surrounded by the **pyloric sphincter**, which is a group of thickened circular smooth muscles and controls the **rate of discharge** of stomach contents into the duodenum. The sphincter is constricted by sympathetic stimulation and relaxed by parasympathetic action.
- Receives blood from the right and left gastric, right and left gastroepiploic, and short gastric arteries.
- Undergoes contraction, which is characterized by the appearance of longitudinal folds of mucous membrane, the **rugae**. The **gastric canal**, a grooved channel along the lesser curvature formed by the rugae, directs fluids toward the pylorus.
- Produces mucus, hydrochloric acid, pepsin, and the hormone gastrin. **Mucus** protects the stomach from self-digestion, **hydrochloric acid** destroys many organisms and provides the required acid environment for pepsin activity, **pepsin** converts proteins to polypeptides, and **gastrin** produced in the stomach stimulates gastric acid secretion. Parasympathetic fibers in the vagus nerve stimulate gastric secretion.

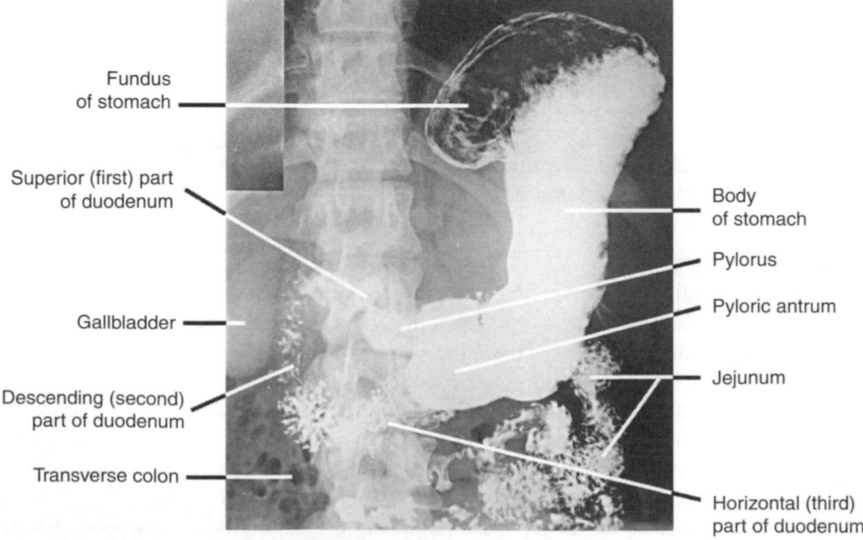

FIGURE 4.7. Radiograph of the stomach and small intestines.

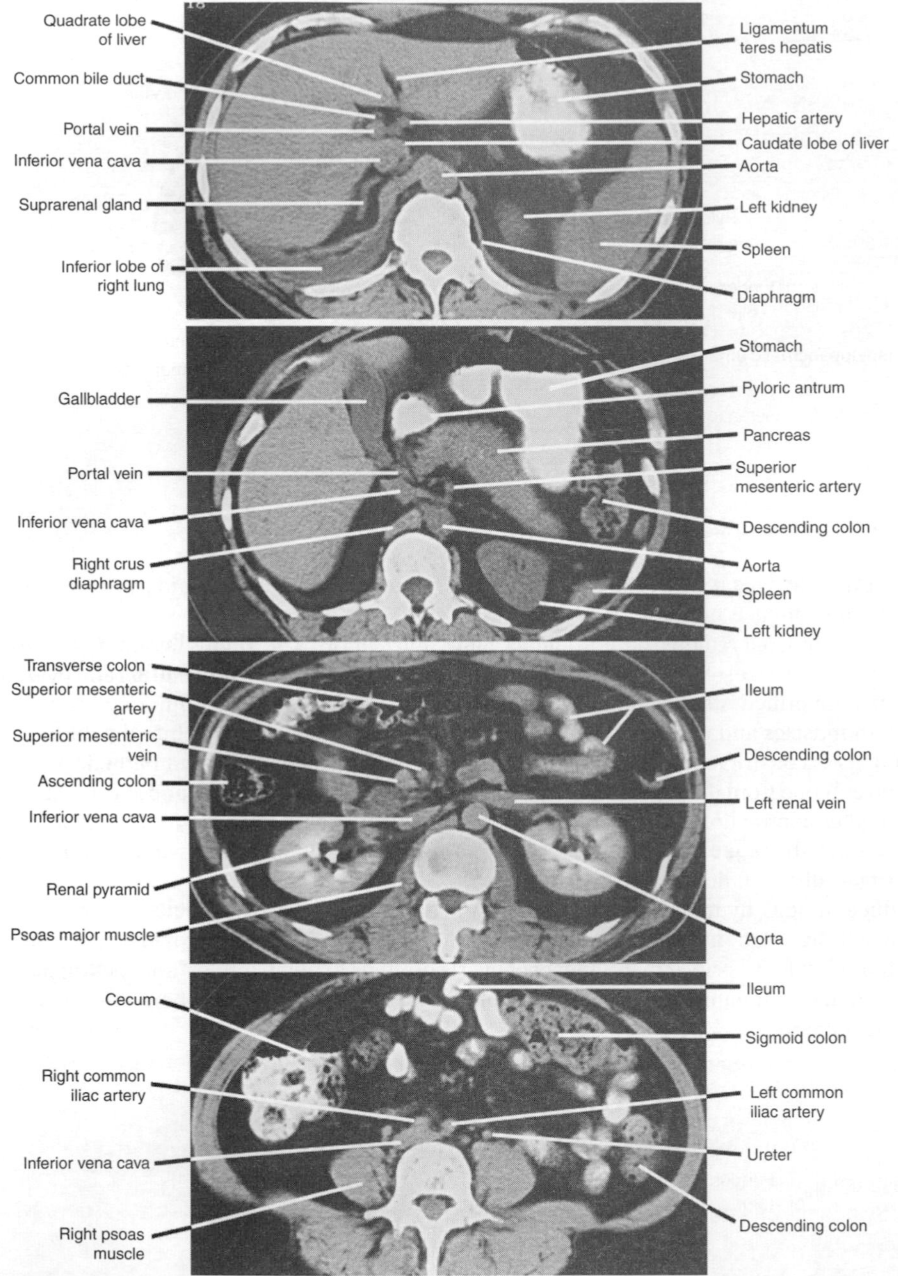

FIGURE 4.8. Computed tomography scans of the abdomen at different levels.

CLINICAL CORRELATES

Peptic ulcer is erosion in the lining of the stomach or duodenum. It is commonly caused by an infection with a bacterium called ***Helicobacter pylori*** but is also caused by stress, acid, and pepsin. It occurs most commonly in the pyloric region of the stomach (**gastric ulcer**) or the first part of the duodenum (**duodenal ulcer**). Symptoms of peptic ulcer are epigastric pain (burning, cramping, or aching), abdominal indigestion, nausea, vomiting, loss of appetite, weight loss, and fatigue. It may be treated with antibiotics or surgical intervention, including a partial gastrectomy and vagotomy. **Gastric ulcers** may perforate into the lesser sac and erode the pancreas and the splenic artery, causing fatal hemorrhage. **Duodenal ulcers** may erode the pancreas or the gastroduodenal artery, causing burning and cramping epigastric pain, and are three times more common than gastric ulcers.

III. SMALL INTESTINE (See Figures 4.6, 4.7, and 4.8)

- Extends from the pyloric opening to the ileocecal junction.
- Is the location of **complete digestion and absorption** of most of the products of digestion and water, electrolytes, and minerals such as calcium and iron.
- Consists of the **duodenum**, **jejunum**, and **ileum**.

A. Duodenum

- Is a **C-shaped tube** surrounding the head of the pancreas and is the shortest (25 cm [10 in.] long or 12 fingerbreadths in length) but widest part of the small intestine.
- Is retroperitoneal except for the beginning of the first part, which is connected to the liver by the **hepatoduodenal ligament** of the lesser omentum.
- Receives blood from the celiac (foregut) and superior mesenteric (midgut) artery.
- Is divided into four parts:

1. Superior (First) Part

- Has a mobile or free section, termed the **duodenal cap** (because of its appearance on radiographs), into which the pylorus invaginates.

2. Descending (Second) Part

- Contains the junction of the foregut and midgut, where the common bile and main pancreatic ducts open.
- Contains the **greater papilla**, on which terminal openings of the bile and main pancreatic ducts are located, and the **lesser papilla**, which lies 2 cm above the greater papilla and marks the site of entry of the **accessory pancreatic duct**.

3. Transverse (Third) Part

- Is the longest part and crosses the IVC, aorta, and vertebral column to the left.
- Is crossed anteriorly by the superior mesenteric vessels.

4. Ascending (Fourth) Part

- Ascends to the left of the aorta to the level of the second lumbar vertebra and terminates at the duodenojejunal junction, which is fixed in position by the **suspensory ligament (of Treitz)**, a surgical landmark. This fibromuscular band is attached to the right crus of the diaphragm.

CLINICAL CORRELATES

Small bowel obstruction is caused by postoperative adhesions, tumors, Crohn's disease, hernias, peritonitis, gallstones, volvulus, congenital malrotation, stricture, and intussusception (invagination of one part of the intestine into another). Strangulated obstructions are surgical emergencies and may cause death, if untreated, because the arterial occlusion leads to bowel ischemia and necrosis. Symptoms include colicky abdominal pain and cramping, nausea and vomiting, constipation, dizziness, abdominal distention, and high-pitched bowel sounds. **Inflammatory bowel disease** includes Crohn's disease and ulcerative colitis. **Crohn's disease** usually occurs in the ileum (ileitis or enteritis), but it may occur in any part of the digestive tract. Symptoms include diarrhea, rectal bleeding, anemia, weight loss, and fever. **Ulcerative colitis** involves the colon and the rectum, causing ulcers in the lining (mucosa) of the organs, and patients with prolonged ulcerative colitis are at increased risk for developing colon cancer.

Celiac disease is an **immune reaction to** eating **gluten** (protein of wheat, barley, and rye). Gluten ingestion triggers an immune system response which may produce inflammation that **damages the lining of the small intestine**, causing **malabsorption** of nutrients, constipation, diarrhea, vitamin and mineral deficiencies, fatigue, and weight loss.

B. Jejunum

- Makes up the proximal two-fifths of the small intestine (the ileum makes up the distal three-fifths).
- Is emptier, larger in diameter, and thicker walled than the ileum.
- Has the **plicae circulares** (circular folds), which are tall and closely packed.
- Contains no Peyer patches (aggregations of lymphoid tissue).
- Has translucent areas called **windows** between the blood vessels of its mesentery.
- Has less prominent **arterial arcades** (anastomotic loops) in its mesentery compared with the ileum.
- Has longer **vasa recta** (straight arteries, or arteriae rectae) compared with the ileum.

C. Ileum

- Is longer than the jejunum and occupies the **false pelvis** in the right lower quadrant of the abdomen.
- Is characterized by the presence of **Peyer patches** (lower portion), shorter plicae circulares and vasa recta, and more mesenteric fat and arterial arcades when compared with the jejunum.
- The ileocecal fold is the bloodless fold of Treves (surgeon at the London Hospital who drained the appendix abscess of King Edward VII in 1902).

CLINICAL CORRELATES **Meckel's diverticulum** is an **outpouching** (fingerlike pouch) of the **ileum**, derived from an unobliterated vitelline duct and located **2 ft** proximal to the ileocecal junction on the **antimesenteric side**. It is approximately **2 in**. long, occurs in approximately **2%** of the population, may contain **two types** of ectopic tissues (gastric and pancreatic), presents in the first **two decades** of life and more often in the first **2 years**, and is found **two times** as frequently in boys as in girls. It represents persistent portions of the **embryonic yolk stalk** (vitelline or omphalomesenteric duct) and may be free or connected to the umbilicus via a fibrous cord or a fistula. The diverticulum may cause diverticulitis, ulceration, **bleeding**, perforation, bowel obstruction, abdominal pain and discomfort, vomiting, fever, and constipation.

IV. LARGE INTESTINE (See Figures 4.8 and 4.14)

- Extends from the ileocecal junction to the anus and is approximately 1.5 m (5 ft) long.
- Consists of the **cecum**, **appendix**, **colon**, **rectum**, and **anal canal**.
- Functions to convert the liquid contents of the ileum into semisolid feces by **absorbing water**, **salts**, and **electrolytes**. It also stores and **lubricates** feces with mucus.

A. Colon

- Has **ascending** and **descending** colons that are retroperitoneal and **transverse** and **sigmoid** colons that are surrounded by peritoneum (they have their own mesenteries, the **transverse mesocolon** and the **sigmoid mesocolon**, respectively). The ascending and transverse colons are supplied by the superior mesenteric artery and the vagus nerve; the descending and sigmoid colons are supplied by the inferior mesenteric artery and the pelvic splanchnic nerves.
- Is characterized by the following:
  1. **Teniae coli**: three narrow bands of the outer longitudinal muscular coat.
  2. **Sacculations or haustra**: produced by the teniae, which are slightly shorter than the gut.
  3. **Epiploic appendages**: peritoneum-covered sacs of fat, attached in rows along the teniae.

CLINICAL CORRELATES **Diverticulitis** is inflammation of diverticula (external evaginations) of the intestinal wall, commonly found in the colon, especially the sigmoid colon, and the **diverticula** develop as a result of high pressure within the colon. Symptoms are abdominal pain usually in the left lower abdomen (but can be anywhere), chills, fever, nausea, and constipation. Risk factors include older age and a low-fiber diet, and diverticulitis can be treated with rest, high-fiber diet, and antibiotics. Complications may include bleeding, perforations, peritonitis, and stricture or fistula formation.

Sigmoid volvulus is a twisting of the sigmoid colon around its mesentery, creating a colonic obstruction and may cause intestinal ischemia that may progress to infarction and necrosis, peritonitis, and abdominal distension. It may occur when the sigmoid colon and its mesentery are abnormally long. Symptoms include vomiting, abdominal pain, constipation, bloody diarrhea, and hematemesis.

Megacolon (Hirschsprung disease) is caused by the **absence of enteric ganglia** (cell bodies of parasympathetic postganglionic fibers) in the lower part of the colon, which leads to dilation of the colon proximal to the inactive segment. It is of congenital origin, results from failure of neural crest cells to migrate and form the myenteric plexus, and is usually diagnosed during infancy and childhood. Symptoms are constipation or diarrhea, abdominal distention, vomiting, and a lack of appetite.

Colostomy is the most effective treatment; the surgeon removes the affected part of the colon, and the proximal part of the colon is then connected to a surgically created hole, called a stoma, on the abdomen. After the lower part of the colon heals, the surgeon reconnects the colon inside the body and closes the stoma.

B. Cecum

- Is the **blind pouch of the large intestine**. It lies in the right iliac fossa and is usually surrounded by peritoneum but has no mesentery.

C. Appendix

- Is a **narrow**, **hollow**, **muscular tube** with large aggregations of lymphoid tissue in its wall.
- Is suspended from the terminal ileum by a small mesentery, the **mesoappendix**, which contains the appendicular vessels.
- Causes **spasm** and **distention when inflamed**, resulting in **pain** that is referred to the periumbilical region and moves down and to the right.
- Has a base that lies deep to **McBurney point**, which occurs at the junction of the lateral one-third of the line between the right anterior superior iliac spine and the umbilicus. This is the site of maximum tenderness in **acute appendicitis**.

CLINICAL CORRELATES

Acute appendicitis is an acute inflammation of the appendix, usually resulting from bacteria or viruses that are trapped by an obstruction of the lumen by feces. Symptoms include rebound tenderness, periumbilical pain that may move to the right iliac fossa on McBurney point, accompanied by loss of appetite, nausea, vomiting, fever, diarrhea, and constipation. Its rupture may cause peritonitis, leading rapidly to septicemia and eventually death, if untreated. Appendicitis can be treated by appendectomy.

CLINICAL CORRELATES

Colonoscopy is an internal examination of the colon, using a flexible colonoscope with a small camera. The colon must be completely empty, the patient lies on his or her side, and the colonoscope is inserted through the anus and gently advanced to the terminal small intestine. Since better views are obtained during withdrawal than during insertion, a careful examination is done during withdrawal of the scope, looking for bleeding, ulcers, diverticulitis, polyps, colon cancer, and inflammatory bowel diseases. Tissue biopsy may be taken.

D. Rectum and Anal Canal

- Extend from the sigmoid colon to the anus.
- Are described as **pelvic organs** (see Pelvis: VIII, Chapter 5).

V. ACCESSORY ORGANS OF THE DIGESTIVE SYSTEM

A. Liver (Figures 4.8 and 4.9)

- Is the **largest visceral organ** and the **largest gland** in the human body.
- Plays an important role in **production and secretion of bile** (used in emulsification of fats); **detoxification** (by filtering the blood to remove bacteria and foreign particles that have gained entrance from the intestine); **storage** of carbohydrate as **glycogen** (to be broken down later to glucose); production and storage of lipids as **triglycerides**; **plasma protein synthesis** (albumin and globulin); **production** of blood **coagulants** (fibrinogen and prothrombin), **anticoagulants** (heparin), and **bile pigments** (bilirubin and biliverdin) from the breakdown of hemoglobin; **reservoir** for blood and platelets; and **storage** of certain vitamins, iron, and copper. In the fetus, the liver is important in the manufacture of red blood cells.
- Is surrounded by the peritoneum and is attached to the diaphragm by the **coronary and falciform ligaments** and the right and left **triangular** ligaments.

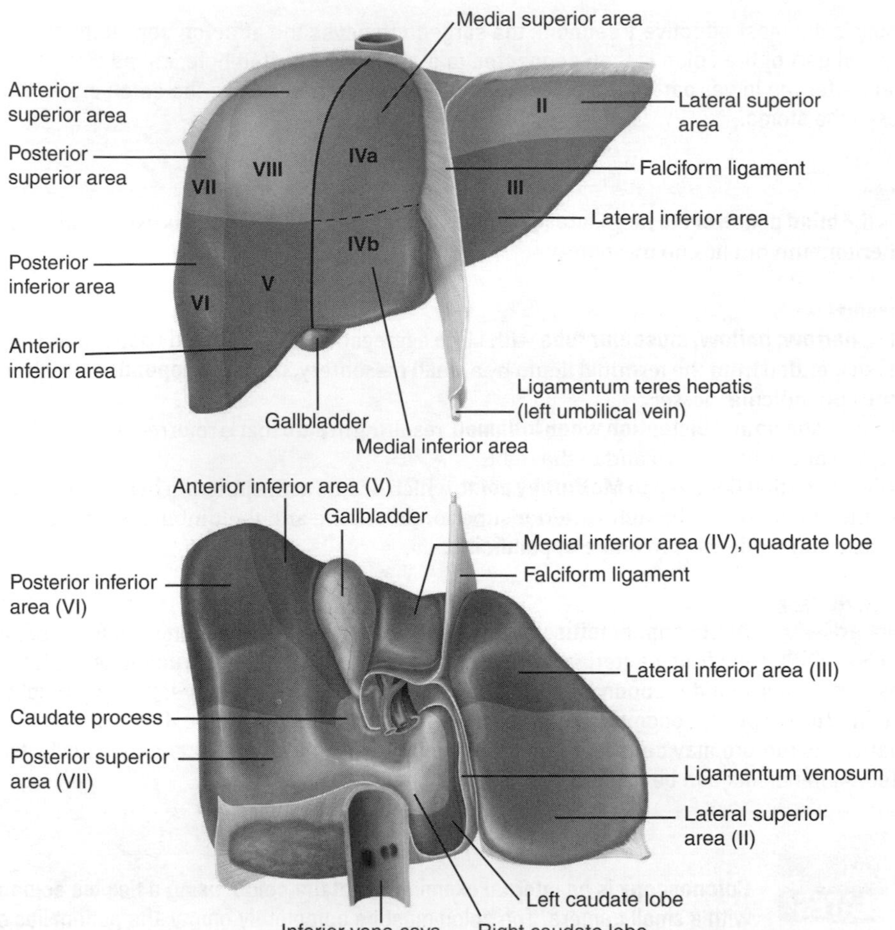

FIGURE 4.9. Anterior and visceral surface of the liver, and divisions of the liver based on hepatic drainage and blood supply.

- Has a **bare area** on the diaphragmatic surface, which is limited by layers of the coronary ligament but is devoid of peritoneum.
- Receives oxygenated blood from the **hepatic artery** and deoxygenated, nutrient-rich, sometimes toxic blood from the **portal vein**; its venous blood is drained by the **hepatic veins** into the IVC.
- Contains the **portal triad**, which is a group of the branches of the **portal vein**, **hepatic artery**, and **bile duct** at every corner of the lobule, surrounded by a connective tissue sheath, the perivascular fibrous capsule.
- Is divided, based on hepatic drainage and blood supply, into the **right and left lobes** by the fossae for the gallbladder and the IVC. (These lobes correspond to the functional units or hepatic segments.)

1. Lobes of the Liver (See Figure 4.9)

- Right and left lobes are further divided into eight functionally independent segments (Couinaud, 1957). Each segment can be identified numerically or by name.

(a) Right Lobe

- Is divided into **anterior** and **posterior segments**, each of which is subdivided into superior and inferior areas or segments.

(b) Left Lobe

- Is divided into **medial** and **lateral segments**, each of which is subdivided into superior and inferior areas (segments).
- Includes the **medial superior (caudate lobe)**, **medial inferior (quadrate lobe)**, **lateral superior**, and **lateral inferior segments**. The **quadrate lobe** receives blood from the left hepatic artery and drains bile into the left hepatic duct, whereas the **caudate lobe** receives blood from the right and left hepatic arteries and drains bile into both right and left hepatic ducts.

2. **Fissures and Ligaments of the Liver** (See Figure 4.9)
   - Include an H-shaped group of fissures:
     (a) Fissure for the round ligament **(ligamentum teres hepatis)**, located between the lateral portion of the left lobe and the quadrate lobe.
     (b) Fissure for the **ligamentum venosum**, located between the caudate lobe and the lateral portion of the left lobe.
     (c) Fossa for the **gallbladder**, located between the quadrate lobe and the major part of the right lobe.
     (d) Fissure for the **IVC**, located between the caudate lobe and the major part of the right lobe.
     (e) **Porta hepatis.** This **transverse fissure on the visceral surface** of the liver between the quadrate and caudate lobes lodges the hepatic ducts, hepatic arteries, branches of the **portal vein**, hepatic nerves, and lymphatic vessels.

CLINICAL CORRELATES

Liver cirrhosis is a condition in which liver cells are progressively destroyed and replaced by fatty and fibrous tissue that surrounds the intrahepatic blood vessels and biliary radicals, impeding the circulation of blood through the liver. It is caused by chronic alcohol abuse (alcoholism); viral hepatitis and ingestion of poisons. Liver cirrhosis causes **portal hypertension**, resulting in **esophageal varices** (dilated veins in the lower part of the esophagus), **hemorrhoids** (dilated veins around the anal canal), **caput medusa** (dilated veins around the umbilicus), **spider nevi** or **spider angioma** (small, red, spiderlike arterioles in the cheeks, neck, and shoulder), **ascites** (accumulation of fluid in the peritoneal cavity), **edema** in the legs (lower albumin levels facilitate water retention), **jaundice** (yellow eyes or skin resulting from bile duct disease failing to remove bilirubin), **hepatic encephalopathy** (shunted blood bypassing the liver contains toxins that reach the brain), **splenomegaly** (enlarged spleen resulting from venous congestion causing sequestered blood cells that lead to **thrombocytopenia**, a low platelet count, and easy bruising), **hepatomegaly** (due to fatty changes and fibrosis), **palmar erythema** (persistent redness of the palms), **testicular atrophy**, **gynecomastia**, and **pectoral alopecia** (loss of hair).

Liver biopsy is performed percutaneously by needle puncture, which commonly goes through the right 8th or 9th (perhaps 7th to 10th) intercostal space in the right midaxillary line under ultrasound or computed tomography (CT) scan guidance. While taking the biopsy, the patient is asked to hold his or her breath in full expiration to reduce the costodiaphragmatic recess and to lessen the possibility of damaging the lung and causing pneumothorax. **Transjugular liver biopsy** is also accomplished by inserting a catheter into the right internal jugular vein and guiding it through the superior vena cava, IVC, and right hepatic vein. A biopsy needle is inserted through a catheter into the liver where a biopsy sample is obtained.

B. Gallbladder (See Figures 4.8, 4.9, and 4.10)
- Is located at the junction of the right ninth costal cartilage and lateral border of the rectus abdominis, which is the site of maximum tenderness in acute inflammation of the gallbladder.
- Is a **pear-shaped sac** lying on the inferior surface of the liver in a fossa between the right and quadrate lobes with a capacity of approximately 30 to 50 mL and is in contact with the **duodenum** and **transverse colon**.
- Consists of the fundus, body, and neck: the **fundus** is the rounded blind end located at the tip of the right ninth costal cartilage in the midclavicular line and contacts the transverse colon; the **body** is the major part and rests on the upper part of the duodenum and the transverse colon; the **neck** is the narrow part and gives rise to the **cystic duct** with **spiral valves** (Heister valves).
- Receives bile, concentrates it (by absorbing water and salts), stores it, and releases it during digestion.
- **Contracts to expel bile** as a result of stimulation by the hormone **cholecystokinin**, which is produced by the duodenal mucosa or by parasympathetic stimulation when food arrives in the duodenum.

- Receives blood from the cystic artery, which arises from the right hepatic artery within the **cystohepatic triangle (of Calot)**, which is formed by the visceral surface of the liver superiorly, the cystic duct inferiorly, and the common hepatic duct medially.
- May have an abnormal conical pouch (**Hartmann pouch**) in its neck, and the pouch is also called the ampulla of the gallbladder.

CLINICAL CORRELATES **Gallstones (choleliths or cholelithiasis)** are formed by solidification of bile constituents and composed chiefly of **cholesterol crystals**, usually mixed with bile pigments and calcium. Bile crystallizes and forms sand, gravel, and finally stones. Gallstones present commonly in **f**at, **f**ertile (multiparous) **f**emales who are older than **f**orty (40) years (**4-F** individuals). Stones may become lodged in the (a) **fundus of the gallbladder**, where they may ulcerate through the wall of the fundus of the gallbladder into the transverse colon or through the wall of the body of the gallbladder into the duodenum (in the former case, they are passed naturally to the rectum, but in the latter case, they may be held up at the **ileocecal junction**, producing an **intestinal** obstruction); (b) **bile duct**, where they obstruct bile flow to the duodenum, leading to **jaundice**; and (c) **hepatopancreatic ampulla**, where they block both the biliary and the pancreatic duct systems. In this case, bile may enter the pancreatic duct system, causing aseptic or noninfectious **pancreatitis**.

CLINICAL CORRELATES **Cholecystitis** is an inflammation of the gallbladder, caused by obstruction of the cystic duct by gallstones. It causes pain in the upper right quadrant and the epigastric region, fever, nausea, and vomiting. The pain may radiate to the back or right shoulder region.

Cholecystectomy is surgical removal of the gallbladder resulting from inflammation or presence of gallstones in the gallbladder. It can be performed via open surgical or laparoscopic techniques.

C. Pancreas (See Figures 4.8 and 4.10)

- Lies largely in the floor of the lesser sac in the epigastric and left hypochondriac regions, where it forms a major portion of the stomach bed.
- Is a retroperitoneal organ except for a small portion of its **tail**, which lies in the **lienorenal** (splenorenal) **ligament**.
- Has a **head** that lies within the C-shaped concavity of the duodenum. If tumors are present in the head, bile flow is obstructed, resulting in **jaundice**. Bile pigments accumulate in the blood, giving the skin and eyes a characteristic yellow coloration.
- Has an **uncinate process**, which is a projection of the lower part of the head to the left behind the superior mesenteric vessels. The **tail** projects toward the hilum of the spleen.
- Receives blood from branches of the splenic artery and from the superior and inferior pancreaticoduodenal arteries.
- Is both an **exocrine gland**, which produces digestive enzymes that help digest fats, proteins, and carbohydrates, and an **endocrine gland** (islets of Langerhans), which secretes the hormones insulin and glucagon, which help the body to use glucose for energy, and also secretes somatostatin. Insulin lowers blood sugar levels by stimulating glucose uptake and glycogen formation and storage. Glucagon enhances blood sugar levels by promoting conversion of glycogen to glucose. Somatostatin suppresses insulin and glucagon secretion.
- Has two ducts, the **main pancreatic duct** and the **accessory pancreatic duct**.

1. Main Pancreatic Duct (Duct of Wirsung)

- Begins in the tail, runs to the right along the entire pancreas, and carries pancreatic juice containing enzymes.
- Joins the bile duct to form the **hepatopancreatic ampulla (ampulla of Vater)** before entering the second part of the duodenum at the greater papilla.

2. Accessory Pancreatic Duct (Santorini Duct)

- Begins in the lower portion of the head and drains a small portion of the head and body.
- Empties at the lesser duodenal papilla approximately 2 cm above the greater papilla.

CLINICAL CORRELATES **Pancreatitis** is an inflammation of the pancreas and is caused by gallstones or alcohol abuse. Symptoms include upper abdominal pain (which may be severe and constant and may present as back pain), nausea, vomiting, weight loss, fatty stools, mild jaundice, diabetes, low blood pressure, heart failure, and kidney failure.

Pancreatic cancer frequently causes severe back pain, has the potential to invade into the adjacent organs, and is extremely difficult to treat. Cancer of the pancreatic head often compresses and obstructs the bile duct, usually causing a painless obstructive jaundice and surgical resection called a pancreaticoduodenectomy (Whipple procedure) can be curative in this particular instance. Cancer of the pancreatic neck and body may cause portal or IVC obstruction because the pancreas overlies these large veins.

CLINICAL CORRELATES **Diabetes mellitus** is characterized by hyperglycemia that is caused by an **inadequate production** of insulin or **inadequate action** of insulin on body tissues. There are two types of diabetes: **type I** diabetes (also known as insulin-dependent diabetes), in which the pancreas (β cells) produces an **insufficient amount** of insulin; and **type II** diabetes, which results from **insulin resistance** of target tissues (a condition in which the body fails to properly use insulin or fails to respond properly to the insulin action). Diabetes causes diabetic retinopathy, neuropathy, kidney failure, heart disease, stroke, and limb disease. It has symptoms of polyuria (excessive secretion of urine), polydipsia (thirst), weight loss, tiredness, infections of urinary tract, and blurring of vision.

D. Duct System for Bile Passage (See Figure 4.10)

1. Right and Left Hepatic Ducts

- Are formed by union of the **intrahepatic ductules** from each lobe of the liver and drain bile from the corresponding halves of the liver.

2. Common Hepatic Duct

- Is formed by union of the right and left hepatic ducts.
- Is accompanied by the proper hepatic artery and the portal vein.

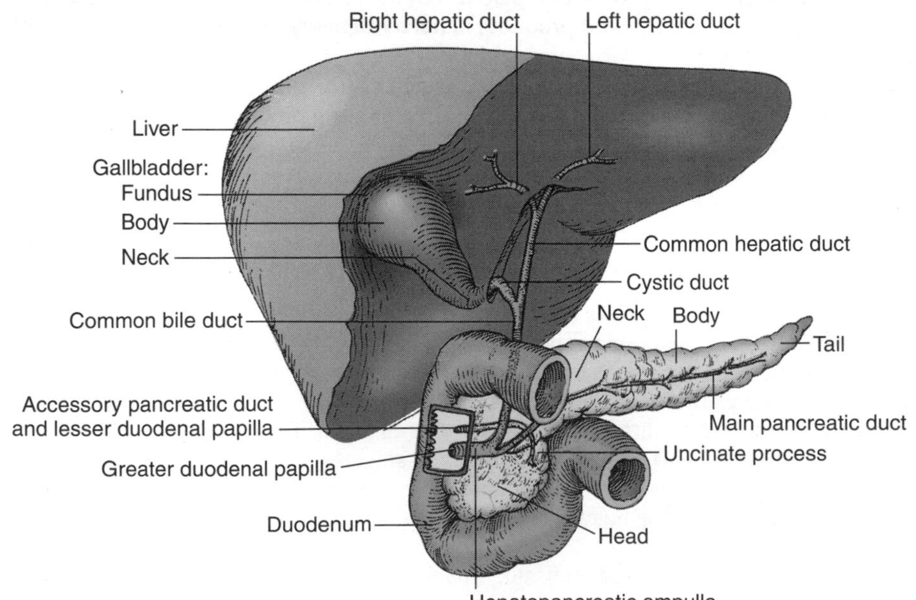

FIGURE 4.10. Extrahepatic bile passages and pancreatic ducts.

3. Cystic Duct

- Has spiral folds (valves) to keep it constantly open, and thus bile can pass upward into the **gallbladder** when the common bile duct is closed.
- Runs alongside the hepatic duct before joining the common hepatic duct.
- Is a common site of **impaction** of **gallstones.**

4. Common Bile Duct (Ductus Choledochus)

- Is formed by union of the common hepatic duct and the cystic duct.
- Is located lateral to the proper hepatic artery and anterior to the portal vein in the right free margin of the lesser omentum.
- Descends behind the first part of the duodenum and runs through the head of the pancreas.
- Joins the main pancreatic duct to form the **hepatopancreatic duct (hepatopancreatic ampulla)**, which enters the second part of the duodenum at the greater papilla.
- Contains the **sphincter of Boyden**, which is a circular muscle layer around the lower end of the duct.

5. Hepatopancreatic Duct or Ampulla (Ampulla of Vater)

- Is formed by the union of the common bile duct and the main pancreatic duct and enters the second part of the duodenum at the greater papilla. This represents the junction of the embryonic foregut and midgut.
- Contains the **sphincter of Oddi**, which is a circular muscle layer around it in the greater duodenal papilla.

VI. SPLEEN (See Figures 4.6, 4.8, and 4.12)

- Is a large **vascular lymphatic organ** lying against the diaphragm and ribs 9 to 11 in the left hypochondriac region, covered by peritoneum except at the hilum, and supported by the **lienogastric (splenogastric)** and **lienorenal (splenorenal) ligaments.**
- Is developed as a thickening of the mesenchyme in the dorsal mesogastrium and supplied by the splenic artery and drained by the splenic vein.
- Is composed of **white pulp**, which consists of primarily lymphatic tissue around the central arteries and is the primary site of immune and phagocytic action, and **red pulp**, which consists of venous sinusoids and splenic cords and is the primary site of filtration.
- **Filters blood** (removes damaged and worn-out erythrocytes and platelets by macrophages); acts as a **blood reservoir**, storing blood and platelets in the red pulp; provides the **immune response** (protection against infection); and produces **mature lymphocytes**, macrophages, and **antibodies** chiefly in the white pulp.
- Is **hematopoietic** in early life and later destroys aged (i.e., worn-out) red blood cells in the red pulp and sets free the hemoglobin. The **hemoglobin**, a respiratory protein of erythrocytes, is degraded into (a) the **globin** (protein part), which is hydrolyzed to amino acid and reused in protein synthesis; (b) the **iron** released from the heme, which is transported to the bone marrow and reused in erythropoiesis; and (c) the iron-free **heme**, which is metabolized to bilirubin in the liver and excreted in the bile.

CLINICAL CORRELATES

Splenomegaly is caused by venous congestion resulting from thrombosis of the splenic vein or portal hypertension, which causes sequestering of blood cells, leading to thrombocytopenia (a low platelet count) and easy bruising. It has symptoms of fever, diarrhea, bone pain, weight loss, and night sweats.

Rupture of the spleen occurs frequently by fractured ribs or severe blows to the left hypochondrium and causes profuse bleeding. The ruptured spleen is difficult to repair; consequently, **splenectomy** is performed to prevent the person from bleeding to death. The spleen may be removed surgically with minimal effect on body function because its functions are assumed by other reticuloendothelial organs.

Lymphoma is a cancer of lymphoid tissue. **Hodgkin's lymphoma** is a malignancy characterized by painless, progressive enlargement of the lymph nodes, spleen, and other lymphoid tissue, accompanied by night sweats, fever (Pel-Ebstein fever), and weight loss.

VII. DEVELOPMENT OF DIGESTIVE SYSTEM (Figure 4.11)

A. Primitive Gut Tube

- Is a tube of endoderm that is covered by splanchnic mesoderm and is formed from the yolk sac during craniocaudal and lateral folding of the embryo.
- The endoderm forms the epithelial lining and glands of the gut tube mucosa, whereas the splanchnic mesoderm forms all other layers.
- Opens to the yolk sac through the vitelline duct that divides the embryonic gut into the foregut, midgut, and hindgut.

B. Foregut

1. Foregut Derivatives

- Are supplied by the celiac artery.

2. Esophagus

- Develops from the narrow part of the foregut that is divided into the esophagus and trachea by the tracheoesophageal septum.

3. Stomach

- Develops as a fusiform dilation of the foregut during week 4. The primitive stomach rotates 90 degrees clockwise during its formation, causing the formation of the lesser peritoneal sac.

4. Duodenum

- Develops from the distal end of the foregut (upper duodenum) and the proximal segment of the midgut (lower duodenum).
- The junction of the foregut and midgut is at the opening of the common bile duct.

5. Liver

- Develops as an endodermal outgrowth of the foregut, the hepatic diverticulum, and is involved in hematopoiesis from week 6 and begins bile formation in week 12.
- Liver parenchymal cells and the lining of the biliary ducts are endodermal derivatives of the hepatic diverticulum, whereas the sinusoids and other blood vessels are mesodermal derivatives of the septum transversum.

(a) Hepatic Diverticulum

- Grows into the mass of splanchnic mesoderm called the septum transversum and proliferates to form the liver parenchyma and sends hepatic cell cords to surround the vitelline veins, which form hepatic sinusoids.

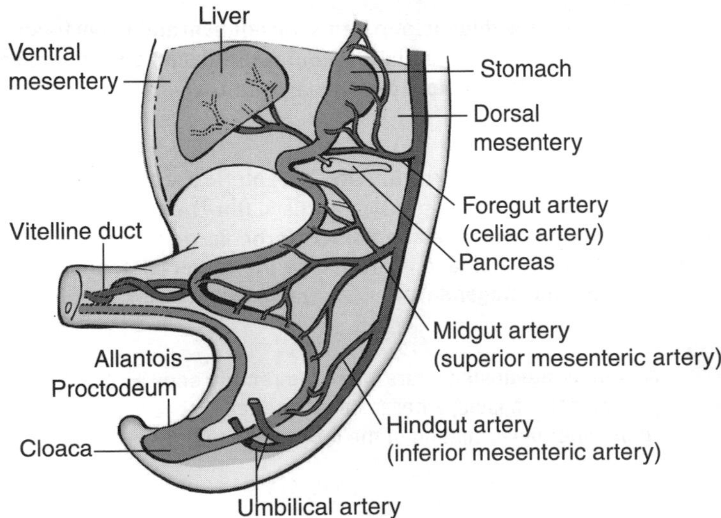

FIGURE 4.11. Formation of the midgut loop and the foregut, midgut, and hindgut arteries.

(Reprinted with permission from Langman J. *Medical embryology.* 4th ed. Baltimore, MD: Williams & Wilkins; 1981:150.)

(b) **Septum Transversum**

- Is a mesodermal mass between the developing pericardial and peritoneal cavities; gives rise to Kupffer cells and hematopoietic cells; and central tendon of the diaphragm.

6. **Gallbladder**

- Develops from the hepatic diverticulum as a solid outgrowth of cells. The end of the outgrowth expands to form the gallbladder, and the narrow portion forms the **cystic duct**. The connection between the hepatic diverticulum and foregut narrows to form the **bile duct**.

7. **Pancreas**

- Arises from the ventral and dorsal pancreatic buds from endoderm of the caudal foregut and is formed by migration of the ventral bud (head of the pancreas) to fuse with the dorsal bud (rest of the pancreas).
- The ventral pancreatic bud forms the uncinate process and part of the head of the pancreas, and the dorsal pancreatic bud forms the remaining part of the head, body, and tail of the pancreas.
- Main pancreatic duct is formed by fusion of the duct of the ventral bud with the distal part of the duct of the dorsal bud.
- Accessory pancreatic duct is formed from the proximal part of the duct of the dorsal bud.

CLINICAL CORRELATES

Annular pancreas occurs when the ventral and dorsal pancreatic buds form a ring around the duodenum, thereby obstructing it.

8. **Spleen**

- Arises from mesoderm of the dorsal mesogastrium in week 5 and is not an embryologic derivative of the foregut. It is a hematopoietic organ until week 15.

C. **Midgut**

1. **Midgut Derivatives**

- Are supplied by the superior mesenteric artery.

2. **Lower Duodenum**

- Arises from the upper portion of the midgut.

3. **The Midgut Loop**

- Is formed by rapid lengthening of the gut tube, communicates with yolk sac by way of the vitelline duct or yolk stalk, and herniates through the umbilicus during the physiologic umbilical herniation.
- Rotates 270 degrees counterclockwise around the superior mesenteric artery as it returns to the abdominal cavity.
  (a) The cranial limb of the midgut loop forms the **jejunum** and **ileum** (cranial portion).
  (b) The caudal limb forms the caudal portion of the **ileum**, **cecum**, **appendix**, **ascending colon**, and the **transverse colon** (proximal two-thirds).

D. **Hindgut**

1. **Hindgut derivatives** are supplied by the inferior mesenteric artery.
2. **Cranial end** of the hindgut forms the transverse (distal third), descending, and sigmoid colons.
3. **Caudal end** of the hindgut joins the **allantois** (diverticulum of yolk sac into body stalk) and forms the **cloaca**. The dilated **cloaca** is divided by the **urorectal septum** into the **rectum** and **anal canal** dorsally and the **urogenital sinus** ventrally, which forms the urinary bladder.

CLINICAL CORRELATES

Anorectal agenesis occurs when the rectum ends as a blind sac above the puborectalis muscle, whereas **anal agenesis** occurs when the anal canal ends as a blind sac because of abnormal formation of the urorectal septum.

E. **Proctodeum**

- Is an invagination of the ectoderm of the terminal part of the hindgut, which gives rise to the lower anal canal and the urogenital external orifice.

F. Mesenteries

- The primitive gut tube is suspended within the peritoneal cavity of the embryo by the ventral and dorsal mesenteries, from which all adult mesenteries are derived.
- **Ventral mesentery** forms the lesser omentum, falciform, coronary, and triangular ligaments.
- **Dorsal mesentery** forms the greater omentum, mesentery of the small intestine, mesoappendix, transverse mesocolon, and sigmoid mesocolon.

VIII. CELIAC AND MESENTERIC ARTERIES

A. Celiac Trunk (Figures 4.12 and 4.13)

- Arises from the front of the abdominal aorta immediately below the aortic hiatus of the diaphragm, between the right and left crura.
- Divides into the left gastric, splenic, and common hepatic arteries.

1. Left Gastric Artery

- Is the **smallest branch** of the celiac trunk.
- Runs upward and to the left toward the cardia, giving rise to **esophageal** and **hepatic branches** and then turns to the right and runs along the lesser curvature within the lesser omentum to anastomose with the right gastric artery.

2. Splenic Artery

- Is the **largest branch** of the celiac trunk and runs a highly tortuous course along the superior border of the pancreas and enters the lienorenal ligament.
- Gives rise to the following:
  - **(a)** A number of pancreatic branches, including the **dorsal pancreatic artery**.
  - **(b)** A few **short gastric arteries**, which pass through the lienogastric ligament to reach the fundus of the stomach.
  - **(c)** The **left gastroepiploic (gastro–omental) artery**, which reaches the greater omentum through the lienogastric ligament and runs along the greater curvature of the stomach to distribute to the stomach and greater omentum.

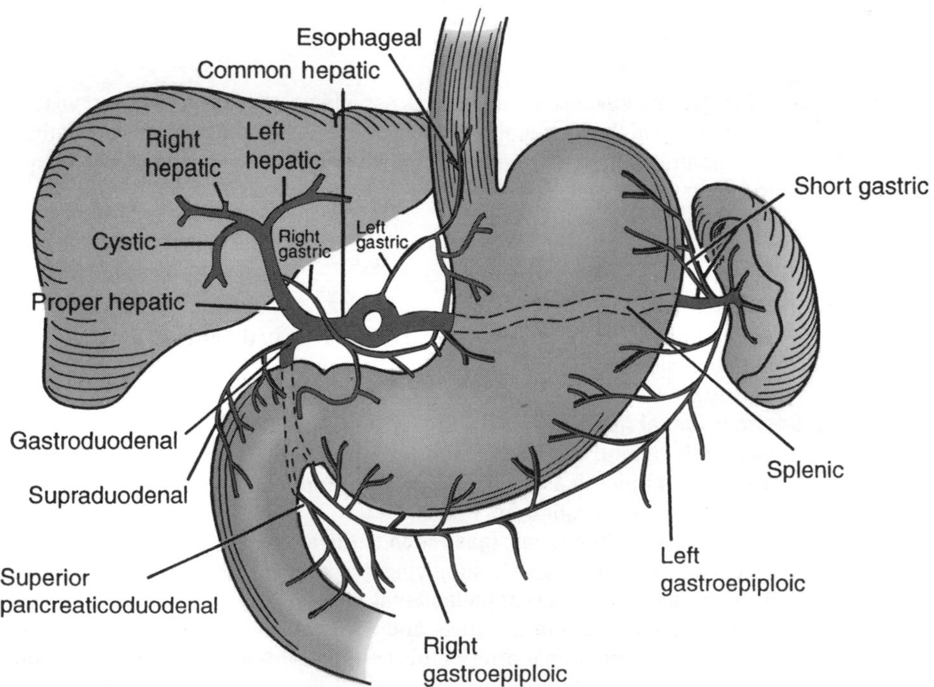

FIGURE 4.12. Branches of the celiac trunk.

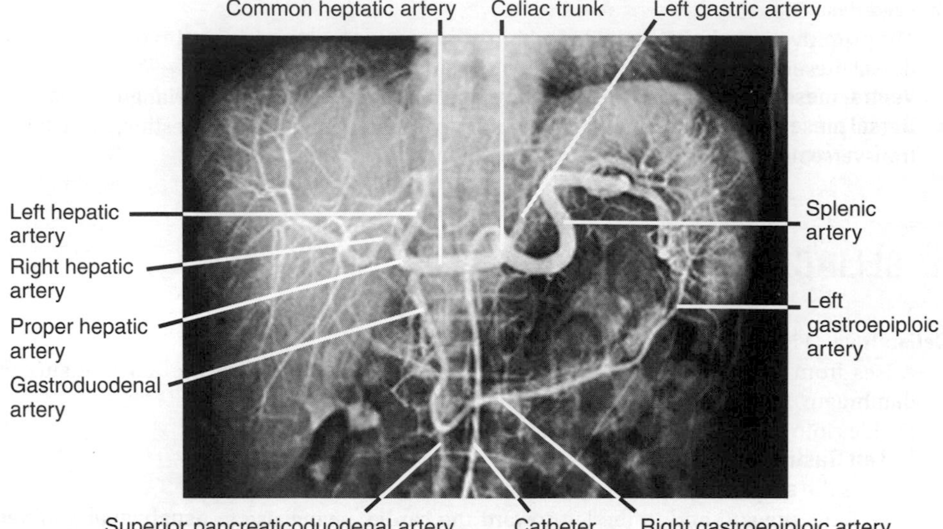

FIGURE 4.13. Celiac angiogram showing its three major branches.

(Reprinted with permission from Agur AMR, Darley AF. *Grant's Atlas of Anatomy.* 12th ed. Philadelphia, PA: Lippincott Williams & Wilkins; 2009:131.)

3. Common Hepatic Artery

- Runs to the right along the upper border of the pancreas and divides into the proper hepatic artery, the gastroduodenal artery, and possibly the right gastric artery.

(a) Proper Hepatic Artery

- Ascends in the free edge of the lesser omentum and divides, near the porta hepatis, into the **left** and **right hepatic arteries**; the right hepatic artery gives rise to the **cystic artery** in the **cystohepatic triangle of Calot** (bounded by the common hepatic duct, cystic duct, and inferior surface of the liver).
- Gives rise, near its beginning, to the **right** gastric artery.

CLINICAL CORRELATES

Pringle maneuver is a temporary cross-clamping (intermittent soft vascular clamping) of the hepatoduodenal ligament containing portal triads at the foramen of Winslow for control of hepatic bleeding during liver surgery or donor hepatectomy for living donor liver transplantation.

(b) Right Gastric Artery

- Arises from the proper hepatic or common hepatic artery, runs to the pylorus and then along the lesser curvature of the stomach, and anastomoses with the left gastric artery.

(c) Gastroduodenal Artery

- Descends behind the first part of the duodenum, giving off the supraduodenal artery to its superior aspect and a few retroduodenal arteries to its inferior aspect.
- Divides into two major branches:
  1. The **right gastroepiploic (gastro–omental) artery** runs to the left along the greater curvature of the stomach, supplying the stomach and the greater omentum.
  2. The **superior pancreaticoduodenal artery** passes between the duodenum and the head of the pancreas and further divides into the anterior–superior pancreaticoduodenal artery and the posterior–superior pancreaticoduodenal artery.

B. **Superior Mesenteric Artery** (Figure 4.14)

- Arises from the aorta behind the neck of the pancreas.
- Descends across the uncinate process of the pancreas and the third part of the duodenum and then enters the root of the mesentery behind the transverse colon to run to the right iliac fossa.
- Gives rise to the following branches:

1. **Inferior Pancreaticoduodenal Artery**

- Passes to the right and divides into the anterior-inferior pancreaticoduodenal artery and the posterior-inferior pancreaticoduodenal artery, which anastomose with the corresponding branches of the superior pancreaticoduodenal artery.

2. **Middle Colic Artery**

- Enters the transverse mesocolon and divides into the **right branch**, which anastomoses with the right colic artery, and the **left branch**, which anastomoses with the ascending branch of the left colic artery. The branches of the mesenteric arteries form an anastomotic channel, the **marginal artery**, along the large intestine.

3. **Right Colic Artery**

- Arises from the superior mesenteric artery or the ileocolic artery.
- Runs to the right behind the peritoneum and divides into **ascending and descending branches**, distributing to the ascending colon.

4. **Ileocolic Artery**

- Descends behind the peritoneum toward the right iliac fossa and ends by dividing into the **ascending colic artery**, which anastomoses with the right colic artery, **anterior and posterior cecal arteries**, the **appendicular artery**, and **ileal branches.**

5. **Intestinal Arteries**

- Are 12 to 15 in number and supply the jejunum and ileum.
- Branch and anastomose to form a series of arcades in the mesentery.

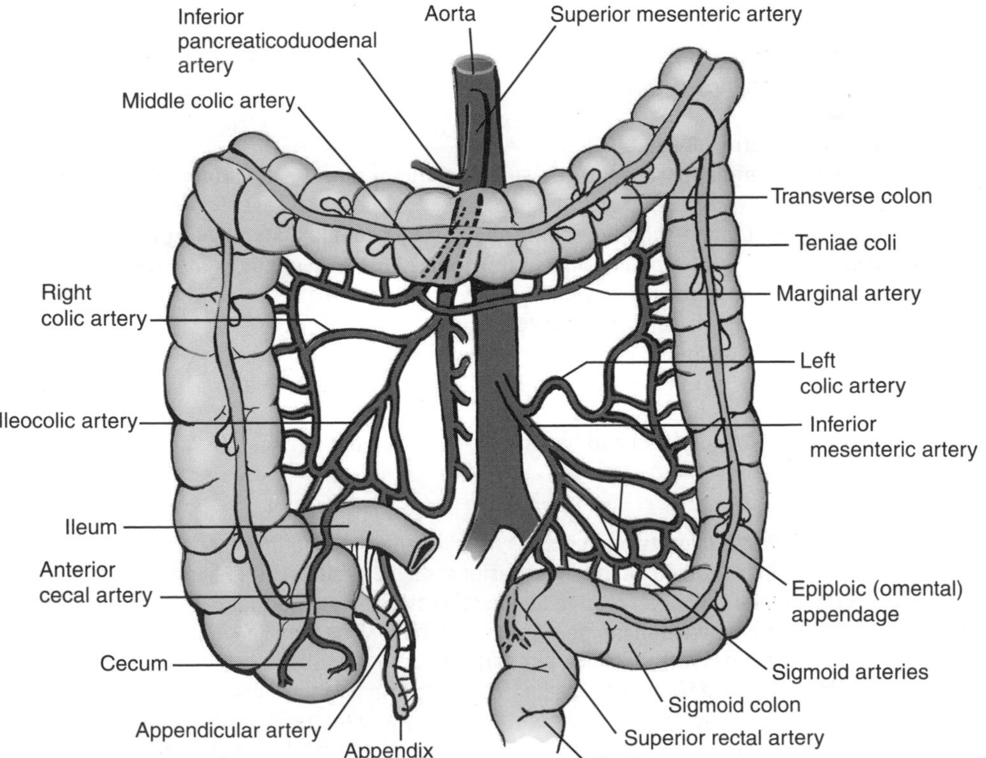

FIGURE 4.14. Branches of the superior and inferior mesenteric arteries.

CLINICAL CORRELATES **Superior mesenteric artery obstruction** is caused by a thrombus, an embolus, atherosclerosis, an aortic aneurysm, a tumor in the uncinate process of the pancreas, compression by the third part of the duodenum, or surgical scar tissue. The obstruction leads to small and large intestinal ischemia, resulting in necrosis of all or part of the involved intestinal segment. Symptoms are abdominal pain, nausea, vomiting, diarrhea, and electrolyte imbalance.

C. Inferior Mesenteric Artery (See Figure 4.14)

- Passes to the left behind the peritoneum and distributes to the descending and sigmoid colons and the upper portion of the rectum.
- Gives rise to:

1. Left Colic Artery

- Runs to the left behind the peritoneum toward the descending colon and divides into **ascending and descending branches.**

2. Sigmoid Arteries

- Are two to three in number, run toward the sigmoid colon in its mesentery, and divide into ascending and descending branches.

3. Superior Rectal Artery

- Is the **termination of the inferior mesenteric artery**, descends into the pelvis, divides into two branches that follow the sides of the rectum, and anastomoses with the middle and inferior rectal arteries. (The middle and inferior rectal arteries arise from the internal iliac and internal pudendal arteries, respectively.)

IX. HEPATIC PORTAL VENOUS SYSTEM

- Is a system of vessels in which blood collected from one capillary bed (of intestine) passes through the portal vein and then through a second capillary network (liver sinusoids) before reaching the IVC (systemic circulation).

A. Portal Vein (See Figures 4.8 and 4.15)

- Drains the abdominal part of the gut, spleen, pancreas, and gallbladder and is 8 cm (3.2 in.) long.
- Is formed by the union of the **splenic vein** and the **superior mesenteric vein** posterior to the neck of the pancreas. The **inferior mesenteric vein** joins either the splenic or the superior mesenteric vein or the junction of these two veins.
- Receives the **left gastric (or coronary) vein.**
- Carries deoxygenated blood containing nutrients.
- Carries three times as much blood as the hepatic artery and maintains a higher blood pressure than in the IVC.
- Ascends behind the bile duct and hepatic artery within the free margin of the lesser omentum.

CLINICAL CORRELATES **Portal hypertension** results from liver cirrhosis or thrombosis in the portal vein, forming **esophageal varices, caput medusae**, and **hemorrhoids**. It can be treated by diverting blood from the portal to the caval system by the **portacaval shunt**, achieved by creating a communication between the portal vein and the IVC, as they lie close together below the liver, or by the **splenorenal** (Warren) **shunt**, accomplished by anastomosing the splenic vein to the left renal vein. Portal hypertension can also be treated by **transjugular intrahepatic portosystemic shunt** (TIPS), in which a catheter is placed percutaneously into the right internal jugular vein through which an intrahepatic shunt is created between a hepatic vein and a branch of the portal vein within the liver, followed by placement of an expandable stent in the created tract or channel, and thus blood flows from the portal vein into the hepatic vein and then into IVC.

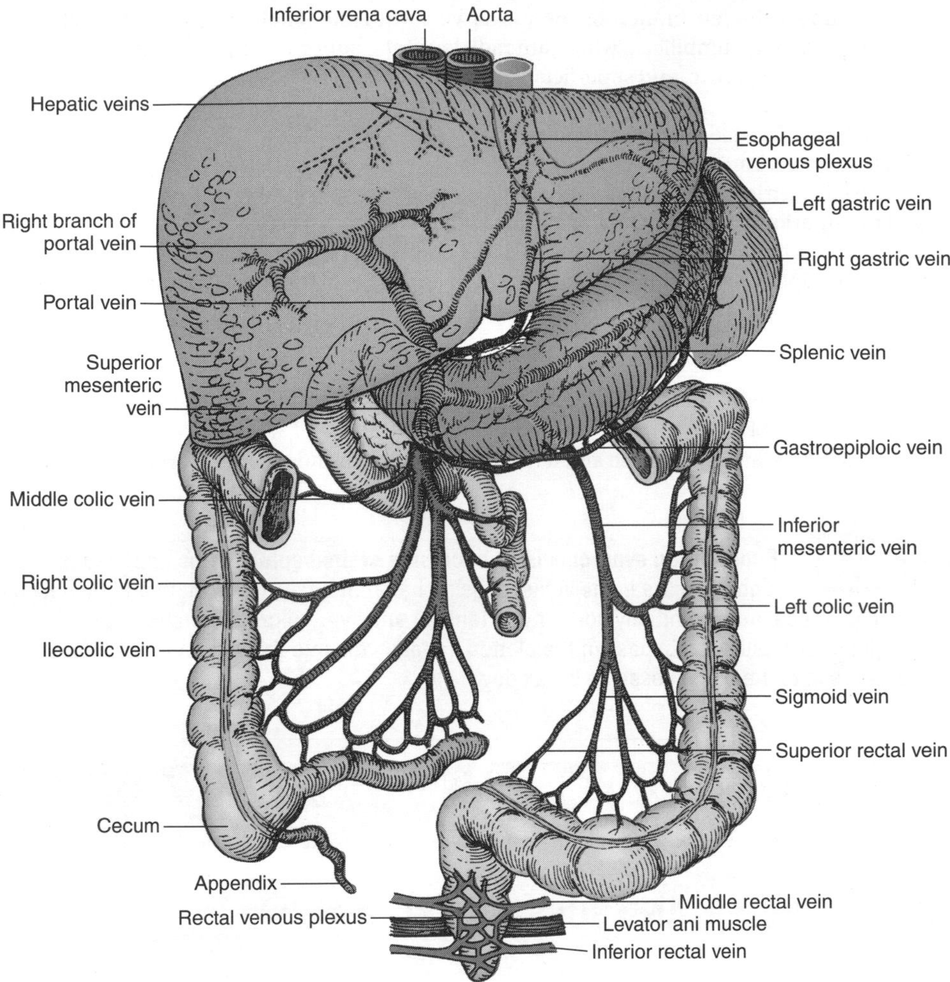

FIGURE 4.15. Portal venous system.

1. **Superior Mesenteric Vein**
   - Accompanies the superior mesenteric artery on its right side in the root of the mesentery.
   - Crosses the third part of the duodenum and the uncinate process of the pancreas and terminates posterior to the neck of the pancreas by joining the splenic vein, thereby forming the portal vein.
   - Has tributaries that are some of the veins that accompany the branches of the superior mesenteric artery.
2. **Splenic Vein**
   - Is formed by the union of tributaries from the spleen.
   - Receives the short gastric, left gastroepiploic, and pancreatic veins.
3. **Inferior Mesenteric Vein**
   - Is formed by the union of the superior rectal and sigmoid veins.
   - Receives the left colic vein and usually drains into the splenic vein, but it may drain into the superior mesenteric vein or the junction of the superior mesenteric and splenic veins.
4. **Left Gastric (Coronary) Vein**
   - Drains normally into the portal vein.
   - Has **esophageal tributaries** that anastomose with the esophageal veins of the azygos system at the lower part of the esophagus and thereby enter the systemic venous system.
5. **Paraumbilical Veins**
   - Are found in the **falciform ligament** and are virtually closed; however, they dilate in **portal hypertension**.

- Connect the left branch of the portal vein with the small subcutaneous veins in the region of the umbilicus, which are radicles of the superior epigastric, inferior epigastric, thoracoepigastric, and superficial epigastric veins.

B. Important Portal–Caval (Systemic) Anastomoses

- These structures are located between:
  1. The left gastric vein and the esophageal vein of the azygos system.
  2. The superior rectal vein and the middle and inferior rectal veins.
  3. The paraumbilical veins and radicles of the epigastric (superficial and inferior) veins.
  4. The retroperitoneal veins draining the colon and twigs of the renal, suprarenal, and gonadal veins.

C. Hepatic Veins

- Consist of the right, middle, and left hepatic veins that lie in the intersegmental planes and converge on the IVC.
- Have no valves, and the middle and left veins frequently unite before entering the vena cava.

CLINICAL CORRELATES **Budd–Chiari syndrome** is an **occlusion of the hepatic veins** and results in high pressure in the veins, causing hepatomegaly, upper right abdominal pain, ascites, mild jaundice, and eventually portal hypertension and liver failure. It can be treated by balloon angioplasty or surgical bypass of the clotted hepatic vein into the vena cava or infusion of thrombolytics in to the blood vessel to break down clot.

RETROPERITONEAL VISCERA, DIAPHRAGM, AND POSTERIOR ABDOMINAL WALL

I. KIDNEY, URETER, AND SUPRARENAL GLAND

A. Kidney (See Figures 4.8 and 4.16)

- Is retroperitoneal and extends from T12 to L3 vertebrae in the erect position. The right kidney lies a little lower than the left because of the large size of the right lobe of the liver. The right kidney usually is related to rib 12 posteriorly, whereas the left kidney is related to ribs 11 and 12 posteriorly.
- Is invested by a firm, fibrous **renal capsule** and is surrounded by the renal fascia, which divides the fat into two regions. The **perirenal (perinephric) fat** lies in the **perinephric space** between the renal capsule and renal fascia, and the **pararenal (paranephric) fat** lies external to the renal fascia.
- Has an indentation—the **hilus**—on its medial border, through which the ureter, renal vessels, and nerves enter or leave the organ.
- Consists of the **medulla** and **cortex**, containing 1 to 2 million **nephrons** (in each kidney), which are the anatomic and functional units of the kidney. Each nephron consists of a **renal corpuscle** (found only in the cortex), **a proximal convoluted tubule**, **Henle loop**, and **a distal convoluted tubule**.
- Has arterial segments, including the **superior**, **anterosuperior**, **anteroinferior**, **inferior**, and **posterior segments**, which are of surgical importance.
- Filters blood to **produce urine**; reabsorbs nutrients, essential ions, and water; **excretes urine** (by which metabolic [toxic] waste products are eliminated) and foreign substances; **regulates the salt, ion (electrolyte)**, and **water balance**; and **produces erythropoietin**.
- Also **produces renin** by juxtaglomerular cells (in the wall of the afferent arterioles), which converts plasma protein angiotensinogen to angiotensin I (inactive decapeptide), which is converted to angiotensin II (potent vasoconstrictor) by enzymes in the lung endothelial cells. The angiotensin II increases blood pressure and volume and stimulates aldosterone production by the suprarenal cortex, thereby regulating the salt, ion, and water balance between the blood and urine.

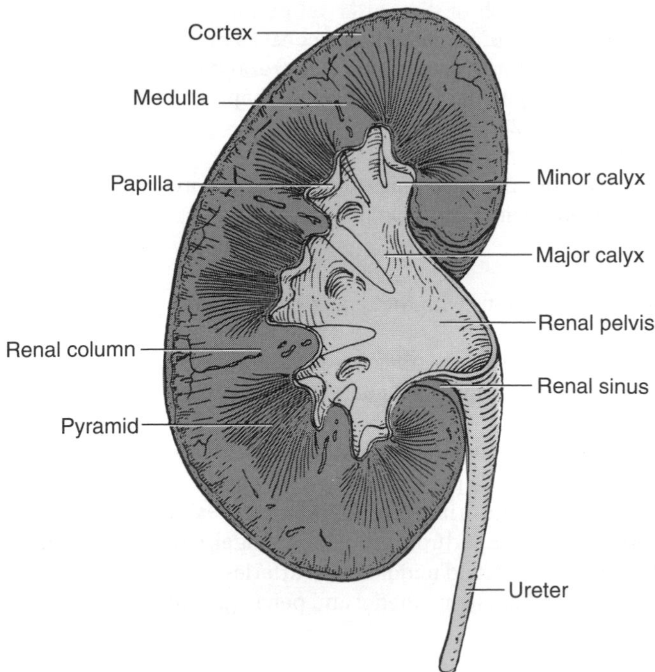

FIGURE 4.16. Frontal section of the kidney.

CLINICAL CORRELATES

Pelvic kidney is an **ectopic kidney** that occurs when kidneys fail to ascend and thus remain in the pelvis. Two pelvic kidneys may fuse to form a solid lobed organ because of fusion of the renal anlagen, called a **cake (rosette) kidney**.

Horseshoe kidney develops as a result of fusion of the lower poles of two kidneys and may obstruct the urinary tract by its impingement on the ureters.

Nephroptosis is downward displacement of the kidney, **dropped kidney**, or **floating kidney** caused by loss of supporting fat. The kidney moves freely in the abdomen and even into the pelvis. It may cause a kink in the ureter or compression of the ureter by an aberrant inferior polar artery, resulting in hydronephrosis.

Polycystic kidney disease is a genetic disorder characterized by numerous cysts filled with fluid in the kidney; the cysts can slowly replace much of normal kidney tissues, reducing kidney function and leading to kidney failure. It is caused by a failure of the collecting tubules to join a distal convoluted tubule, which causes dilations of the loops of Henle, resulting in progressive renal dysfunction. This kidney disease has symptoms of high blood pressure, pain in the back and side, headaches, and blood in the urine. It may be treated by hemodialysis or peritoneal dialysis and kidney transplantation.

CLINICAL CORRELATES

Kidney stone (renal calculus or nephrolith) is formed by combination of a high level of calcium with oxalate, phosphate, urea, uric acid, and cystine. Crystals and subsequently stones are formed in the urine and collected in calyces of the kidney or in the ureter. The kidney stone varies in size from a grain of sand to the size of a golf ball and produces severe **colicky pain** while traveling down through the ureter from the kidney to the bladder. Common signs of kidney stones include nausea and vomiting, urinary frequency and urgency, and pain during urination.

1. **Cortex**
   - Forms the outer part of the kidney and also projects into the medullary region between the renal pyramids as **renal columns**.
   - Contains renal corpuscles and proximal and distal convoluted tubules. The **renal corpuscle** consists of the **glomerulus** (a tuft of capillaries) surrounded by a **glomerular (Bowman) capsule**, which is the invaginated blind end of the nephron.

2. Medulla

- Forms the inner part of the kidney and consists of 8 to 12 **renal pyramids** (of Malpighi), which contain straight tubules (**Henle loops**) and **collecting tubules**. An apex of the renal pyramid, the **renal papilla**, fits into the cup-shaped **minor calyx** on which the collecting tubules open (10 to 25 openings).

3. Minor Calyces

- Receive urine from the collecting tubules and empty into two or three **major calyces**, which in turn empty into an upper dilated portion of the ureter, the **renal pelvis**.

B. Ureter

- Is a **muscular tube** that begins with the renal pelvis, extending from the kidney to the **urinary bladder**.
- Is retroperitoneal, descends on the transverse processes of the lumbar vertebrae and the psoas muscle, is crossed anteriorly by the gonadal vessels, and crosses the bifurcation of the common iliac artery.
- May be obstructed by renal calculi (kidney stones) where it joins the renal pelvis (**ureteropelvic junction**), where it crosses the pelvic brim over the distal end of the common iliac artery, or where it enters the wall of the urinary bladder (**ureterovesicular junction**).
- Receives blood from the aorta and from the renal, gonadal, common, and internal iliac, umbilical, superior and inferior vesical, and middle rectal arteries.
- Is innervated by the lumbar (sympathetic) and pelvic (parasympathetic) splanchnic nerves.

CLINICAL CORRELATES

Obstruction of the ureter occurs by renal calculi or kidney stones where the ureter joins the renal pelvis (ureteropelvic junction), where it crosses the pelvic brim, or where it enters the wall of the urinary bladder (ureterovesicular junction). Kidney stones at these narrow points result in hydroureter and hydronephrosis.

Hydronephrosis is a **fluid-filled enlargement of the renal pelvis** and **calyces** as a result of obstruction of the ureter. It is due to an obstruction of urine flow by kidney stones in the ureter, by compression on the ureter by abnormal blood vessels, or by the developing fetus at the pelvic brim. It has symptoms of nausea and vomiting, urinary tract infection, fever, dysuria (painful or difficult urination), urinary frequency, and urinary urgency.

C. Suprarenal (Adrenal) Gland (Figure 4.17)

- Is a retroperitoneal organ lying on the superomedial aspect of the kidney. It is surrounded by a capsule and renal fascia.

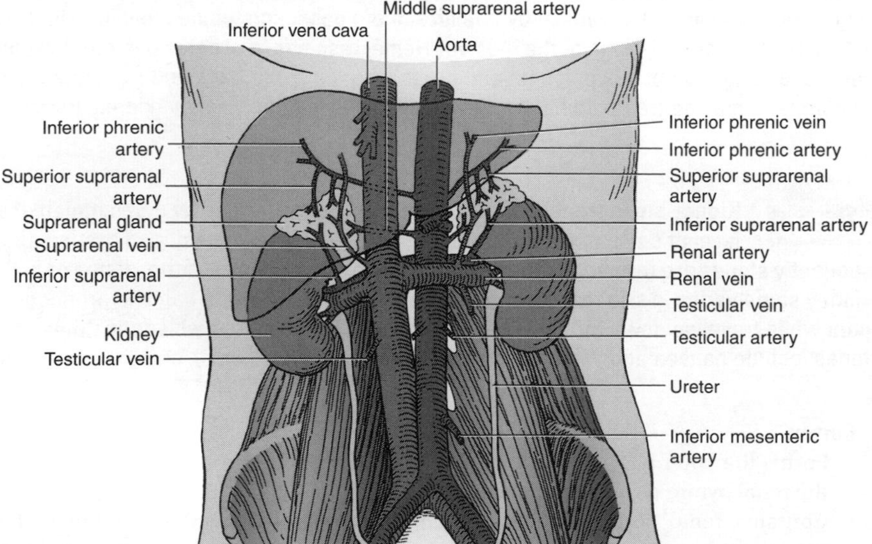

FIGURE 4.17. Suprarenal glands, kidneys, and abdominal aorta and its branches.

- Is **pyramidal** on the right and **semilunar** on the left.
- Has a **cortex** that is essential to life and produces three types of steroid hormones. The outer zona glomerulosa produces mineralocorticoids, mainly aldosterones ('**s**alt' steroids); the middle zona fasciculata produces glucocorticoids, mainly cortisol and corticosterone ('**e**nergy' steroids); and the inner zona reticularis produces androgens ('se**x**' steroids); thus, the mnemonic is **SEX**. Aldosterone controls electrolyte (sodium, potassium, etc.) and water balance; cortisol controls glucose regulation and suppresses immune response; and androgen controls sexual development (maleness).
- Has a **medulla** that is derived from embryonic neural crest cells, receives preganglionic sympathetic nerve fibers directly, and secretes epinephrine and norepinephrine.
- Receives arteries from three sources: the superior suprarenal artery from the **inferior phrenic artery**, the middle suprarenal artery from the abdominal **aorta**, and the inferior suprarenal artery from the **renal artery**.
- Is drained via the suprarenal vein, which empties into the **IVC** on the right and the **renal vein** on the left.

CLINICAL CORRELATES

Addison's disease is a disorder caused by an **adrenocortical insufficiency** (insufficient production of cortisol and, in some cases, aldosterone) caused by autoimmune destruction of the suprarenal cortex or tuberculosis. Symptoms include muscle weakness, loss of appetite, weight loss, fatigue, low blood pressure, and darkening of the skin, as well as nausea, vomiting, and diarrhea.

Disorders of the suprarenal cortex are caused by an excess production of glucocorticoids (**Cushing syndrome**) or aldosterone (**Conn syndrome**) or by androgens (**hirsutism**) associated with hyperplasia or tumor of the suprarenal cortex or the anterior pituitary gland. Signs and symptoms are trunk obesity, moon face, muscle weakness, high blood pressure, high blood sugar, and kyphosis for Cushing syndrome; hypertension, headache, muscle cramps, fatigue, polyuria, and polydipsia for Conn syndrome; and excess hair growth in both males and females but a male pattern of hair distribution in females for hirsutism.

II. DEVELOPMENT OF KIDNEY, URINARY BLADDER, AND SUPRARENAL GLAND

- Kidney and suprarenal cortex develop from mesoderm, but suprarenal medulla develops from neural crest cells.

A. Kidney

- Develops from the intermediate mesoderm that forms the nephrogenic cord in longitudinal ridge.
- Develops from the last of three sets of kidneys: pronephros, mesonephros, and metanephros.
  1. The **pronephros** appears early, degenerates rapidly, and never forms functional nephrons.
  2. The **mesonephros** largely degenerates but forms the **mesonephric (Wolffian) duct**, which forms the **ureteric bud** and contributes to the **male reproductive tract**.
  3. The **metanephros** develops from the ureteric bud and forms the permanent kidney, which ascends from the sacral region to the upper lumbar region.
     - **(a)** Ureteric bud forms the ureter, which dilates at its upper end to form the renal pelvis. The renal pelvis repeatedly divides to form the major calyces, the minor calyces, and collecting tubules.
     - **(b)** Metanephric mesoderm forms the nephrons of adult kidney (glomerulus, renal capsule, proximal convoluted tubules, and loop of Henle), distal convoluted tubules, and collecting tubules forms from ureteric bud as stated above under (a).
  4. The **urogenital** sinus forms from the hindgut. The urorectal septum divides the cloaca into the rectum and anal canal posteriorly and the urogenital sinus anteriorly, which forms the bladder and part of the urethra.

B. Urinary Bladder

- Develops from the upper end of the **urogenital sinus**, which is continuous with the allantois.
  1. The **allantois** degenerates and forms a fibrous cord in the adult called the urachus.
  2. The **trigone** of the bladder is formed by the incorporation of the lower end of **the** mesonephric ducts into the posterior wall of the urogenital sinus.

C. Suprarenal Gland

1. The **cortex** forms as a result of two waves of **mesoderm** proliferation.
   - **(a)** The first wave of the coelomic mesothelial cells forms the fetal cortex.
   - **(b)** The second wave of cells surrounds the fetal cortex and forms the adult cortex.
2. The **medulla** forms from **neural crest cells**, which migrate to the fetal cortex and differentiate into chromaffin cells.

III. POSTERIOR ABDOMINAL BLOOD VESSELS AND LYMPHATICS

A. Aorta (See Figures 4.8 and 4.17)

- Passes through the **aortic hiatus** in the diaphragm at the level of T12, descends anterior to the vertebral bodies, and bifurcates into the **right and left common iliac arteries** anterior to L4.
- Gives rise to the following:

1. **Inferior Phrenic Arteries**
   - Arise from the aorta immediately below the aortic hiatus, supply the diaphragm, and give rise to the **superior suprarenal arteries.**
   - Diverge across the crura of the diaphragm, with the left artery passing posterior to the esophagus and the right artery passing posterior to the IVC.
2. **Middle Suprarenal Arteries**
   - Arise from the aorta and run laterally on the crura of the diaphragm just superior to the renal arteries.
3. **Renal Arteries**
   - Arise from the aorta inferior to the origin of the superior mesenteric artery. The right artery is longer and a little lower than the left and passes posterior to the IVC; the left artery passes posterior to the left renal vein.
   - Give rise to the inferior suprarenal and ureteric arteries.
   - Divide into the superior, anterosuperior, anteroinferior, inferior, and posterior segmental branches.
4. **Testicular or Ovarian Arteries**
   - Descend retroperitoneally and run laterally on the psoas major muscle and across the ureter.
     - **(a)** The **testicular artery** accompanies the ductus deferens into the scrotum, where it supplies the spermatic cord, epididymis, and testis.
     - **(b)** The **ovarian artery** enters the suspensory ligament of the ovary, supplies the ovary, and anastomoses with the ovarian branch of the uterine artery.
5. **Lumbar Arteries**
   - Consist of four or five pairs that arise from the back of the aorta.
   - Run posterior to the sympathetic trunk, the IVC (on the right side), the psoas major muscle, the lumbar plexus, and the quadratus lumborum.
   - Divide into smaller anterior branches (to supply adjacent muscles) and larger posterior branches, which accompany the dorsal primary rami of the corresponding spinal nerves and divide into spinal and muscular branches.
6. **Middle Sacral Artery**
   - Arises from the back of the aorta, just above its bifurcation; descends on the front of the sacrum; and ends in the coccygeal body.
   - Supplies the rectum and anal canal, and anastomoses with the lateral sacral and superior and inferior rectal arteries.

B. Inferior Vena Cava

- Is formed on the right side of L5 by the union of the two **common iliac veins**, below the bifurcation of the aorta.
- Is longer than the abdominal aorta and ascends along the right side of the aorta.
- Passes through the **opening for the IVC** in the central tendon of the diaphragm at the level of T8 and enters the right atrium of the heart.
- Receives the right gonadal, suprarenal, and inferior phrenic veins. On the left side, these veins usually drain into the left renal vein.
- Also receives the three (left, middle, and right) **hepatic veins**. The middle and left hepatic veins frequently unite for approximately 1 cm before entering the vena cava.
- Receives the right and left renal veins. The left renal vein runs posterior to the superior mesenteric artery and anterior to the abdominal aorta.

C. Cisterna Chyli

- Is the lower dilated end of the **thoracic duct** and lies just to the right and posterior to the aorta, usually between two crura of the diaphragm.
- Is formed by the **intestinal and lumbar lymph trunks.**

D. Lymph Nodes Related to the Aorta

1. Preaortic Nodes

- Include the celiac, superior mesenteric, and inferior mesenteric nodes; drain the lymph from the GI tract, spleen, pancreas, gallbladder, and liver; and their efferent vessels form the intestinal trunk.

2. Para-aortic, Lumbar, or Lateral Aortic Lymph Nodes

- Drain lymph from the kidneys, suprarenal glands, testes or ovaries, uterus, and uterine tubes; receive lymph from the common, internal, or external iliac; and their efferent vessels form the right and left lumbar trunks.

IV. NERVES OF THE POSTERIOR ABDOMINAL WALL

A. Lumbar Plexus (See Figure 4.18)

- Is formed by the union of the ventral rami of the first three lumbar nerves and a part of the fourth lumbar nerve.
- Lies anterior to the transverse processes of the lumbar vertebrae within the substance of the psoas muscle.

1. Subcostal Nerve (T12)

- Runs behind the lateral lumbocostal arch and in front of the quadratus lumborum.
- Penetrates the transverse abdominal muscle to run between it and the internal oblique muscle.
- Innervates the **external oblique**, **internal oblique**, **transverse**, **rectus abdominis**, and **pyramidalis muscles**.

2. Iliohypogastric Nerve (L1)

- Emerges from the lateral border of the psoas muscle and runs in front of the quadratus lumborum.
- Pierces the transverse abdominal muscle near the iliac crest to run between this muscle and the internal oblique muscle.
- Pierces the internal oblique muscle and then continues medially deep to the external oblique muscle.
- Innervates the internal oblique and transverse muscles of the abdomen and divides into an **anterior cutaneous branch**, which innervates the skin above the pubis, and a **lateral cutaneous branch**, which innervates the skin of the gluteal region.

3. Ilioinguinal Nerve (L1)

- Runs in front of the quadratus lumborum, piercing the transverse and then the internal oblique muscle to run between the internal and external oblique aponeuroses.
- Accompanies the **spermatic cord (or the round ligament of the uterus)**, continues through the inguinal canal, and emerges through the superficial inguinal ring (see Figure 4.3).

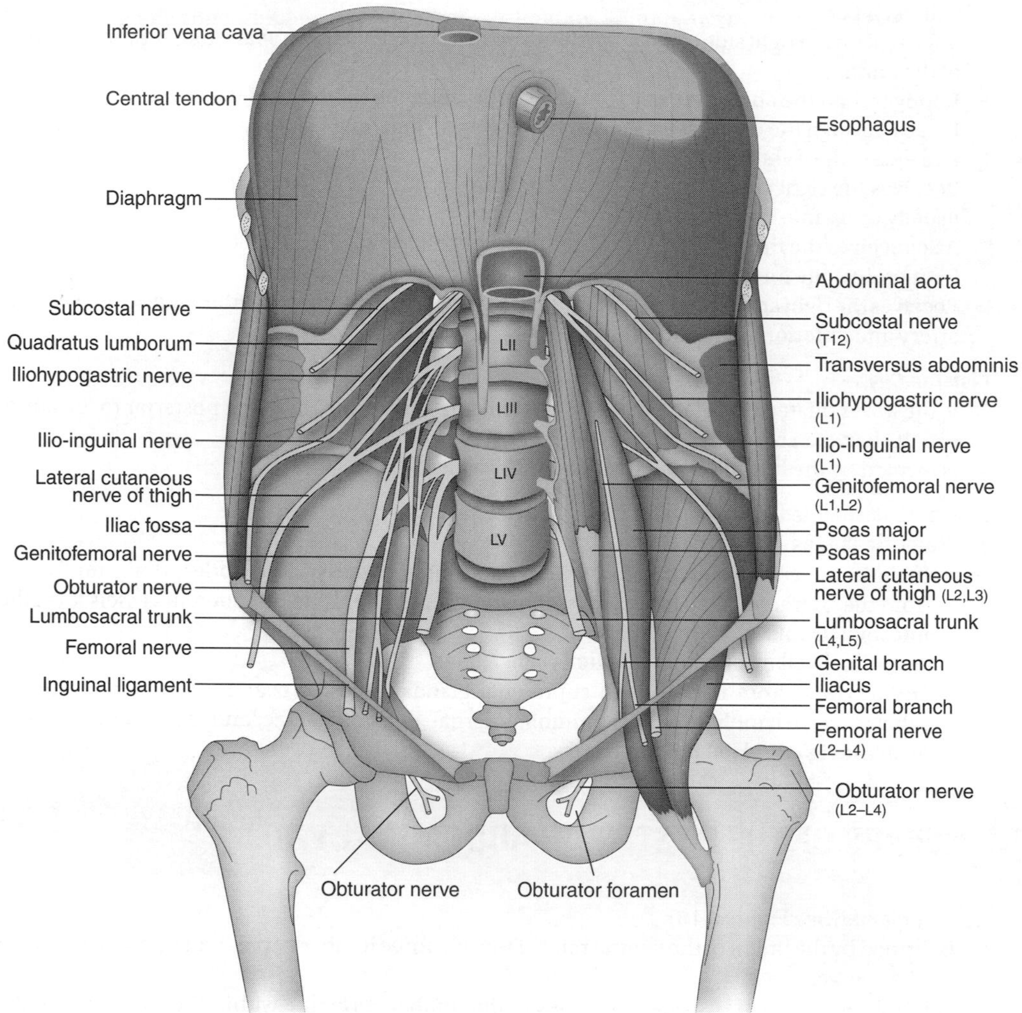

FIGURE 4.18. Lumbar plexus, diaphragm, and posterior abdominal wall.

- Innervates the internal oblique and transverse muscles and gives off **femoral cutaneous branches** to the upper medial part of the thigh and **anterior scrotal or labial branches**.

4. **Genitofemoral Nerve (L1–L2)**
   - Emerges on the front of the psoas muscle and descends on its anterior surface.
   - Divides into a **genital branch**, which enters the inguinal canal through the deep inguinal ring to reach the spermatic cord and supply the cremaster muscle and the scrotum (or labium majus), and a **femoral branch**, which supplies the skin of the femoral triangle.
5. **Lateral Femoral Cutaneous Nerve (L2–L3)**
   - Emerges from the lateral side of the psoas muscle and runs in front of the iliacus and behind the inguinal ligament.
   - Innervates the skin of the anterior and lateral thigh.
6. **Femoral Nerve (L2–L4)**
   - Emerges from the lateral border of the psoas major and descends in the groove between the psoas and iliacus.
   - Enters the femoral triangle deep to the inguinal ligament and lateral to the femoral vessels, outside the femoral sheath, and divides into numerous branches.
   - Innervates the skin of the thigh and leg, the muscles of the front of the thigh, and the hip and knee joints.
   - Innervates the quadriceps femoris, pectineus, and sartorius muscles and gives rise to the **anterior femoral cutaneous nerve** and the **saphenous nerve**.

7. Obturator Nerve (L2–L4)

- Arises from the second, third, and fourth lumbar nerves and descends along the medial border of the psoas muscle. It runs forward on the lateral wall of the pelvis and enters the thigh through the **obturator foramen**.
- Divides into **anterior** and **posterior branches** and innervates the adductor group of muscles, the pectineus, the hip and knee joints, and the skin of the medial side of the thigh.

8. Accessory Obturator Nerve (L3–L4)

- Is present in approximately 9% of the population.
- Descends medial to the psoas muscle, passes over the superior pubic ramus, and supplies the hip joint and the pectineus muscle.

9. Lumbosacral Trunk (L4–L5)

- Is formed by the lower part of the fourth lumbar nerve and all of the fifth lumbar nerve, which enters into the formation of the sacral plexus.

B. Autonomic Nerves in the Abdomen (See Figure 4.19)

1. Autonomic Ganglia

(a) Sympathetic Chain (Paravertebral) Ganglia

- Are composed primarily of ascending and descending preganglionic sympathetic general visceral efferent (GVE) fibers and general visceral afferent (GVA) fibers with cell bodies located in the dorsal root ganglia.
- Also contain cell bodies of the postganglionic sympathetic fibers.

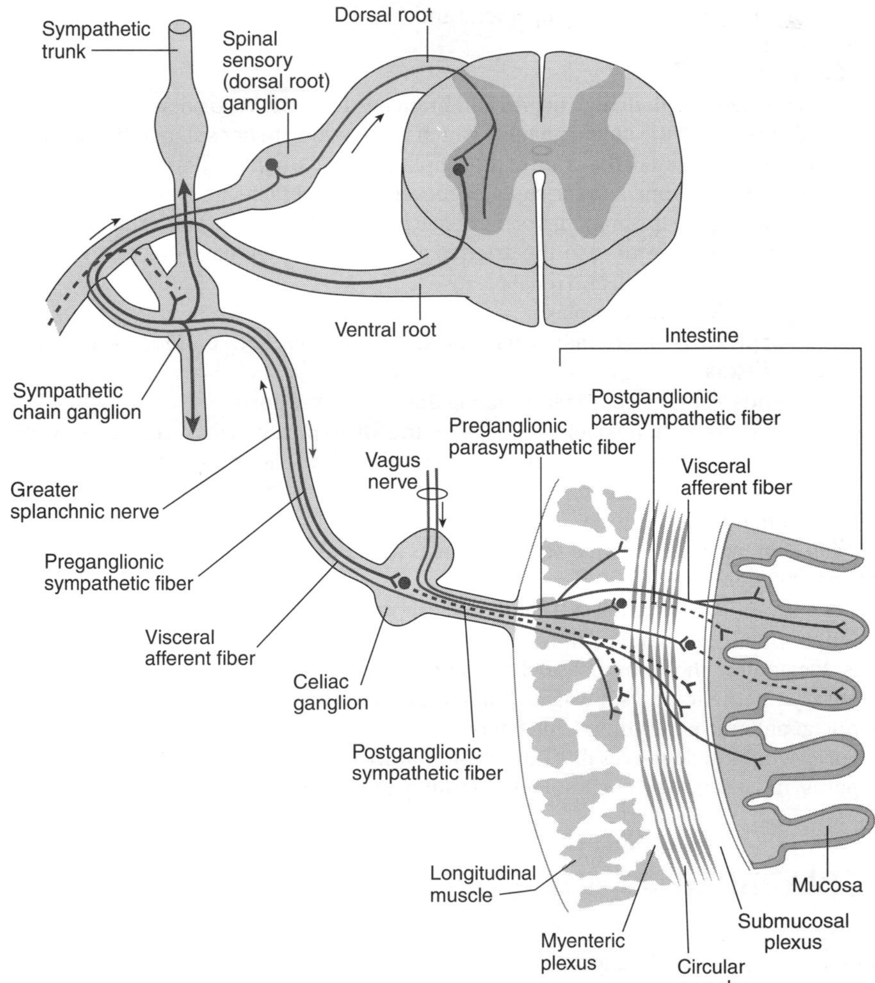

FIGURE 4.19. Nerve supply to the viscera.

(b) Collateral (Prevertebral) Ganglia

- Include the celiac, superior mesenteric, aorticorenal, and inferior mesenteric ganglia, usually located near the origin of the respective arteries.
- Are formed by cell bodies of the postganglionic sympathetic fibers.
- Receive preganglionic sympathetic fibers by way of the **greater**, **lesser**, and **least splanchnic nerves.**

(c) Para-aortic Bodies

- Are also called aortic bodies, Zuckerkandl bodies, **organs of Zuckerkandl**, or aortic glomera.
- Are small masses of chromaffin cells found near the sympathetic chain ganglia along the abdominal aorta and serve as chemoreceptors responsive to lack of oxygen, excess of carbon dioxide, and increased hydrogen ion concentration that help to control respiration.

2. Splanchnic Nerves

(a) Thoracic Splanchnic Nerves

- Contain preganglionic sympathetic (GVE) fibers, with cell bodies located in the lateral horn (intermediolateral cell column) of the spinal cord, and GVA fibers, with cell bodies located in the dorsal root ganglia.
- The greater splanchnic nerve enters the celiac ganglion, the lesser splanchnic nerve enters the aorticorenal ganglion, and the least splanchnic nerve joins the renal plexus.

(b) Lumbar Splanchnic Nerves

- Arise from the lumbar sympathetic trunks and join the celiac, mesenteric, aortic, and superior hypogastric plexuses.
- Contain preganglionic sympathetic and GVA fibers.

3. Autonomic Plexuses

(a) Celiac Plexus

- Is formed by splanchnic nerves and branches from the vagus nerves.
- Also contains the **celiac ganglia**, which receive the greater splanchnic nerves.
- Lies on the front of the crura of the diaphragm and on the abdominal aorta at the origins of the celiac trunk and the superior mesenteric and renal arteries.
- Extends along the branches of the celiac trunk and forms the **subsidiary plexuses**, which are named according to the arteries along which they pass, such as gastric, splenic, hepatic, suprarenal, and renal plexuses.
- Is also called the solar plexus.
- Solar plexus is the combined nerve plexus of the celiac and superior mesenteric plexuses.

(b) Aortic Plexus

- Extends from the celiac plexus along the front of the aorta.
- Extends its branches along the arteries and forms plexuses that are named accordingly—superior mesenteric, testicular (or ovarian), and inferior mesenteric.
- Continues along the aorta and forms the **superior hypogastric plexus** just below the bifurcation of the aorta.

(c) Superior and Inferior Hypogastric Plexuses (See Pelvis: X. B. Autonomic Nerves, Chapter 5)

4. Enteric Division

- Consists of **the myenteric (Auerbach) plexus**, which is located chiefly between the longitudinal and circular muscle layers, and the **submucosal (Meissner) plexus**, which is located in the submucosa. Both parts consist of preganglionic and postganglionic parasympathetic fibers, postganglionic sympathetic fibers, GVA fibers, and cell bodies of postganglionic parasympathetic fibers.
- Have sympathetic nerves that inhibit GI motility and secretion and constrict GI sphincters; parasympathetic nerves stimulate GI motility and secretion and relax GI sphincters.

V. THE DIAPHRAGM AND ITS OPENINGS

A. Diaphragm (See Figures 4.18 and 4.20)

- Arises from the xiphoid process (sternal part), lower six costal cartilages (costal part), medial and lateral lumbocostal arches (lumbar part), vertebrae L1 to L3 for the right crus, and vertebrae L1 to L2 for the left crus.

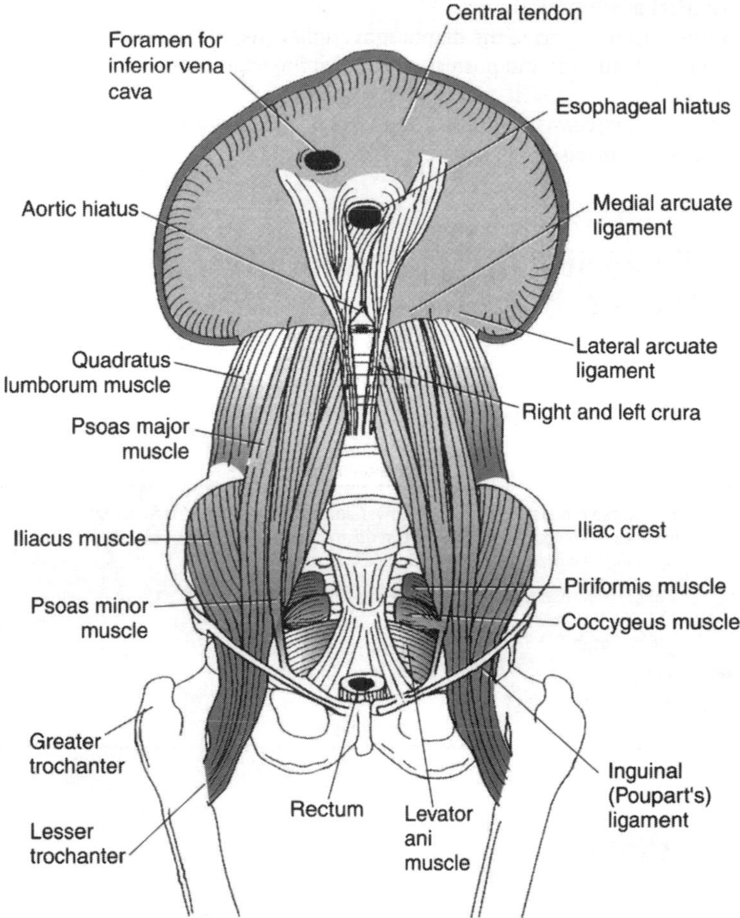

FIGURE 4.20. Diaphragm and Muscles of the Posterior Abdominal Wall

- Inserts into the **central tendon** and is the principal muscle of inspiration.
- Receives somatic motor fibers solely from the phrenic nerve; its **central part** receives sensory fibers from the phrenic nerve, whereas the **peripheral part** receives sensory fibers from the intercostal nerves.
- Receives blood from the musculophrenic, pericardiophrenic, superior phrenic, and inferior phrenic arteries.
- Descends when it contracts, causing an increase in thoracic volume by increasing the vertical diameter of the thoracic cavity and thus decreasing intrathoracic pressure.
- Ascends when it relaxes, causing a decrease in thoracic volume with an increased thoracic pressure.

1. Right Crus

- Is larger and longer than the left crus.
- Originates from vertebrae L1 to L3 (the left crus originates from L1 to L2).
- Splits to enclose the esophagus.

2. Medial Arcuate Ligament (Medial Lumbocostal Arch)

- Extends from the body of L1 to the transverse process of L1 and passes over the psoas muscle and the sympathetic trunk.

3. Lateral Arcuate Ligament (Lateral Lumbocostal Arch)

- Extends from the transverse process of L1 to rib 12 and passes over the quadratus lumborum.

B. Apertures through the Diaphragm

1. Vena Caval Hiatus (Vena Caval Foramen)

- Lies in the central tendon of the diaphragm at the level of T8 and transmits the IVC and occasionally the right phrenic nerve.

2. Esophageal Hiatus

- Lies in the muscular part of the diaphragm (right crus) at the level of T10 and transmits the esophagus and anterior and posterior trunks of the vagus nerves.

3. Aortic Hiatus

- Lies behind or between two crura at the level of T12 and transmits the aorta, thoracic duct, azygos vein, and occasionally greater splanchnic nerve.

VI. MUSCLES OF THE POSTERIOR ABDOMINAL WALL (Table 4.2)

table 4.2 Muscles of the Posterior Abdominal Wall

Muscle	Origin	Insertion	Nerve	Action
Quadratus lumborum	Transverse processes of L3–L5; iliolumbar ligament; iliac crest	Lower border of last rib; transverse processes of L1–L3	Subcostal; L1–L3	Depresses rib 12; flexes trunk laterally
Psoas major	Transverse processes, intervertebral disks and bodies of T12–L5	Lesser trochanter	L2–L3	Flexes thigh and trunk
Psoas minor	Bodies and intervertebral disks of T12–L1	Pectineal line; iliopectineal eminence	L1	Aids in flexing of trunk

HIGH-YIELD TOPICS

- The **inguinal triangle** is bounded by the lateral edge of the rectus abdominis (linea semilunaris), the inferior epigastric vessels, and the inguinal ligament. The **superficial inguinal ring** is in the aponeurosis of the external abdominal oblique muscle and lies just lateral to the pubic tubercle. The **deep inguinal ring** lies in the transversalis fascia, just **lateral** to the inferior epigastric vessels. **The inguinal canal** transmits the spermatic cord or the round **ligament** of the uterus and the genital branch of the genitofemoral nerve.
- The **spermatic cord** contains the ductus deferens, testicular, cremasteric, and deferential arteries; pampiniform plexus of testicular veins; genital branch of the genitofemoral and cremasteric nerves; the testicular sympathetic plexus; and lymph vessels. The **spermatic cord** is covered by the **external spermatic fascia** derived from the aponeurosis of the external oblique abdominal muscle, the **cremasteric fascia** (cremaster muscle and fascia) derived from the internal oblique abdominal muscle, and the **internal spermatic fascia** derived from the transversalis fascia.
- **Inguinal hernia** arises when a portion of intestine protrudes through a weak spot in the inguinal canal or in the inguinal triangle. It occurs superior to the inguinal ligament and lateral to the pubic tubercle. In a **reducible hernia**, the contents of the hernial sac can be returned to their normal position. **Incarcerated hernia** is an irreducible hernia where the hernial sac is entrapped or stuck in the groin. **Strangulated hernia** is an irreducible hernia in which the intestine becomes tightly trapped or twisted; thus, the circulation is arrested, and gangrene (death of tissue) occurs unless relief is prompt.
- **Indirect inguinal hernia** passes through the deep inguinal ring, inguinal canal, and superficial inguinal ring and descends into the scrotum. Indirect hernias lie lateral to the inferior epigastric vessels, are **congenital** (present at birth), derived from persistence of the processus vaginalis, and covered by the peritoneum and the coverings of the spermatic cord (Figure 4.3).
- **Direct inguinal hernia** occurs in the inguinal triangle directly through the abdominal wall muscles (posterior wall of the inguinal canal), lateral to the edge of the conjoint tendon (falx inguinalis),

and rarely descends into the scrotum. Located medial to the inferior epigastric vessels, the hernia protrudes forward to (but rarely through) the superficial inguinal ring. It is **acquired** (develops after birth) and has a sac formed by peritoneum and occasionally transversalis fascia.

- **Cremasteric reflex** is a **drawing up of the testis** by contraction of the cremaster muscle when the skin on the upper medial side of the thigh is stroked. The efferent limb of the reflex arc is the **genital branch of the genitofemoral nerve**; the afferent limb is a **femoral branch of the genitofemoral nerve** and also of the ilioinguinal nerve.
- **Peritonitis** is inflammation and infection of the peritoneum. Common causes include leakage of feces from a burst appendix, a penetrating wound to the abdomen, a perforating ulcer that leaks stomach contents into the peritoneal cavity (lesser sac), or poor sterile technique during abdominal surgery.
- **Paracentesis (abdominal tap)** is a procedure in which a needle is inserted 1 to 2 in. through the abdominal wall into the peritoneal cavity to obtain a sample or drain fluid while the patient's body is elevated at a 45-degree angle. The puncture site is midline at approximately 2 cm below the umbilicus or lateral to McBurney point, avoiding the inferior epigastric vessels.
- **Epigastric hernia** is a protrusion of extraperitoneal fat or a small piece of greater omentum through a defect in the linea alba above the umbilicus and may contain a small portion of intestine.
- The **median umbilical fold** or ligament contains the fibrous remnant of the obliterated **urachus**, the **medial umbilical fold** contains the fibrous remnant of the obliterated **umbilical artery**, and the **lateral umbilical fold** contains the **inferior epigastric vessels**.
- The **lesser omentum** contains the right and left gastric vessels, and its right free margin contains the proper hepatic artery, bile duct, and portal vein, forming the anterior wall of the epiploic foramen.
- The greater **omentum** contains the right and left gastroepiploic vessels. The **mesentery proper** contains the superior mesenteric vessels and branches and tributaries. The **transverse mesocolon** contains the middle colic vessels. The **sigmoid mesocolon** contains the sigmoid vessels, and the **mesoappendix** contains the appendicular vessels.
- The **lienogastric** (gastrosplenic) ligament contains the short gastric and left gastroepiploic vessels, and the **lienorenal** (splenorenal) ligament contains the splenic vessels and tail of the pancreas.
- The free margin of the **falciform ligament** contains the **ligamentum teres hepatis**, which is the fibrous remnant of the left umbilical vein, and the **paraumbilical vein**, which connects the left branch of the portal vein with the subcutaneous veins in the region of the umbilicus.
- Retroperitoneal structures include the duodenum (second, third, and fourth parts), pancreas except a small portion of its tail, ascending colon, descending colon, kidney, ureter, suprarenal gland, renal and suprarenal vessels, gonadal vessels, abdominal aorta, IVC, and so forth.
- **Umbilical hernia** may occur due to failure of the midgut to return to the abdomen early in fetal life, and it occurs as a protrusion of intestines and other organs through a defect in the abdominal wall at the umbilicus. The hernia is covered by subcutaneous tissue and skin, is not usually treated surgically, but it closes spontaneously. In contrast, an **omphalocele** is a persistence of the herniation of abdominal contents that remain outside the abdominal cavity, are covered only by the amniotic membrane, and thus immediate surgical repair is required. **Gastroschisis** is a protrusion of intestines and other organs through a defect in the abdominal wall on the right side of the umbilicus without involving the umbilical cord.
- **Gastroesophageal reflux disease** (**GERD**) is caused by a lower esophageal sphincter dysfunction (relaxation or weakness) and hiatal hernia, causing reflux of stomach contents. Symptoms include heartburn or acid indigestion, painful swallowing, burping, and feeling of fullness in the chest.
- **Hiatal or esophageal hernia** is a herniation of a part of the stomach through the esophageal hiatus into the thoracic cavity. The hernia is caused by an abnormally large esophageal hiatus by a relaxed and weakened lower esophageal sphincter, or by an increased pressure in the abdomen, resulting from coughing, vomiting, straining, and constipation.
- The stomach is divided into the cardia, fundus, body, pyloric antrum, and pyloric canal. The **rugae** are longitudinal folds of mucous membrane and form the gastric canals along the lesser curvature that direct fluids toward the pylorus.
- The stomach produces mucus, **hydrochloric acid** (which destroys many organisms in food and drink), **pepsin** (which converts proteins to polypeptides), and **gastrin** (which is produced in its pyloric antrum and stimulates gastric acid secretion).

- **Peptic ulcer** is erosion in the lining of the stomach or duodenum. It is commonly caused by an infection with ***Helicobacter pylori***, but is also caused by stress, acid, and pepsin. It occurs most commonly in the pyloric region of the stomach (**gastric ulcer**) or the first part of the duodenum (**duodenal ulcer**). Symptoms of peptic ulcer are epigastric pain (burning, cramping, or aching), abdominal indigestion, nausea, vomiting, loss of appetite, weight loss, and fatigue. **Gastric ulcers** may perforate into the lesser sac and erode the pancreas and the splenic artery, causing fatal hemorrhage. **Duodenal ulcers** may erode the pancreas or the gastroduodenal artery, and are three times more common than gastric ulcers.
- The **duodenum** is a C-shaped small intestine surrounding the head of the pancreas and is retroperitoneal except for the beginning of the first part. Its descending (second) part contains the junction of the foregut and midgut, where the bile duct and main pancreatic ducts open at the greater papilla. The duodenojejunal junction is fixed in position by the suspensory ligament of Treitz, a surgical landmark.
- The **jejunum** constitutes the proximal two-fifths of the small intestine. It has tall, closely packed plicae circulares, is emptier, larger in diameter, and thicker walled than the ileum. The **ileum** is longer than the jejunum, and its mesentery contains more prominent arterial arcades and shorter vasa recta. Its lower part contains Peyer patches (aggregations of lymphoid tissue).
- **Small bowel obstruction** is caused by postoperative adhesions, tumors, Crohn disease, hernias, peritonitis, gallstones, volvulus, congenital malrotation, stricture, and intussusception. Strangulated obstructions occluding the arterial supply are surgical emergencies causing death, if untreated. Sign and symptoms include colicky abdominal pain, cramping, nausea and vomiting, constipation, dizziness, abdominal distention, and high-pitched bowel sounds.
- **Inflammatory bowel disease** includes Crohn disease and ulcerative colitis. **Crohn disease** usually occurs in the ileum (ileitis or enteritis), but may occur in any part of the digestive tract. Symptoms include diarrhea, rectal bleeding, anemia, weight loss, and fever. **Ulcerative colitis** involves the colon and the rectum, causing ulcers in the lining (mucosa) of the organs. Patients with prolonged ulcerative colitis are at increased risk for developing colon cancer.
- **Celiac disease** is an **immune reaction to** eating **gluten** (protein of wheat, barley, and rye). Gluten ingestion triggers an immune response resulting in inflammation that **damages the lining of the small intestine**. Celiac disease causes **malabsorption** of nutrients, constipation, diarrhea, vitamin and mineral deficiencies, fatigue, and weight loss.
- **Meckel diverticulum** is an **outpouching** (fingerlike pouch) of the **ileum**, derived from an unobliterated vitelline duct, located **2 ft** proximal to the ileocecal junction on the **antimesenteric side**. It is approximately **2 in**. long, occurs in approximately **2%** of the population, may contain **two types** of ectopic tissues (gastric and pancreatic), presents in the first **two decades** of life (more often in the first **2 years**), and is found **two times** as frequently in boys as in girls.
- The **large intestine** consists of the cecum, appendix, colon, rectum, and anal canal and functions to convert the liquid contents of the ileum into semisolid feces by absorbing water and electrolytes such as sodium and potassium.
- The **colon** includes the ascending and descending colons, which are retroperitoneal, and transverse and sigmoid colons, which are surrounded by peritoneum. The ascending and transverse colons are supplied by the superior mesenteric artery and the vagus nerve; the descending and sigmoid colons are supplied by the inferior mesenteric artery and the pelvic splanchnic nerves. The colons are characterized by presence of **teniae coli**, sacculations or **haustra**, and **epiploic appendages**.
- The **appendix** has large aggregations of lymphoid tissue, and its base lies deep to **McBurney point**. Maximum tenderness in **acute appendicitis** occurs at the point which is located one-third the distance along a line connecting the right anterior–superior iliac spine and the umbilicus.
- **Diverticulitis** is inflammation of diverticula (external evaginations) of the intestinal wall, commonly found in the colon, especially the sigmoid colon, developing as a result of high pressure within the colon. Symptoms are abdominal pain usually in the left lower abdomen, chills, fever, nausea, and constipation.
- **Sigmoid volvulus** is a twisting of the sigmoid colon around its mesentery creating a colonic obstruction. Volvulus can cause intestinal ischemia that may progress to infarction, necrosis, peritonitis, and abdominal distension. Symptoms include vomiting, abdominal pain, constipation, bloody diarrhea, and hematemesis.

- **Megacolon (Hirschsprung disease)** is caused by the **absence of enteric ganglia** (cell bodies of parasympathetic postganglionic fibers) in the lower part of the colon, which leads to dilation of the colon proximal to the inactive segment. It is of congenital origin, results from failure of neural crest cells to migrate and form the myenteric plexus, and is usually diagnosed during infancy and childhood. Symptoms are constipation or diarrhea, abdominal distention, vomiting, and a lack of appetite.
- The **liver** is the largest visceral organ and plays an important role in bile production and secretion, detoxification, storage of carbohydrate as glycogen, protein synthesis, production of heparin and bile pigments from breakdown of hemoglobin, and storage of vitamins, iron, and copper.
- The liver is divided, based on hepatic drainage and blood supply, into the right and left lobe by the fossae for the gallbladder and the IVC. On the visceral surface of the liver, there is an **H-shaped group** of fissures, including fissures for the ligamentum teres hepatis, the ligamentum venosum, **gallbladder**, and the IVC. The **porta hepatis** is a transverse fissure between the **quadrate** and **caudate lobes** that transmits the hepatic ducts, hepatic arteries, branches of the portal vein, hepatic nerves, and lymphatic vessels.
- The liver contains the portal triad, which consists of (a) branches of the hepatic artery bringing oxygen and nutrients to the liver, (b) branches of the portal vein bringing nutrient-rich and oxygen-poor blood to the liver, and (c) hepatic ducts that carry bile in the opposite direction of the blood flow. Bile emulsifies fat in the digestive system.
- **Liver cirrhosis** is a disease in which liver cells are progressively destroyed and replaced by fatty and fibrous tissue that surrounds the intrahepatic blood vessels and biliary radicles, thus impeding the circulation of blood through the liver. Causes include chronic alcohol abuse (alcoholism); hepatitis B, C, and D; and ingestion of poisons. Liver cirrhosis may cause **portal hypertension**, resulting in **esophageal varices** (dilated veins in the lower part of the esophagus), **hemorrhoids** (dilated veins around the anal canal), **caput medusa** (dilated veins around the umbilicus), **spider nevi** or **spider angioma** (small, red, spiderlike arterioles in the cheeks, neck, and shoulder), **ascites** (accumulation of fluid in the peritoneal cavity), **edema** in the legs (lower albumin levels lead to decreased oncotic pressure and increased fluid into tissues surrounding blood vessels), **jaundice** (yellow eyes or skin resulting from bile duct disease failing to remove bilirubin), **splenomegaly** (enlarged spleen resulting from venous congestion causing sequestered blood cells that lead to **thrombocytopenia**, a low platelet count, and easy bruising), **palmar erythema** (persistent redness of the palms), and **pectoral alopecia** (loss of hair).
- The **gallbladder** with its fundus, body, and neck (that contains Hartmann pouch and joins the cystic duct) lies on the visceral surface of the liver and has a capacity of 30 to 50 mL. It receives bile, concentrates it (by absorbing water and salts), stores it, and releases it. It receives blood from the cystic artery arising from the right hepatic artery within the **cystohepatic triangle (of Calot)**, which is formed by the visceral surface of the liver, the cystic duct, and the common hepatic duct.
- **Gallstones (choleliths or cholelithiasis)** are formed by solidification of bile constituents and composed chiefly of **cholesterol crystals**, usually mixed with bile pigments and calcium. Bile crystallizes and forms sand, gravel, and finally stones. Gallstones present commonly in **f**at, **f**ertile (multiparous) **f**emales who are older than **f**orty (40) years **(4-F/5-F** individuals).
- **Cholecystitis** is an inflammation of the gallbladder, caused by obstruction of the cystic duct by gallstones. Symptoms are pain in the upper right quadrant and the epigastric region, fever, nausea, and vomiting. The pain may radiate to the back or right shoulder region.
- **Bile** flows from the liver through the right and left hepatic ducts, which unite to form the common hepatic duct. This is joined by the cystic duct to form the bile duct. The bile duct descends behind the first part of the duodenum and runs through the head of the pancreas and joins the main pancreatic duct to form the hepatopancreatic duct, which enters the second part of the duodenum at the greater papilla.
- The **pancreas** is a retroperitoneal organ except for a small portion of its tail, which lies in the lienorenal (splenorenal) ligament. It is divided into the head, neck, body, and tail. The head lies within the C-shaped concavity of the duodenum, and its lower portion projects to the left behind the superior mesenteric vessels as the **uncinate process**. The tail projects toward the hilum of the spleen. The pancreas is both an **exocrine gland**, which produces digestive enzymes, and an **endocrine gland**, which secretes insulin, glucagon, and somatostatin.
- **Pancreatitis** is an inflammation of the pancreas commonly caused by gallstones or alcohol abuse. Symptoms include upper abdominal pain (which may be severe and constant and may reach to the

back), nausea, vomiting, weight loss, fatty stools, mild jaundice, diabetes, low blood pressure, heart failure, and kidney failure.

- **Pancreatic cancer** frequently causes severe back pain, has the potential to invade into the adjacent organs, and is extremely difficult to treat. Surgical resection called a pancreaticoduodenectomy or **Whipple procedure** may extend life. Cancer of the pancreatic head often compresses and obstructs the bile duct, causing obstructive jaundice. Cancer of the pancreatic neck and body may cause portal or IVC obstruction because the pancreas overlies these large veins.
- **Diabetes mellitus** is characterized by hyperglycemia caused by an **inadequate production** of insulin or **inadequate action** of insulin on body tissues. There are two types of diabetes: **type I** diabetes (also known as insulin-dependent diabetes), in which the pancreas (β cells) produces an **insufficient amount** of insulin, and **type II** diabetes, which results from **insulin resistance** of target tissues. Diabetes causes **diabetic retinopathy**, neuropathy, kidney failure, heart disease, stroke, and limb disease. It has symptoms of polyuria (excessive secretion of urine), polydipsia (thirst), weight loss, tiredness, infections of urinary tract, and blurring of vision.
- **Annular pancreas** occurs when the ventral and dorsal pancreatic buds form a ring around the duodenum, thereby obstructing it.
- The **spleen** is a large vascular lymphatic organ that develops in the dorsal mesogastrium. It is supported by the lienogastric (splenogastric) and lienorenal (splenorenal) ligaments.
- The spleen contains **white pulp**, which consists of diffuse and nodular lymphoid tissue and provides the immune function, and **red pulp**, which consists of venous sinusoids and splenic cords. It is hematopoietic in early life, and later **destroys and removes aged** (or worn-out) **red blood cells.**
- The spleen **filters blood** (lymph nodes **filter the lymph**), **stores blood** and platelets, **produces lymphocytes and antibodies**, and is involved in body defense against foreign particles (removal of blood-borne antigens as its immune function).
- The spleen metabolizes **hemoglobin** into (a) **globin** (protein part), which is hydrolyzed to amino acids that are reused for protein synthesis; (b) **iron**, which is released from heme and transported to the bone marrow where it is reused in erythropoiesis; and (c) iron-free **heme**, which is metabolized to bilirubin in the liver and excreted in the bile.
- **Splenomegaly** is caused by venous congestion resulting from thrombosis of the splenic vein or portal hypertension, causing sequestering of blood cells, leading to thrombocytopenia (a low platelet count) and easy bruising.
- **Rupture of the spleen** occurs frequently by fractured ribs or severe blows to the left hypochondrium and causes profuse bleeding. The ruptured spleen is difficult to repair; consequently, **splenectomy** is performed to prevent the person from bleeding to death.
- **Lymphoma** is a cancer of lymphoid tissue. **Hodgkin's lymphoma** is a malignancy characterized by painless, progressive enlargement of the lymph nodes, spleen, and other lymphoid tissue, accompanied by night sweats, fever, and weight loss.
- **Superior mesenteric artery obstruction** is caused by a thrombus, an embolus, atherosclerosis, an aortic aneurysm, a tumor in the uncinate process of the pancreas, compression by the third part of the duodenum, or surgical scar tissue. The obstruction leads to small and large intestinal ischemia, resulting in necrosis of all or part of the involved intestinal segment.
- The **portal vein** is formed by the union of the splenic vein and the superior mesenteric vein and receives the right and left gastric vein. The inferior mesenteric vein joins the splenic vein or the superior mesenteric vein or the junction of these veins. The portal vein carries deoxygenated blood containing nutrients and toxins and carries three times as much blood as the hepatic artery.
- The important **portal–caval (systemic) anastomoses** occur between (a) the left gastric vein and the esophageal vein of the azygos vein; (b) the superior rectal vein and the middle and inferior rectal veins; (c) the paraumbilical veins and radicles of the epigastric (superficial and inferior) veins; and (d) the retrocolic veins and twigs of the renal, suprarenal, and gonadal veins.
- **Portal hypertension** results from liver cirrhosis or thrombosis in the portal vein, forming **esophageal varices**, **caput medusae**, and **hemorrhoids**. It can be treated by diverting blood from the portal to the caval system using a **portacaval shunt** achieved by creating a communication between the portal vein and the IVC as they lie close together below the liver, or by the **splenorenal (Warren) shunt** accomplished by anastomosing the splenic vein to the left renal vein.

- **Portal Budd–Chiari or Chiari syndrome** is an **occlusion of the hepatic veins** and results in high pressure in the veins, causing hepatomegaly, upper right abdominal pain, ascites, mild jaundice, and eventually portal hypertension and liver failure.
- The **kidney** is retroperitoneal in position and extends from T12 to L3, with the right kidney a little lower than the left. It is invested by a fibrous renal capsule and is surrounded by the renal fascia that divides the fat into two regions. The **perirenal fat** lies between the renal capsule and renal fascia, and the **pararenal fat** lies external to the renal fascia.
- The kidney consists of the medulla and cortex, containing 1 to 2 million nephrons, which are the anatomic and functional units. Each **nephron** consists of a **renal corpuscle**, a proximal convoluted tubule, Henle loop, and a distal convoluted tubule. The **renal corpuscle** consists of a **glomerulus** (tuft of capillaries), surrounded by a **glomerular capsule**, which is the invaginated blind end of the nephron.
- The kidney produces and excretes urine (by which metabolic waste products are eliminated), **maintains electrolyte** (ionic) balance and pH, and **produces renin** and erythropoietin. The cortex contains renal corpuscles and proximal and distal convoluted tubules.
- The **medulla** consists of 8 to 12 renal pyramids, which contain straight tubules (Henle loops) and collecting tubules. The apex of the renal pyramid, the renal papilla, fits into the cup-shaped minor calyx on which the collecting tubules open.
- The **minor calyces** receive urine from the collecting tubules and empty into two or three **major calyces**, which in turn empty into the renal pelvis.
- The right **renal artery** arises from the abdominal aorta, is **longer** and a little lower than the left, and passes posterior to the IVC; the left artery passes posterior to the left renal vein.
- The **ureter** is a muscular tube that extends from the kidney to the urinary bladder. It may be obstructed by **renal calculi** (kidney stones) where it joins the renal pelvis (**ureteropelvic junction**), where it crosses the **pelvic brim** over the distal end of the common iliac artery, or where it enters the wall of the urinary bladder (**ureterovesicul junction**).
- **Pelvic kidney** is an **ectopic kidney** that occurs when kidneys fail to ascend and thus remain in the pelvis. Two pelvic kidneys may fuse to form a solid lobed organ called a **cake (rosette) kidney**.
- **Horseshoe kidney** develops as a result of **fusion of the lower poles of two kidneys** and may obstruct the urinary tract by its **impingement on the ureters**.
- **Nephroptosis** is a downward displacement of the kidney, **dropped kidney**, or **floating kidney** caused by loss of supporting perirenal fascia. It may cause intermittent ureteric obstruction or kinking of a renal artery, resulting in hydronephrosis.
- **Polycystic kidney disease** is a genetic disorder characterized by numerous cysts filled with fluid in the kidney. The cysts can slowly replace much of normal kidney tissues, reducing kidney function and leading to kidney failure.
- **Kidney stone (renal calculus or nephrolith)** is composed of calcium oxalate or calcium phosphate, urea, uric acid, or cystine. Crystals and subsequently stones are formed in the urine and collected in calyces of the kidney or in the ureter.
- **Obstruction of the ureter** occurs by renal calculi or kidney stones and result in hydroureter and hydronephrosis.
- **Hydronephrosis** is a **fluid-filled enlargement of the renal pelvis** and **calyces** as a result of obstruction of the ureter.
- The **suprarenal (adrenal) gland** is a retroperitoneal organ lying on the superomedial aspect of the kidney and is surrounded by a capsule and renal fascia.
- Its cortex is essential to life and produces steroid hormones. The medulla is derived from embryonic neural crest cells, receives preganglionic sympathetic nerve fibers directly, and secretes epinephrine and norepinephrine.
- The gland receives arteries from three sources: the superior suprarenal artery from the inferior phrenic artery, the middle suprarenal from the abdominal aorta, and the inferior suprarenal artery from the renal artery. It drains via the suprarenal vein, which empties into the IVC on the right and the renal vein on the left.
- **Addison's disease** is a disorder caused by an adrenocortical insufficiency (insufficient production of cortisol and, in some cases, aldosterone) caused by autoimmune destruction of the suprarenal cortex or tuberculosis.

- **Disorders of the suprarenal cortex** also include an excess production of glucocorticoids (**Cushing syndrome**) or aldosterone (**Conn syndrome**) or by androgens (**hirsutism**).
- The **suprarenal** and **gonadal veins** drain into the IVC on the right and the renal vein on the left. The azygos vein is connected to the IVC, while the hemiazygos vein is connected to the left renal vein.
- The **cisterna chyli** is the lower dilated end of the thoracic duct and lies just to the right and posterior to the aorta, usually between two crura of the diaphragm. It is formed by the intestinal and lumbar lymph trunks.
- The **diaphragm** arises from the xiphoid process, lower six costal cartilages, and medial and lateral lumbocostal arches and vertebrae, and inserts into the **central tendon**. It is the principal muscle of inspiration and receives somatic motor fibers solely from the phrenic nerve. Its central part receives sensory fibers from the phrenic nerve, whereas the peripheral part receives sensory fibers from the intercostal nerves.
- It has (a) the **vena caval hiatus**, which lies in the central tendon at the level of T8 and transmits the IVC and the right phrenic nerve; (b) the **esophageal hiatus**, which lies in the muscular part of the diaphragm at the level of T10 and transmits the esophagus and vagus nerves; and (c) the **aortic hiatus**, which lies between the two crura at the level of T12 and transmits the aorta, thoracic duct, azygos vein, and sometimes greater splanchnic nerve.
- Autonomic nerve functions in the abdomen:

	Functions of Autonomic Nerves	
	Sympathetic Nerve	**Parasympathetic Nerve**
Gastrointestinal tract	Inhibits motility and secretion; contracts sphincters	Stimulates motility and secretion; relaxes sphincters
Liver and gallbladder	Promotes breakdown of glycogen to glucose	Promotes glycogen storage; increases bile secretion
Suprarenal medulla	Promotes epinephrine and norepinephrine secretion	No effect
Kidney	Constricts renal arteries, reducing urine formation	May cause vasodilation of renal vascular bed

Review Test

Directions: Each of the numbered items or incomplete statements in this section is followed by answers or by completions of the statement. Select the **one**-lettered answer or completion that is **best** in each case.

1. A 63-year-old man comes to the emergency department with back pain, weakness, and shortness of breath. On examination, he has an aneurysm of the abdominal aorta at the aortic hiatus of the diaphragm. Which of the following pairs of structures would most likely be compressed?

(A) Vagus nerve and azygos vein
(B) Esophagus and vagus nerve
(C) Azygos vein and thoracic duct
(D) Thoracic duct and vagus nerve
(E) Inferior vena cava (IVC) and phrenic nerve

2. A 36-year-old woman with yellow pigmentation of the skin and sclerae presents at the outpatient clinic. Which of the following conditions most likely is the cause of her obstructive jaundice?

(A) Aneurysm of the splenic artery
(B) Perforated ulcer of the stomach
(C) Obstruction of the main pancreatic duct
(D) Cancer in the head of the pancreas
(E) Cancer in the body of the pancreas

3. A 2-year-old boy presents with pain in his groin that has been increasing in nature over the past few weeks. He is found to have a degenerative malformation of the transversalis fascia during development. Which of the following structures on the anterior abdominal wall is likely defective?

(A) Superficial inguinal ring
(B) Deep inguinal ring
(C) Inguinal ligament
(D) Sac of a direct inguinal hernia
(E) Anterior wall of the inguinal canal

4. A 29-year-old man comes to a local hospital with duodenal peptic ulcer and complains of cramping epigastric pain. Which of the following structures harbors the cell bodies of abdominal pain fibers?

(A) Lateral horn of the spinal cord
(B) Anterior horn of the spinal cord
(C) Dorsal root ganglion
(D) Sympathetic chain ganglion
(E) Celiac ganglion

5. A 42-year-old obese woman with seven children is brought to a local hospital by her daughter. Physical examination and her radiograph reveal that large gallstones have ulcerated through the posterior wall of the fundus of the gallbladder into the intestine. Which of the following parts of the intestine is most likely to initially contain gallstones?

(A) Cecum
(B) Ascending colon
(C) Transverse colon
(D) Descending colon
(E) Sigmoid colon

6. A 35-year-old woman comes to a local hospital with abdominal tenderness and acute pain. On examination, her physician observes that an abdominal infection has spread retroperitoneally. Which of the following structures is most likely affected?

(A) Stomach
(B) Transverse colon
(C) Jejunum
(D) Descending colon
(E) Spleen

7. During an annual health examination of a 46-year-old woman, a physician finds hypersecretion of norepinephrine from her suprarenal medulla. Which of the following types of nerve fibers are most likely overstimulated?

(A) Preganglionic sympathetic fibers
(B) Postganglionic sympathetic fibers
(C) Somatic motor fibers
(D) Postganglionic parasympathetic fibers
(E) Preganglionic parasympathetic fibers

8. A 6-year-old girl comes to her pediatrician with constipation, abdominal distention, and vomiting. After thorough examination, she is diagnosed as having Hirschsprung disease (aganglionic megacolon), which is a congenital disease and leads to dilation of the colon. This condition is caused by an absence of which of the following kinds of neural cell bodies?

(A) Sympathetic preganglionic neuron cell bodies
(B) Sympathetic postganglionic neuron cell bodies
(C) Parasympathetic preganglionic neuron cell bodies
(D) Parasympathetic postganglionic neuron cell bodies
(E) Sensory neuron cell bodies

9. A pediatric surgeon is resecting a possible malignant mass from the liver of a neonate with cerebral palsy. The surgeon divides the round ligament of the liver during surgery. A fibrous remnant of which of the following fetal vessels is severed?

(A) Ductus venosus
(B) Ductus arteriosus
(C) Left umbilical vein
(D) Right umbilical vein
(E) Umbilical artery

10. A 27-year-old woman has suffered a gunshot wound to her midabdomen. After examining the patient's angiogram, a trauma surgeon locates the source of bleeding from pairs of veins that typically terminate in the same vein. Which of the following veins are damaged?

(A) Left and right ovarian veins
(B) Left and right gastroepiploic veins
(C) Left and right colic veins
(D) Left and right suprarenal veins
(E) Left and right hepatic veins

11. A 43-year-old man complains of abdominal pain just above his umbilicus. On examination, a tumor is found anterior to the IVC. Which of the following structures would most likely be compressed by this tumor?

(A) Right sympathetic trunk
(B) Left third lumbar artery
(C) Third part of the duodenum
(D) Left renal artery
(E) Cisterna chyli

12. A 33-year-old man with a perforated gastric ulcer complains of excruciating pain in his stomach. It is observed that the pain comes from peritoneal irritation by gastric contents in the lesser sac. Which of the following nerves contain sensory nerve fibers that convey this sharp, stabbing pain?

(A) Vagus nerves
(B) Greater splanchnic nerves
(C) Lower intercostal nerves
(D) White rami communicantes
(E) Gray rami communicantes

13. A young boy is brought to the hospital after a bicycle accident and possible pelvic fracture. While awaiting a computed tomography (CT) scan of his pelvis, a physician proceeds with a focal neurologic examination. In testing the child's reflexes, which of the following nerves would carry afferent impulses of the cremasteric reflex?

(A) Subcostal nerve
(B) Lateral femoral cutaneous nerve
(C) Genitofemoral nerve
(D) Iliohypogastric nerve
(E) Femoral nerve

14. A 21-year-old man receives a penetrating knife wound in the abdomen and is injured in both the superior mesenteric artery and the vagus nerve. Which portion of the colon would most likely be impaired by this injury?

(A) Ascending and descending colons
(B) Transverse and sigmoid colons
(C) Descending and sigmoid colons
(D) Ascending and transverse colons
(E) Transverse and descending colons

15. A 42-year-old man with portal hypertension secondary to cirrhosis of the liver and subsequent massive ascites presents to the emergency department. He refuses to have a transjugular intrahepatic portosystemic shunt (TIPS) procedure and prefers surgery. Which of the following surgical connections is involved in the most practical method of shunting portal blood around the liver?

(A) Superior mesenteric vein to the inferior mesenteric vein
(B) Portal vein to the superior vena cava
(C) Portal vein to the left renal vein
(D) Splenic vein to the left renal vein
(E) Superior rectal vein to the left colic vein

16. A 78-year-old man is suffering from ischemia of the suprarenal glands. This condition results from rapid occlusion of direct branches of which of the following arteries?

(A) Aorta, splenic, and inferior phrenic arteries
(B) Renal, splenic, and inferior mesenteric arteries
(C) Aorta, inferior phrenic, and renal arteries
(D) Superior mesenteric, inferior mesenteric, and renal arteries
(E) Aorta and hepatic and renal arteries

17. A radiograph of a 32-year-old woman reveals a perforation in the posterior wall of the stomach in which the gastric contents have spilled into the lesser sac. The general surgeon has opened the lienogastric (gastrosplenic) ligament to reach the lesser sac and notes erosion of the ulcer into an artery. Which of the following vessels is most likely involved?

(A) Splenic artery
(B) Gastroduodenal artery
(C) Left gastric artery
(D) Right gastric artery
(E) Left gastroepiploic artery

18. A 35-year-old woman with a history of cholecystectomy arrives in the emergency department with intractable hiccups most likely caused by an abdominal abscess secondary to surgical infection. Which of the following nerves carries pain sensation caused by irritation of the peritoneum on the central portion of the inferior surface of the diaphragm?

(A) Vagus nerve
(B) Lower intercostal nerve
(C) Phrenic nerve
(D) Greater splanchnic nerve
(E) Subcostal nerve

19. A 16-year-old boy with a ruptured spleen comes to the emergency department for splenectomy. Soon after ligation of the splenic artery just distal to its origin, a surgical resident observes that the patient is healing normally. Normal blood flow would occur in which of the following arteries?

(A) Short gastric arteries
(B) Dorsal pancreatic artery
(C) Inferior pancreaticoduodenal artery
(D) Left gastroepiploic artery
(E) Artery in the lienorenal ligament

20. A 9-year-old boy was admitted to the emergency department complaining of nausea, vomiting, fever, and loss of appetite. On examination, he was found to have tenderness and pain on the right lower quadrant. Based on signs and symptoms, the diagnosis of acute appendicitis was made. During an appendectomy performed at McBurney point, which of the following structures is most likely to be injured?

(A) Deep circumflex femoral artery
(B) Inferior epigastric artery
(C) Iliohypogastric nerve
(D) Genitofemoral nerve
(E) Spermatic cord

21. A 54-year-old man with a long history of alcohol abuse presents to the emergency department with rapidly increasing abdominal distention most likely resulting from an alteration in portal systemic blood flow. Which of the following characteristics is associated with the portal vein or the portal venous system?

(A) Lower blood pressure than in the IVC
(B) Least risk of venous varices because of portal hypertension
(C) Distention of the portal vein resulting from its numerous valves
(D) Caput medusae and hemorrhoids caused by portal hypertension
(E) Less blood flow than in the hepatic artery

22. While examining radiographs and angiograms of a 52-year-old patient, a physician is trying to distinguish the jejunum from the ileum. He has observed that the jejunum has:

(A) Fewer plicae circulares
(B) Fewer mesenteric arterial arcades
(C) Less digestion and absorption of nutrients
(D) Shorter vasa recta
(E) More fat in its mesentery

23. A 67-year-old woman with a long history of liver cirrhosis was seen in the emergency department. In this patient with portal hypertension, which of the following veins is most likely to be dilated?

(A) Right colic vein
(B) Inferior epigastric vein
(C) Inferior phrenic vein
(D) Suprarenal vein
(E) Ovarian vein

24. A 26-year-old patient is admitted to a local hospital with a retroperitoneal infection. Which of the following arteries is most likely to be infected?

(A) Left gastric artery
(B) Proper hepatic artery
(C) Middle colic artery
(D) Sigmoid arteries
(E) Dorsal pancreatic artery

25. A pediatric surgeon has resected a structure that is a fibrous remnant of an embryonic or fetal artery in a 5-year-old child. Which of the following structures is most likely to be divided?

(A) Lateral umbilical fold
(B) Medial umbilical fold
(C) Median umbilical fold
(D) Ligamentum teres hepatis
(E) Ligamentum venosum

26. A 57-year-old patient has a tumor in the body of the pancreas that obstructs the inferior mesenteric vein just before joining the splenic vein. Which of the following veins is most likely to be enlarged?

(A) Middle colic vein
(B) Left gastroepiploic vein
(C) Inferior pancreaticoduodenal vein
(D) Ileocolic vein
(E) Left colic vein

27. An elderly man with prostatic hypertrophy returns to his urologist with another case of epididymitis. An acute infection involving the dartos muscle layer of the scrotum most likely leads to an enlargement of which of the following lymph nodes?

(A) Preaortic nodes
(B) Lumbar nodes
(C) External iliac nodes
(D) Superficial inguinal nodes
(E) Common iliac nodes

28. A patient with cirrhosis is scheduled for liver transplant surgery. During the operation rounds, the transplant physician explains to his residents that one of the reasons a surgeon must pay close attention to the anatomic location of the liver is that this organ:

(A) Receives blood only from the hepatic arteries
(B) Manufactures red blood cells in an adult
(C) Drains bile from the quadrate lobe into the right hepatic duct
(D) Drains venous blood into the hepatic veins
(E) Functions to concentrate and store bile

29. A 41-year-old woman is brought to the emergency department by her family because of acute onset of right upper quadrant pain, nausea, and vomiting. For this case, it is important to remember that the bile duct:

(A) Drains bile into the second part of the duodenum
(B) Can be blocked by cancer in the body of the pancreas
(C) Joins the main pancreatic duct, which carries hormones
(D) Is formed by union of the right and left hepatic duct
(E) Lies posterior to the portal vein in the right free edge of the lesser omentum

30. A patient with diverticulosis of the colon presents for follow-up to his primary care physician with ongoing complaints of left lower quadrant pain and occasionally bloody stools. His physician begins workup with appropriating test by recalling that the sigmoid colon:

(A) Is drained by systemic veins
(B) Is a retroperitoneal organ
(C) Receives parasympathetic fibers from the vagus nerve
(D) Receives its blood from the superior mesenteric artery
(E) Has teniae coli and epiploic appendages

31. A 19-year-old man with a ruptured appendix is sent to the emergency department for surgery. To cut off the blood supply to the appendix (if collateral circulation is discounted), a surgeon should ligate which of the following arteries?

(A) Middle colic artery
(B) Right colic artery
(C) Ileocolic artery
(D) Inferior mesenteric artery
(E) Common iliac artery

32. Because of an inflammatory bowel disease (Crohn disease) and a small bowel obstruction leading to bowel ischemia, an elderly woman requires bypass of her ileum and jejunum and is scheduled for a gastrocolostomy. The surgeon will ligate all arteries that send branches to the stomach. Which of the following arteries may be spared?

(A) Splenic artery
(B) Gastroduodenal artery
(C) Inferior pancreaticoduodenal artery
(D) Left gastroepiploic artery
(E) Proper hepatic artery

33. A 38-year-old woman with peptic ulcer disease of the stomach experiences severe abdominal pain. Which of the following nervous structures is most likely involved?

(A) Greater splanchnic nerve
(B) Ventral roots of the spinal nerve
(C) Lower intercostal nerve
(D) Vagus nerve
(E) Gray ramus communicans

34. A 3-year-old boy is diagnosed as having a persistent processus vaginalis in its middle portion. Which of the following conditions is most likely to be associated with this developmental anomaly?

(A) Direct inguinal hernia
(B) Gubernaculum testis
(C) Hematocele
(D) Hydrocele
(E) Cryptorchidism

35. Examination of a 54-year-old man reveals an isolated tumor located at the porta hepatis. This tumor most likely compresses which of the following structures?

(A) Cystic duct
(B) Hepatic veins
(C) Common hepatic artery
(D) Left gastric artery
(E) Branches of the portal vein

36. A patient is rushed to the operating room for an emergent cholecystectomy (resection of a gallbladder) because of cholecystitis. While locating landmarks before surgical resection of an infected gallbladder, the surgeon recalls a portal–caval anastomosis. Which of the following pairs of veins form a portal–caval anastomosis?

(A) Hepatic veins and IVC
(B) Superior and middle rectal vein
(C) Left and right gastric vein
(D) Inferior and superficial epigastric veins
(E) Suprarenal and renal veins

37. Mrs. Jones is undergoing a routine colonoscopy for colon cancer prevention. The gastroenterologist finds a Meckel diverticulum. Which of the following statements is true about the diverticulum?

(A) It is found 2 ft distal to the ileocecal junction
(B) It is located on the mesenteric side of the ileum
(C) It occurs in approximately 20% of the population
(D) It is a persistent remnant of the embryonic yolk stalk
(E) It may contain renal and suprarenal tissues

38. A 54-year-old man comes to a hospital with abdominal pain, jaundice, loss of appetite, and weight loss. On examination of his radiograms and CT scans, a physician finds a slowly growing tumor in the uncinate process of the pancreas. Which of the following structures is most likely compressed by this tumor?

(A) Main pancreatic duct
(B) Splenic artery
(C) Portal vein
(D) Superior mesenteric artery
(E) Superior pancreaticoduodenal artery

39. A 6-year-old boy comes to his pediatrician with a lump in the groin near the thigh and pain in the groin. On examination, the physician makes a diagnosis of a direct inguinal hernia because the herniated tissue:

(A) Enters the deep inguinal ring
(B) Lies lateral to the inferior epigastric artery
(C) Is covered by spermatic fasciae
(D) Descends into the scrotum
(E) Develops after birth

40. A 21-year-old man developed a hernia after lifting heavy boxes while moving into his new house. During the repair of his resulting hernia, the urologist recalls that the genitofemoral nerve:

(A) Runs in front of the quadratus lumborum
(B) Is a branch of the femoral nerve
(C) Supplies the testis
(D) Passes through the deep inguinal ring
(E) Gives rise to an anterior scrotal branch

41. An oncologist is reviewing a CT scan of a 74-year-old man with newly diagnosed hepatocellular carcinoma. He locates the affected quadrate lobe of the liver that:

(A) Lies between the IVC and ligamentum venosum
(B) Receives blood from the right hepatic artery
(C) Drains bile into the left hepatic duct
(D) Is a medial superior segment
(E) Is functionally a part of the right lobe

42. A 58-year-old man is presented with edema of the lower limb and enlarged superficial veins of the abdominal wall. Examination of radiographs and angiograms reveals obstruction of the IVC just proximal to the entrance of the renal vein. This venous blockage may result in dilation of which of the following veins?

(A) Left suprarenal vein
(B) Right inferior phrenic vein
(C) Right hepatic vein
(D) Left gastric vein
(E) Portal vein

43. A physical fitness trainer for a young Hollywood movie star explains the reasons for 100 stomach crunches a day. The young star, a medical student before 'hitting it big,' reaffirms to his trainer that the lateral margin of the rectus abdominis, the muscle responsible for a washboard stomach, defines which of the following structures?

(A) Linea alba
(B) Linea semilunaris
(C) Linea semicircularis
(D) Transversalis fascia
(E) Falx inguinalis

44. During surgical treatment of portal hypertension in a 59-year-old man with liver cirrhosis, a surgeon inadvertently lacerates the dilated paraumbilical veins. The veins must be repaired to allow collateral flow. Which of the following ligaments is most likely severed?

(A) Lienorenal ligament
(B) Lienogastric ligament
(C) Gastrophrenic ligament
(D) Ligamentum teres hepatis
(E) Ligamentum venosum

45. A 43-year-old woman is admitted to the hospital because of deep abdominal pain in her epigastric region. On examination, it is observed that a retroperitoneal infection erodes an artery that runs along the superior border of the pancreas. Which of the following arteries is likely injured?

(A) Right gastric artery
(B) Left gastroepiploic artery
(C) Splenic artery
(D) Gastroduodenal artery
(E) Dorsal pancreatic artery

46. A 19-year-old young woman with a long history of irritable bowel syndrome presents for the possibility of surgical resection of the gastrointestinal (GI) tract where the vagal parasympathetic innervation terminates. Which of the following sites is most appropriate for surgical resection?

(A) Duodenojejunal junction
(B) Ileocecal junction
(C) Right colic flexure
(D) Left colic flexure
(E) Anorectal junction

47. A 58-year-old man is admitted to the hospital with severe abdominal pain, nausea, and vomiting resulting in dehydration. Emergency CT scan reveals a tumor located between the celiac trunk and the superior mesenteric artery. Which of the following structures is likely compressed by this tumor?

(A) Fundus of the stomach
(B) Neck of the pancreas
(C) Transverse colon
(D) Hepatopancreatic ampulla
(E) Duodenojejunal junction

48. An emergent hernia repair is scheduled. As the attending physician is driving to the hospital, the medical student assisting on the case quickly reviews his anatomy atlas and is trying to commit to memory that the internal oblique abdominis muscle contributes to the formation of which of the following structures?

(A) Inguinal ligament
(B) Deep inguinal ring
(C) Falx inguinalis (conjoint tendon)
(D) Internal spermatic fascia
(E) Reflected inguinal ligament

49. A 9-year-old girl has crashed into her neighbor's brick fence while riding her bike and is brought to the emergency department with a great deal of abdominal pain. Her radiogram and angiogram show laceration of the superior mesenteric artery immediately distal to the origin of the middle colic artery. If collateral circulation is discounted, which of the following organs may become ischemic?

(A) Descending colon
(B) Duodenum
(C) Pancreas
(D) Ascending colon
(E) Transverse colon

50. A 53-year-old woman with known kidney disease presents to a hospital because her pain has become increasingly more severe. A physician performing kidney surgery must remember that:

(A) The left kidney lies a bit lower than the right one
(B) The perirenal fat lies external to the renal fascia
(C) The renal fascia does not surround the suprarenal gland
(D) The left renal vein runs anterior to both the aorta and the left renal artery
(E) The right renal artery is shorter than the left renal artery

51. A neonatal baby was born with diabetes mellitus due to an inadequate production of insulin. Cells in the endocrine portion of the pancreas that secrete insulin, glucagon, and somatostatin are derived from which of the following?

(A) Ectoderm
(B) Mesoderm
(C) Endoderm
(D) Proctodeum
(E) Neural crest cells

52. During development, the midgut artery appears to be markedly narrowed at its origin. Which of the following structures is derived from the midgut and may receive inadequate blood supply?

(A) Gallbladder
(B) Stomach
(C) Descending colon
(D) Ascending colon
(E) Rectum

53. A 3-year-old boy is admitted to the children's hospital with complaints of restlessness, abdominal pain, and fever. An MRI examination reveals that he has a double ureter. Which of the following embryonic structures is most likely failed to develop normally?

(A) Mesonephric (Wolffian) duct
(B) Paramesonephric (Müllerian) duct
(C) Ureteric bud
(D) Metanephros
(E) Pronephros

54. A neonate has a small reducible protrusion through a defined ring at the umbilicus. His pediatrician indicates to the parents that this will likely close spontaneously. Which of the following congenital malformations is present?

(A) Umbilical hernia
(B) Symptomatic patent urachus
(C) Patent omphalomesenteric duct
(D) Omphalocele
(E) Gastroschisis

Questions 55 to 59: Choose the appropriate lettered structure in this CT scan of the abdomen (see Figure below) at the level of the 12th thoracic vertebra.

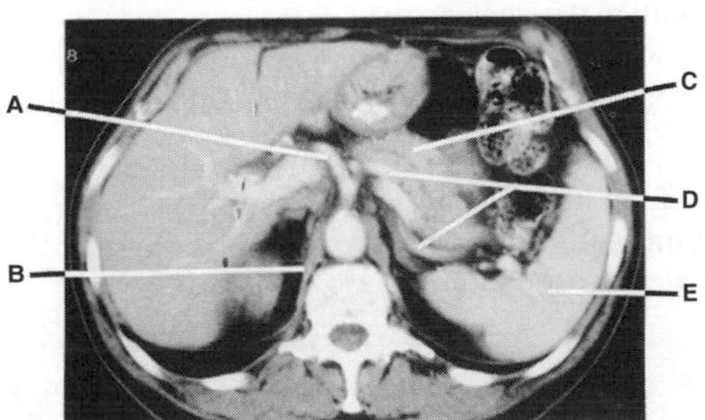

55. Which structure is hematopoietic in early life and later destroys worn-out red blood cells?

56. Which structure runs along the superior border of the pancreas and enters the lienorenal ligament?

57. Which structure is divided into the proper hepatic and gastroduodenal arteries?

58. Which structure provides an attachment of the suspensory muscle of the duodenum (ligament of Treitz)?

59. Which structure is retroperitoneal in position and receives blood from the splenic artery?

Questions 60 to 64: Choose the appropriate lettered structure in this CT scan of the abdomen (see Figure below) at the level of the upper lumbar vertebra.

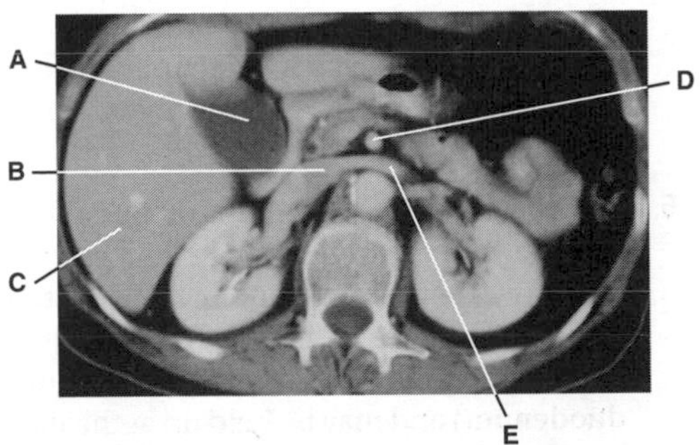

60. Which structure is a direct branch of the aorta and supplies blood to the ascending and transverse colons?

61. Which structure receives blood from the liver and kidney and enters the thorax by piercing the central tendon of the diaphragm?

62. Which structure receives bile, concentrates it by absorbing water and salt, and stores it?

63. Which structure receives blood from the left gonad and suprarenal gland?

64. Which structure receives blood from the portal vein?

Answers and Explanations

1. **The answer is C.** The aortic hiatus of the diaphragm transmits the azygos vein and thoracic duct. The vagus nerve passes through the esophageal hiatus, and the right phrenic nerve may run through the vena caval hiatus.

2. **The answer is D.** Because the bile duct traverses the head of the pancreas, cancer in the head of the pancreas obstructs the bile duct, resulting in jaundice. Aneurysm of the splenic artery, obstruction of the main pancreatic duct, a stomach ulcer, and cancer in the body of the pancreas are not closely associated with the bile duct. The tail of the pancreas is located at the hilus of the spleen, which lies far from the bile duct.

3. **The answer is B.** The deep inguinal ring lies in the transversalis fascia, just lateral to the inferior epigastric vessels. The superficial inguinal ring is in the aponeurosis of the external oblique muscle. The inguinal ligament and the anterior wall of the inguinal canal are formed by the aponeurosis of the external oblique muscle. The sac of a direct inguinal hernia is formed by the peritoneum.

4. **The answer is C.** Cell bodies of the abdominal pain fibers are located in the dorsal root ganglion. The lateral horn of the spinal cord contains cell bodies of sympathetic preganglionic nerve fibers; the anterior horn contains cell bodies of general somatic efferent (GSE) fibers. The sympathetic chain ganglion contains cell bodies of sympathetic postganglionic fibers, which supply blood vessels, sweat glands, and hair follicles. The celiac ganglion contains cell bodies of sympathetic postganglionic fibers, which supply the visceral organs such as stomach and intestine.

5. **The answer is C.** The fundus of the gallbladder is in contact with the transverse colon, and thus, gallstones erode through the posterior wall of the gallbladder and enter the transverse colon. They are passed naturally to the rectum through the descending colon and sigmoid colon. Gallstones lodged in the body of the gallbladder may ulcerate through the posterior wall of the body of the gallbladder into the duodenum (because the gallbladder body is in contact with the duodenum) and may be held up at the ileocecal junction, producing an intestinal obstruction.

6. **The answer is D.** The descending colon is a retroperitoneal organ. The rest of the organs are surrounded by peritoneum.

7. **The answer is A.** The suprarenal medulla is the only organ that receives preganglionic sympathetic fibers. No other nerve fibers are involved in secretion of norepinephrine from the suprarenal medulla.

8. **The answer is D.** Aganglionic megacolon (Hirschsprung disease) is caused by the absence of enteric ganglia (parasympathetic postganglionic neuron cell bodies) in the lower part of the colon, which leads to dilatation of the colon proximal to the inactive segment, resulting in an inability to evacuate the bowels. The other neuron cell bodies listed are not involved in this condition.

9. **The answer is C.** The left umbilical vein becomes the round ligament of the liver after birth. The right umbilical vein did not leave a fibrous remnant because it was degenerated during the early embryonic period. The ductus venosus forms the ligamentum venosum; the ductus arteriosus forms the ligamentum arteriosum; the umbilical artery forms the medial umbilical ligament.

10. **The answer is E.** The right and left hepatic veins drain into the inferior vena cava (IVC). The right gastroepiploic vein drains into the superior mesenteric vein, but the left one drains into the splenic vein. The right gonadal and suprarenal veins drain into the IVC, whereas the left

ones drain into the left renal vein. The right colic vein ends in the superior mesenteric vein, but the left one terminates in the inferior mesenteric vein.

11. **The answer is C.** The third part of the duodenum (transverse portion) crosses anterior to the IVC. The other structures do not cross the IVC anteriorly.

12. **The answer is C.** Pain sensation originating from peritoneal irritation by gastric contents in the lesser sac is carried by lower intercostals nerves. The vagus nerves carry sensory fibers associated with reflexes in the gastrointestinal (GI) tract. The greater splanchnic nerves and white rami communicantes carry pain (general visceral afferent [GVA]) fibers from the wall of the stomach and other areas of the GI tract. The gray rami communicantes contains no sensory fibers but contain sympathetic postganglionic fibers.

13. **The answer is C.** Stimulation of the cremaster muscle draws the testis up from the scrotum toward the superficial inguinal ring. The efferent limb of the reflex arc is the genital branch of the genitofemoral nerve, whereas the afferent limb is the femoral branch of the genitofemoral nerve. The other nerves are not involved in the cremasteric reflex.

14. **The answer is D.** The ascending and transverse colons receive blood from the superior mesenteric artery and parasympathetic nerve fibers from the vagus nerve. However, the descending and sigmoid colons receive blood from the inferior mesenteric artery and the parasympathetic nerve fibers from the pelvic splanchnic nerve arising from sacral spinal nerves (S2–S4).

15. **The answer is D.** Portal hypertension can be reduced by diverting blood from the portal to the caval system. This is accomplished by connecting the splenic vein to the left renal vein or by creating a communication between the portal vein and the IVC. A connection between a hepatic vein and a branch of the portal vein can be accomplished by the transjugular intrahepatic portosystemic shunt (TIPS) procedure in the treatment of bleeding esophageal varices.

16. **The answer is C.** The suprarenal gland receives arteries from three sources. The superior suprarenal artery arises from the inferior phrenic artery, the middle suprarenal artery arises from the abdominal aorta, and the inferior suprarenal artery arises from the renal artery. The hepatic, superior mesenteric, inferior mesenteric, and splenic arteries do not supply the suprarenal gland.

17. **The answer is E.** The left gastroepiploic artery runs through the lienogastric ligament, and hence, it is the artery most likely injured. The splenic artery is found in the lienorenal ligament. The right and left gastric arteries run within the lesser omentum. The gastroduodenal artery descends between the duodenum and the head of the pancreas.

18. **The answer is C.** The diaphragm receives somatic motor fibers solely from the phrenic nerves. However, the peritoneum on the central part of the diaphragm receives sensory fibers from the phrenic nerve, and the peripheral part of the diaphragm receives such fibers from the lower intercostal nerves. The subcostal nerve supplies the peritoneum inferior to the diaphragm. The vagus and greater splanchnic nerves do not carry pain fibers from the peritoneum.

19. **The answer is C.** The inferior pancreaticoduodenal artery is a branch of the superior mesenteric artery. All of other arteries are branches of the splenic artery.

20. **The answer is C.** The iliohypogastric nerve runs medially and inferiorly between the internal oblique and transverse abdominal muscles near the McBurney point, the point at the junction of the lateral one-third of the line between the anterior superior iliac spine and the umbilicus. Other structures are not found near the McBurney point.

21. **The answer is D.** Portal hypertension can cause esophageal varices, caput medusa, and hemorrhoids. The portal vein has higher pressure than systemic veins; the vein and its tributaries have no valves, or, if present, they are insignificant. In addition, the portal vein carries two to three times as much blood as the hepatic artery.

22. **The answer is B.** The jejunum has fewer mesenteric arterial arcades but longer vasa recta than the ileum. The plicae circulares (circular folds) are tall and closely packed in the jejunum and

are low and sparse in the ileum, and the lower part of the ileum has no plicae circulares. More digestion and absorption of nutrients occurs in the jejunum than in the ileum, and less fat is found in the mesentery of the jejunum.

23. **The answer is A.** The right colic vein belongs to the portal venous system and empties into the superior mesenteric vein, which joins the splenic vein to form the portal vein. The inferior epigastric, inferior phrenic, suprarenal, and ovarian veins belong to the systemic (or caval) venous system and drain directly or indirectly into the IVC.

24. **The answer is E.** The pancreas is a retroperitoneal organ, except for a small portion of its tail. The dorsal pancreatic artery would be the infected artery because it arises from the splenic artery and runs retroperitoneally along the superior border of the pancreas behind the peritoneum. The other arteries run within layers of the peritoneum. The left gastric arteries run within the lesser omentum; the proper hepatic artery runs within the free margin of the lesser omentum; the middle colic artery runs within the transverse mesocolon; the sigmoid arteries run within the sigmoid mesocolon.

25. **The answer is B.** The medial umbilical fold or ligament contains a fibrous remnant of the umbilical artery. The median umbilical fold contains a fibrous remnant of the urachus. The lateral umbilical fold (ligament) contains the inferior epigastric artery and vein, which are adult blood vessels. The ligamentum venosum contains a fibrous remnant of the ductus venosus, and the ligamentum teres hepatic contains a fibrous remnant of the left umbilical vein.

26. **The answer is E.** The left colic vein is a tributary of the inferior mesenteric vein. The middle colic, inferior pancreaticoduodenal, and ileocolic veins drain into the superior mesenteric vein. The left gastroepiploic vein empties into the splenic vein.

27. **The answer is D.** The superficial inguinal lymph nodes receive lymph from the scrotum, penis, buttocks, and lower part of the anal canal, and their efferent vessels enter primarily to the external iliac nodes and ultimately to the lumbar (aortic) nodes. The deep inguinal nodes receive lymph from the testis and upper parts of the vagina and anal canal, and their efferent vessels enter the external iliac nodes.

28. **The answer is D.** The liver receives blood from the hepatic artery and portal vein and drains its venous blood into the hepatic veins. The liver manufactures red blood cells in the fetus. The liver plays important roles in bile production and secretion. The quadrate lobe drains bile into the left hepatic duct, not the right hepatic duct, whereas the caudate lobe drains bile into the right and left hepatic ducts. The gallbladder functions to concentrate and store bile.

29. **The answer is A.** The bile duct is formed by union of the common hepatic and cystic ducts, lies lateral to the proper hepatic artery and anterior to the portal vein in the right free margin of the lesser omentum, traverses the head of the pancreas, and drains bile into the second part of the duodenum at the greater papilla. The endocrine part of the pancreas secretes the hormones insulin and glucagon, which are transported through the bloodstream. The main pancreatic duct carries pancreatic juice containing enzymes secreted from the exocrine part of the pancreas.

30. **The answer is E.** The sigmoid colon has teniae coli and epiploic appendages. The sigmoid colon receives blood from the inferior mesenteric artery, drains its venous blood through the portal tributaries, has its own mesentery (sigmoid mesocolon, therefore, is not a retroperitoneal organ), and receives parasympathetic preganglionic fibers from the pelvic splanchnic nerve.

31. **The answer is C.** The appendicular artery is a branch of the ileocolic artery. The other arteries do not supply the appendix. The middle colic and right colic arteries are branches of the superior mesenteric artery. The inferior mesenteric artery passes to the left behind the peritoneum and distributes to the descending and sigmoid colons and the upper portion of the rectum. The common iliac arteries are bifurcations from the aorta.

32. **The answer is C.** The inferior pancreaticoduodenal artery does not supply the stomach. All of the other arteries supply the stomach. Gastrocolostomy is used to establish a communication between the stomach and colon, bypassing the small intestine when the patient has Crohn disease (inflammation disease) and small bowel obstruction.

33. **The answer is A**. The greater splanchnic nerve carries pain fibers from the upper GI tract. Neither the ventral roots of the spinal nerves nor the gray rami communicantes contain sensory nerve fibers. The vagus nerve contains sensory fibers associated with reflexes, but it does not contain pain fibers. The lower intercostal nerves carry general somatic afferent (GSA) pain fibers from the diaphragm, abdominal wall, and peritoneum but not GVA pain fibers from the GI tract.

34. **The answer is D**. If a middle portion of the processus vaginalis persists, it forms a congenital hydrocele. If the entire processus vaginalis persists, it develops a congenital indirect inguinal hernia. Gubernaculum testis is the fetal ligament that connects the bottom of the fetal testis to the developing scrotum. Hematocele is an effusion of blood into the cavity of the tunica vaginalis. Cryptorchidism is failure of the testis to descend from the abdomen to the scrotum.

35. **The answer is E**. The porta hepatis is the transverse fissure (doorway) in the liver and contains the hepatic ducts, hepatic arteries, and branches of the portal vein. The other structures are not found in the porta hepatis.

36. **The answer is B**. Portal–caval anastomoses occur between the left gastric vein and esophageal vein of the azygos, the superior rectal and middle or inferior rectal veins, paraumbilical and superficial epigastric veins, and retrocolic veins and twigs of the renal vein. The hepatic veins and the IVC are systemic or caval veins. The left and right gastric veins belong to the portal venous system. The inferior and superficial epigastric veins and the suprarenal and renal veins are systemic veins.

37. **The answer is D**. The Meckel diverticulum is a persistent remnant of the yolk stalk (vitelline duct) and located 2 ft proximal to the ileocecal junction on the antimesenteric border of the ileum. It is approximately 2 in. long, occurs in approximately 2% of the population, and contains two types of mucosal (gastric and pancreatic) tissues in its wall.

38. **The answer is D**. The uncinate process of the pancreas is a projection of the lower part of its head to the left behind the superior mesenteric vessels. The superior pancreaticoduodenal artery runs between the duodenum and the head of the pancreas. The main pancreatic duct runs transversely through the entire pancreas superior to the uncinate process. The splenic artery runs along the superior border of the pancreas. The portal vein runs behind the neck of the pancreas.

39. **The answer is E**. A direct hernia is acquired (develops after birth), whereas an indirect inguinal hernia is congenital. The direct hernia does not enter the deep inguinal ring but occurs through the posterior wall of the inguinal canal, lies medial to the inferior epigastric artery, is covered only by peritoneum, and does not descend into the scrotum.

40. **The answer is D**. The genitofemoral nerve descends on the anterior surface of the psoas muscle and gives rise to a genital branch, which enters the inguinal canal through the deep inguinal ring to supply the cremaster muscle, and a femoral branch, which supplies the skin of the femoral triangle. The genitofemoral nerve is not a branch of the femoral nerve but arises from the lumbar plexus and does not supply the testis. It is the ilioinguinal nerve that gives rise to an anterior scrotal branch.

41. **The answer is C**. The quadrate lobe of the liver drains bile into the left hepatic duct and receives blood from the left hepatic artery. It lies between the gallbladder fossa and the ligamentum teres hepatic, is a medial inferior segment, and is a part of the left lobe.

42. **The answer is A**. The veins distal to obstruction are dilated, but the veins proximal to obstruction are not dilated but have low blood pressure. The suprarenal vein drains into the left renal vein and thus is dilated because of high pressure. The right phrenic and right hepatic veins drain into the IVC above the obstruction. The left gastric vein joins the portal vein, which enters the liver.

43. **The answer is B**. The linea semilunaris is a curved line along the lateral border of the rectus abdominis. The linea alba is a tendinous median raphe between the two rectus abdominis muscles. The linea semicircularis is an arcuate line of the rectus sheath, which is the lower limit of the posterior layer of the rectus sheath. The falx inguinalis (conjoint tendon) is formed by

aponeuroses of the internal oblique and transverse abdominal muscles (otherwise known as the transversalis fascia).

44. The answer is D. The paraumbilical veins and the ligamentum teres hepatis are contained in the free margin of the falciform ligament. The lienorenal ligament contains the splenic vessels and a small portion of the tail of the pancreas. The lienogastric ligament contains the left gastroepiploic and short gastric vessels. The gastrophrenic ligament contains no named structures. The hepatoduodenal ligament, a part of the lesser omentum, contains the bile duct, proper hepatic artery, and portal vein in its free margin.

45. The answer is C. The splenic artery arises from the celiac trunk, runs along the superior border of the pancreas, and enters the spleen through the lienorenal ligament and the hilus of the spleen. The right gastric artery runs along the lesser curvature of the stomach, and the left gastroepiploic artery runs along the greater curvature of the stomach. The gastroduodenal artery runs behind the first part of the duodenum. The dorsal pancreatic artery descends behind the neck of the pancreas and divides into right and left branches to supply the pancreas.

46. The answer is D. The vagus nerve supplies parasympathetic nerve fibers to the GI tract and terminates approximately at the left colic flexure (junction of the transverse colon and the descending colon). The duodenojejunal junction, ileocecal junction, and right colic flexure are supplied by the vagus nerve. The descending colon, sigmoid colon, rectum, anal canal, and anorectal junction are supplied by the pelvic splanchnic nerve for parasympathetic innervation.

47. The answer is B. The pyloric canal and the neck of the pancreas are situated anterior to the abdominal aorta between the origin of the celiac trunk and the superior mesenteric artery. The transverse colon passes anterior to the superior mesenteric artery and the third part of the duodenum. The other structures are not located in front of the aorta.

48. The answer is C. The falx inguinalis (conjoint tendon) is formed by the aponeuroses of the internal oblique and transverse muscles of the abdomen. The inguinal ligament is formed by aponeurosis of the external oblique abdominal muscle, and the reflected inguinal ligament is formed by certain fibers of the inguinal ligament reflected from the pubic tubercle upward toward the linea alba. The deep inguinal ring lies in the transversalis fascia, and the internal spermatic fascia is formed by the transversalis fascia.

49. The answer is D. The right colic and ileocolic arteries arise from the superior mesenteric artery distal to the origin of the middle colic artery. The right colic artery may arise from the ileocolic artery and supplies the ascending colon. The duodenum and pancreas receive blood from the inferior pancreaticoduodenal artery and superior pancreaticoduodenal artery. The pancreas is also supplied by the splenic artery of the celiac trunk. The transverse colon receives blood from the middle colic artery. The descending colon is supplied by the left colic artery, which is a branch of the inferior mesenteric artery.

50. The answer is D. The left renal vein runs anterior to both the aorta and the left renal artery. The renal fascia lies external to the perirenal fat and internal to the pararenal fat, and it also surrounds the suprarenal gland. The right renal artery runs behind the IVC and is longer than the left renal artery. Because of the large size of the right lobe of the liver, the right kidney lies a little lower than the left kidney.

51. Answer is C. Cells in the islets of Langerhans, an endocrine portion of the pancreas, are derived from the endoderm of the caudal foregut (from the liver diverticulum). Proctodeum is an invagination of the ectoderm of the terminal part of the hindgut.

52. **Answer is D**. The ascending colon is derived from the midgut. The gallbladder and stomach are derived from the foregut, and the descending colon and rectum are derived from the hindgut.

53. **Answer is C**. The ureteric bud is an outgrowth of the mesonephric duct and develops into the ureter, renal pelvis, calyces, and collecting tubules. However, a bifurcated ureteric bud results in a partial duplication (bifid) of the ureter, whereas two separate ureteric buds result in a complete duplication. Mesonephric duct forms efferent ductules, epididymal duct, ductus deferens, ejaculatory duct, and seminal vesicles. Paramesonephric duct regress and its vestigial remnants form the appendix testis. Metanephros develops into the adult kidney. Pronephros degenerates and never forms functional nephrons.

54. **The answer is A**. In most case, an umbilical hernia closes spontaneously by age 4 and requires no surgery unless there is incarceration. A symptomatic patent urachus (drainage of urine at the umbilicus) is typically surgically excised. A patent omphalomesenteric duct (Meckel diverticulum) is promptly repaired to minimize the potential for intestinal obstruction or prolapse. Omphalocele and gastroschisis are defects that require surgical repair.

55. **The answer is E**. The spleen lies in the left hypochondriac region, is hematopoietic in early life, and later functions in worn-out red blood cell destruction. It filters blood, stores red blood cells, and produces lymphocytes and antibodies.

56. **The answer is D**. The splenic artery is a branch of the celiac trunk, follows a tortuous course along the superior border of the pancreas, and divides into several branches that run through the lienorenal ligament.

57. **The answer is A**. The common hepatic artery is divided into the proper hepatic and gastroduodenal arteries.

58. **The answer is B**. The duodenojejunal flexure is supported by a fibromuscular band called the suspensory ligament of the duodenum (ligament of Treitz), which is attached to the right crus of the diaphragm.

59. **The answer is C**. The pancreas is an endocrine and exocrine gland; is retroperitoneal in position; and receives blood from the splenic, gastroduodenal, and superior mesenteric arteries.

60. **The answer is D**. The superior mesenteric artery, a direct branch of the aorta, supplies blood to the ascending and transverse colons.

61. **The answer is B**. The IVC, which receives blood from the liver, kidneys, and other abdominal structures, enters the thorax through the vena caval foramen to empty into the right atrium.

62. **The answer is A**. The gallbladder receives bile, concentrates it by absorbing water and salt, and stores it.

63. **The answer is E**. The left renal vein runs anterior to the aorta but posterior to the superior mesenteric artery and receives blood from the gonad and suprarenal gland.

64. **The answer is C**. The liver receives venous blood from the portal vein and arterial blood from the hepatic arteries.

chapter 5 Perineum and Pelvis

PERINEAL REGION

I. PERINEUM

- Is a **diamond-shaped space** that has the same boundaries as the inferior aperture of the pelvis.
- Is bounded by the **pubic symphysis** anteriorly, the **ischiopubic rami** anterolaterally, the **ischial tuberosities** laterally, the **sacrotuberous ligaments** posterolaterally, and the **tip of the coccyx** posteriorly.
- Has a floor that is composed of skin and fascia and a roof formed by the **pelvic diaphragm** with its fascial covering.
- Is divided into an anterior **urogenital triangle** and a posterior **anal triangle** by a line connecting the two **ischial tuberosities**.

II. UROGENITAL TRIANGLE (Figures 5.1 to 5.2)

A. Superficial Perineal Space (Pouch)

- Lies between the **inferior fascia of the urogenital diaphragm (perineal membrane)** and the membranous layer of the superficial perineal fascia **(Colles fascia)**.
- Contains the superficial transverse perineal muscle, the ischiocavernosus muscles and crus of the penis or clitoris, the bulbospongiosus muscles and the bulb of the penis or the vestibular bulbs, the central tendon of the perineum, the greater vestibular glands (in the female), branches of the internal pudendal vessels, and the perineal nerve and its branches.

1. Colles Fascia

- Is the **deep membranous layer** of the superficial perineal fascia and forms the inferior boundary of the superficial perineal pouch.
- Is continuous with the **dartos tunic** of the scrotum, with the **superficial fascia** of the penis, and with the **Scarpa fascia** of the anterior abdominal wall.

CLINICAL CORRELATES **Extravasated urine** may result from **rupture** of the bulbous portion of the **spongy urethra** below the urogenital diaphragm; the urine may pass into the superficial perineal space and spread inferiorly into the scrotum, anteriorly around the penis, and superiorly into the lower part of the abdominal wall. The urine cannot spread laterally into the thigh because the inferior fascia of the urogenital diaphragm (the perineal membrane) and the superficial fascia of the perineum are firmly attached to the ischiopubic rami and are connected with the deep fascia of the thigh (fascia lata). It cannot spread posteriorly into the anal region (ischiorectal fossa) because the perineal membrane and Colles fascia are continuous with each other around the superficial transverse perineal muscles. If the membranous part of the urethra is ruptured, urine escapes into the deep perineal space and can extravasate upward around the prostate and bladder or downward into the superficial perineal space.

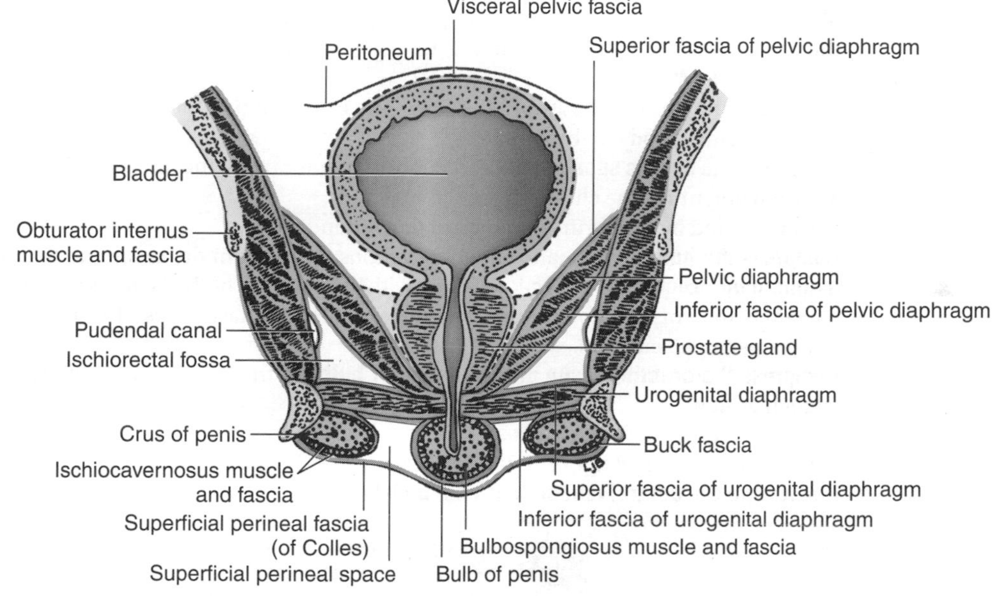

FIGURE 5.1. Frontal section of the male perineum and pelvis.

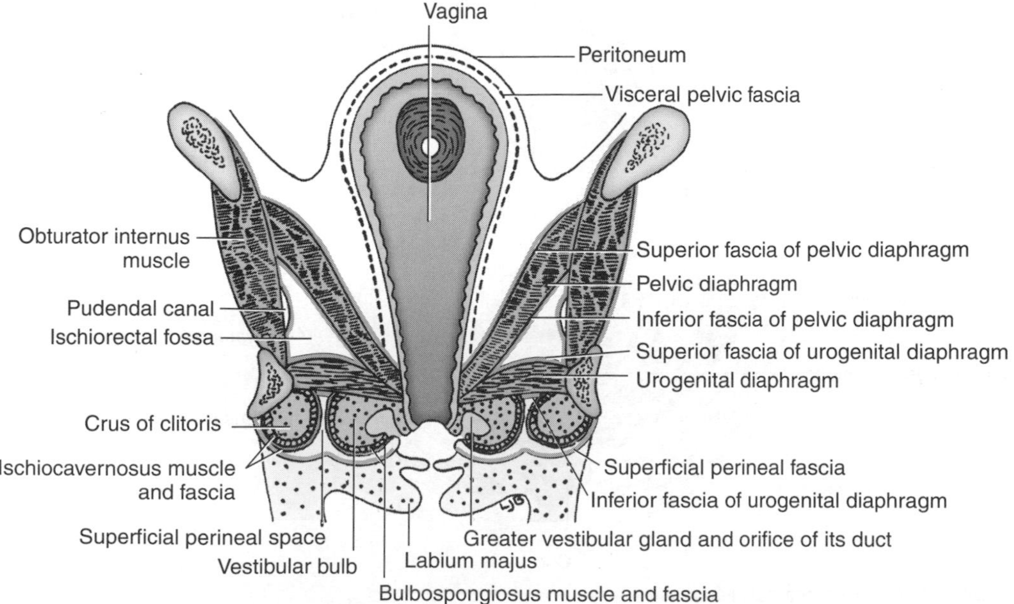

FIGURE 5.2. Frontal section of the female perineum and pelvis.

2. Perineal Membrane

- Is the **inferior fascia of the urogenital diaphragm** that forms the inferior boundary of the deep perineal pouch and the superior boundary of the superficial pouch.
- Lies between the urogenital diaphragm and the external genitalia, is perforated by the urethra, and is attached to the posterior margin of the urogenital diaphragm and the ischiopubic rami.
- Is thickened anteriorly to form the transverse ligament of the perineum, which spans the subpubic angle just behind the deep dorsal vein of the penis.

3. Muscles of the Superficial Perineal Space (Figures 5.3 to 5.4)

(a) Ischiocavernosus Muscles

- Arise from the inner surface of the ischial tuberosities and the ischiopubic rami.
- Insert into the **corpus cavernosum** (the crus of the penis or clitoris).
- Are innervated by the perineal branch of the pudendal nerve.
- **Maintain erection** of the penis by compressing the crus and the deep dorsal vein of the penis, thereby retarding venous return.

(b) Bulbospongiosus Muscles

- Arise from the perineal body and fibrous raphe of the bulb of the penis in the male and the perineal body in the female.
- Insert into the **corpus spongiosum** and perineal membrane in the male and the pubic arch and dorsum of the clitoris in the female.
- Are innervated by the perineal branch of the pudendal nerve.
- **Compress the bulb** in the male, impeding venous return from the penis and thereby **maintaining erection**. Contraction (along with contraction of the ischiocavernosus) constricts the corpus spongiosum, thereby expelling the last drops of urine or the final semen in ejaculation.
- **Compress the erectile tissue of the vestibular bulbs** in the female and **constrict the vaginal orifice**.

(c) Superficial Transverse Perineal Muscle

- Arises from the ischial rami and tuberosities.
- Inserts into the **central tendon (perineal body)**.

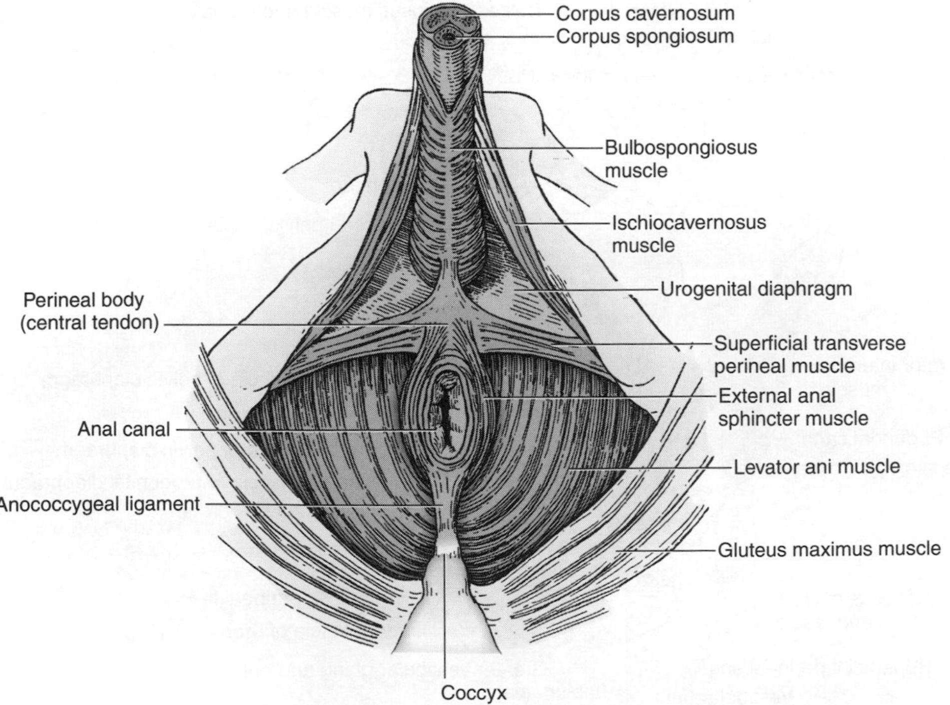

FIGURE 5.3. Muscles of the male perineum.

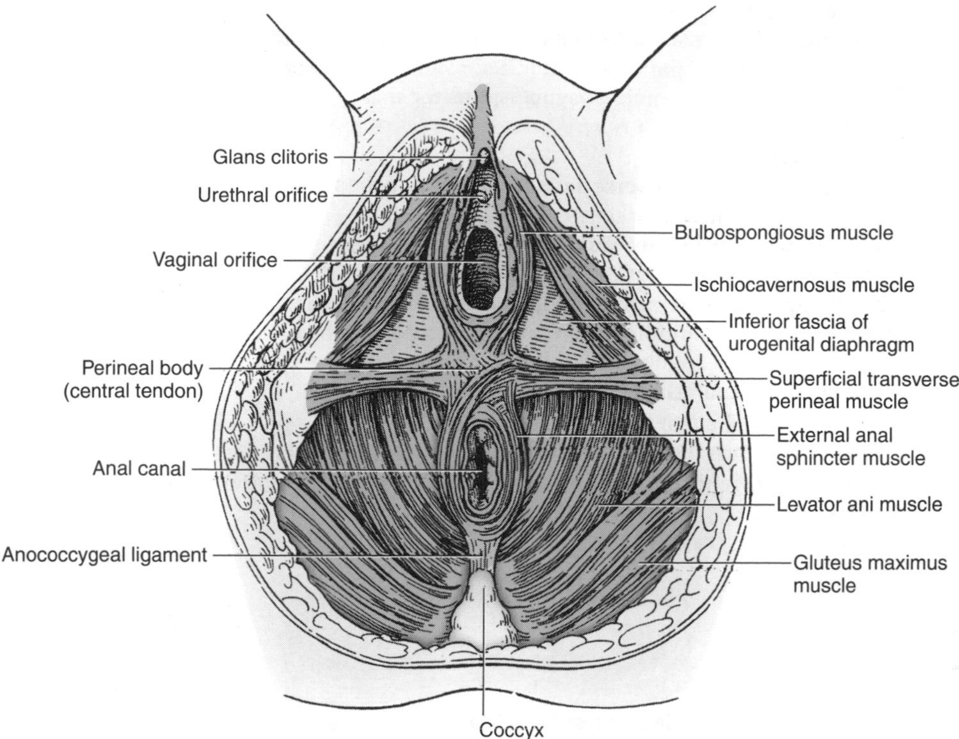

FIGURE 5.4. Muscles of the female perineum.

- Is innervated by the perineal branch of the **pudendal nerve**.
- **Stabilizes the central tendon.**

4. Perineal Body (Central Tendon of the Perineum)

- Is a **fibromuscular mass** located in the center of the perineum between the anal canal and the vagina (or the bulb of the penis).
- Serves as a site of attachment for the superficial and deep transverse perineal, bulbospongiosus, levator ani, and external anal sphincter muscles.

5. Greater Vestibular (Bartholin) Glands

- Lie in the superficial perineal space deep to the vestibular bulbs in the female.
- Are homologous to the **bulbourethral glands** in the male.
- Are compressed during coitus and secrete mucus that **lubricates the vagina**. Ducts open into the vestibule between the **labium minora** below the **hymen**.

B. Deep Perineal Space (Pouch)

- Lies between the superior and inferior fasciae of the urogenital diaphragm.
- Contains the deep transverse perineal muscle and sphincter urethrae, the membranous part of the urethra, the bulbourethral glands (in the male), and branches of the internal pudendal vessels and pudendal nerve.

1. Muscles of the Deep Perineal Space

(a) Deep Transverse Perineal Muscle

- Arises from the inner surface of the **ischial rami**.
- Inserts into the medial tendinous raphe and the perineal body; in the female, it also inserts into the wall of the vagina.
- Is innervated by the perineal branches of the pudendal nerve.
- Stabilizes the perineal body and **supports the prostate gland or the vagina**.

(b) Sphincter Urethrae

- Arise from the inferior pubic ramus.
- Insert into the median raphe and perineal body.

- Are innervated by the perineal branch of the pudendal nerve.
- **Encircle** and **constrict the membranous urethra** in the male.
- Have an inferior part that is attached to the anterolateral wall of the vagina in the female, forming a urethrovaginal sphincter that compresses both the urethra and vagina.

2. Urogenital Diaphragm

- Consists of the deep transverse perineal muscle and the sphincter urethrae and is invested by superior and inferior fasciae.
- Stretches between the two pubic rami and ischial rami but does not reach the pubic symphysis anteriorly.
- Has inferior fascia that provides attachment to the **bulb of the penis.**
- Is pierced by the membranous urethra in the male and by the urethra and the vagina in the female.

3. Bulbourethral (Cowper) Glands

- Lie among the fibers of the sphincter urethrae in the deep perineal pouch in the male, on the posterolateral sides of the membranous urethra. Ducts pass through the inferior fascia of the urogenital diaphragm to open into the bulbous portion of the **spongy (penile) urethra.**

III. ANAL TRIANGLE

A. Ischiorectal (Ischioanal) Fossa (See Figures 5.1 to 5.2)

- Is the potential space on either side of the anorectum and is separated from the pelvis by the levator ani and its fasciae.
- Contains **ischioanal fat**, which allows distention of the anal canal during defecation; the **inferior rectal nerves and vessels**, which are branches of the internal pudendal vessels and the pudendal nerve; and **perineal branches** of the posterior femoral cutaneous nerve (which communicates with the inferior rectal nerve).
- Contains the **pudendal (Alcock) canal** on its lateral wall. This is a fascial canal formed by a split in the obturator internus fascia and transmits the pudendal nerve and internal pudendal vessels.
- Is occasionally the site of an abscess that can extend to other fossa by way of the communication over the anococcygeal raphe.
- Has the following **boundaries**:
  1. **Anterior:** the sphincter urethrae and deep transverse perineal muscles
  2. **Posterior:** the gluteus maximus muscle and the sacrotuberous ligament
  3. **Superomedial:** the sphincter ani externus and levator ani muscles
  4. **Lateral:** the obturator fascia covering the obturator internus muscle
  5. **Floor:** the skin over the anal triangle

B. Muscles of the Anal Triangle (Figure 5.5)

1. Obturator Internus

- Arises from the inner surface of the **obturator membrane.**
- Has a tendon that passes around the lesser sciatic notch to insert into the medial surface of the greater trochanter of the femur.
- Is innervated by the nerve to the obturator.
- **Laterally rotates the thigh.**

2. Sphincter Ani Externus

- Arises from the tip of the coccyx and the anococcygeal ligament, inserts into the central tendon of the perineum, is innervated by the inferior rectal nerve, and **closes the anus.**
- Is composed of three parts: subcutaneous, superficial (main part, attached to the coccyx and central tendon), and deep. **Corrugator cutis ani** muscle is a thin stratum of smooth-muscle fibers radiating from the superficial part of the sphincter to the deep aspect of the perianal skin, causing puckering of that skin, which contributes to the air-/water-tight seal of the anal canal.

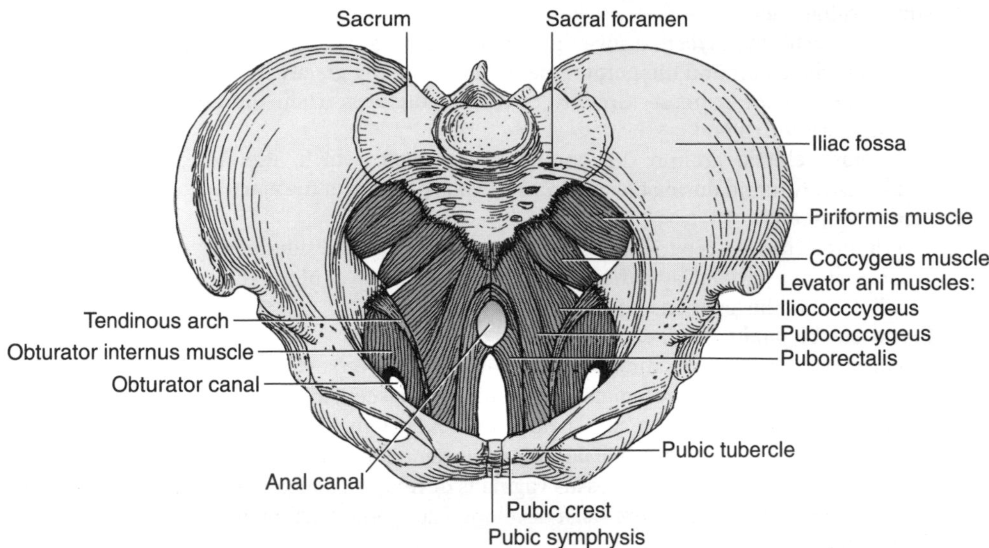

FIGURE 5.5. Muscles of the perineum and pelvis.

3. Levator Ani Muscle

- Arises from the body of the pubis, the arcus tendineus of the levator ani (a thickened part of the obturator fascia), and the ischial spine.
- Inserts into the coccyx and the anococcygeal raphe or ligament.
- Is innervated by the branches of the anterior rami of sacral nerves S3 and S4 and the perineal branch of the pudendal nerve.
- **Supports and raises the pelvic floor.**
- Consists of the puborectalis, pubococcygeus, and iliococcygeus.
- Has as its most anterior fibers, which are also the most medial, the levator prostate or pubovaginalis.

4. Coccygeus

- Arises from the ischial spine and the sacrospinous ligament.
- Inserts into the coccyx and the lower part of the sacrum.
- Is innervated by branches of the fourth and fifth sacral nerves.
- **Supports and raises the pelvic floor.**

C. Anal Canal (See Pelvis: VIII. B.)

IV. EXTERNAL GENITALIA AND ASSOCIATED STRUCTURES

A. Fasciae and Ligaments

1. Fundiform Ligament of the Penis

- Arises from the linea alba and the membranous layer of the superficial fascia of the abdomen.
- Splits into left and right parts, **encircles the body of the penis**, and blends with the superficial penile fascia.
- Enters the septum of the scrotum.

2. Suspensory Ligament of the Penis (or the Clitoris)

- Arises from the pubic symphysis and the arcuate pubic ligament and inserts into the deep fascia of the penis or into the body of the clitoris.
- Lies deep to the fundiform ligaments.

3. Deep Fascia of the Penis (Buck Fascia)

- Is a continuation of the deep perineal fascia.
- Is continuous with the fascia covering the external oblique muscle and the rectus sheath.

4. Tunica Albuginea

- Is a **dense fibrous layer** that envelops both the corpora cavernosa and the corpus spongiosum.
- Is **very dense** around the **corpora cavernosa**, thereby greatly impeding venous return and resulting in the extreme turgidity of these structures when the erectile tissue becomes engorged with blood.
- Is **more elastic** around the **corpus spongiosum**, which, therefore, does not become excessively turgid during erection and permits passage of the ejaculate.

5. Tunica Vaginalis

- Is a serous sac of the peritoneum that covers the front and sides of the testis and epididymis.
- Consists of a parietal layer that forms the innermost layer of the scrotum and a visceral layer adherent to the testis and epididymis.

6. Processus Vaginalis

- Is an embryonic diverticulum of the peritoneum that traverses the inguinal canal, accompanying the round ligament in the female or the testis in its descent into the scrotum and closes forming the tunica vaginalis in the male. If it does not close in females, it forms the **canal of Nuck**, which is an abnormal patent pouch of peritoneum extending into the labia majora.
- Persistence of the entire processus vaginalis develops a congenital indirect **inguinal hernia**, but if its middle portion persists, it develops a congenital **hydrocele**.

7. Gubernaculum

- Is a fibrous cord that connects the fetal testis to the floor of the developing scrotum, and its homologues in the female are the ovarian and round ligaments.
- Appears to play a role in testicular descent by pulling the testis down as it migrates.

B. Male External Genitalia

1. Scrotum

- Is a cutaneous pouch consisting of **thin skin** and the underlying **dartos**, which is continuous with the superficial penile fascia and superficial perineal fascia. The dartos muscle is responsible for wrinkling the scrotal skin, and the cremaster muscle is responsible for elevating the testis.
- Is covered with sparse hairs and has **no fat**, which is important in maintaining a temperature lower than the rest of the body for sperm production.
- Contains the **testis** and its covering and the **epididymis**.
- Is contracted and wrinkled when cold (or sexually stimulated) to increase its thickness and reduce heat loss, bringing the testis into close contact with the body to conserve heat; is relaxed when warm and hence is flaccid and distended to dissipate heat.
- Receives blood from the external pudendal arteries and the posterior scrotal branches of the internal pudendal arteries.
- Is innervated by the anterior scrotal branch of the **ilioinguinal nerve**, the genital branch of the **genitofemoral nerve**, the posterior scrotal branch of the perineal branch of the **pudendal nerve**, and the perineal branch of the **posterior femoral cutaneous nerve**.

2. Testes (See Pelvis: VII. A; Anterior Abdominal Wall: V. D, Chapter 4)

CLINICAL CORRELATES

Hydrocele is an **accumulation of fluid** in the cavity of the **tunica vaginalis** (two layers of the tunica vaginalis) of the testis or along the spermatic cord due to an infection or injury to the testis or partial occlusion of a processus vaginalis. **Hematocele** is a hemorrhage into the cavity of the tunica vaginalis due to injury to the spermatic vessels.

Varicocele is an **enlargement of the pampiniform venous plexus** of the spermatic cord that appears like a "bag of worms" in the scrotum. A varicocele may cause dragging like pain, atrophy of the testis, and/or infertility. It is more common on the left side and can be treated surgically by removing the varicose veins.

If a man wants to have children, it is recommended that he does not wear tight underwear or tight jeans because tight clothing holds the testes close to the body wall, where higher temperatures inhibit sperm production. Under cold conditions, the testes are pulled up toward the warm body wall, and the scrotal skin wrinkles to increase its thickness and reduce heat loss.

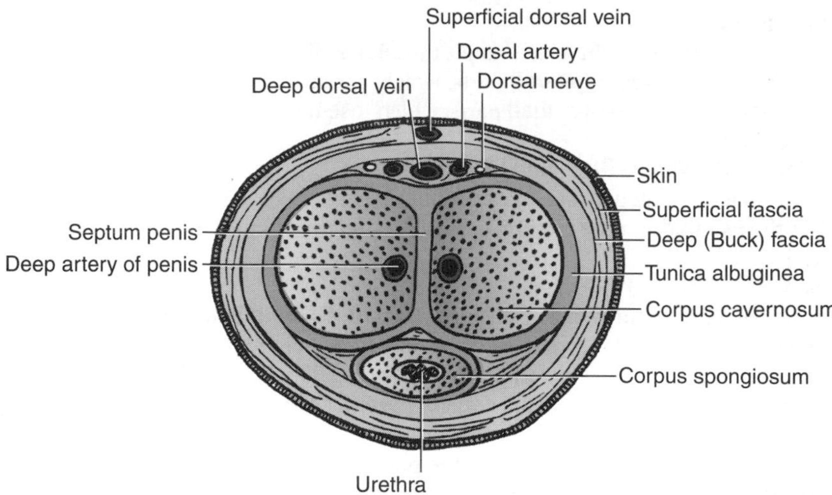

FIGURE 5.6. Cross section of the penis.

3. **Penis** (Figure 5.6)
   - Consists of three masses of **vascular erectile tissue**; these are the paired corpora cavernosa and the midline corpus spongiosum, which are bounded by tunica albuginea.
   - Consists of a **root**, which includes two crura and the bulb of the penis, and the **body**, which contains the single corpus spongiosum and the paired corpora cavernosa.
   - Has a head called the **glans penis**, which is formed by the terminal part of the **corpus spongiosum** and is covered by a free fold of skin, the **prepuce**. The **frenulum** of the prepuce is a median ventral fold passing from the deep surface of the prepuce. The prominent margin of the glans penis is the **corona**, the median slit near the tip of the glans is the **external urethral orifice**, and the terminal dilated part of the urethra in the glans is the **fossa navicularis**.
   - **Preputial glands** are small sebaceous glands of the corona, the neck of the glans penis, and the inner surface of the prepuce, which secrete an odoriferous substance called smegma.

CLINICAL CORRELATES

Epispadias is a congenital malformation in which the spongy urethra opens as a groove on the dorsum of the penis, frequently associated with the **bladder exstrophy** (congenital eversion or turning inside out of an organ, as the bladder). **Hypospadias** is a congenital malformation in which the urethra opens on the underside of the penis because of a failure of the two urethral folds to fuse completely. It is frequently associated with **chordee**, which is a ventral curvature of the penis.

Circumcision is the removal of the foreskin (prepuce) that covers the glans of the penis. It is performed as a therapeutic medical procedure for pathologic phimosis, chronic inflammations of the penis, and penile cancer. It is also performed for cultural, religious, and medical reasons.

Phimosis is a condition in which the foreskin (prepuce) cannot be fully retracted to reveal the glans due to a narrow opening of the prepuce. A very tight foreskin around the tip of the penis may interfere with urination or sexual function. **Paraphimosis** is a painful constriction of the glans penis caused by a tight band of constricted and retracted phimotic foreskin behind the corona. This ring of tissue causes penile ischemia and vascular engorgement, swelling, and edema, leading to penile gangrene.

C. Female External Genitalia

1. **Labia Majora**
   - Are two **longitudinal folds of skin** that run downward and backward from the **mons pubis** and are joined anteriorly by the **anterior labial commissure**.
   - Are homologous to the **scrotum** of the male. Their outer surfaces are covered with pigmented skin, and after puberty, the labia majora are covered with hair.
   - Contain the terminations of the round ligaments of the uterus.

2. Labia Minora

- Are hairless and contain no fat, unlike the labia majora.
- Are divided into **upper (lateral)** parts, which, above the clitoris, fuse to form the **prepuce of the clitoris**, and **lower (medial)** parts, which fuse below the clitoris to form the **frenulum of the clitoris**.

3. Vestibule of the Vagina (Urogenital Sinus)

- Is the space or cleft between the labia minora.
- Has the **openings** for the urethra, the vagina, and the ducts of the greater vestibular glands in its floor.

4. Clitoris

- Is homologous to the **penis** in the male, consists of **erectile tissue**, is enlarged as a result of engorgement with blood, and is not perforated by the urethra.
- Consists of two crura, two corpora cavernosa, and a glans but **no corpus spongiosum**. The **glans clitoris** is derived from the **corpora cavernosa** and is covered by a sensitive epithelium.

5. Bulbs of the Vestibule

- Are the homologues of the bulb of the penis of the corpus spongiosum, a paired mass of erectile tissue on each side of the vaginal orifice.
- Are covered by the bulbospongiosus muscle, and each bulb is joined to one another and to the undersurface of the glans clitoris by a narrow band of erectile tissue.

V. NERVE SUPPLY OF THE PERINEAL REGION (Figure 5.7)

A. Pudendal Nerve (S2–S4)

- Passes through the greater sciatic foramen between the piriformis and coccygeus muscles.

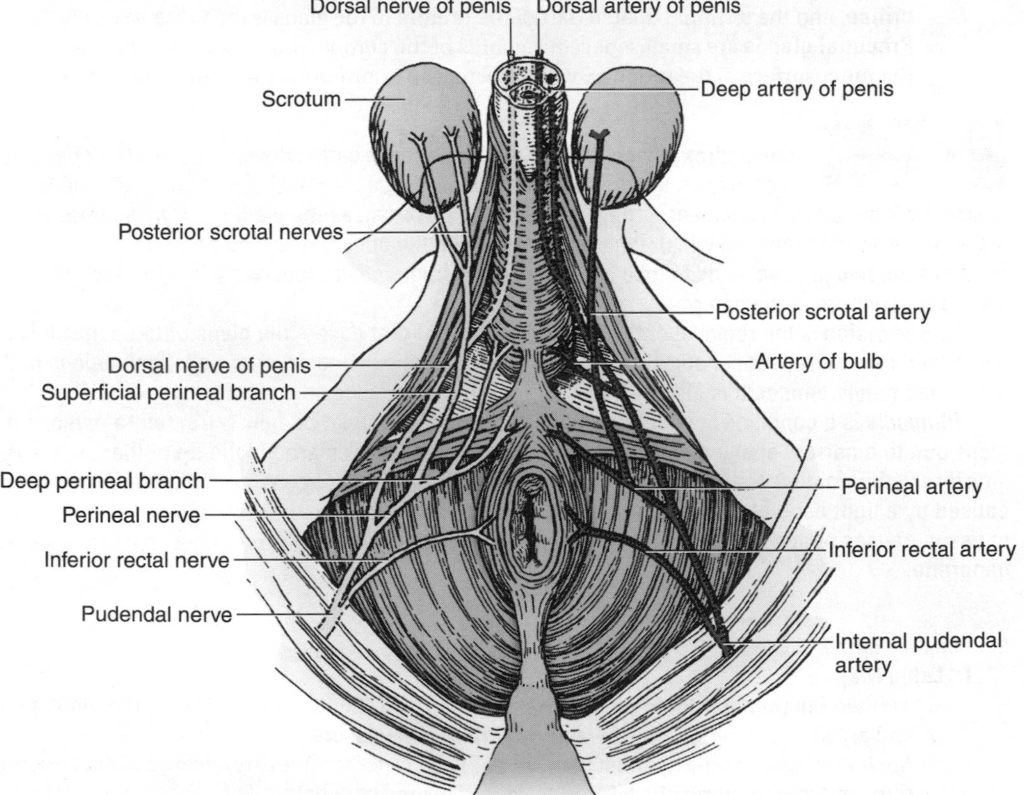

FIGURE 5.7. Internal pudendal artery and pudendal nerve and branches.

- Crosses the ischial spine and enters the perineum with the internal pudendal artery through the lesser sciatic foramen.
- Enters the **pudendal canal**, gives rise to the inferior rectal nerve and the perineal nerve, and terminates as the **dorsal nerve of the penis (or clitoris)**.

CLINICAL CORRELATES **Pudendal nerve block** is performed by injecting a local anesthetic near the pudendal nerve. It is accomplished by inserting a needle through the posterolateral vaginal wall, just beneath the pelvic diaphragm and toward the ischial spine, thus placing the needle around the pudendal nerve. (A finger is placed on the ischial spine and the needle is inserted in the direction of the tip of the finger on the spine.) Pudendal block can be done subcutaneously through the buttock by inserting the needle on the medial side of the ischial tuberosity to deposit the anesthetic near the pudendal nerve.

1. Inferior Rectal Nerve

- Arises within the pudendal canal, divides into several branches, crosses the ischiorectal fossa, and innervates the sphincter ani externus and the skin around the anus.
- Communicates in the ischiorectal fossa with perineal branch of the posterior femoral cutaneous nerve, which supplies the scrotum or labium majus.

2. Perineal Nerve

- Arises within the pudendal canal and divides into a **deep branch**, which supplies all of the perineal muscles, and a **superficial (posterior scrotal or labial) branch**, which supplies the scrotum or labia majora.

3. Dorsal Nerve of the Penis (or Clitoris)

- Pierces the perineal membrane, runs between the two layers of the suspensory ligament of the penis or clitoris, and runs deep to the deep fascia on the dorsum of the penis or clitoris to innervate the skin, prepuce, and glans.

VI. BLOOD SUPPLY OF THE PERINEAL REGION (See Figure 5.7)

A. Internal Pudendal Artery

- Arises from the internal iliac artery.
- Leaves the pelvis by way of the greater sciatic foramen between the piriformis and coccygeus and immediately enters the perineum through the lesser sciatic foramen by hooking around the ischial spine.
- Is accompanied by the pudendal nerve during its course.
- Passes along the lateral wall of the ischiorectal fossa in the pudendal canal.
- Gives rise to the following:

1. Inferior Rectal Artery

- Arises within the pudendal canal, pierces the wall of the pudendal canal, and breaks into several branches, which cross the ischiorectal fossa to **muscles and skin around the anal canal**.

2. Perineal Arteries

- Supply the superficial perineal muscles and give rise to transverse perineal branches and posterior scrotal (or labial) branches.

3. Artery of the Bulb

- Arises within the deep perineal space, pierces the perineal membrane, and supplies the bulb of the penis and the bulbourethral glands (in the male) and the vestibular bulbs and the greater vestibular gland (in the female).

4. Urethral Artery

- Pierces the perineal membrane, enters the corpus spongiosum of the penis, and continues to the **glans penis.**

5. Deep Arteries of the Penis or Clitoris

- Are terminal branches of the internal pudendal artery.
- Pierce the perineal membrane, run through the center of the **corpus cavernosum** of the penis or clitoris, and supply its erectile tissue.

6. Dorsal Arteries of the Penis or Clitoris

- Pierce the perineal membrane and pass through the suspensory ligament of the penis or clitoris.
- Run along its dorsum on each side of the deep dorsal vein and deep to the deep fascia (Buck fascia) and superficial to the tunica albuginea to supply the **glans** and prepuce.

B. External Pudendal Artery

- Arises from the femoral artery, emerges through the saphenous ring, and passes medially over the spermatic cord or the round ligament of the uterus to supply the **skin above the pubis, penis, and scrotum or labium majus.**

C. Veins of the Penis

1. Deep Dorsal Vein of the Penis

- Is an unpaired vein that lies in the dorsal midline deep to the deep (Buck) fascia and superficial to the tunica albuginea.
- Leaves the perineum through the gap between the **arcuate pubic ligament** and the **transverse perineal ligament** and drains into the prostatic and pelvic venous plexuses.

2. Superficial Dorsal Vein of the Penis

- Runs toward the pubic symphysis between the superficial and deep fasciae and terminates in the **external (superficial) pudendal veins,** which drain into the greater saphenous vein.

D. Lymph Nodes and Vessels (Figure 5.8)

1. Lymphatic Drainage of the Perineum

- Occurs via the superficial inguinal lymph nodes, which receive lymph from the lower abdominal wall, buttocks, penis, scrotum, labium majus, and lower parts of the vagina and

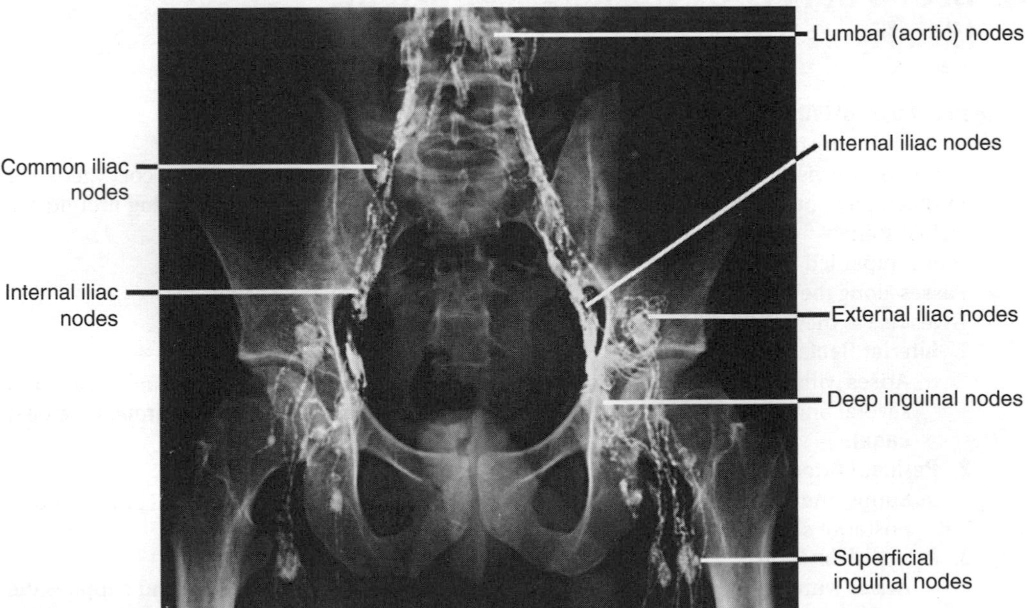

FIGURE 5.8. Lymphograph of the pelvis and lumbar region.

anal canal. These nodes have efferent vessels that drain primarily into the **external iliac nodes** and ultimately to the **lumbar (aortic) nodes.**

- Lymph vessels from the glans penis (or clitoris) and labium minus pass to the deep inguinal and external iliac nodes.

2. Lymphatic Drainage of the Pelvis

- Follows the internal iliac vessels to the internal iliac nodes and subsequently to the lumbar (aortic) nodes.
  1. Internal iliac nodes receive lymph from the upper part of the rectum and vagina and other pelvic organs, and they drain into the common iliac and then to the lumbar (aortic) nodes. However, lymph from the uppermost part of the rectum drains into the inferior mesenteric nodes and then to the aortic nodes.
  2. Lymph from the testis and epididymis or ovary drains along the gonadal vessels directly into the aortic nodes.

PELVIS

I. BONY PELVIS (Figures 5.9 to 5.11)

A. Pelvis

- Is the **basin-shaped ring of bone** formed by the two **hip bones**, the **sacrum**, and the **coccyx**. (The hip or coxal bone consists of the ilium, ischium, and pubis.)
- Is divided by the **pelvic brim** or iliopectineal line into the **pelvis major (false pelvis)** above and the **pelvis minor (true pelvis)** below.
- Has an outlet that is closed by the coccygeus and levator ani muscles, which form the **floor of the pelvis**.
- Is normally tilted in anatomic position. Thus:
  1. The anterior–superior iliac spine and the pubic tubercles are in the same vertical plane.
  2. The coccyx is in the same horizontal plane as the upper margin of the pubic symphysis.
  3. The axis of the pelvic cavity running through the central point of the inlet and the outlet almost parallels the curvature of the sacrum.

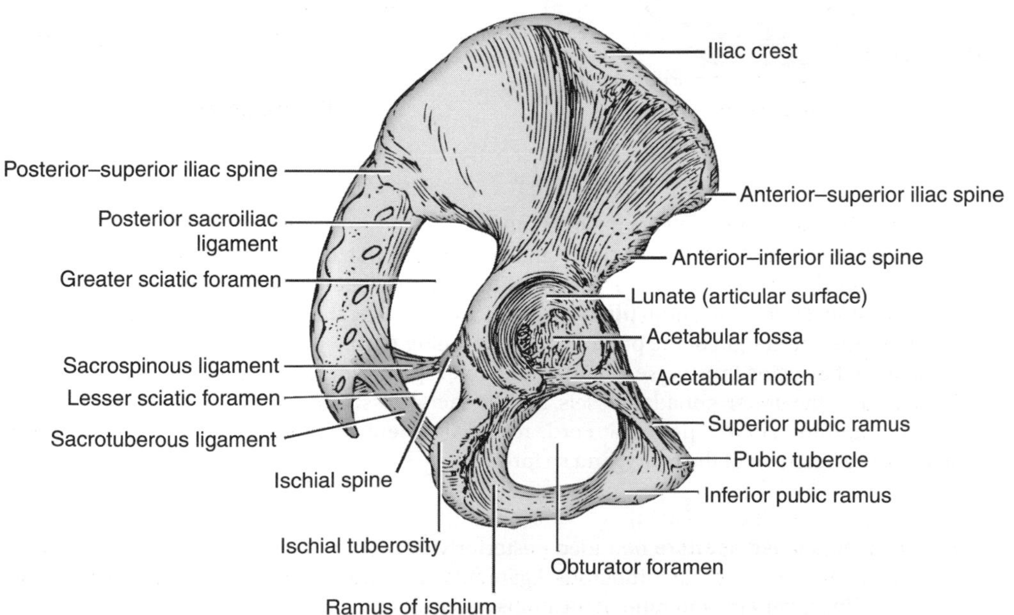

FIGURE 5.9. Lateral view of the hip bone.

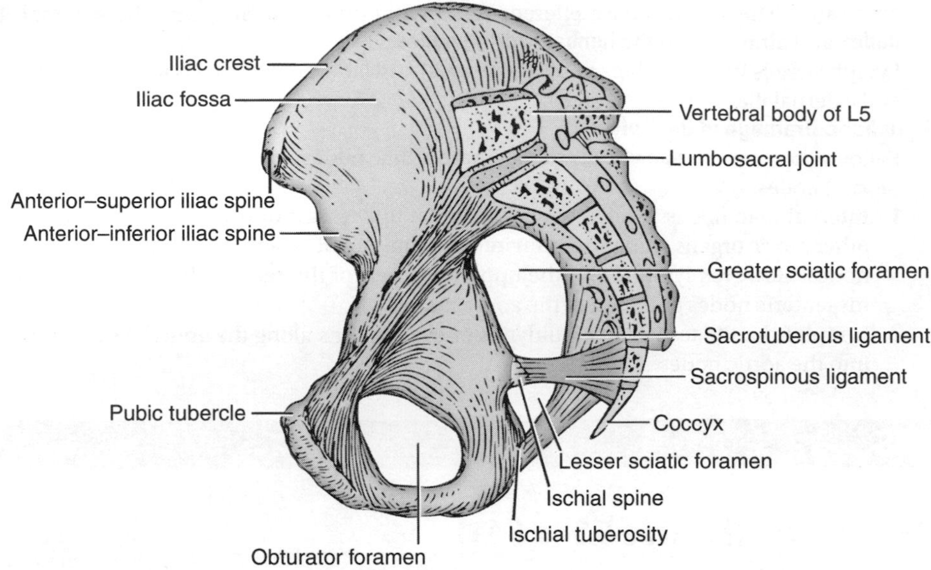

FIGURE 5.10. Medial view of the hip bone.

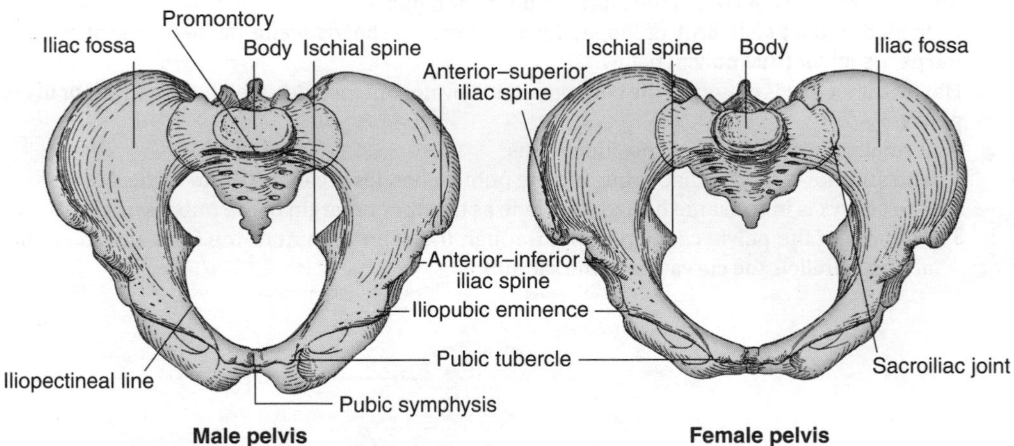

FIGURE 5.11. Male and female pelvic bones.

B. Upper Pelvic Aperture (Pelvic Inlet or Pelvic Brim)

- Is the **superior rim of the pelvic cavity** and is bounded posteriorly by the promontory of the sacrum and the anterior border of the ala of the sacrum **(sacral part)**, laterally by the arcuate or iliopectineal line of the ilium **(iliac part)** and anteriorly by the pectineal line, the pubic crest, and the superior margin of the pubic symphysis **(pubic part)**.
- Is measured by using transverse, oblique, and anteroposterior (conjugate) diameters.
- Is crossed by the ureter, gonadal vessels, middle sacral vessels, iliolumbar vessels, lumbosacral trunk, obturator nerve, spermatic cord, round ligament of the uterus, sympathetic trunk, suspensory ligament of the ovary, and so forth.

C. Lower Pelvic Aperture (Pelvic Outlet)

- Is a **diamond-shaped aperture** bounded posteriorly by the sacrum and coccyx; laterally by the ischial tuberosities and sacrotuberous ligaments; and anteriorly by the pubic symphysis, arcuate pubic ligament, and rami of the pubis and ischium.
- Is closed by the pelvic and urogenital diaphragms.

table 5.1 Differences between the Female and Male Pelvis

	Female	Male
Bones	Smaller, lighter, thinner	Larger, heavier, thicker
Inlet	Transversely oval	Heart-shaped
Outlet	Larger	Smaller
Cavity	Wider, shallower	Narrower, deeper
Subpubic angle	Larger, greater	Smaller, lesser
Sacrum	Shorter, wider	Longer, narrower
Obturator foramen	Oval or triangular	Round

D. Pelvis Major (False Pelvis)

- Is the expanded portion of the bony pelvis above the pelvic brim.

E. Pelvis Minor (True Pelvis)

- Is the cavity of the pelvis below the pelvic brim (or superior aperture) and above the pelvic outlet (or inferior aperture).
- Has an outlet that is closed by the coccygeus and levator ani muscles and the perineal fascia, which form the floor of the pelvis.

F. Differences between the Female and Male Pelvis (Table 5.1)

- The **bones** of the female pelvis are usually **smaller**, lighter, and thinner than those of the male.
- The **inlet** is transversely **oval** in the female and **heart-shaped** in the male.
- The **outlet** is **larger** in the female than in the male because of the everted ischial tuberosities in the female.
- The **cavity** is **wider** and **shallower** in the female than in the male.
- The **subpubic angle** or pubic arch is **larger** and **the greater sciatic notch** is **wider** in the female than in the male.
- The female sacrum is shorter and wider than the male sacrum.
- The **obturator foramen** is **oval** or triangular in the female and round in the male.

II. JOINTS OF THE PELVIS (See Figures 5.10 to 5.11)

A. Lumbosacral Joint

- Is the joint between vertebra L5 and the base of the sacrum, joined by an intervertebral disk and supported by the iliolumbar ligaments.

B. Sacroiliac Joint

- Is a **synovial joint** of an irregular plane type between the articular surfaces of the sacrum and ilium.
- Is covered by cartilage and is supported by the anterior, posterior, and interosseous sacroiliac ligaments.
- **Transmits the weight of the body to the hip bone**.

C. Sacrococcygeal Joint

- Is a **cartilaginous joint** between the sacrum and coccyx, reinforced by the anterior, posterior, and lateral sacrococcygeal ligaments.

D. Pubic Symphysis

- Is a **cartilaginous** or **fibrocartilaginous** joint between the pubic bones in the median plane.

III. PELVIC DIAPHRAGM (See Figure 5.5)

- Forms the **pelvic floor** and **supports all of the pelvic viscera.**
- Is formed by the **levator ani** and **coccygeus** muscles and their fascial coverings.
- Lies posterior and deep to the urogenital diaphragm and medial and deep to the ischiorectal fossa.
- On contraction, **raises the entire pelvic floor.**
- Flexes the anorectal canal during defecation and helps the voluntary control of micturition.
- Helps direct the fetal head toward the birth canal at **parturition.**

IV. LIGAMENTS OR FOLDS AND POUCHES OF THE PELVIS

A. Broad Ligament of the Uterus (Figures 5.12 to 5.13)

- Consists of **two layers of peritoneum**, extends from the lateral margin of the uterus to the lateral pelvic wall, and serves to hold the uterus in position.
- Contains the uterine tube, uterine vessels, round ligament of the uterus, ovarian ligament, ureter (lower part), uterovaginal nerve plexus, and lymphatic vessels.

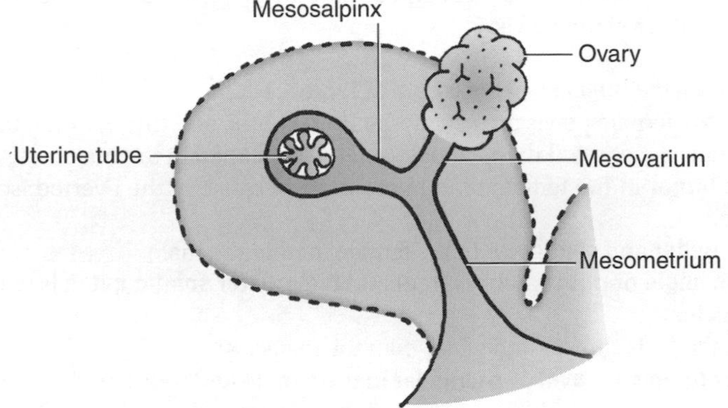

FIGURE 5.12. Sagittal section of the broad ligament.

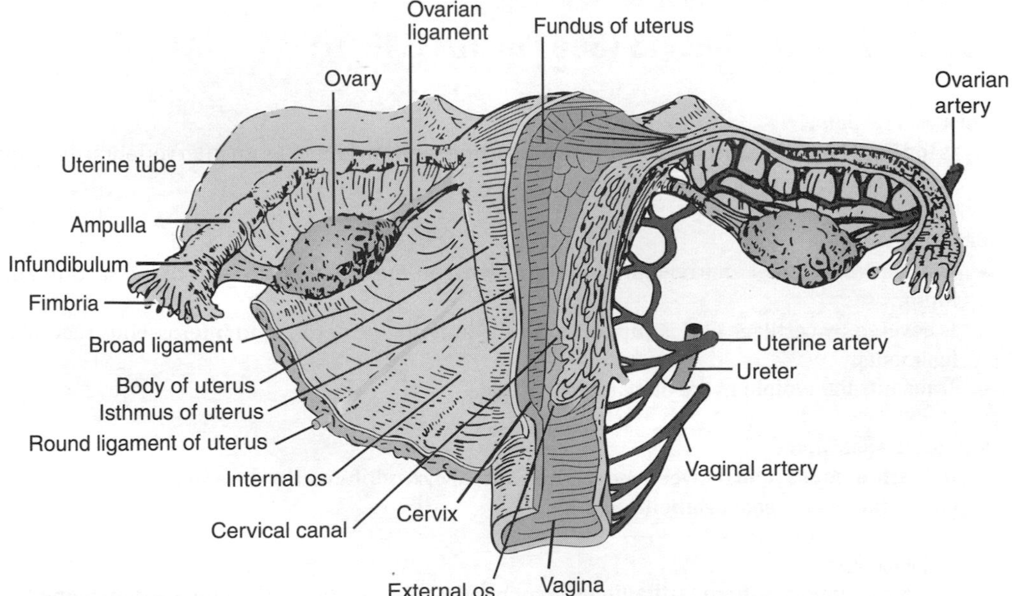

FIGURE 5.13. Female reproductive organs.

- Does not contain the ovary but gives attachment to the ovary through the **mesovarium**.
- Has a posterior layer that curves from the isthmus of the uterus (the **rectouterine fold**) to the posterior wall of the pelvis alongside the rectum.

1. **Mesovarium**
   - Is a fold of peritoneum that connects the anterior surface of the **ovary** with the posterior layer of the broad ligament.
2. **Mesosalpinx**
   - Is a fold of the broad ligament that suspends the **uterine tube**.
3. **Mesometrium**
   - Is a major part of the broad ligament below the mesosalpinx and mesovarium.

B. Round Ligament of the Uterus

- Is attached to the uterus in front of and below the attachment of the uterine tube and represents the remains of the lower part of the **gubernaculum**.
- Runs within the layers of the broad ligament, contains smooth-muscle fibers, and holds the fundus of the uterus forward, keeping the uterus anteverted and anteflexed.
- Enters the inguinal canal at the deep inguinal ring, emerges from the superficial inguinal ring, and becomes lost in the subcutaneous tissue of the labium majus.

C. Ovarian Ligament

- Is a **fibromuscular cord** that extends from the ovary to the uterus below the uterine tube, running within the layers of the broad ligament.

D. Suspensory Ligament of the Ovary

- Is a **band of peritoneum** that extends upward from the ovary to the pelvic wall and transmits the ovarian vessels, nerves, and lymphatics.

E. Lateral or Transverse Cervical (Cardinal or Mackenrodt) Ligaments of the Uterus

- Are **fibromuscular condensations** of pelvic fascia from the cervix and the vagina to the pelvic walls, extend laterally below the base of the broad ligament, and support the uterus.

F. Pubocervical Ligaments

- Are firm bands of connective tissue that extend from the posterior surface of the pubis to the cervix of the uterus.

G. Pubovesical (Female) or Puboprostatic (Male) Ligaments

- Are condensations of the pelvic fascia that extend from the neck of the bladder (or the prostate gland in the male) to the pelvic bone.

H. Sacrocervical Ligaments

- Are firm fibromuscular bands of pelvic fascia that extend from the lower end of the sacrum to the cervix and the upper end of the vagina.

I. Inferior Pubic (Arcuate Pubic) Ligament

- Arches across the inferior aspect of the pubic symphysis and attaches to the medial borders of the inferior pubic rami.

J. Rectouterine (Sacrouterine) Ligaments

- **Hold the cervix back and upward** and sometimes elevate a shelflike fold of peritoneum **(rectouterine fold)**, which passes from the isthmus of the uterus to the posterior wall of the pelvis lateral to the rectum. It corresponds to the **sacrogenital (rectoprostatic) fold** in the male.

K. Rectouterine Pouch (Cul-de-sac of Douglas)

- Is a sac or recess formed by a fold of the peritoneum dipping down between the rectum and the uterus.
- Lies behind the posterior fornix of the vagina and contains peritoneal fluid and some of the small intestine.

L. Rectovesical Pouch

- Is a peritoneal recess between the bladder and the rectum in males, and the **vesicouterine pouch** is a peritoneal sac between the bladder and the uterus in females.

CLINICAL CORRELATES

Culdocentesis is aspiration of fluid from the cul-de-sac of Douglas (rectouterine pouch) by a needle puncture of the posterior vaginal fornix near the midline between the uterosacral ligaments; because the rectouterine pouch is the lowest portion of the peritoneal cavity, it can collect fluid. This procedure is done when pain occurs in the lower abdomen and pelvic regions and a ruptured ectopic pregnancy or ovarian cyst is suspected.

V. URETER AND URINARY BLADDER (Figures 5.14 to 5.16)

A. Ureter

- Is a **muscular tube** that **transmits urine** by peristaltic waves.
- Has **three constrictions** along its course: at its origin where the pelvis of the ureter joins the ureter, where it crosses the pelvic brim, and at its junction with the bladder.
- Crosses the **pelvic brim** in front of the bifurcation of the common iliac artery; descends retroperitoneally on the lateral pelvic wall; and runs medial to the umbilical artery and the obturator vessels and posterior to the ovary, forming the posterior boundary of the ovarian fossa.
- In females, it is accompanied in its course by the uterine artery, which runs above and anterior to it in the base of the broad ligament of the uterus. Because of its location, the ureter is in danger of being injured in the process of hysterectomy. It can be remembered by the mnemonic device, "water (ureter) runs under the bridge (uterine artery)."
- Passes posterior and inferior to the ductus deferens and lies in front of the seminal vesicle before entering the posterolateral aspect of the bladder in males.
- Enters obliquely through the base of the bladder and opens by a slitlike orifice that acts as a valve, and the circular fibers of the intramural part of the ureter act as a sphincter. When the bladder is distended, the valve and sphincter actions prevent the reflux of urine from the urinary bladder into the ureter.
- Receives blood from the aorta and the renal, gonadal, common and internal iliac, umbilical, superior and inferior vesical, and middle rectal arteries.

CLINICAL CORRELATES

Damage of the ureter: In the female, damage may occur during a hysterectomy or surgical repair of a prolapsed uterus because it runs under the uterine artery. The ureter is inadvertently clamped, ligated, or divided during a hysterectomy when the uterine artery is being ligated to control uterine bleeding.

B. Urinary Bladder

- Is situated below the peritoneum and is slightly lower in the female than in the male.
- Extends upward above the pelvic brim as it fills; may reach as high as the umbilicus if fully distended.
- Has the **apex** at the anterior end and the **fundus** or **base** as its posteroinferior triangular portion.
- Has a neck, which is the area where the fundus and the inferolateral surfaces come together, leading into the **urethra**.
- Has a **uvula**, which is a small eminence at the apex of its trigone, projecting into the orifice of the urethra. The **trigone** is bounded by the two orifices of the ureters and the internal urethral orifice, around which is a thick circular layer called the **internal sphincter** (sphincter vesicae).

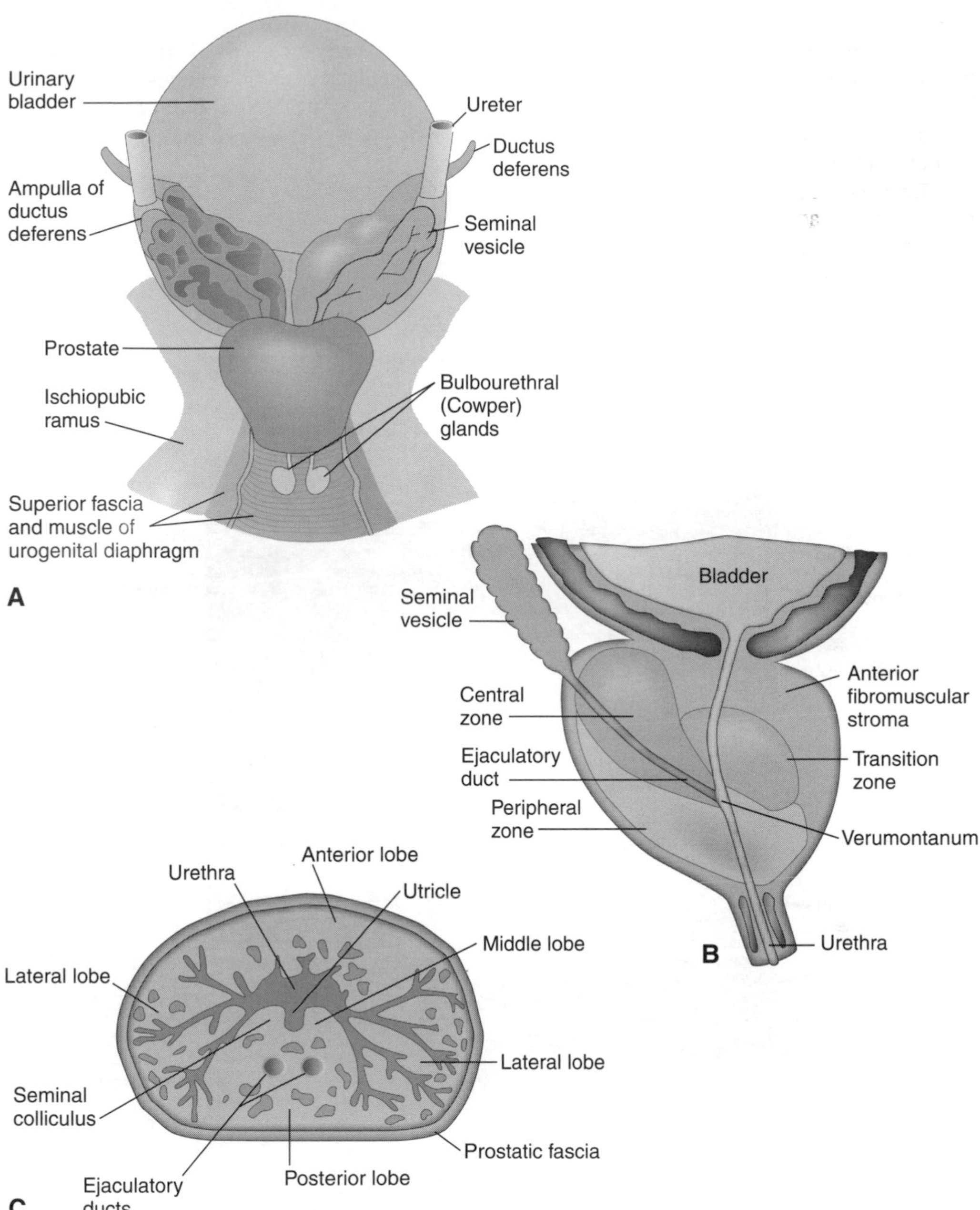

FIGURE 5.14. Male urogenital organs **A:** posterior view of the bladder and male accessory organs. **B:** midsaggital view of the prostate gland showing prostatic zones. **C:** cross section of the prostate showing lobes and internal prostatic structures.

- Has bundles of smooth-muscle fibers that, as a whole, are known as the **detrusor muscle of the bladder**.
- Receives blood from the superior and inferior vesical arteries (and from the vaginal artery in females). Its venous blood is drained by the **prostatic (or vesical) plexus** of veins, which empties into the internal iliac vein.
- Is innervated by nerve fibers from the vesical and prostatic plexuses. The **parasympathetic nerve** (pelvic splanchnic nerve originating from S2–S4) stimulates to contract the musculature (detrusor) of the bladder wall, relaxes the internal urethral sphincter, and promotes emptying. The **sympathetic nerve** relaxes the detrusor of the bladder wall and constricts the internal urethral sphincter.

CLINICAL CORRELATES

Bladder cancer usually originates in cells lining the inside of the bladder (epithelial cells). The most common symptom is blood in the urine (hematuria). Other symptoms include frequent urination and pain upon urination (dysuria). This cancer may be induced by organic carcinogens that are deposited in the urine after being absorbed from the environment and also by cigarette smoking.

Tenesmus is a constant feeling of the desire to empty the bladder or bowel, accompanied by pain, cramping, and straining due to a spasm of the urogenital diaphragm.

Interstitial cystitis is a chronic inflammatory condition of the bladder that causes frequent, urgent, and painful urination.

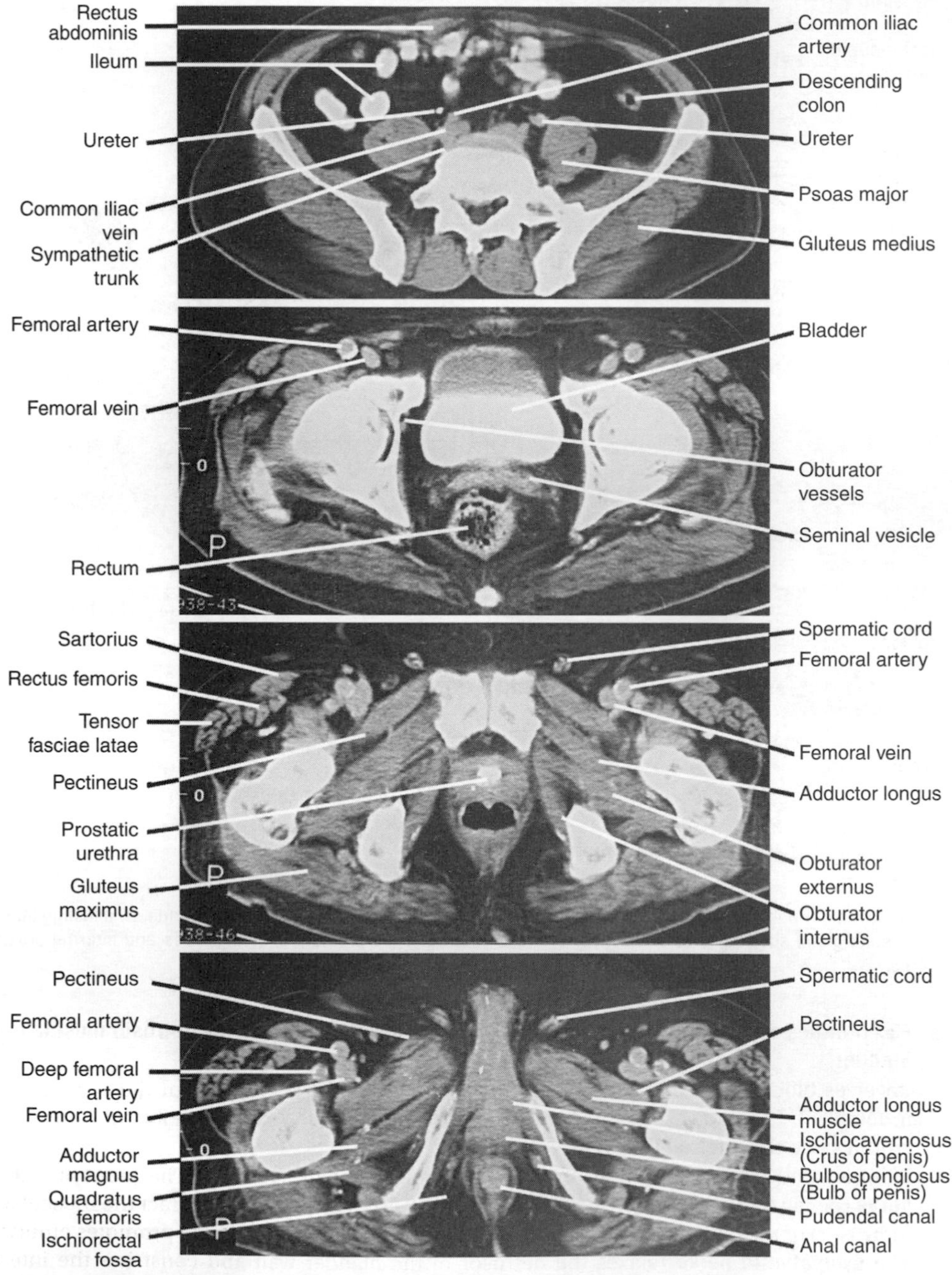

FIGURE 5.15. Computed tomography scans of the male pelvis and perineum.

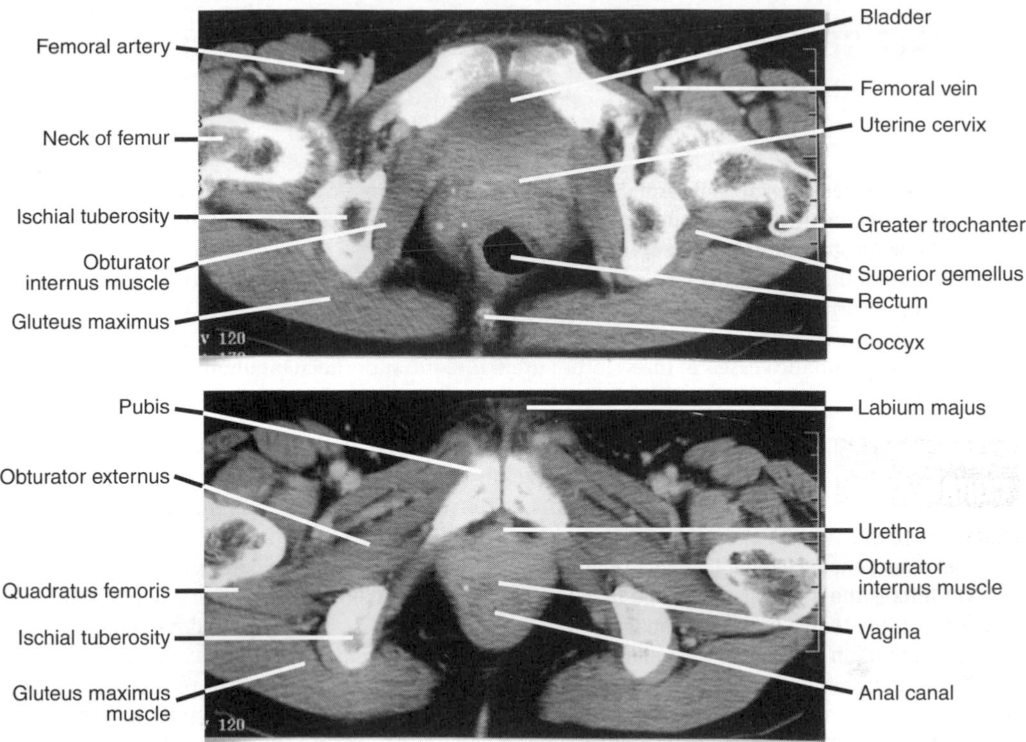

FIGURE 5.16. Computed tomography scans of the female pelvis and perineum.

C. Urethra

- It serves as a passage for urine from the urinary bladder to the exterior, but in men, it also serves as a passage for semen.
- Male urethra is approximately 20 cm long and consists of three parts: prostatic, membranous, and spongy. The lowest part of the membranous urethra is susceptible to rupture or to penetration by a catheter.
- Female urethra is approximately 4 cm long, and its external urethral orifice is situated between the labia minora, in front of the vaginal opening but behind the glans clitoris.

D. Micturition (Urination)

- Is initiated by stimulating **stretch receptors in the detrusor muscle** in the bladder wall by the increasing volume (approximately 300 mL for adults) of urine.
- Can be assisted by contraction of the abdominal muscles, which increases the intra-abdominal and pelvic pressures.
- Involves the following processes:
  1. **Sympathetic** (general visceral efferent [GVE]) fibers induce relaxation of the bladder wall and constrict the internal sphincter, **inhibiting emptying**. (They may also activate the detrusor to prevent the reflux of semen into the bladder during ejaculation.)
  2. **General visceral afferent (GVA)** impulses arise from stretch receptors in the bladder wall and enter the spinal cord (S2–S4) via the pelvic splanchnic nerves.
  3. **Parasympathetic** preganglionic (GVE) fibers in the pelvic splanchnic nerves synapse in the pelvic (inferior hypogastric) plexus; postganglionic fibers to the bladder musculature induce a reflex contraction of the detrusor muscle and relaxation of the internal urethral sphincter, **enhancing the micturition**.
  4. **General somatic efferent (GSE)** fibers in the pudendal nerve cause voluntary relaxation of the external urethral sphincter, and the bladder begins to void.
  5. At the end of micturition, the external urethral sphincter contracts, and bulbospongiosus muscles in the male expel the last few drops of urine from the urethra.

VI. MALE GENITAL ORGANS (Figures 5.17 to 5.18; See Figures 5.14 to 5.15)

A. Testis

- Develops retroperitoneally and descends into the scrotum retroperitoneally.
- Is covered by the **tunica albuginea**, which lies beneath the visceral layer of the **tunica vaginalis**.
- **Produces spermatozoa** and **secretes sex hormones**.
- Is supplied by the testicular artery from the abdominal aorta and is drained by veins of the pampiniform plexus.
- Has lymph vessels that ascend with the testicular vessels and drain into the lumbar (aortic) nodes; lymphatic vessels in the scrotum drain into the superficial inguinal nodes.

CLINICAL CORRELATES

Testicular torsion is twisting of a testis such that the spermatic cord becomes twisted, obstructing blood supply to the testis, and causing sudden urgent pain and swelling of the scrotum or nausea and vomiting. It is most common during adolescence and may be caused by trauma or a spasm of the cremaster muscle. Testicular torsion requires emergency treatment, and if not untwisted, testicular necrosis will occur.

Orchitis is the inflammation of the testis and is marked by pain, swelling, and a feeling of heaviness in the testis. It may be caused by the mumps, gonorrhea, syphilis, or tuberculosis. If testicular infection spreads to the epididymis, it is called **epididymo-orchitis**.

Testicular cancer develops commonly from the rapidly dividing early state spermatogenic cells (seminoma or germ-cell tumor). Tumor also develops from Leydig cells, which produce androgen (Leydig-cell tumor), and Sertoli cells, which support and nourish germ cells and produce androgen-binding protein and the hormone inhibin (Sertoli-cell tumor). Signs and symptoms include a painless mass or lump, testicular swelling, hardness, and a feeling of heaviness or aching in the scrotum or lower abdomen. The cause of cancer is unknown, but the major risk factors are cryptorchidism and Klinefelter syndrome (47, XXY sex chromosome, seminiferous tubule dysgenesis, gynecomastia, and infertility). Metastasis occurs via lymph and blood vessels. It can be treated by the surgical removal of the affected testis and spermatic cord (orchiectomy), radiotherapy, and/or chemotherapy.

Cryptorchidism is a congenital condition in which the testis fails to descend into the scrotum during fetal development. Undescended testes are associated with reduced fertility, increased risk of testicular cancer, and higher susceptibility to testicular torsion and inguinal hernias. Undescended testes are brought down into the scrotum in infancy by a surgical procedure called an orchiopexy or orchidopexy.

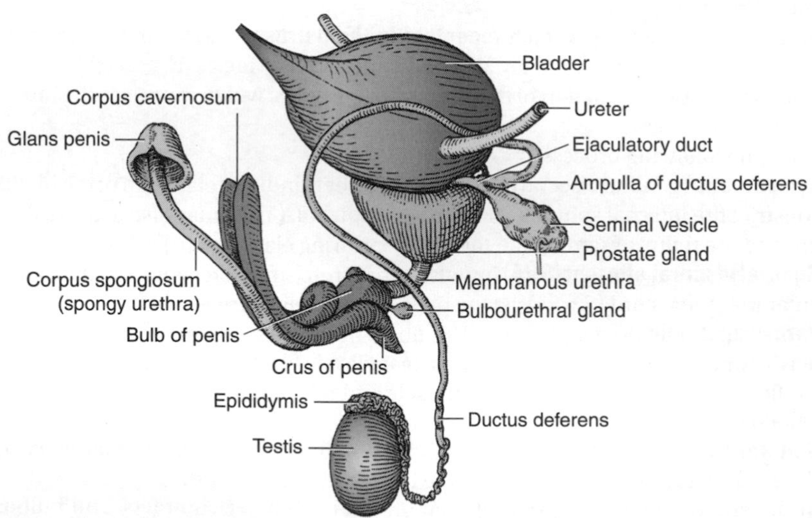

FIGURE 5.17. Male reproductive organs.

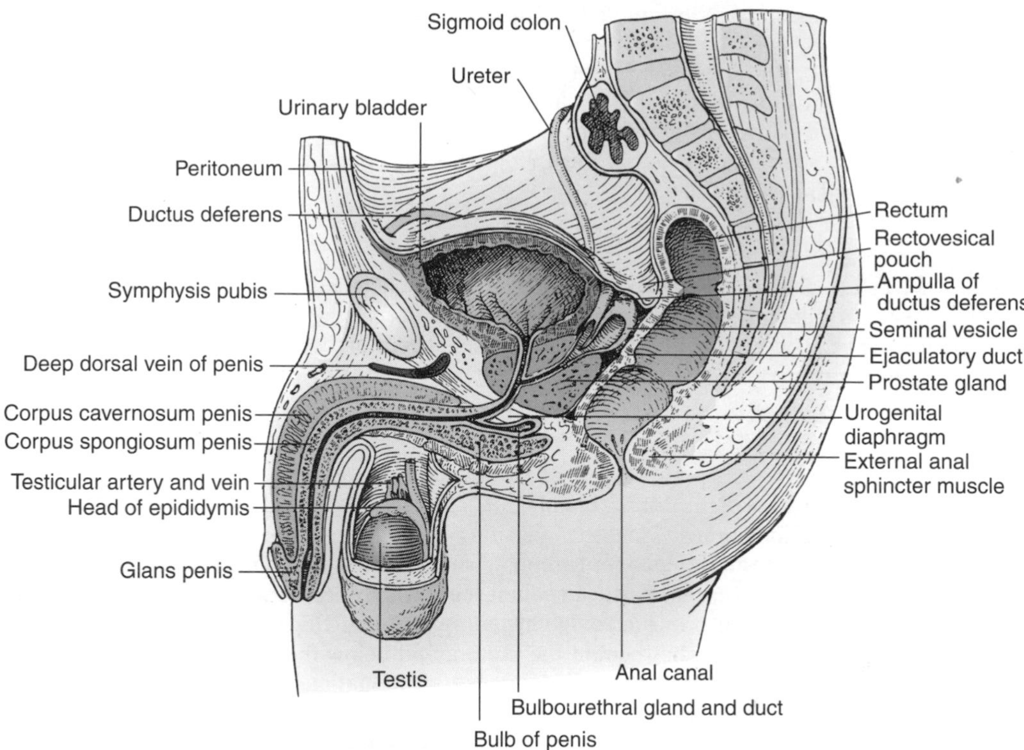

FIGURE 5.18. Sagittal section of the male pelvis.

B. Epididymis

- Consists of a head, body, and tail, and contains a **convoluted duct** approximately 6 m (20 ft) long.
- Functions in the **maturation and storage of spermatozoa** in the head and body and **propulsion of the spermatozoa** into the ductus deferens.

C. Ductus Deferens

- Is a thick-walled tube that enters the pelvis at the deep inguinal ring at the lateral side of the inferior epigastric artery.
- Crosses the medial side of the umbilical artery and obturator nerve and vessels, passes superior to the ureter near the wall of the bladder, and is dilated to become the **ampulla** at its terminal part.
- Contains fructose, which is nutritive to spermatozoa, and receives innervation primarily from sympathetic nerves of the hypogastric plexus and parasympathetic nerves of the pelvic plexus.

CLINICAL CORRELATES

Vasectomy is the surgical excision of a portion of the vas deferens (ductus deferens) through the scrotum. It stops the passage of spermatozoa but neither reduces the amount of ejaculate greatly nor diminishes sexual desire.

D. Ejaculatory Ducts

- Are formed by the union of the ductus deferens with the ducts of the seminal vesicles. Peristaltic contractions of the muscular layer of the ductus deferens and the ejaculatory ducts propel spermatozoa with seminal fluid into the urethra.
- Open into the prostatic urethra on the **seminal colliculus** just lateral to the blind **prostatic utricle** (see the section on urethral crest).

E. Seminal Vesicles

- Are enclosed by dense endopelvic fascia and are **lobulated glandular structures** that are diverticula of the ductus deferens.

- Lie inferior and lateral to the ampullae of the ductus deferens against the fundus (base) of the bladder.
- Produce the alkaline constituent of the **seminal fluid**, which contains **fructose** and **choline**.
- Have lower ends that become narrow and form ducts, which join the ampullae of the ductus deferens to form the **ejaculatory ducts**.
- Do not store spermatozoa, as was once thought; this is done by the epididymis, the ductus deferens, and its ampulla.

CLINICAL CORRELATES **Seminal vesicles** produce the alkaline constituent of the seminal fluid, which contains fructose and choline. **Fructose** provides a **forensic determination** for occurrence of **rape**, whereas **choline** crystals provide the basis for the determination of the presence of **semen (Florence test)**.

F. Prostate Gland

- Is located at the base of the urinary bladder and consists chiefly of glandular tissue mixed with smooth muscle and fibrous tissue.
- Has five lobes: the **anterior lobe** (or isthmus), which lies in front of the urethra and is devoid of glandular substance; the **middle (median) lobe**, which lies between the urethra and the ejaculatory ducts and is prone to **benign hypertrophy** obstructing the internal urethral orifice; the **posterior lobe**, which lies behind the urethra and below the ejaculatory ducts, contains glandular tissue, and is prone to **carcinomatous transformation**; and the **right and left lateral lobes**, which are situated on either side of the urethra and form the main mass of the gland.
- Secretes a fluid that produces the characteristic **odor of semen**. This fluid, the secretion from the seminal vesicles and the bulbourethral glands, and the spermatozoa constitute the **semen or seminal fluid**.
- Secretes **prostate-specific antigen (PSA)**, prostaglandins, citric acid and acid phosphatase, and proteolytic enzymes.
- Has ducts that open into the **prostatic sinus**, a groove on either side of the **urethral crest**.
- Receives the **ejaculatory duct**, which opens into the urethra on the **seminal colliculus** just lateral to the blind **prostatic utricle**.

CLINICAL CORRELATES **Hypertrophy of the prostate** is a benign enlargement of the prostate that affects older men and occurs most often in the **middle lobe**, obstructing the internal urethral orifice and thus leading to **nocturia** (excessive urination at night), **dysuria** (difficulty or pain in urination), and **urgency** (sudden desire to urinate). Cancer occurs most often in the posterior lobe. **T**rans**u**rethral **r**esection of the **p**rostate **(TURP)** is the surgical removal of the prostate by means of a cystoscope passed through the urethra. **Prostatitis is the inflammation of the prostate.**

Prostate cancer is a slow-growing cancer that occurs particularly in the posterior lobe. It is usually symptomless in the early stages, but it can impinge on the urethra in the late stage. Prostate cancer spreads to the bony pelvis, pelvic lymph nodes, vertebral column, and skull via the vertebral venous plexus, producing pain in the pelvis, the lower back, and the bones. This cancer also metastasizes to the heart and lungs through the prostatic venous plexus, internal iliac veins, and into the inferior vena cava. It can be detected by digital rectal examination, ultrasound imaging with a device inserted into the rectum, or PSA test. PSA concentration in the blood of normal males is less than 4.0 ng/mL.

Prostatectomy is the **surgical removal** of a part or all of the prostate gland. Perineal prostatectomy is removal of the prostate through an incision in the perineum. Radical prostatectomy is removal of the prostate with seminal vesicles, ductus deferens, some pelvic fasciae, and pelvic lymph nodes through the retropubic or the perineal route. A careful dissection of the pelvic and prostatic nerve plexuses is required during prostatectomy to avoid loss of erection and ejaculation.

G. Urethral Crest

- Is located on the posterior wall of the **prostatic urethra** and has numerous openings for the prostatic ducts on either side.
- Has an ovoid-shaped enlargement called the **seminal colliculus (verumontanum)**, on which the two ejaculatory ducts and the **prostatic utricle** open. At the summit of the colliculus is the prostatic utricle, which is an invagination (a blind pouch) approximately 5 mm deep; it is analogous to the uterus and vagina in the female.

H. Prostatic Sinus

- Is a groove between the urethral crest and the wall of the prostatic urethra and receives the ducts of the prostate gland.

I. Erection

- Depends on **stimulation of parasympathetics** from the pelvic splanchnic nerves, which dilates the arteries supplying the erectile tissue, and thus causes engorgement of the corpora cavernosa and corpus spongiosum, compressing the veins and thus impeding venous return and causing full erection.
- Is also maintained by **contraction of the bulbospongiosus and ischiocavernosus muscles**, which compresses the erectile tissues of the bulb and the crus.
- Is often described using a popular mnemonic: **p**oint (erection by **p**arasympathetic) and **s**hoot (ejaculation by **s**ympathetic).

J. Ejaculation

- Begins with nervous stimulation. Friction to the glans penis and other sexual stimuli result in **excitation of sympathetic fibers**, leading to contraction of the smooth muscle of the epididymal ducts, the ductus deferens, the seminal vesicles, and the prostate in turn.
- Occurs as a result of contraction of the smooth muscle, thus pushing spermatozoa and the secretions of both the seminal vesicles and prostate into the prostatic urethra, where they join secretions from the bulbourethral and penile urethral glands. All of these secretions are **ejected** together from the penile urethra because of the rhythmic contractions of the bulbospongiosus, which compresses the urethra.
- Involves contraction of the sphincter of the bladder, preventing the entry of urine into the prostatic urethra and the reflux of the semen into the bladder.

VII. FEMALE GENITAL ORGANS (Figure 5.19; See Figures 5.13 and 5.16)

A. Ovaries

- Lie on the posterior aspect of the **broad ligament** on the side wall of the pelvic minor and are bounded by the external and internal iliac vessels.
- Are not covered by the peritoneum, and thus, the ovum or oocyte is expelled into the peritoneal cavity and then into the uterine tube.
- Are not enclosed in the broad ligament, but their anterior surface is attached to the posterior layer of the broad ligament by the **mesovarium**.
- Have a surface that is covered by **germinal (columnar) epithelium**, which is modified from the developmental peritoneal covering of the ovary.
- Are supplied primarily by the ovarian arteries, which are contained in the suspensory ligament and anastomose with branches of the uterine artery.
- Are drained by the ovarian veins; the right ovarian vein joins the inferior vena cava, and the left ovarian vein joins the left renal vein.

CLINICAL CORRELATES

Ovarian cancer develops from germ cells that produce ova or eggs, stromal cells that produce estrogen and progesterone, and epithelial cells that cover the outer surface of the ovary. Its symptoms include a feeling of pressure in the pelvis or changes in bowel or bladder habits. Diagnosis involves feeling a mass during a pelvic examination, visualizing it by using an ultrasound probe placed in the vagina, or using a blood test for a protein associated with ovarian cancer (CA-125). Some germ-cell cancers release certain protein markers, such as human chorionic gonadotropin and α-fetoprotein, into the blood. Cancer signs and symptoms include unusual vaginal bleeding, postmenopausal bleeding, bleeding after intercourse and pain during intercourse, pelvic pressure, abdominal and pelvic pain, back pain, indigestion, and loss of appetite.

B. Uterine Tubes

- Extend from the uterus to the uterine end of the ovaries and **connect the uterine cavity to the peritoneal cavity**.
- Are each subdivided into four parts: the **uterine part**, the **isthmus**, the **ampulla** (the longest and widest part), and the **infundibulum** (the funnel-shaped termination formed of **fimbriae**).
- **Convey the fertilized or unfertilized oocytes to the uterus** by ciliary action and muscular contraction, which takes 3 to 4 days.
- Transport spermatozoa in the opposite direction (toward the eggs); **fertilization** takes place within the tube, usually in the **infundibulum** or **ampulla**. Fertilization is the process beginning with penetration of the secondary oocyte by the sperm and completed by fusion of the male and female pronuclei.

C. Uterus

- Is the organ of gestation in which the fertilized oocyte normally becomes embedded and the developing organism grows until its birth.
- Is normally **anteverted** (i.e., angle of 90 degrees at the junction of the vagina and cervical canal) and **anteflexed** (i.e., angle of 160 to 170 degrees at the junction of the cervix and body).
- Is supported by the pelvic diaphragm; the urogenital diaphragm; the round, broad, lateral, or transverse cervical (cardinal) ligaments; and the pubocervical, sacrocervical, and rectouterine ligaments.
- Is supplied primarily by the uterine artery and secondarily by the ovarian artery.
- Has an anterior surface that rests on the posterosuperior surface of the bladder.
- Is divided into four parts for the purpose of description:

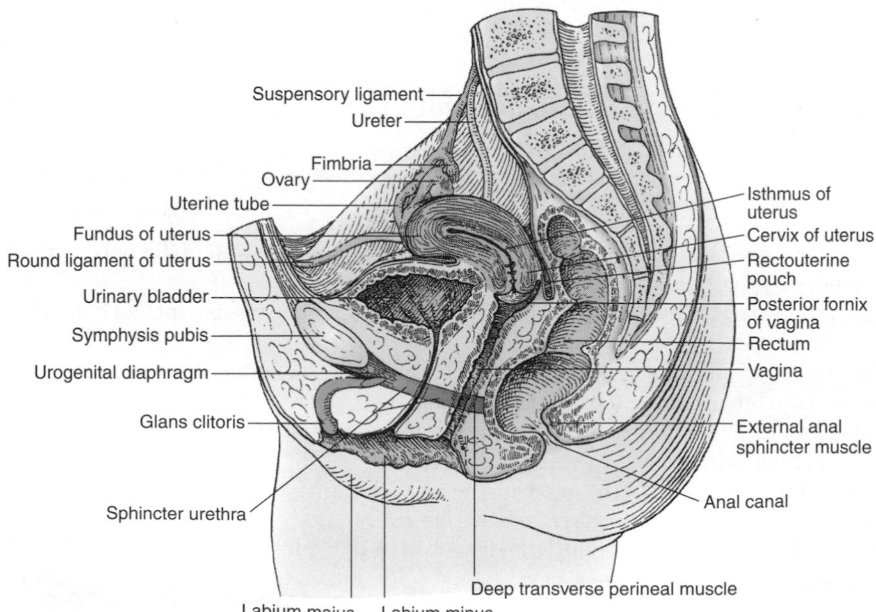

FIGURE 5.19. Sagittal section of the female pelvis.

1. **Fundus**
   - Is the **rounded part** of the uterus located superior and anterior to the plane of the entrance of the uterine tube.
2. **Body**
   - Is the main part of the uterus located inferior to the fundus and superior to the isthmus. The uterine cavity is triangular in the coronal section and is continuous with the lumina of the uterine tube and with the internal os.
3. **Isthmus**
   - Is the **constricted part** of the uterus located between the body and cervix of the uterus. It corresponds to the internal os.
4. **Cervix**
   - Is the inferior narrow part of the uterus that projects into the vagina and divides into the following regions:
     1. **Internal os:** the junction of the cervical canal with the uterine body.
     2. **Cervical canal**: the cavity of the cervix between the internal and external ostia.
     3. **External os**: the opening of the cervical canal into the vagina.

CLINICAL CORRELATES

Uterine prolapse is the protrusion of the cervix of the uterus into the lower part of the vagina close to the vestibule and causes a **bearing-down sensation** in the womb and an increased frequency of and burning sensation on urination. The prolapse occurs as a result of advancing age and menopause and results from **weakness of the muscles, ligaments, and fasciae of the pelvic floor** such as the pelvic diaphragm, urogenital diaphragm, ovarian and cardinal (transverse cervical) ligaments, and broad and round ligaments of the uterus that constitute the support of the uterus and other pelvic viscera. The vagina may prolapse too. Symptoms include the pelvic heaviness, pelvic pain, lower back pain, constipation, difficulty urinating, urinary frequency, and painful sexual intercourse. Treatments include special (Kegel) exercises to strengthen the muscles, estrogen-replacement therapy, and surgical correction and reconstruction for weakened and stretched ligaments and muscles of the pelvic floor.

CLINICAL CORRELATES

Fibromyoma or **leiomyoma** is the most common benign neoplasm of the female genital tract derived from smooth muscle. It may cause urinary frequency, dysmenorrhea, abortion, or obstructed labor. A **fibroid** is a benign uterine tumor made of smooth-muscle cells and fibrous connective tissue in the wall of the uterus. A large fibroid can cause bleeding, pressure, and pain in the pelvis, heavy menstrual periods, and infertility.

Endometriosis is a benign disorder in which a mass of endometrial tissue (stroma and glands) occurs aberrantly in various locations, including the uterine wall, ovaries, or other extraendometrial sites. It frequently forms cysts containing altered blood.

Endometrial cancer is the most common type (approximately 90%) of uterine cancer and develops from the endometrium of the uterus usually from the uterine glands. Its main symptom is vaginal bleeding, which allows for early detection; other symptoms are clear vaginal discharge, lower abdominal pain, and pelvic cramping. Risk factors include obesity, nulliparity, infertility, early menarche (onset of menstruation), late menopause (cessation of menstruation), and postmenopausal estrogen-replacement therapy because estrogens stimulate the growth and division of endometrial cells.

Cervical cancer is a slow-growing cancer that develops from the epithelium covering the cervix. The major risk factor for development of cervical cancer is human papillomavirus infection. Cancer cells grow upward to the endometrial cavity, downward to the vagina, and lateral to the pelvic wall, invading the bladder and rectum directly. A **Papanicolaou (Pap) smear** or cervical smear test is effective in detecting cervical cancer early. This cancer metastasizes to extrapelvic lymph nodes, liver, lung, and bone, and can be treated by the surgical removal of the cervix or by a hysterectomy.

Hysterectomy is the **surgical removal of the uterus**, performed either through the abdominal wall or through the vagina. It may result in injury to the ureter, which lies in the transverse cardinal ligament beneath the uterine artery.

D. Vagina

- Extends between the vestibule and the cervix of the uterus.
- Is located at the lower end of the birth canal.
- Serves as the **excretory channel** for the products of menstruation; also serves to receive the penis during coitus.
- Has a **fornix** that forms the recess between the cervix and the wall of the vagina.
- Opens into the vestibule and is partially closed by a membranous crescentic fold, the **hymen**.
- Is supported by the levator ani; the transverse cervical, pubocervical, and sacrocervical ligaments (upper part); the urogenital diaphragm (middle part); and the perineal body (lower part).
- Receives blood from the vaginal branches of the uterine artery and of the internal iliac artery.
- Has lymphatic drainage in two directions: the lymphatics from the upper three-fourths drain into the internal iliac nodes, and the lymphatics from the lower one-fourth, below the hymen, drain downward to the perineum and thus into the superficial inguinal nodes.
- Is innervated by nerves derived from the uterovaginal plexus for the upper three-fourths and by the deep perineal branch of the pudendal nerve for the lower one-fourth.

CLINICAL CORRELATES

Vaginismus is a painful spasm of the vagina resulting from involuntary contraction of the vaginal musculature, preventing sexual intercourse. It may be caused by organic or psychogenic factors or traumatic experiences such as rape and sexual abuse.

Mediolateral episiotomy is a **surgical incision through the posterolateral vaginal wall,** just lateral to the perineal body, to enlarge the birth canal and thus prevent uncontrolled tearing during parturition. The mediolateral episiotomy allows greater expansion of the birth canal into the ischiorectal fossa. However, the incision is more difficult to close layer by layer, and there is an increased risk of infection because of contamination of the ischiorectal fossa. In a **median episiotomy**, the incision is carried posteriorly in the midline through the posterior vaginal wall and the central tendon (perineal body). The median episiotomy is relatively bloodless and painless, but this incision provides a limited expansion of the birth canal with a slight possibility of tearing the anal sphincters.

VIII. RECTUM AND ANAL CANAL

A. Rectum (See Figure 5.15)

- Is the part of the **large intestine** that extends from the sigmoid colon to the anal canal and follows the curvature of the sacrum and coccyx.
- Has a lower dilated part called the **ampulla**, which lies immediately above the pelvic diaphragm and **stores the feces.**
- Has a peritoneal covering on its anterior, right, and left sides for the proximal third; only on its front for the middle third; and no covering for the distal third.
- Has a mucous membrane and a circular muscle layer that forms three permanent transverse folds **(Houston valves)**, which appear to support the fecal mass.
- Receives blood from the superior, middle, and inferior rectal arteries and the middle sacral artery. (The superior rectal artery pierces the muscular wall and courses in the submucosal layer and anastomoses with branches of the inferior rectal artery. The middle rectal artery supplies the posterior part of the rectum.)
- Has venous blood that returns to the portal venous system via the superior rectal vein and to the caval (systemic) system via the middle and inferior rectal veins. (The middle rectal vein drains primarily the muscular layer of the lower part of the rectum and upper part of the anal canal.)
- Receives parasympathetic nerve fibers by way of the pelvic splanchnic nerve.

CLINICAL CORRELATES **Ulcerative colitis** is chronic ulceration of the colon and rectum with cramping abdominal pain, rectal bleeding, diarrhea, and loose discharge of pus and mucus with scanty fecal particles. Complications include hemorrhoids, abscesses, anemia, electrolyte imbalance, perforation of the colon, and carcinoma.

Diverticulitis is the inflammation of an abnormal pouch (diverticulum) in the intestinal wall, commonly found in the colon, especially the sigmoid colon. Diverticula develop as a result of high pressure within the colon. Symptoms are abdominal pain (usually in the left lower abdomen but can be anywhere), chills, fever, nausea, and constipation. Risk factors include older age and a low-fiber diet, and it can be treated with rest, high-fiber diet, and antibiotics. Complications may include bleeding, perforations, peritonitis, and stricture or fistula formation.

CLINICAL CORRELATES **Rectal or digital (finger) examination** is performed by inserting a gloved, lubricated finger into the rectum; using the other hand to press on the lower abdomen or pelvic area; and palpating for lumps, tumors, enlargements, tissue hardening, hemorrhoids, rectal carcinoma, prostate cancer, seminal vesicle, ampulla of the ductus deferens, bladder, uterus, cervix, ovaries, anorectal abscesses, polyps, chronic constipation, and other abnormalities.

Colorectal cancer develops in the epithelial cells lining the lumen of the colon and rectum. Cancer risk factors include high fat intake, a family history, and polyps. Its symptoms include fatigue, weakness, weight loss, change in bowel habits, diarrhea or constipation, and red or dark blood in stool. Cancer can be detected by **colonoscopy**, which is an examination of the inside of the colon and rectum using a colonoscope (an elongated, flexible, lighted endoscope) inserted into the rectum. Suspicious areas are photographed for future reference, and a polyp or other abnormal tissue can be obtained during the procedure for pathologic examination. Rectal cancer may spread along lymphatic vessels and through the venous system. The superior rectal vein is a tributary of the portal vein, and thus, rectal cancer may metastasize to the liver. Rectal cancer may penetrate posteriorly the rectal wall and invade the sacral plexus, producing sciatica, and invade laterally the ureter and anteriorly the vagina, uterus, bladder, prostate, or seminal vesicles.

B. Anal Canal (See Figure 5.15)

- Lies below the pelvic diaphragm and ends at the **anus**.
- Is divided into an upper two-thirds **(visceral portion)**, which belongs to the intestine, and a lower one-third **(somatic portion)**, which belongs to the perineum with respect to mucosa, blood supply, and nerve supply.
- Has **anal columns**, which are 5 to 10 longitudinal folds of mucosa in its upper half (each column contains a small artery and a small vein).
- Has **anal valves**, which are crescent-shaped mucosal folds that connect the lower ends of the anal columns.
- Has **anal sinuses**, which are a series of pouchlike recesses at the lower end of the anal column in which the anal glands open.
- The **internal anal sphincter** (a thickening of the circular smooth muscle in the lower part of the rectum) is separated from the **external anal sphincter** (skeletal muscle that has three parts: subcutaneous, superficial, and deep) by the intermuscular (intersphincteric) groove called **Hilton white line**.
- Has a point of demarcation between visceral and somatic portions called the **pectinate (dentate) line**, which is a serrated line following the anal valves and crossing the bases of the anal columns (see Table 5.2).
  1. The epithelium is **columnar** or **cuboidal** above the pectinate line and stratified squamous below it.
  2. Venous drainage above the pectinate line goes into the **portal venous system** mainly via the superior rectal vein; below the pectinate line, it goes into the **caval system** via the middle and inferior rectal veins.

table 5.2 Divisions of the Pectinate Line

	Above Pectinate Line	Below Pectinate Line
Epithelium	Columnar or cuboidal	Stratified squamous
Venous drainage	Portal venous system	Caval venous system
Lymphatics	Internal iliac nodes	Superficial inguinal nodes
Sensory innervation	Visceral sensory	Somatic sensory
Hemorrhoids	Internal hemorrhoids	External hemorrhoids

3. The lymphatic vessels drain into the **internal iliac nodes** above the line and into the **superficial inguinal nodes** below it.
4. The sensory innervation above the line is through fibers from the pelvic plexus and thus is of the visceral type; the sensory innervation below it is by somatic nerve fibers of the pudendal nerve (which are very sensitive).
5. **Internal hemorrhoids** occur above the pectinate line, and **external hemorrhoids** occur below it.

CLINICAL CORRELATES **Hemorrhoids** are dilated internal and external venous plexuses around the rectum and anal canal. **Internal hemorrhoids** occur above the pectinate line and are covered by mucous membrane; their pain fibers are carried by GVA fibers of the sympathetic nerves. **External hemorrhoids** are situated below the pectinate line, are covered by skin, and are more painful than internal hemorrhoids because their pain fibers are carried by GSA fibers of the inferior rectal nerves.

C. Defecation

- Is initiated by **distention of the rectum**, which has filled from the sigmoid colon, and afferent impulses transmitted to the spinal cord by the pelvic splanchnic nerve. The pelvic splanchnic nerve increases peristalsis (contracts smooth muscles in the rectum), whereas the sympathetic nerve causes a decrease in peristalsis, maintains tone in the internal sphincter, and contains vasomotor and sensory (pain) fibers.
- Involves the following:
  1. The intra-abdominal pressure is increased by holding the breath and contracting the diaphragm, the abdominal muscles, and the levator ani, thus facilitating the expulsion of feces.
  2. The **puborectalis** relaxes, which decreases the angle between the ampulla of the rectum and the upper portion of the anal canal, thus aiding defecation.
  3. The smooth muscle in the wall of the rectum contracts, the internal anal sphincter relaxes, and the external anal sphincter relaxes to pass the feces.
  4. After evacuation, the contraction of the puborectalis and the anal sphincters closes the anal canal.

IX. BLOOD VESSELS OF THE PELVIS (Figure 5.20)

A. Internal Iliac Artery

- Arises from the bifurcation of the common iliac artery, in front of the sacroiliac joint, and is crossed in front by the ureter at the pelvic brim.
- Is commonly divided into a **posterior division**, which gives rise to the iliolumbar, lateral sacral, and superior gluteal arteries, and an **anterior division**, which gives rise to the inferior gluteal, internal pudendal, umbilical, obturator, inferior vesical, middle rectal, and uterine arteries.

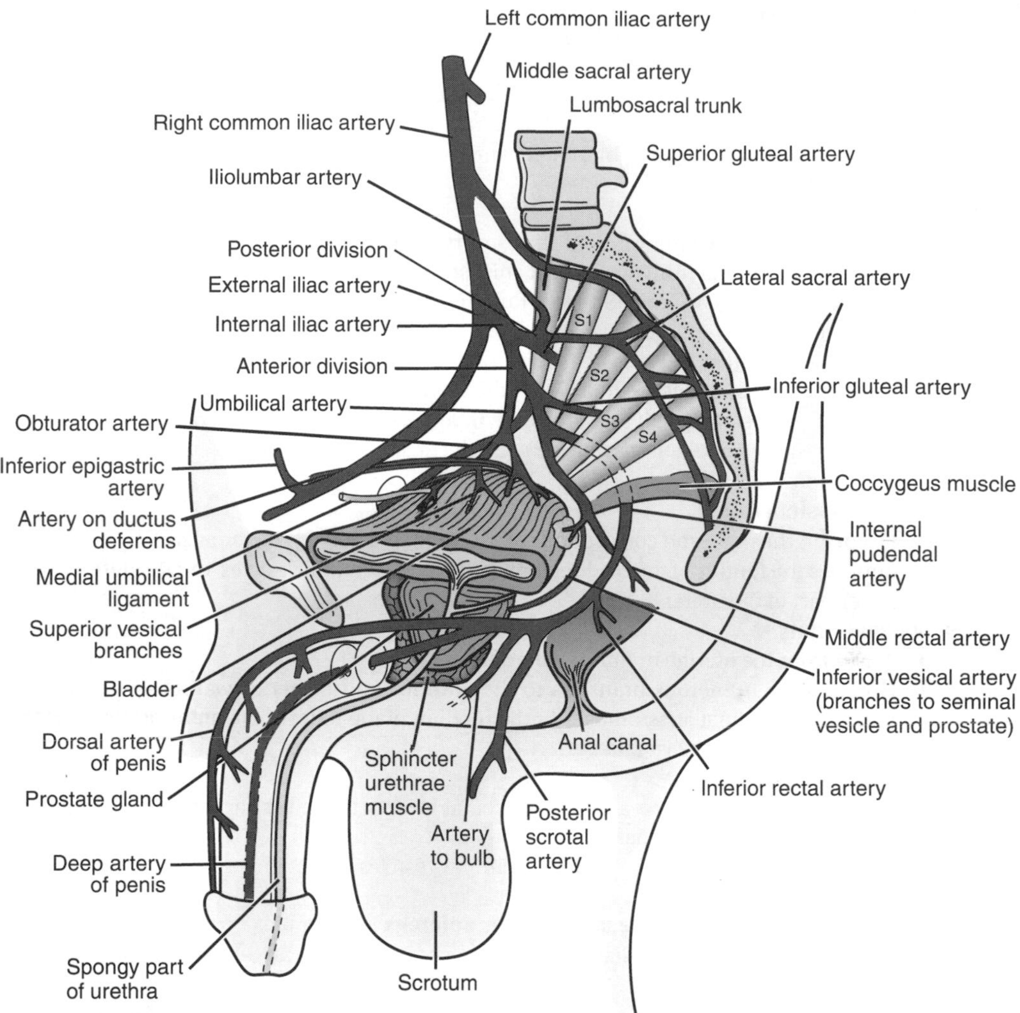

FIGURE 5.20. Branches of the internal iliac artery.

1. **Iliolumbar Artery**
   - Runs superolaterally to the iliac fossa, deep to the psoas major.
   - Divides into an **iliac branch** supplying the iliacus muscle and the ilium and a **lumbar branch** supplying the psoas major and quadratus lumborum muscles.
2. **Lateral Sacral Artery**
   - Passes medially in front of the sacral plexus, giving rise to **spinal branches**, which enter the anterior sacral foramina to supply the spinal meninges and the roots of the sacral nerves and then emerge through the posterior sacral foramina to supply the muscles and skin overlying the sacrum.
3. **Superior Gluteal Artery**
   - Usually runs between the lumbosacral trunk and the first sacral nerve.
   - Leaves the pelvis through the **greater sciatic foramen** above the piriformis muscle to supply muscles in the buttocks.
4. **Inferior Gluteal Artery**
   - Runs between the first and second or between the second and third sacral nerves.
   - Leaves the pelvis through the **greater sciatic foramen**, inferior to the piriformis.
5. **Internal Pudendal Artery**
   - Leaves the pelvis through the greater sciatic foramen, passing between the piriformis and coccygeus muscles, and enters the perineum through the **lesser sciatic foramen**.

6. **Umbilical Artery**
   - Runs forward along the lateral pelvic wall and along the side of the bladder.
   - Has a proximal part that gives rise to the **superior vesical artery** to the superior part of the bladder and, in the male, to the **artery of the ductus deferens**, which supplies the ductus deferens, the seminal vesicles, the lower part of the ureter, and the bladder.
   - Has a distal part that is obliterated and continues forward as the **medial umbilical ligament.**
7. **Obturator Artery**
   - Usually arises from the internal iliac artery, but in approximately 20% to 30% of the population, it arises from the inferior epigastric artery. It then passes close to or across the femoral canal to reach the obturator foramen and hence is susceptible to damage during hernia operations.
   - Runs through the upper part of the obturator foramen, divides into **anterior and posterior branches**, and supplies the muscles of the thigh.
   - Forms a **posterior branch** that gives rise to an acetabular branch, which enters the joint through the acetabular notch and reaches the head of the femur by way of the ligamentum capitis femoris.
8. **Inferior Vesical Artery**
   - Occurs in the male and corresponds to the **vaginal artery** in the female.
   - Supplies the fundus of the bladder, prostate gland, seminal vesicles, ductus deferens, and lower part of the ureter.
9. **Vaginal Artery**
   - Arises from the uterine or internal iliac artery.
   - Gives rise to numerous branches to the anterior and posterior wall of the vagina and makes longitudinal anastomoses in the median plane to form the **anterior and posterior azygos arteries of the vagina.**
10. **Middle Rectal Artery**
    - Runs medially to supply mainly the muscular layer of the lower part of the rectum and the upper part of the anal canal.
    - Also supplies the prostate gland and seminal vesicles (or vagina) and the ureter.
11. **Uterine Artery**
    - Is homologous to the **artery of the ductus deferens** in the male.
    - Arises from the internal iliac artery or in common with the vaginal or middle rectal artery.
    - Runs medially in the base of the broad ligament to reach the junction of the cervix and the body of the uterus, runs in front of and above the ureter near the lateral fornix of the vagina, then ascends along the margin of the uterus, and ends by anastomosing with the ovarian artery.
    - Divides into a large **superior branch**, supplying the body and fundus of the uterus, and a smaller **vaginal branch**, supplying the cervix and vagina.

B. Median Sacral Artery

- Is an unpaired artery arising from the posterior aspect of the abdominal aorta just before its bifurcation.
- Descends in front of the sacrum, supplying the posterior portion of the rectum, and ends in the **coccygeal body**, which is a small cellular and vascular mass located in front of the tip of the coccyx.

C. Superior Rectal Artery

- Is the direct continuation of the inferior mesenteric artery.

D. Ovarian Artery

- Arises from the abdominal aorta, crosses the proximal end of the external iliac artery to enter the pelvic minor, and reaches the ovary through the suspensory ligament of the ovary.

E. Veins of the Pelvis

- Generally correspond to arteries.

CLINICAL CORRELATES **Cancer cells in the pelvis** may metastasize from pelvic organs to the vertebral column, spinal cord, and brain via connections of the pelvic veins with the vertebral venous plexus and cranial dural sinus. Prostatic or uterine cancer can spread to the heart and lungs via the internal iliac veins draining from the prostatic or vesical venous plexus into the inferior vena cava.

F. Lymphatic Vessels

- Follow the internal iliac vessels to the internal iliac nodes, to the common iliac nodes, and then to the aortic nodes.
- Drain lymph from the rectum (upper part) along the superior rectal vessels, inferior mesenteric nodes, and then aortic nodes. Lymph vessels from the ovary, uterine tube, and fundus follow the ovarian artery and drain into the paraaortic nodes. Lymph vessels from the uterine body and cervix and bladder drain into the internal and external iliac nodes. Lymph vessels from the prostate and rectum (lower part) drain into the internal iliac nodes.

X. NERVE SUPPLY TO THE PELVIS

A. Sacral Plexus

- Is formed by the fourth and fifth lumbar ventral rami (the lumbosacral trunk) and the first four sacral ventral rami.
- Lies largely on the internal surface of the piriformis muscle in the pelvis.

1. Superior Gluteal Nerve (L4–S1)

- Leaves the pelvis through the greater sciatic foramen above the piriformis.
- Innervates the gluteus medius, gluteus minimus, and tensor fascia lata muscles.

2. Inferior Gluteal Nerve (L5–S2)

- Leaves the pelvis through the greater sciatic foramen below the piriformis.
- Innervates the gluteus maximus muscle.

3. Sciatic Nerve (L4–S3)

- Is the **largest nerve in the body** and is composed of **peroneal** and **tibial** parts.
- Leaves the pelvis through the greater sciatic foramen below the piriformis.
- Enters the thigh in the hollow between the ischial tuberosity and the greater trochanter of the femur.

4. Nerve to the Obturator Internus Muscle (L5–S2)

- Leaves the pelvis through the greater sciatic foramen below the piriformis.
- Enters the perineum through the lesser sciatic foramen.
- Innervates the obturator internus and superior gemellus muscles.

5. Nerve to the Quadratus Femoris Muscle (L5–S1)

- Leaves the pelvis through the greater sciatic foramen below the piriformis.
- Descends deep to the gemelli and obturator internus muscles and ends in the deep surface of the quadratus femoris, supplying the quadratus femoris and the inferior gemellus muscles.

6. Posterior Femoral Cutaneous Nerve (S1–S3)

- Leaves the pelvis through the greater sciatic foramen below the piriformis.
- Lies alongside the sciatic nerve and descends on the back of the knee.
- Gives rise to several **inferior cluneal nerves** and **perineal branches**.

7. Pudendal Nerve (S2–S4)

- Leaves the pelvis through the greater sciatic foramen below the piriformis.
- Enters the perineum through the lesser sciatic foramen and the pudendal canal in the lateral wall of the ischiorectal fossa.
- Its branches are described in the section on the nerves of the perineal region.

8. Branches Distributed to the Pelvis

- Include the nerve to the piriformis muscle (S1–S2), the nerves to the levator ani and coccygeus muscles (S3–S4), the nerve to the sphincter ani externus muscle, and the pelvic splanchnic nerves (S2–S4).

B. Autonomic Nerves

1. Superior Hypogastric Plexus

- Is the continuation of the aortic plexus below the aortic bifurcation and receives the lower two lumbar splanchnic nerves.
- Lies behind the peritoneum, descends in front of the fifth lumbar vertebra, and ends by bifurcation into the **right and left hypogastric nerves** in front of the sacrum.
- Contains preganglionic and postganglionic sympathetic fibers, visceral afferent fibers, and few, if any, parasympathetic fibers, which may run a recurrent course through the inferior hypogastric plexus.

2. Hypogastric Nerve

- Is the lateral extension of the superior hypogastric plexus and lies in the extraperitoneal connective tissue lateral to the rectum.
- Provides branches to the sigmoid colon and the descending colon.
- Is joined by the pelvic splanchnic nerves to form the inferior hypogastric or pelvic plexus.

3. Inferior Hypogastric (Pelvic) Plexus

- Is formed by the union of **hypogastric, pelvic splanchnic, and sacral splanchnic nerves** and lies against the posterolateral pelvic wall, lateral to the rectum, vagina, and base of the bladder.
- Contains **pelvic ganglia**, in which both sympathetic and parasympathetic preganglionic fibers synapse. Hence, it consists of preganglionic and postganglionic sympathetic fibers, preganglionic and postganglionic parasympathetic fibers, and visceral afferent fibers.
- Gives rise to subsidiary plexuses, including the middle rectal plexus, uterovaginal plexus, vesical plexus, differential plexus, and prostatic plexus.

4. Sacral Splanchnic Nerves

- Consist primarily of preganglionic sympathetic fibers that come off the chain and synapse in the inferior hypogastric (pelvic) plexus.

5. Pelvic Splanchnic Nerves (Nervi Erigentes)

- Arise from the sacral segment of the spinal cord (S2–S4) and are the only splanchnic nerves that carry parasympathetic fibers. (All other splanchnic nerves are sympathetic.)
- Contribute to the formation of the pelvic (or inferior hypogastric) plexus, and supply the descending colon, sigmoid colon, and other viscera in the pelvis and perineum.

XI. DEVELOPMENT OF THE LOWER GASTROINTESTINAL TRACT AND URINARY ORGANS (Figure 5.21)

A. Hind Gut

- Sends off a diverticulum, the allantois, and terminates as a blind sac of endoderm called the cloaca, which is in contact with an ectodermal invagination called the proctodeum.

B. Endodermal Cloaca

- Is divided by the urorectal septum into an anterior part, which becomes the **primitive bladder** and the **urogenital sinus**, and a posterior part called the anorectal canal, which forms the rectum and the upper half of the anal canal. The lower half of the anal canal forms from the ectoderm of the proctodeum.
- The primitive bladder is divided into an upper dilated portion, the **bladder**, and a lower narrow portion, the **urethra**.

C. Mesonephric (Wolffian) Duct

- Gives origin to the ureteric bud, which forms the **ureter**, renal pelvis, major and minor calyces, and collecting tubules.
- Forms the epididymal duct, **vas deferens**, ejaculatory ducts, and seminal vesicles in the male, but in the female, it largely degenerates, and small remnants persist as the duct of epoophoron (Gärtner) and the duct of the paroophoron.

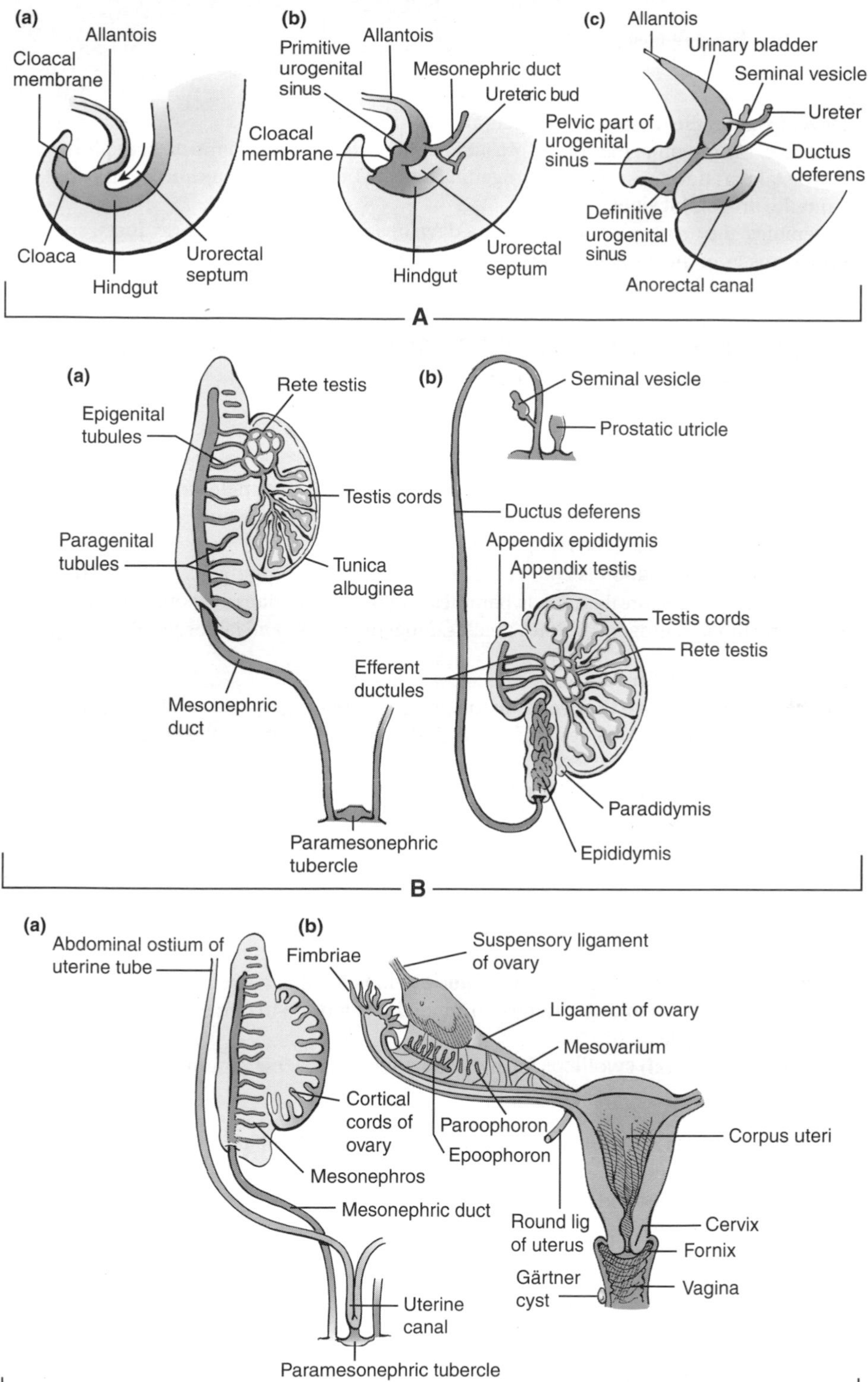

FIGURE 5.21. Development of the urogenital and reproductive systems. **A:** Development of the urogenital systems. **B:** Development of the male reproductive system. **C:** Development of the female reproductive system. **Aa:** The urorectal septum arises between the allantois and the hindgut. **Ab:** The cloaca divides into the urogenital sinus and anorectal canal, the mesonephric duct, and the ureteric bud. **Ac:** The urogenital sinus develops into the urinary bladder, and the seminal vesicles are formed by an outbudding of the ductus deferens. **Ba:** The paramesonephric duct has degenerated except for the appendix testis and the prostatic utricle. **Bb:** The genital duct after descent of the testis, showing the testis cords, the rete testis, and efferent ductules. **Ca:** The paramesonephric tubercle and uterine canal are formed. **Cb:** The genital ducts after descent of the ovary, showing the ligament of the ovary and the round ligament of the uterus. The mesonephric systems are degenerated except epoophoron, paroophoron, and Gärtner cyst.

D. Urethra

- Develops from the mesonephric ducts and the urogenital sinus.
- In males, the proximal part of the prostatic urethra develops from the **mesonephric ducts**, and the distal part develops from the urogenital sinus. The membranous and penile urethrae form from the **urogenital sinus**.
- In females, the upper part of the urethra develops from the mesonephric ducts, and the lower end forms from the urogenital sinus.

XII. DEVELOPMENT OF THE REPRODUCTIVE SYSTEM (See Figure 5.21)

A. Indifferent Embryo

- **Genotype of the embryo** is established at fertilization, but male and female embryos are phenotypically indistinguishable between weeks 1 and 6. Male and female characteristics of the external genitalia can be recognized by week 12.
- **Phenotypic differentiation** is completed by week 20. The components that will form the adult reproductive systems are the gonads, paramesonephric (Müllerian) ducts, mesonephric (Wolffian) ducts and tubules, urogenital sinus, phallus, urogenital folds, and labioscrotal swellings.

B. Development of Genital Organs

- **Indifferent gonads** form the ovaries in the presence of estrogen and the absence of testosterone in females and form **testes**, seminiferous tubules, and rete testes in the presence of testosterone in males.
- **Paramesonephric (Müllerian) ducts** form **uterine tubes** and the **uterus**, cervix, and upper vagina in females and form the prostatic utricle and appendix of testes in males.
- **Mesonephric (Wolffian)** ducts form the epoophoron (vestigial) in females and efferent ductules, epididymal duct, **ductus deferens**, ejaculatory duct, and seminal vesicles in males.
- **Urogenital sinus** forms the urinary bladder, urethra, urethral glands, greater vestibular glands, and lower vagina in females and urinary **bladder**, urethra, **prostate**, and bulbourethral glands in males.
- **Genital tubercle or phallus forms the clitoris in females and the penis in males.**
- **Urogenital (urethral) folds (or ridges)** form the **labia minora** in females and the spongy urethra of the penis in males.
- **Labioscrotal (genital) swellings** form the **labia majora** in females and **scrotum** in males.

C. Descent of the Ovaries and Testes

- **Ovaries and testes** develop within the abdominal cavity but later descend into the pelvis and scrotum, respectively. The gubernaculum and the processus vaginalis are involved in the descent of the ovaries and testes.
- **Gubernaculum** forms the ovarian ligament and round ligament of the uterus in females and gubernaculum testes in males.
- **Processus vaginalis** forms no adult structures in females and the tunica vaginalis testis in males.

HIGH-YIELD TOPICS

- The **perineum** is a diamond-shaped space bounded by the pubic symphysis, ischiopubic rami, ischial tuberosities, sacrotuberous ligaments, and the tip of the coccyx. It is divided into urogenital and anal triangles.
- The **superficial perineal space** (pouch) lies between the **inferior fascia** of the urogenital diaphragm (perineal membrane) and the **superficial perineal fascia** (Colles fascia). It contains perineal muscles, crus of the penis or clitoris, bulb of the penis or vestibule, the perineal body, **greater vestibular glands** (female), branches of the internal pudendal vessels, and the pudendal nerve.

- The **deep perineal space** (pouch) lies between the **superior and inferior fasciae of the urogenital diaphragm**. It contains the urogenital diaphragm, the membranous part of the urethra, the **bulbourethral glands** in the male, and branches of the internal pudendal vessels and pudendal nerve.
- The **ischiorectal fossa** is separated from the pelvis by the levator ani and its fasciae and is bounded by the urogenital diaphragm (anteriorly), the gluteus maximus and sacrotuberous ligament (posteriorly), the sphincter ani externus and levator ani (superomedially), the obturator fascia (laterally), and the skin (floor). It contains the **inferior rectal neurovascular structures and fat**.
- The **scrotum** is a sac of skin with **no fat** and the **dartos muscle** (fascia), which is continuous with the superficial penile fascia and superficial perineal fascia. It contains the **testis** and **epididymis** and receives blood from the external and internal pudendal arteries. Innervation is by the anterior scrotal branch of the **ilioinguinal nerve**, genital branch of the **genitofemoral nerve**, **posterior scrotal branch** of the perineal branch of the **pudendal nerve**, and the perineal branch of the **posterior femoral cutaneous nerve**. Scrotal lymphatics drain into the **superficial inguinal nodes**. The dartos muscle, cremaster muscle, and pampiniform plexus help regulate the temperature of the testes; the dartos muscle is responsible for wrinkling the scrotal skin, whereas the cremaster muscles are responsible for elevating the testes. The **scrotal skin wrinkles** to increase its thickness and reduce heat loss.
- The **penis** consists of a root (two crura and the bulb of the penis) and the body, which is formed by the **single corpus spongiosum** and **paired corpora cavernosa**. Its head is called the **glans penis**, which is the terminal part of the **corpus spongiosum**.
- **Extravasated urine** may result from **rupture** of the bulbous portion of the **spongy urethra** below the urogenital diaphragm; urine may pass into the superficial perineal space and **spread** inferiorly into the **scrotum**, anteriorly around the **penis**, and superiorly into the lower part of the **abdominal wall**.
- **Hydrocele** is an abnormal accumulation of serous **fluid between the two layers of the tunica vaginalis**. Causes include infection or injury to the testis or incomplete closure of the processus vaginalis. **Hematocele** is a **hemorrhage** into the cavity of the tunica vaginalis due to injury to the spermatic vessels.
- **Varicocele** is an enlargement of the pampiniform venous plexus that appears like a "**bag of worms**" in the scrotum. A varicocele may cause dragginglike pain, atrophy of the testis, and/or infertility.
- **Epispadias** is a congenital malformation in which the **spongy urethra opens** as a groove **on the dorsum** of the penis. **Hypospadias** is a congenital malformation in which the **urethra opens on the ventral surface** of the penis due to failure of the urethral folds to fuse completely.
- **Phimosis** is the **inability to** fully **retract the foreskin** (prepuce) over the glans due to a narrow opening of the prepuce. A very tight foreskin around the tip of the penis may interfere with urination or sexual function.
- The **labia majora** are two longitudinal folds of skin that are **homologous to the scrotum** and contain the terminations of the round ligaments of the uterus. The **labia minora** are **hairless** and contain **no fat.** They are divided into an upper (lateral) part, which fuses above the clitoris to form the **prepuce** of the clitoris, and a lower (medial) part, which fuses below the clitoris to form the **frenulum** of the clitoris. The vestibule of the vagina is the space between the labia minora and has openings for the urethra, vagina, and ducts of the greater vestibular glands.
- The **clitoris is homologous to the penis** and consists of **two crura**, **two corpora cavernosa**, and a glans but **no corpus spongiosum**. The glans clitoris is derived from the **corpora cavernosa** and is covered by a sensitive epithelium.
- The **pudendal nerve** (S2–S4) passes through the **greater sciatic foramen** between the piriformis and coccygeus muscles and enters the perineum with the internal pudendal vessels through the **lesser sciatic foramen**. The pudendal nerve enters the pudendal canal, gives rise to the inferior rectal and perineal nerves, and terminates as the dorsal nerve of the penis (or clitoris).
- The **inferior rectal nerve** innervates the sphincter ani externus and the skin around the anus.
- The **perineal nerve** divides into a deep branch, which supplies all of the perineal muscles, and a superficial (posterior scrotal or labial) branch, which supplies the scrotum or labia majora.
- The **dorsal nerve** of the penis or clitoris runs between the two layers of the suspensory ligament of the penis or clitoris and runs deep to the deep fascia on the dorsum of the penis or clitoris to innervate the skin, prepuce, and glans.
- The **internal pudendal artery** is accompanied by the pudendal nerve during its course, leaving the pelvis by way of the greater sciatic foramen and entering the perineum through the lesser sciatic foramen.

- The **internal pudendal vein** arises from the lower part of the **prostatic venous plexus** in the male or the vesical plexus in the female and usually empties into the internal iliac vein.
- The **deep dorsal vein** of the penis is an **unpaired vein** that begins behind the glans and lies in the dorsal midline deep to the deep fascia and superficial to the tunica albuginea, leaves the perineum through the gap between the arcuate pubic ligament and the transverse perineal ligament, and drains into the prostatic and pelvic venous plexuses. The superficial dorsal vein of the penis runs toward the pubic symphysis and terminates in the external (superficial) pudendal veins, which drain into the greater saphenous vein. The deep dorsal vein of the clitoris is small but also runs in the median plane between the left and right dorsal arteries and ends in the lower part of the vesical venous plexus.
- The **pelvis** is a basin-shaped ring of bone formed by the two **hip bones**, the **sacrum**, and the **coccyx.** The hip or coxal bone consists of the ilium, ischium, and pubis. The pelvis major (false pelvis) lies above the pelvic brim, while the pelvis minor (true pelvis) lies below.
- The **pelvic diaphragm** is formed by the **levator ani** and **coccygeus**, forms the pelvic floor, and supports all of the pelvic viscera. It flexes the anorectal canal during defecation, helps the voluntary control of micturition, and also helps direct the fetal head toward the birth canal at parturition.
- The **broad ligament** extends from the uterus to the lateral pelvic wall and serves to **hold the uterus** in position. It contains the uterine tube, uterine vessels, round ligament of the uterus, ovarian ligament, ureter, nerve plexus, and lymphatic vessels. It **does not contain the ovary** but is attached to the ovary through the mesovarium.
- The **round ligament** of the uterus is the remains of the **lower part of the gubernaculum**, runs within the broad ligament, and keeps the uterus anteverted and anteflexed. It enters the inguinal canal at the deep inguinal ring, emerges from the superficial inguinal ring, and becomes lost in the labium majus. The ovarian ligament extends from the ovary to the uterus below the uterine tube within the layers of the broad ligament.
- The **lateral or transverse cervical** (**cardinal** or Mackenrodt) ligament supports the uterus and extends from the cervix and vagina to the pelvic wall. It is a condensation of **endopelvic fascia** and contains the **uterine vessels.**
- **Pudendal nerve block** is accomplished by inserting a needle through the posterolateral vaginal wall, just beneath the pelvic diaphragm and toward the ischial spine, thus placing the local anesthetic around the pudendal nerve.
- **Culdocentesis** is aspiration of fluid from the cul-de-sac of Douglas (rectouterine pouch) by a needle puncture of the posterior vaginal fornix near the midline between the uterosacral ligaments.
- The **ureter has three constrictions** along its course: **at the origin** where the pelvis of the ureter joins the ureter, where it crosses the **pelvic brim**, and at its **junction with the urinary bladder**. Distally, the ureter is in close proximity to the uterine artery and thus is sometimes injured by a clamp during surgical procedures and may be ligated and sectioned by mistake during a hysterectomy. The **ureter passes under the uterine artery** to reach the bladder. This relationship can be remembered using the mnemonic device, "**water (ureter) runs under the bridge** (uterine artery)."
- The **trigone** of the urinary bladder is bounded by the two orifices of the ureters and the internal urethral orifice. The uvula is a small rounded elevation just behind the **urethral orifice at the apex of the trigone**. The musculature of the bladder (bundles of smooth-muscle fibers) is known as the detrusor muscle. The urethral orifice is encircled by a circular layer of smooth muscle called the internal sphincter (sphincter vesicae). The bladder receives blood from the superior and inferior vesical arteries, and venous blood drains to the prostatic or vesical plexus of veins, which empty into the internal iliac vein. The bladder is innervated by nerve fibers from the vesical and prostatic plexuses.
- **Micturition** (urination) is initiated when increasing volume of urine stimulates stretch receptors in the detrusor muscle in the bladder wall. Afferent (GVA) impulses arise from the stretch receptors in the bladder wall and enter the spinal cord (S2–S4) via the pelvic splanchnic nerves. Sympathetic fibers induce relaxation of the bladder wall and constrict the internal sphincter, inhibiting emptying. Parasympathetic fibers in the pelvic splanchnic nerve induce contraction of the detrusor muscle and relaxation of the internal sphincter, enhancing the urge to void. Somatic motor fibers in the pudendal nerve cause voluntary relaxation of the external urethral sphincter, allowing the bladder to void. At the end of micturition, the external urethral sphincter contracts and bulbospongiosus muscles in the male expel the last few drops of urine from the urethra.

- **Bladder cancer** usually originates in cells lining the inside of the bladder (**epithelial cells**). The most common symptom is **blood in the urine** (hematuria). Other symptoms include **frequent urination** and **pain upon urination** (dysuria).
- **Vesicle tenesmus** is the continuing **urge to void** after urination due to spasm of the urogenital diaphragm.
- **Interstitial cystitis** is a chronic inflammation of the bladder that causes frequent, urgent, and painful urination.
- **Seminal vesicles** produce the alkaline constituent of the seminal fluid, which contains fructose and choline. It also contains a substance that causes the semen to clot after ejaculation. Fructose provides a forensic **determination for occurrence of rape**, while choline crystals can **detect the presence of semen (Florence test)**.
- The **ductus deferens** transports and stores spermatozoa, is dilated distally to become the ampulla, and joins the duct of the seminal vesicle to form the ejaculatory duct, which empties into the prostatic urethra **on the seminal colliculus**.
- **Erection and ejaculation** are often described using a popular mnemonic device: **point (erection by parasympathetic)** and **shoot (ejaculation by sympathetic)**.
- **Vasectomy** is the surgical excision of a portion of the vas deferens (ductus deferens) through the scrotum. It stops the passage of spermatozoa but neither reduces the amount of ejaculate greatly nor diminishes sexual desire.
- The **prostate gland** is located at the base of the urinary bladder, and its secretion **liquefies the semen** that was clotted by the seminal fluid. It has **five lobes**, including the anterior lobe, **middle lobe (prone to benign hypertrophy)**, lateral lobes, and **posterior lobe (prone to carcinomatous transformation)**.
- **Benign prostatic hypertrophy** (BPH) is the **enlargement** of the prostate that affects older men and occurs most often in the **middle lobe**, obstructing the internal urethral orifice. Hypertrophy can result in **nocturia, dysuria**, and **urgency**. Transurethral resection of the prostate (**TURP**) is the surgical removal of excess prostatic tissue using a cystoscope passed through the urethra. Prostatitis is the inflammation of the prostate.
- **Prostate cancer** is a slow-growing cancer that occurs particularly in the **posterior lobe**. Prostate cancer spreads to the bony pelvis, pelvic lymph nodes, vertebral column, and skull via the vertebral venous plexus, producing pain in the pelvis, the lower back, and the bones. This cancer also metastasizes to the heart and lungs through the prostatic venous plexus, internal iliac veins, and into the inferior vena cava. It can be detected by digital rectal examination, ultrasound imaging with a device inserted into the rectum, or PSA test. **PSA** concentration in the blood of normal males is **less than 4.0 ng/mL.**
- **Prostatectomy** is the surgical removal of a part or all of the prostate gland. Perineal prostatectomy is removal of the prostate through an incision in the perineum. Radical prostatectomy is removal of the prostate with seminal vesicles, ductus deferens, some pelvic fasciae, and pelvic lymph nodes through the retropubic or the perineal route.
- The **testis** develops in the posterior abdomen and descends into the scrotum retroperitoneally. The germ cells produce **sperm**; sustentacular (Sertoli) cells secrete **androgen-binding protein** and the hormone **inhibin**; interstitial (Leydig) cells secrete **sex hormones**; and myoid cells help to squeeze sperm through the tubules.
- The **epididymis** is a convoluted duct consisting of a head, body, and tail. It functions in **maturation and storage of spermatozoa** in the head and body and the propulsion of the spermatozoa into the ductus deferens.
- **Testicular torsion** is rotation of a testis such that the **spermatic cord becomes twisted, obstructing blood supply** to the testis. It may be caused by trauma or a spasm of the cremaster muscle resulting in sudden urgent pain, swelling of the scrotum, nausea, and vomiting. Testicular torsion requires emergency treatment and if not corrected, testicular necrosis will occur.
- **Orchitis** is the **inflammation** of the testis and is marked by pain, swelling, and a feeling of heaviness in the testis. It is commonly associated with the mumps, but can also have bacterial origins such as gonorrhea, syphilis, or tuberculosis.
- **Testicular cancer** commonly develops from rapidly dividing spermatogenic cells (**seminoma** or **germ-cell tumor**). More rarely, tumors can arise from Leydig cells (**Leydig-cell tumor**), which

produce androgen, or Sertoli cells. Signs and symptoms include a painless mass or lump, testicular swelling, hardness, and a feeling of heaviness or aching in the scrotum or lower abdomen.

- **Cryptorchidism** is a congenital condition in which the **testis fails to descend** into the scrotum during fetal development. Undescended testes are brought down into the scrotum in infancy by a surgical procedure called an orchiopexy or orchidopexy.
- The **ovaries** are almond-shaped structures that lie on the lateral walls of the pelvic cavity, are suspended by suspensory and round ligaments, and **produce oocytes** or **ova and steroid hormones**. The ovarian cycle includes the follicular phase, ovulation phase, and luteal phase.
- The **uterine tube** extends from the uterus to the ovary and consists of the isthmus, ampulla, and infundibulum. The fimbriated distal end creates currents, helping **draw an ovulated oocyte into the uterine tube.**
- The **uterus** contains a fundus, body, isthmus, and cervix and is supported by the broad, transverse cervical (cardinal) and round ligaments, urogenital diaphragm, and muscles of the pelvic floor, which provide the most important support. The uterine wall consists of the **perimetrium, myometrium**, and **endometrium**; the uterine cycle includes the menstrual, proliferative, and secretory phases; the first two phases are a shedding and then a rebuilding of endometrium in the 2 weeks before ovulation, and the third phase prepares the **endometrium to receive an embryo in the 2 weeks after ovulation.**
- The **vagina** extends between the vestibule and the cervix of the uterus, serves as the **excretory channel** for the products of menstruation, **receives the penis** and **semen** during coitus, and acts as the **birth canal**. The vaginal fornix is a ringlike recess around the tip of the cervix.
- **Ovarian cancer** develops from germ cells that produce ova, stromal cells that produce estrogen and progesterone, and epithelial cells that cover the outer surface of the ovary. Diagnosis involves feeling a mass during a pelvic examination, visualizing it by transvaginal ultrasound, or using a blood test for a protein associated with ovarian cancer (CA-125). Cancer signs and symptoms include unusual vaginal bleeding, postmenopausal bleeding, **bleeding after intercourse, pain during intercourse**, pelvic pressure, abdominal and pelvic pain, **back pain**, indigestion, and loss of appetite.
- **Uterine prolapse** is the **protrusion of the cervix** of the uterus into the lower part of the vagina close to the vestibule and causes a **bearing-down sensation** in the womb and an increased frequency of and burning sensation on urination. The prolapse occurs as a result of advancing age and menopause and results from weakness of the muscles, ligaments, and fasciae of the pelvic floor that constitute the support of the uterus and other pelvic viscera.
- **Fibromyoma** or **leiomyoma** is the most common **benign neoplasm** of the female genital tract derived from smooth muscle. It may cause urinary frequency, dysmenorrhea, abortion, or obstructed labor. A **fibroid** is a benign uterine tumor made of smooth-muscle cells and fibrous connective tissue in the wall of the uterus. A large fibroid can cause bleeding, pressure, and pain in the pelvis, heavy menstrual periods, and infertility.
- **Endometriosis** is a benign disorder in which a **mass of endometrial tissue** (stroma and glands) occurs aberrantly in various locations, including the uterine wall, ovaries, or other extraendometrial sites.
- **Endometrial cancer** is the most common type (approximately **90%**) of **uterine cancer** and develops from the endometrium of the uterus usually from the uterine glands. Its main symptom is vaginal bleeding, which allows for early detection; other symptoms are clear vaginal discharge, lower abdominal pain, and pelvic cramping.
- **Cervical cancer** is a slow-growing cancer that develops from the **epithelium** covering the cervix. Cancer cells grow upward to the endometrial cavity, downward to the vagina, and laterally to the pelvic wall, invading the bladder and rectum directly.
- **Hysterectomy** is the surgical removal of the uterus, performed either through the abdominal wall or through the vagina. It may result in **injury to the ureter**, which lies in the transverse cardinal ligament beneath the uterine artery.
- **Vaginismus** is a **painful spasm of the vagina** resulting from involuntary contraction of the vaginal musculature, preventing sexual intercourse. It may be caused by organic or psychogenic factors or traumatic experiences such as rape and sexual abuse.
- **Mediolateral episiotomy** is a surgical incision through the posterolateral vaginal wall, just lateral to the perineal body, to enlarge the birth canal and thus prevent uncontrolled tearing during

parturition. The mediolateral episiotomy **allows greater expansion of the birth canal** into the ischiorectal fossa. The midline episiotomy is also commonly used.

- The **rectum** extends from the sigmoid colon to the anal canal; receives blood from the superior, middle, and inferior rectal arteries; and **drains its venous blood into the portal venous system** via the superior rectal vein and **into the caval system** via the middle and inferior rectal veins. The feces are stored in the ampulla, which is the lower dilated part of the rectum that lies above the pelvic diaphragm.
- The **anal canal** divides into an upper two-thirds (visceral portion), which belongs to the intestine, and a **lower one-third** (somatic portion), which belongs to the perineum. A point of **demarcation** between visceral and somatic portions is called the **pectinate line**, which is a serrated line following the anal valves. **Hilton white line** is the **intermuscular** (intersphincteric) **groove** between the lower border of the internal anal sphincter and the subcutaneous part of the external anal sphincter (Table 5.2).
- **Rectal tenesmus** is the **urge to evacuate** the bowel with little to no stool passage, accompanied by pain, cramping, and straining.
- **Inflammatory bowel disease** (IBD) is the chronic inflammation of the intestines. The most common forms of IBD are **ulcerative colitis** and **Crohn's disease**. Symptoms include cramping abdominal pain, bloody stool, diarrhea, and passage of mucus. Ulcerative colitis is chronic ulceration of the colon and rectum, while Crohn disease can occur anywhere in the digestive tract.
- **Diverticulitis** is the inflammation of an abnormal pouch (diverticulum) in the intestinal wall, commonly found in the colon, especially the **sigmoid colon**. Diverticula develop as a result of high pressure within the colon. Symptoms are abdominal pain (usually in the left lower abdomen but can be anywhere), chills, fever, nausea, and constipation.
- **Rectal or digital (finger) examination** is performed by inserting a gloved, lubricated finger into the rectum; using the other hand to press on the lower abdomen or pelvic area; and palpating for tumors, hemorrhoids, rectal carcinoma, prostate cancer, seminal vesicle, bladder, uterus, cervix, ovaries, polyps, and other abnormalities.
- **Colorectal (colon) cancer** develops in the **epithelial cell lining** of the lumen of the colon and rectum. Cancer risk factors include high fat intake, a family history, and polyps. Its symptoms include fatigue, weakness, weight loss, change in bowel habits, diarrhea or constipation, and red or dark blood in stool. Cancer can be detected by colonoscopy. Colorectal cancer may spread along lymphatic vessels and through the venous system, and it may **metastasize to the liver, the vagina, uterus, bladder, prostate, or seminal vesicles**.
- **Hemorrhoids** are dilated internal and external venous plexuses around the rectum and anal canal. **Internal hemorrhoids occur above the pectinate line** and are covered by mucous membrane; their pain fibers are carried by **GVA fibers** of the sympathetic nerves. **External hemorrhoids are situated below the pectinate line**, are covered by skin, and are more painful than internal hemorrhoids because their pain fibers are carried by **GSA fibers** of the inferior rectal nerves.
- **Cancer cells in the pelvis** may metastasize from pelvic organs **to the vertebral column, spinal cord, and brain** via connections of the pelvic veins with the vertebral venous plexus and cranial dural sinus. Prostatic or uterine cancer can spread to the heart and lungs via the internal iliac veins draining from the prostatic or vesical venous plexus into the inferior vena cava.
- Autonomic nerve functions in the pelvis:

Functions of Autonomic Nerves

	Sympathetic Nerve	Parasympathetic Nerve
Urinary bladder	Contracts sphincter vesicae; inhibits detrusor muscle; inhibits voiding	Relaxes sphincter vesicae; contracts detrusor muscle; promotes voiding
Genital organs	Causes vasoconstriction and ejaculation; contracts uterus	Vasodilation and erection; relaxes uterus

Review Test

Directions: Each of the numbered items or incomplete statements in this section is followed by answers or by completions of the statement. Select the **one**-lettered answer or completion that is **best** in each case.

1. A 68-year-old woman with uterine carcinoma undergoes surgical resection. This cancer can spread directly to the labia majora in lymphatics that follow which of the following structures?

(A) Pubic arcuate ligament
(B) Suspensory ligament of the ovary
(C) Cardinal (transverse cervical) ligament
(D) Suspensory ligament of the clitoris
(E) Round ligament of the uterus

2. A 17-year-old boy suffers a traumatic groin injury during a soccer match. The urologist notices tenderness and swelling of the boy's left testicle that may be produced by thrombosis in which of the following veins?

(A) Left internal pudendal vein
(B) Left renal vein
(C) Inferior vena cava
(D) Left inferior epigastric vein
(E) Left external pudendal vein

3. On a busy Saturday night in Chicago, a 16-year-old boy presents to the emergency department with a stab wound from a knife that entered the pelvis above the piriformis muscle. Which of the following structures is most likely to be damaged?

(A) Sciatic nerve
(B) Internal pudendal artery
(C) Superior gluteal nerve
(D) Inferior gluteal artery
(E) Posterior femoral cutaneous nerve

4. A 22-year-old woman receives a deep cut in the inguinal canal 1 in. lateral to the pubic tubercle. Which of the following ligaments is lacerated within the inguinal canal?

(A) Suspensory ligament of the ovary
(B) Ovarian ligament
(C) Mesosalpinx
(D) Round ligament of the uterus
(E) Rectouterine ligament

5. A 29-year-old carpenter sustains severe injuries of the pelvic splanchnic nerve by a deep puncture wound, which has become contaminated. The injured parasympathetic preganglionic fibers in the splanchnic nerve are most likely to synapse in which of the following ganglia?

(A) Ganglia in or near the viscera or pelvic plexus
(B) Sympathetic chain ganglia
(C) Collateral ganglia
(D) Dorsal root ganglia
(E) Ganglion impar

6. A 59-year-old woman comes to a local hospital for uterine cancer surgery. As the uterine artery passes from the internal iliac artery to the uterus, it crosses superior to which of the following structures that is sometimes mistakenly ligated during such surgery?

(A) Ovarian artery
(B) Ovarian ligament
(C) Uterine tube
(D) Ureter
(E) Round ligament of the uterus

7. A 29-year-old woman is admitted to a hospital because the birth of her child is several days overdue. Tearing of the pelvic diaphragm during childbirth leads to paralysis of which of the following muscles?

(A) Piriformis
(B) Sphincter urethrae
(C) Obturator internus
(D) Levator ani
(E) Sphincter ani externus

8. A 37-year-old small business manager receives a gunshot wound in the pelvic cavity, resulting in a lesion of the sacral splanchnic nerves. Which of the following nerve fibers would primarily be damaged?

(A) Postganglionic parasympathetic fibers
(B) Postganglionic sympathetic fibers

(C) Preganglionic sympathetic fibers
(D) Preganglionic parasympathetic fibers
(E) Postganglionic sympathetic and parasympathetic fibers

9. A young couple is having difficulty conceiving a child. Their physician at a reproduction and fertility clinic explains to them that

(A) The ovary lies within the broad ligament
(B) The glans clitoris is formed from the corpus spongiosum
(C) Erection of the penis is a sympathetic response
(D) Ejaculation follows parasympathetic stimulation
(E) Fertilization occurs in the infundibulum or ampulla of the uterine tube

10. A 46-year-old woman has a history of infection in her perineal region. A comprehensive examination reveals a tear of the superior boundary of the superficial perineal space. Which of the following structures would most likely be injured?

(A) Pelvic diaphragm
(B) Colles fascia
(C) Superficial perineal fascia
(D) Deep perineal fascia
(E) Perineal membrane

11. A 58-year-old man is diagnosed as having a slowly growing tumor in the deep perineal space. Which of the following structures would most likely be injured?

(A) Bulbourethral glands
(B) Crus of penis
(C) Bulb of vestibule
(D) Spongy urethra
(E) Great vestibular gland

12. An elderly man with a benign enlargement of his prostate experiences difficulty in urination, urinary frequency, and urgency. Which of the following lobes of the prostate gland is commonly involved in benign hypertrophy that obstructs the prostatic urethra?

(A) Anterior lobe
(B) Middle lobe
(C) Right lateral lobe
(D) Left lateral lobe
(E) Posterior lobe

13. A 59-year-old man is diagnosed with prostate cancer following a digital rectal examination. For the resection of prostate cancer, it is important to know that the prostatic ducts open into or on which of the following structures:

(A) Membranous part of the urethra
(B) Seminal colliculus
(C) Spongy urethra
(D) Prostatic sinus
(E) Prostatic utricle

14. A 29-year-old woman with a ruptured ectopic pregnancy is admitted to a hospital for culdocentesis. A long needle on the syringe is most efficiently inserted through which of the following structures?

(A) Anterior fornix of the vagina
(B) Posterior fornix of the vagina
(C) Anterior wall of the rectum
(D) Posterior wall of the uterine body
(E) Posterior wall of the bladder

15. A 37-year-old man is suffering from carcinoma of the skin of the penis. Cancer cells are likely to metastasize directly to which of the following lymph nodes?

(A) External iliac nodes
(B) Internal iliac nodes
(C) Superficial inguinal nodes
(D) Aortic (lumbar) nodes
(E) Deep inguinal nodes

16. A 42-year-old woman who has had six children develops a weakness of the urogenital diaphragm. Paralysis of which of the following muscles would cause such a symptom?

(A) Sphincter urethrae
(B) Coccygeus
(C) Superficial transversus perinei
(D) Levator ani
(E) Obturator internus

17. A 43-year-old man has a benign tumor located near a gap between the arcuate pubic ligament and the transverse perineal ligament. Which of the following structures is most likely compressed by this tumor?

(A) Perineal nerve
(B) Deep dorsal vein of the penis
(C) Superficial dorsal vein
(D) Posterior scrotal nerve
(E) Deep artery of the penis

18. An obstetrician performs a median episiotomy on a woman before parturition to prevent uncontrolled tearing. If the perineal body is damaged, the function of which of the following muscles might be impaired?

(A) Ischiocavernosus and sphincter urethrae
(B) Deep transverse perineal and obturator internus
(C) Bulbospongiosus and superficial transverse perineal
(D) External anal sphincter and sphincter urethrae
(E) Bulbospongiosus and ischiocavernosus

19. A 22-year-old man has a gonorrheal infection that has infiltrated the space between the inferior fascia of the urogenital diaphragm and the superficial perineal fascia. Which of the following structures might be inflamed?

(A) Bulb of the penis
(B) Bulbourethral gland
(C) Membranous part of the male urethra
(D) Deep transverse perineal muscle
(E) Sphincter urethrae

20. A 39-year-old man is unable to expel the last drops of urine from the urethra at the end of micturition because of paralysis of the external urethral sphincter and bulbospongiosus muscles. This condition may occur as a result of injury to which of the following nervous structures?

(A) Pelvic plexus
(B) Prostatic plexus
(C) Pudendal nerve
(D) Pelvic splanchnic nerve
(E) Sacral splanchnic nerve

21. A 21-year-old marine biologist asks about her first bimanual examination, and it is explained to her that the normal position of the uterus is

(A) Anteflexed and anteverted
(B) Retroflexed and anteverted
(C) Anteflexed and retroverted
(D) Retroverted and retroflexed
(E) Anteverted and retroverted

22. After his bath but before getting dressed, a 4-year-old boy was playing with his puppy. The boy's penis was bitten by the puppy, and the deep dorsal vein was injured. The damaged vein

(A) Lies superficial to Buck fascia
(B) Drains into the prostatic venous plexus
(C) Lies lateral to the dorsal artery of the penis
(D) Is found in the corpus spongiosum
(E) Is dilated during erection

23. A 62-year-old man is incapable of penile erection after rectal surgery with prostatectomy. The patient most likely has a lesion of which of the following nerves?

(A) Dorsal nerve of the penis
(B) Perineal nerve
(C) Hypogastric nerve
(D) Sacral splanchnic nerve
(E) Pelvic splanchnic nerve

24. A 23-year-old massage therapist who specializes in women's health attends a lecture at an annual conference on techniques of massage. She asks, "What structure is drained by the lumbar (aortic) lymph nodes?" Which of the following structures is the correct answer to this question?

(A) Perineum
(B) Lower part of the vagina
(C) External genitalia
(D) Ovary
(E) Lower part of the anterior abdominal wall

25. A sexually active adolescent presents with an infection within the ischiorectal fossa. Which of the following structures is most likely injured?

(A) Vestibular bulb
(B) Seminal vesicle
(C) Greater vestibular gland
(D) Inferior rectal nerve
(E) Internal pudendal artery

26. A first-year resident in the urology department reviews pelvic anatomy before seeing patients. Which of the following statements is correct?

(A) The dorsal artery of the penis supplies the glans penis.
(B) The seminal vesicles store spermatozoa.
(C) The duct of the bulbourethral gland opens into the membranous urethra.
(D) The duct of the greater vestibular gland opens into the vagina.
(E) The anterior lobe of the prostate gland is prone to carcinomatous transformation.

27. A 43-year-old woman presents with a prolapsed uterus. Repair of a prolapsed uterus requires knowledge of the supporting structures of the uterus. Which of the following structures plays the most important role in the support of the uterus?

(A) Levator ani
(B) Sphincter urethrae
(C) Uterosacral ligament
(D) Ovarian ligament
(E) Arcuate pubic ligament

28. A 16-year-old boy presents to the emergency department with rupture of the penile urethra. Extravasated urine from this injury can spread into which of the following structures?

(A) Scrotum
(B) Ischiorectal fossa
(C) Pelvic cavity
(D) Testis
(E) Thigh

29. A 23-year-old woman visits her obstetrician for an annual checkup. During vaginal examination, which of the following structures may be palpated?

(A) Apex of the urinary bladder
(B) Fundus of the uterus
(C) Terminal part of the round ligament of the uterus
(D) Body of the clitoris
(E) Uterine cervix

30. A 53-year-old bank teller is admitted to a local hospital for surgical removal of a benign pelvic tumor confined within the broad ligament. There is a risk of injuring which of the following structures that lies in this ligament?

(A) Ovary
(B) Proximal part of the pelvic ureter
(C) Terminal part of the round ligament of the uterus
(D) Uterine tube
(E) Suspensory ligament of the ovary

31. A 72-year-old man comes to his physician for an annual checkup. Which of the following structures is most readily palpated during rectal examination?

(A) Prostate gland
(B) Epididymis
(C) Ejaculatory duct
(D) Ureter
(E) Testis

32. A 48-year-old college football coach undergoes a radical prostatectomy for a malignant tumor in his prostate. Following surgery, he is incapable of achieving an erection. Which of the following nerves is most likely damaged during the surgery?

(A) Sacral splanchnic nerve
(B) Pelvic splanchnic nerve
(C) Pudendal nerve
(D) Dorsal nerve of the penis
(E) Posterior scrotal nerve

33. While performing a pelvic exenteration, the surgical oncologist notices a fractured or ruptured boundary of the pelvic inlet. Which of the following structures is most likely damaged?

(A) Promontory of the sacrum
(B) Anterior–inferior iliac spine
(C) Inguinal ligament
(D) Iliac crest
(E) Arcuate pubic ligament

34. A 32-year-old patient with multiple fractures of the pelvis has no cutaneous sensation in the urogenital triangle. The function of which of the following nerves is most likely to be spared?

(A) Ilioinguinal nerve
(B) Iliohypogastric nerve
(C) Posterior cutaneous nerve of the thigh
(D) Pudendal nerve
(E) Genitofemoral nerve

35. A 22-year-old victim of an automobile accident has received destructive damage to structures that form the boundary of the perineum. Which of the following structures is spared?

(A) Pubic arcuate ligament
(B) Tip of the coccyx
(C) Ischial tuberosities
(D) Sacrospinous ligament
(E) Sacrotuberous ligament

36. A 32-year-old man undergoes vasectomy as a means of permanent birth control. A physician performing the vasectomy by making an incision on each side of the scrotum should remember which of the following statements most applicable to the scrotum?

(A) It is innervated by the ilioinguinal and genitofemoral nerves.
(B) It receives blood primarily from the testicular artery.
(C) Its venous blood drains primarily into the renal vein on the left.
(D) Its lymphatic drainage is primarily into upper lumbar nodes.
(E) Its dartos tunic is continuous with the perineal membrane.

37. A 37-year-old woman complains of a bearing-down sensation in her womb and an increased frequency of and burning sensation on urination. On examination by her gynecologist, she is diagnosed with a uterine prolapse. Which of the following structures provides the primary support for the cervix of the uterus?

(A) External anal sphincter
(B) Broad ligament of the uterus
(C) Cardinal (transverse cervical) ligament
(D) Round ligament of the uterus
(E) Suspensory ligament of the ovary

38. A woman is delivering a breech baby. The obstetrician decides that it is best to perform a mediolateral episiotomy. Which of the following structures should the obstetrician avoid incising?

(A) Vaginal wall
(B) Superficial transverse perineal muscle
(C) Bulbospongiosus
(D) Levator ani
(E) Perineal membrane

39. During pelvic surgery, a surgeon notices severe bleeding from the artery that remains within the true pelvis. Which of the following arteries is most likely to be injured?

(A) Iliolumbar artery
(B) Obturator artery
(C) Uterine artery
(D) Internal pudendal artery
(E) Inferior gluteal artery

40. A neurosurgeon performs a surgical resection of a rare meningeal tumor in the sacral region. He tries to avoid an injury of the nerve that arises from the lumbosacral plexus and remains within the abdominal or pelvic cavity. To which of the following nerves should he pay particular attention?

(A) Ilioinguinal nerve
(B) Genitofemoral nerve
(C) Lumbosacral trunk
(D) Femoral nerve
(E) Lateral femoral cutaneous nerve

41. After repair of a ruptured diverticulum, a 31-year-old patient begins to spike with fever and complains of abdominal pain. An infection in the deep perineal space would most likely damage which of the following structures?

(A) Ischiocavernosus muscles
(B) Superficial transverse perineal muscles
(C) Levator ani
(D) Sphincter urethrae
(E) Bulbospongiosus

42. A radiologist interprets a lymphangiogram for a 29-year-old patient with metastatic carcinoma. Upper lumbar nodes most likely receive lymph from which of the following structures?

(A) Lower part of the anal canal
(B) Labium majus
(C) Clitoris
(D) Testis
(E) Scrotum

43. A 49-year-old woman has a large mass on the pelvic brim. Which of the following structures is most likely compressed by this mass when crossing the pelvic brim?

(A) Deep dorsal vein of the penis
(B) Uterine tube
(C) Ovarian ligament
(D) Uterine artery
(E) Lumbosacral trunk

44. A 26-year-old man comes to a hospital with fever, nausea, pain, and itching in the perineal region. On examination by a urologist, he is diagnosed as having infected bulbourethral (Cowper) glands. Which of the following structures is/are affected by this infection?

(A) Superficial perineal space
(B) Sphincter urethrae
(C) Production of sperm
(D) Testis
(E) Seminal vesicles

45. A 21-year-old man is involved in a high-speed motor vehicle accident. As a result, he has extensive damage to his sphincter urethra. Which of the following best describes the injured sphincter urethra?

(A) Smooth muscle
(B) Innervated by the perineal nerve
(C) Lying between the perineal membrane and Colles fascia
(D) Enclosed in the pelvic fascia
(E) Part of the pelvic diaphragm

46. A 6-month-old male infant is admitted to the children's hospital because he has no testis in his scrotum. During physical examination, the pediatrician palpated the testis in the inguinal canal. What is the diagnosis of this condition?

(A) Male pseudohermaphroditism
(B) Hypospadias

(C) Epispadias
(D) Cryptorchid testis
(E) Chordee

47. An obstetrician is about to perform a pudendal block so a woman can experience less pain when she delivers her child. He recalls what he learned in medical school about this nerve. Which of the following statements is correct?

(A) It passes superficial to the sacrotuberous ligament
(B) It innervates the testis and epididymis in a male
(C) It provides motor fibers to the coccygeus
(D) It can be blocked by injecting an anesthetic near the inferior margin of the ischial spine
(E) It arises from the lumbar plexus

48. A trauma surgeon in the emergency department at a local center examines a 14-year-old boy with extensive pelvic injuries after a hit and run accident. The surgeon inspects the ischiorectal fossa because it

(A) Accumulates urine leaking from rupture of the bulb of the penis
(B) Contains the inferior rectal vessels
(C) Has a pudendal canal along its medial wall
(D) Is bounded anteriorly by the sacrotuberous ligament
(E) Contains a perineal branch of the fifth lumbar nerve

49. An elderly man with prostatitis is seen at an internal medicine clinic. The seminal colliculus of his prostate gland is infected, and its fine openings are closed. Which of the following structures is/are most likely to be disturbed?

(A) Ducts of the prostate gland
(B) Prostatic utricle
(C) Ducts of the bulbourethral glands
(D) Ejaculatory ducts
(E) Duct of the seminal vesicles

50. A general surgeon is giving a lecture to a team of surgery residents. She describes characteristics of structures above the pectinate line of the anal canal, which include

(A) Stratified squamous epithelium
(B) Venous drainage into the caval system
(C) Lymphatic drainage into the superficial inguinal nodes
(D) Visceral sensory innervation
(E) External hemorrhoids

51. A 5-month-old boy is admitted to the children's hospital because of urine being expelled from the dorsal aspect of the penis. Which of the following embryologic structures failed to fuse in this patient?

(A) Labioscrotal swellings or folds
(B) Urogenital sinus
(C) Spongy urethra
(D) Phallus
(E) Urethral folds

52. A 78-year-old man has carcinoma of the rectum. The cancer is likely to metastasize via the veins into which of the following structures?

(A) Spleen
(B) Kidney
(C) Liver
(D) Duodenum
(E) Suprarenal gland

53. During a partial hysterectomy leaving the ovaries in tact, the surgeon detaches the ovary from the uterus by transecting the ovarian ligament. This ligament developed from which embryonic structure?

(A) Mesonephric duct
(B) Urogenital folds
(C) Gubernaculum
(D) Processus vaginalis
(E) Paramesonephric ducts

Questions 54 to 58: Choose the appropriate lettered structure in this magnetic resonance image (see Figure below) of the female perineum and pelvis.

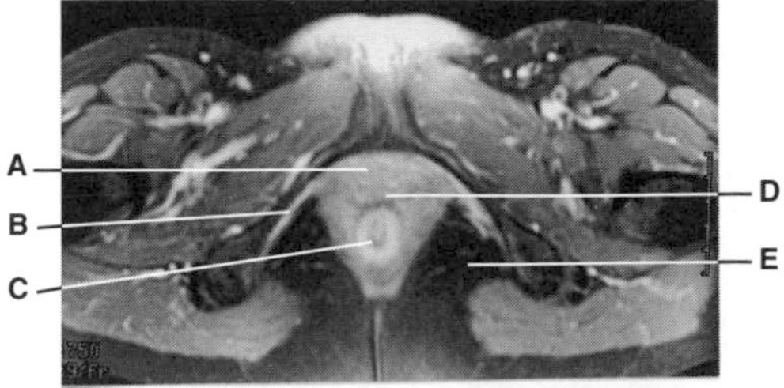

54. Which structure extends between the vestibule and the cervix of the uterus and serves as the excretory channel for the products of menstruation?

55. Which structure in the female is much shorter than the corresponding structure in the male?

56. Into which structure does hemorrhage occur after injury to the inferior rectal vessels?

57. Which structure has a Houston valve or fold, with its venous blood drained by the portal venous system?

58. Which structure is innervated by the nerve passing through both the greater and lesser sciatic foramina?

Questions 59 to 63: Choose the appropriate lettered structure in this computed tomography scan (see Figure below) of the male perineum and pelvis.

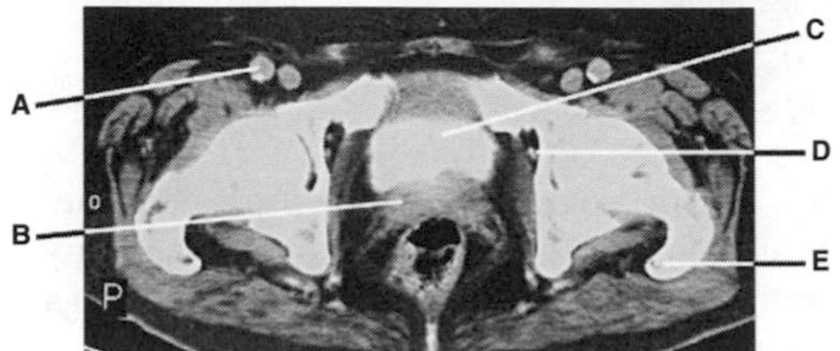

59. Which structure, when fractured, results in paralysis of the obturator internus muscles?

60. Which structure secretes fluid containing fructose, which allows for forensic determination of rape?

61. In which structure would ligation of the external iliac artery reduce blood pressure?

62. A knife wound to the obturator foramen might injure which structure?

63. A stab wound immediately superior to the pubic symphysis on the anterior pelvic wall would most likely injure which visceral organ first?

Answers and Explanations

1. **The answer is E.** The round ligament of the uterus runs laterally from the uterus through the deep inguinal ring, inguinal canal, and superficial inguinal ring and becomes lost in the subcutaneous tissues of the labium majus. Thus, carcinoma of the uterus can spread directly to the labium majus by traveling in lymphatics that follow the ligament.

2. **The answer is B.** A tender swollen left testis may be produced by thrombosis in the left renal vein because the left testicular vein drains into the left renal vein. The right testicular vein drains into the inferior vena cava. The left internal pudendal vein empties into the left internal iliac vein. The left inferior epigastric vein drains into the left external iliac vein, and the left external pudendal vein empties into the femoral vein.

3. **The answer is C.** The superior gluteal nerve leaves the pelvis through the greater sciatic foramen, above the piriformis. The sciatic nerve, internal pudendal vessels, inferior gluteal vessels and nerve, and posterior femoral cutaneous nerve leave the pelvis below the piriformis.

4. **The answer is D.** The round ligament of the uterus is found in the inguinal canal along its course. The other ligaments do not pass through the inguinal canal.

5. **The answer is A.** The pelvic splanchnic nerves carry preganglionic parasympathetic general visceral efferent fibers that synapse in the ganglia of the inferior hypogastric plexus and in terminal ganglia in the muscular walls of the pelvic organs. The sympathetic preganglionic fibers synapse in the sympathetic chain (paravertebral) ganglia or in the collateral (prevertebral) ganglia. The dorsal root ganglia contain cell bodies of general somatic afferent (GSA) and general visceral afferent (GVA) fibers and have no synapsis. The two sympathetic trunks unite and terminate in the ganglion impar (coccygeal ganglion), which is the most inferior, unpaired ganglion located in front of the coccyx.

6. **The answer is D.** The ureter runs under the uterine artery near the cervix; thus, the ureter is sometimes mistakenly ligated during pelvic surgery. The other structures mentioned are not closely related to the uterine artery near the uterine cervix.

7. **The answer is D.** The pelvic diaphragm is formed by the levator ani and coccygeus, whereas the urogenital diaphragm consists of the sphincter urethrae and deep transverse perinei muscles. The piriformis passes through the greater sciatic notch and inserts on the greater trochanter of the femur. The obturator internus forms the lateral wall of the ischiorectal fossa. The sphincter ani externus is composed of three layers, including the subcutaneous (corrugator cutis ani), superficial, and deep portions, and maintains a voluntary tonic contracture.

8. **The answer is C.** The sacral splanchnic nerves consist primarily of preganglionic sympathetic neurons and also contain GVA fibers. None of the other fibers listed are contained in these nerves.

9. **The answer is E.** Fertilization takes place in the infundibulum or ampulla of the uterine tube. The glans clitoris is derived from the corpora cavernosa, whereas the glans penis is the expanded terminal part of the corpus spongiosum. Erection of the penis is caused by parasympathetic stimulation, whereas ejaculation is mediated via the sympathetic nerve. The ovaries are not enclosed in the broad ligament, but their anterior surface is attached to the posterior surface of the broad ligament.

10. **The answer is E.** The superior (deep) boundary of the superficial perineal space is the perineal membrane (inferior fascia of the urogenital diaphragm). Colles fascia is the deep membranous layer of the superficial perineal fascia. The deep perineal fascia essentially divides the superficial perineal space into a superficial and deep compartment. The pelvic diaphragm consists of the levator ani and coccygeus muscles.

11. **The answer is A.** The deep perineal space contains the bulbourethral (Cowper) glands. The crus of the penis, bulb of the vestibule, spongy urethra, and great vestibular gland are found in the superficial perineal space.

12. **The answer is B.** The middle lobe of the prostate gland is commonly involved in benign prostatic hypertrophy, resulting in obstruction of the prostatic urethra, whereas the posterior lobe is commonly involved in carcinomatous transformation. The anterior lobe contains little glandular tissue, and the two lateral lobes on either side of the urethra form the major part of the gland.

13. **The answer is D.** Ducts from the prostate gland open into the prostatic sinus, which is a groove on either side of the urethral crest. The prostate gland receives the ejaculatory duct, which opens into the prostatic urethra on the seminal colliculus (a prominent elevation of the urethral crest) just lateral to the prostatic utricle, which is a small blind pouch. The bulbourethral gland lies on the lateral side of the membranous urethra within the deep perineal space, but its duct opens into the bulbous portion of the spongy (penile) urethra.

14. **The answer is B.** A needle should be inserted through the posterior fornix just below the posterior lip of the cervix while the patient is in the supine position to aspirate abnormal fluid in the cul-de-sac of Douglas (rectouterine pouch). Rectouterine excavation is not most efficiently aspirated by puncture of other structures.

15. **The answer is C.** The superficial inguinal nodes receive lymph from the penis, scrotum, buttocks, labium majus, and the lower parts of the vagina and anal canal. These nodes have efferent vessels that drain primarily into the external iliac and common iliac nodes and ultimately to the lumbar (aortic) nodes. The internal iliac nodes receive lymph from the upper part of the rectum, vagina, uterus, and other pelvic organs, and they drain into the common iliac nodes and then into the lumbar (aortic) nodes. Lymph vessels from the glans penis drain initially into the deep inguinal nodes and then into the external iliac nodes.

16. **The answer is A.** The urogenital diaphragm consists of the sphincter urethrae and deep transverse perineal muscles. Weakness of the muscles, ligaments, and fasciae of the pelvic floor, such as the pelvic diaphragm, urogenital diaphragm, and cardinal (transverse cervical) ligaments, occurs as a result of multiple child delivery, advancing age, and menopause. The pelvic diaphragm is composed of the levator ani and coccygeus muscles. The superficial transversus perinei is one of the superficial perineal muscles, and the obturator internus forms the lateral wall of the ischiorectal fossa.

17. **The answer is B.** The deep dorsal vein, dorsal artery, and dorsal nerve of the penis pass through a gap between the arcuate pubic ligament and the transverse perineal ligament. The perineal nerve divides into a deep branch, which supplies all of the perineal muscles, and superficial branches as posterior scrotal nerves, which supply the scrotum. The superficial dorsal vein of the penis empties into the greater saphenous vein. The deep artery of the penis runs in the corpus cavernosum of the penis.

18. **The answer is C.** The perineal body (central tendon of the perineum) is a fibromuscular node at the center of the perineum. It provides attachment for the bulbospongiosus, the superficial and deep transverse perineal muscles, and the sphincter ani externus muscles. Other muscles (ischiocavernosus, sphincter urethrae, and obturator internus) are not attached to the perineal body.

19. **The answer is A.** The bulb of the penis is located in the superficial perineal space between the inferior fascia of the urogenital diaphragm and the membranous layer of the superficial perineal fascia (Colles fascia). All of the other structures are found in the deep perineal pouch.

20. **The answer is C.** The perineal branch of the pudendal nerve supplies the external urethral sphincter and bulbospongiosus muscles in the male. All other nervous structures do not supply skeletal muscles but supply smooth muscles in the perineal and pelvic organs. The pelvic and prostatic plexuses contain both sympathetic and parasympathetic nerve fibers. The pelvic

splanchnic nerve carries preganglionic parasympathetic fibers, whereas the sacral splanchnic nerve transmits preganglionic sympathetic fibers.

21. **The answer is A.** The normal position of the uterus is anteverted (i.e., angle of 90 degrees at the junction of the vagina and cervical canal) and anteflexed (i.e., angle of 160 to 170 degrees at the junction of the cervix and body).

22. **The answer is B.** The deep dorsal vein of the penis lies medial to the dorsal artery of the penis on the dorsum of the penis and deep to Buck fascia, drains into the prostatic plexus of veins, and is compressed against the underlying deep fascia of the penis during erection.

23. **The answer is E.** The pelvic splanchnic nerve contains preganglionic parasympathetic fibers, whereas the sacral splanchnic nerve contains preganglionic sympathetic fibers. Parasympathetic fibers are responsible for erection, whereas sympathetic fibers are involved with ejaculation. The right and left hypogastric nerves contain primarily sympathetic fibers and visceral sensory fibers. The dorsal nerve of the penis and the perineal nerve provide sensory nerve fibers.

24. **The answer is D.** The lymphatic vessels from the ovary ascend with the ovarian vessels in the suspensory ligament and terminate in the lumbar (aortic) nodes. Lymphatic vessels from the perineum, external genitalia, and lower part of the anterior abdominal wall drain into the superficial inguinal nodes.

25. **The answer is D.** The ischiorectal fossa contains the inferior rectal nerves and vessels and adipose tissue. The bulb of the vestibule and the great vestibular gland are located in the superficial perineal space, whereas the bulbourethral gland is found in the deep perineal space. The internal pudendal artery runs in the pudendal canal, but its branches pass through the superficial and deep perineal spaces.

26. **The answer is A.** The dorsal artery of the penis supplies the glans penis. The seminal vesicles store no spermatozoa. The duct of the bulbourethral gland opens into the bulbous portion of the spongy urethra, whereas the greater vestibular gland opens into the vestibule between the labium minora and the hymen. The anterior lobe of the prostate is devoid of glandular substance, the middle lobe is prone to benign hypertrophy, and the posterior lobe is prone to carcinomatous transformation.

27. **The answer is A.** The pelvic diaphragm, particularly the levator ani, provides the most important support for the uterus, although the urogenital diaphragm and the uterosacral and ovarian ligaments support the uterus. The arcuate pubic ligament arches across the inferior aspect of the pubic symphysis.

28. **The answer is A.** Extravasated urine from the penile urethra below the perineal membrane spreads into the superficial perineal space, scrotum, penis, and anterior abdominal wall. However, it does not spread into the testis, ischiorectal fossa, pelvic cavity, and thigh because Scarpa fascia ends by firm attachment to the fascia lata of the thigh.

29. **The answer is E.** In addition to the uterine cervix, the uterus, uterine tubes, ovaries, and ureters can be palpated. The apex of the urinary bladder is the anterior end of the bladder; thus, it cannot be palpated. The fundus of the uterus is the anterosuperior part of the uterus. The terminal part of the round ligament of the uterus emerges from the superficial inguinal ring and becomes lost in the subcutaneous tissue of the labium majus.

30. **The answer is D.** The uterine tubes lie in the broad ligament. The anterior surface of the ovary is attached to the posterior surface of the broad ligament of the uterus. The ureter descends retroperitoneally on the lateral pelvic wall but is crossed by the uterine artery in the base (in the inferomedial part) of the broad ligament. The terminal part of the round ligament of the uterus becomes lost in the subcutaneous tissue of the labium majus. The suspensory ligament of the ovary is a band of peritoneum that extends superiorly from the ovary to the pelvic wall.

31. **The answer is A.** The prostate gland may be palpated on rectal examination. The ejaculatory duct runs within the prostate gland and cannot be felt. In the male, the pelvic part of the ureter

lies lateral to the ductus deferens and enters the posterosuperior angle of the bladder, where it is situated anterior to the upper end of the seminal vesicle, and thus, it cannot be palpated during rectal examination. However, in the female, the ureter can be palpated during vaginal examination because it runs near the uterine cervix and the lateral fornix of the vagina to enter the posterosuperior angle of the bladder. The testes are examined during a routine annual checkup but obviously not during a rectal examination.

32. The answer is B. Parasympathetic preganglionic fibers in the pelvic splanchnic nerve are responsible for erection of the penis. Sympathetic preganglionic fibers in the sacral splanchnic nerve are responsible for ejaculation. The pudendal nerve supplies the external anal sphincter and perineal muscles and supplies GSA fibers to the perineal region. The dorsal nerve of the penis is a terminal branch of the pudendal nerve and supplies sensation of the penis. The posterior scrotal nerves are superficial branches of the perineal nerve and supply sensory fibers to the scrotum.

33. The answer is A. The pelvic inlet (pelvic brim) is bounded by the promontory and the anterior border of the ala of the sacrum, the arcuate line of the ilium, the pectineal line, the pubic crest, and the superior margin of the pubic symphysis.

34. The answer is B. The iliohypogastric nerve innervates the skin above the pubis. The skin of the urogenital triangle is innervated by the pudendal nerve, perineal branches of the posterior femoral cutaneous nerve, anterior scrotal or labial branches of the ilioinguinal nerve, and the genital branch of the genitofemoral nerve.

35. The answer is D. The sacrospinous ligament forms a boundary of the lesser sciatic foramen. The pubic arcuate ligament, tip of the coccyx, ischial tuberosities, and sacrotuberous ligament all form part of the boundary of the perineum.

36. The answer is A. The scrotum is innervated by branches of the ilioinguinal, genitofemoral, pudendal, and posterior femoral cutaneous nerves. The scrotum receives blood from the posterior scrotal branches of the internal pudendal arteries and the anterior scrotal branches of the external pudendal arteries, but it does not receive blood from the testicular artery. Similarly, the scrotum is drained by the posterior scrotal veins into the internal pudendal vein. The lymph vessels from the scrotum drain into the superficial inguinal nodes, whereas the lymph vessels from the testis drain into the upper lumbar nodes. The dartos tunic is continuous with the membranous layer of the superficial perineal fascia (Colles fascia).

37. The answer is C. The cardinal (transverse cervical) ligament provides the major ligamentous support for the uterus. The sphincter ani externus does not support the uterus. The broad and round ligaments of the uterus provide minor supports for the uterus. The suspensory ligament of the ovary does not support the uterus.

38. The answer is D. An obstetrician should avoid incising the levator ani and the external anal sphincter. The levator ani is the major part of the pelvic diaphragm, which forms the pelvic floor and supports all of the pelvic organs. None of the other choices applies here.

39. The answer is C. Of all the arteries listed, the uterine artery remains within the pelvic cavity.

40. The answer is C. The lumbosacral trunk is formed by part of the ventral ramus of the fourth lumbar nerve and the ventral ramus of the fifth lumbar nerve. This trunk contributes to the formation of the sacral plexus by joining the ventral ramus of the first sacral nerve in the pelvic cavity and does not leave the pelvic cavity. All other nerves leave the abdominal and pelvic cavities.

41. The answer is D. The sphincter urethrae are found in the deep perineal space, whereas the other structures are located in the superficial perineal space.

42. The answer is D. Lymphatic vessels from the testis and epididymis ascend along the testicular vessels in the spermatic cord through the inguinal canal and continue upward in the abdomen to drain into the upper lumbar nodes. The lymph from the other structures drains into the superficial inguinal lymph nodes.

43. **The answer is E.** All of the listed structures do not cross the pelvic brim except the lumbosacral trunk, which arises from L4 and L5, enters the true pelvis by crossing the pelvic brim, and contributes to the formation of the sacral plexus. The deep dorsal vein of the penis enters the pelvic cavity by passing under the symphysis pubis between the arcuate and transverse perineal ligaments.

44. **The answer is B.** The bulbourethral glands lie on either side of the membranous urethra, embedded in the sphincter urethrae. Their ducts open into the bulbous part of the penile urethra. Semen—a thick, yellowish-white, viscous, spermatozoa-containing fluid—is a mixture of the secretions of the testes, seminal vesicles, prostate, and bulbourethral glands. Sperm, or spermatozoa, are produced in the seminiferous tubules of the testis and mature in the head of the epididymis. The seminal vesicles are lobulated glandular structures, produce the alkaline constituent of the seminal fluid that contains fructose and choline, and lie inferior and lateral to the ampullae of the ductus deferens against the fundus (base) of the bladder.

45. **The answer is B.** The sphincter urethra is a striated muscle that lies in the deep perineal space and forms a part of the urogenital diaphragm but not the pelvic diaphragm. It is not enclosed in the pelvic fascia. It is innervated by a deep (muscular) branch of the perineal nerve.

46. **The answer is D.** Cryptorchid testis is called an undescended testis, which is located in the inguinal region. Male pseudohermaphroditism is a condition in which the affected individual is a genetic and gonadal male with genital anomalies. Hypospadias occurs when the spongy urethra opens on the underside of the penis, frequently associated with the chordee, which is a ventral curvature of the penis. Epispadias occurs when the urethra opens on the dorsal surface of the penis.

47. **The answer is D.** The pudendal nerve, which arises from the sacral plexus, provides sensory innervation to the labium majus (or scrotum in a male). It leaves the pelvis through the greater sciatic foramen and enters the perineum through the lesser sciatic foramen near the inferior margin of the ischial spine. Therefore, it can be blocked by injection of an anesthetic near the inferior margin of the ischial spine.

48. **The answer is B.** The ischiorectal fossa is bounded posteriorly by the gluteus maximus and the sacrotuberous ligament. It contains fat, the inferior rectal nerve and vessels, and perineal branches of the posterior femoral cutaneous nerve. The pudendal canal runs along its lateral wall. Urine leaking from a ruptured bulb of the penis does not spread into the ischiorectal fossa because Scarpa fascia ends by firm attachment to the fascia lata of the thigh.

49. **The answer is D.** The ejaculatory ducts, which open onto the seminal colliculus, may be injured. The prostate ducts open into the urethral sinus, the bulbourethral ducts open into the bulbous part of the penile urethra, and the ducts of the seminal vesicle join the ampulla of the ductus deferens to form the ejaculatory duct. The prostatic utricle is a minute pouch on the summit of the seminal colliculus.

50. **The answer is D.** The pectinate line is a point of demarcation between visceral and somatic portions of the anal canal. Characteristics above the pectinate line include columnar epithelium, venous drainage into the portal system, lymphatic drainage into the internal iliac nodes, visceral sensory innervation, and internal hemorrhoids.

51. **The answer is C.** A developmental defect in the spongy urethra results in epispadias, causing the patient to pass urine through an opening on the dorsum of the penis. Labioscrotal swellings form the scrotum in males and the labia majora in females. Urogenital sinus forms the urinary bladder, urethra, prostate, and bulbourethral glands in males, and the bladder, urethra, lower vagina, and greater vestibular glands in females. The phallus (genital tubercle) forms the penis in males and the clitoris in females. Urethral (urogenital) folds form the spongy urethra and a portion of the shaft of the penis in males and the labia minora in females.

52. **The answer is C.** Cancer cells from rectal cancer are likely to metastasize to the liver via the superior rectal, inferior mesenteric, splenic, and portal veins. Cancer cells are not directly spread to the other organs listed. The spleen and duodenum drain their venous blood to the

portal venous system, and the kidney and suprarenal gland empty into the caval (inferior vena cava) system.

53. The answer is C. The ovarian ligament and the round ligament of the uterus are formed by the gubernaculum. The mesonephric duct gives rise only to the vestigial epoophoron in the female. The urogenital folds form the labia minora. The processus vaginalis forms no adult female structures, while the paramesonephric ducts form the uterine tubes, uterus, cervix, and upper vagina.

54. The answer is D. The vagina is the genital canal in the female, extending from the vestibule to the uterine cervix. The vagina transmits the products of menstruation and receives the penis in copulation.

55. The answer is A. In females, the urethra extends from the bladder, runs above the anterior vaginal wall, and pierces the urogenital diaphragm to reach the urethral orifice in the vestibule behind the clitoris. It is approximately 4 cm long. In males, the urethra is approximately 20 cm long.

56. The answer is E. The ischiorectal fossa lies in the anal triangle and is bound laterally by the obturator internus with its fascia and superomedially by the levator ani and external anal sphincter. It contains the inferior rectal vessels. Thus, hemorrhage occurs in the ischiorectal fossa when it is ruptured.

57. The answer is C. The mucous membrane and the circular smooth-muscle layer of the rectum form three transverse folds; the middle one is called Houston valve. The venous blood returns to the portal venous system via the superior rectal vein.

58. The answer is B. The obturator internus muscle and its fascia form the lateral wall of the ischiorectal fossa. This muscle is innervated by the nerve to the obturator internus, which passes through the greater and lesser sciatic foramen.

59. The answer is E. The greater trochanter provides an insertion site for the obturator internus muscle.

60. The answer is B. The seminal vesicle is a lobulated glandular structure and produces the alkaline constituent of the seminal fluid, which contains fructose and choline. Fructose, which is nutritive to spermatozoa, also allows forensic determination of rape, whereas choline crystals are the preferred basis for the determination of the presence of semen.

61. The answer is A. The external iliac artery becomes the femoral artery immediately after passing the inguinal ligament. Therefore, ligation of the external iliac artery reduces blood pressure in the femoral artery.

62. The answer is D. The obturator foramen transmits the obturator nerve and vessels. Therefore, the knife wound in this foramen injures the obturator nerve and vessels.

63. The answer is C. The bladder is situated in the anterior part of the pelvic cavity. Thus, a stab wound superior to the pubic symphysis would injure the bladder.

chapter 6

Lower Limb

BONES OF THE LOWER LIMB

I. HIP (COXAL) BONE (Figures 6.1 to 6.2)

- Is formed by the fusion of the **ilium, pubis**, and **ischium** in the acetabulum.
- Articulates with the sacrum at the sacroiliac joint to form the **pelvic girdle**.

A. Ilium

- Forms the lateral part of the hip bone and consists of the **body**, which joins the pubis and ischium to form the acetabulum, and the **ala** or wing, which forms the iliac crest.
- Comprises also the anterior–superior iliac spine, anterior–inferior iliac spine, posterior iliac spine, **greater sciatic notch, iliac fossa**, and gluteal lines.

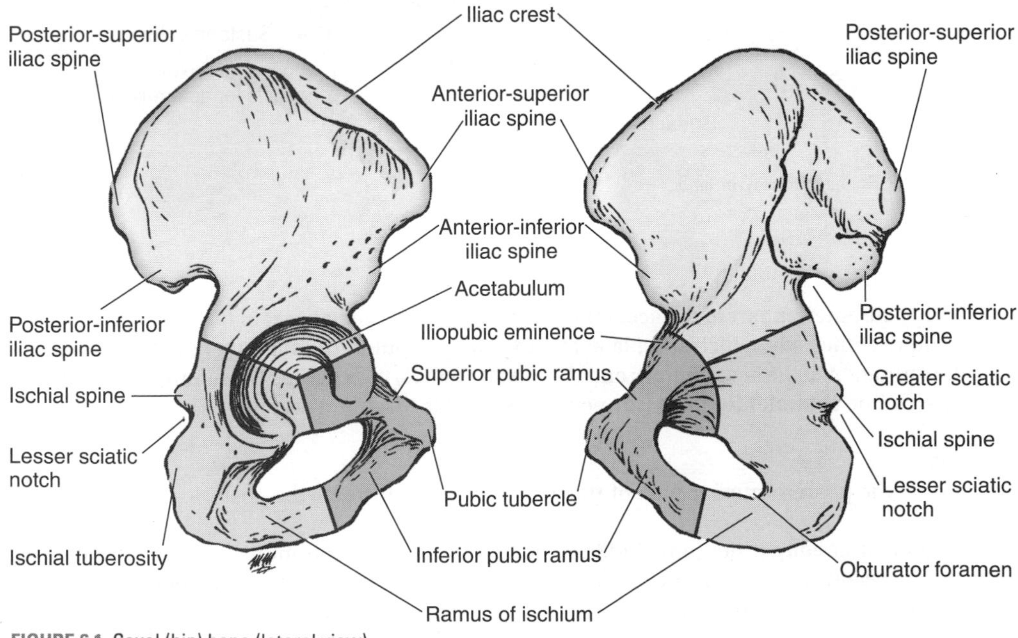

FIGURE 6.1. Coxal (hip) bone (lateral view).

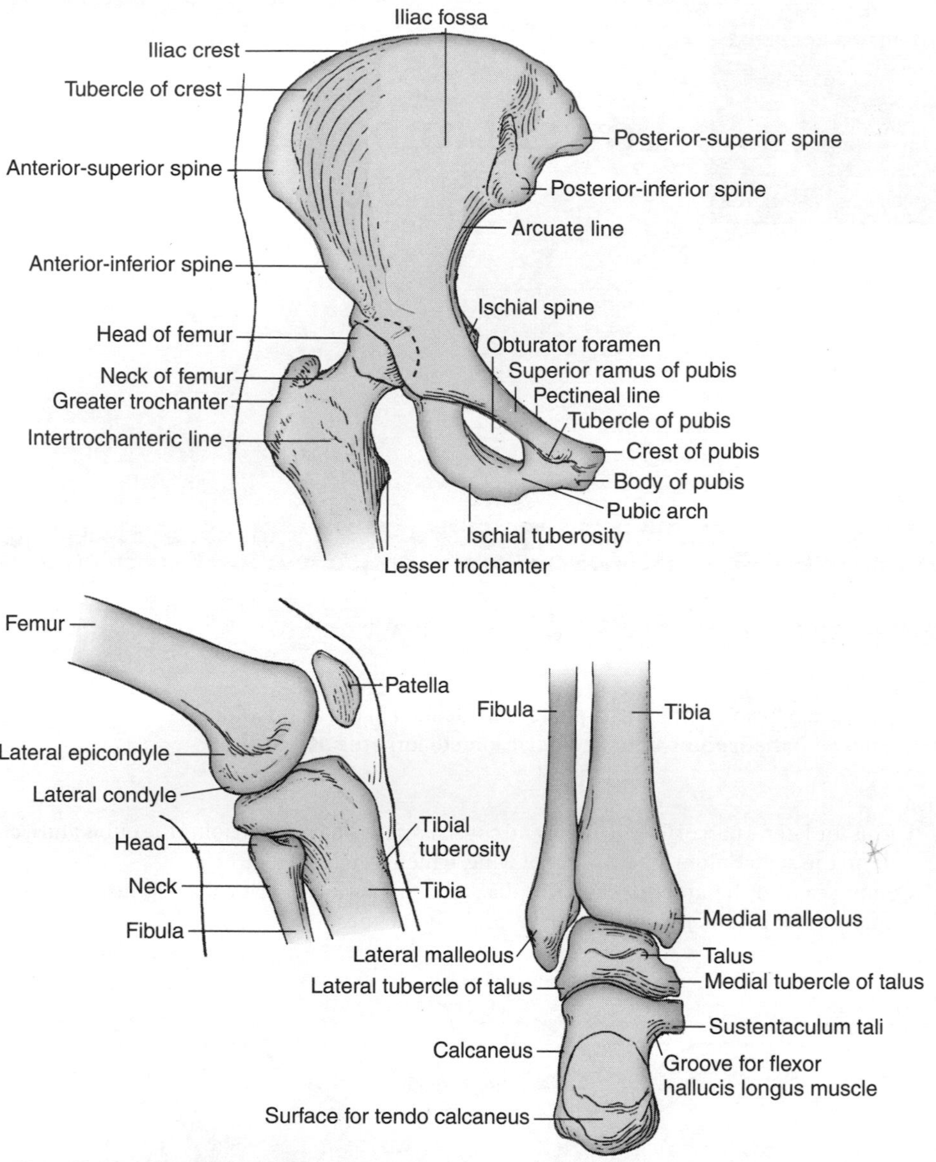

FIGURE 6.2. Bones of the lower limb.

B. Pubis

- Forms the anterior part of the acetabulum and the anteromedial part of the hip bone.
- Comprises the **body**, which articulates at the symphysis pubis; the **superior ramus**, which enters the formation of the acetabulum; and the **inferior ramus**, which joins the ramus of the ischium, a part of the **obturator foramen** (formed by fusion of the ischium and pubis).

C. Ischium

- Forms the posteroinferior part of the acetabulum and the lower posterior part of the hip bone.
- Consists of the **body**, which joins the ilium and superior ramus of the pubis to form the acetabulum, and the **ramus**, which joins the inferior pubic ramus to form the **ischiopubic ramus**.
- Has the ischial spine, ischial tuberosity, and lesser sciatic notch.

D. Acetabulum

- Is an incomplete cup-shaped cavity on the lateral side of the hip bone in which the head of the femur fits.
- Includes the **acetabular notch**, which is bridged by the transverse acetabular ligament.
- Is formed by the **ilium** superiorly, the **ischium** posteroinferiorly, and the **pubis** anteromedially.

II. BONES OF THE THIGH AND LEG (Figures 6.2 to 6.3)

A. Femur

- Is the longest and strongest bone of the body.

1. Head

- Forms about two-thirds of a sphere and is directed medially, upward, and slightly forward to fit into the acetabulum.
- Has a depression in its articular surface, the **fovea capitis femoris**, to which the ligamentum capitis femoris is attached.

CLINICAL CORRELATES

Fracture of the femoral head is a rare injury caused by posterior hip dislocation in advanced age (osteoporosis) and requires hip replacement. It presents as a **shortened lower limb with medial rotation**.

Fracture of the neck of the femur results in ischemic necrosis of the neck and head because of an interruption of blood supply from the root of the femoral neck to the femoral head by the medial femoral circumflex artery, except for its small proximal part. It causes a pull of the distal fragment upward by the quadriceps femoris, adductors, and hamstring muscles so that the affected **lower limb is shortened with lateral rotation.**

Pertrochanteric fracture is a femoral fracture through the trochanters and is a form of the extracapsular hip fracture. The pull of the quadriceps femoris, adductors, and hamstring muscles may produce shortening and lateral rotation of the leg. It is common in elderly women because of an increased incidence of osteoporosis. In **fracture of the middle third of the femoral shaft**, the proximal fragment is pulled by the quadriceps and the hamstrings, resulting in shortening, and the distal fragment is rotated backward by the two heads of the gastrocnemius.

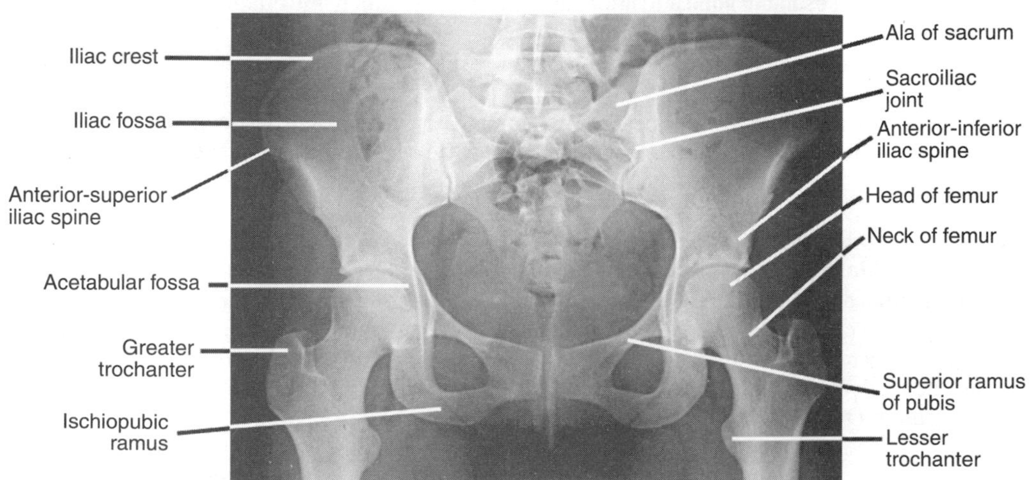

FIGURE 6.3. Radiograph of the hip, thigh, and pelvis.

2. **Neck**
   - Connects the head to the body (shaft), forms an angle of about 125 degrees with the shaft, and is a **common site of fractures**.
   - Is separated from the shaft in front by the **intertrochanteric line**, to which the iliofemoral ligament is attached.
3. **Greater Trochanter**
   - Projects upward from the junction of the neck with the shaft.
   - Provides an insertion for the gluteus medius and minimus, piriformis, and obturator internus muscles.
   - Receives the obturator externus tendon on the medial aspect of the **trochanteric fossa**.
4. **Lesser Trochanter**
   - Lies in the angle between the neck and the shaft.
   - Projects at the inferior end of the **intertrochanteric crest**.
   - Provides an insertion for the iliopsoas tendon.
5. **Linea Aspera**
   - Is the rough line or ridge on the body (shaft) of the femur.
   - Exhibits lateral and medial lips that provide attachments for many muscles and the three intermuscular septa.
6. **Pectineal Line**
   - Runs from the lesser trochanter to the medial lip of the linea aspera.
   - Provides an insertion for the pectineus muscle.
7. **Adductor Tubercle**
   - Is a small prominence at the uppermost part of the medial femoral condyle.
   - Provides an insertion for the adductor magnus muscle.

CLINICAL CORRELATES

A dislocated knee or fractured distal femur may injure the popliteal artery because of its deep position adjacent to the femur and the knee joint capsule.

Transverse patellar fracture results from a blow to the knee or from sudden contraction of the quadriceps muscle. The proximal fragment of the patella is pulled superiorly with the quadriceps tendon, and the distal fragment remains with the patellar ligament.

Bumper fracture is a fracture of the lateral tibial condyle that is caused by an automobile bumper, and it is usually associated with a common peroneal nerve injury.

B. Patella

- Is the **largest sesamoid bone** and is located within the tendon of the quadriceps femoris, which articulates with the femur but not with the tibia.
- Attaches to the tibial tuberosity by a continuation of the quadriceps tendon called the **patellar ligament**.
- Functions to **obviate wear** and attrition on the quadriceps tendon as it passes across the trochlear groove and to increase the angle of pull of the quadriceps femoris, thereby **magnifying its power**.

C. Tibia

- Is the weight-bearing medial bone of the leg.
- Has the **tibial tuberosity** into which the patellar ligament inserts.
- Has medial and lateral condyles that articulate with the condyles of the femur.
- Has a projection called the **medial malleolus** with a **malleolar groove** for the tendons of the tibialis posterior and flexor digitorum longus muscles and another **groove** (posterolateral to the malleolus groove) for the tendon of the flexor hallucis longus muscle. It also provides attachment for the deltoid ligament.

D. Fibula

- Has little or no function in weight-bearing but provides attachment for muscles.
- Has a **head** (apex) that provides attachment for the fibular collateral ligament of the knee joint.

- Has a projection called the **lateral malleolus** that articulates with the trochlea of the talus; lies more inferior and posterior than the medial malleolus; and provides attachment for the anterior talofibular, posterior talofibular, and calcaneofibular ligaments. It also has the **sulcus** for the peroneus longus and brevis muscle tendons.

CLINICAL CORRELATES

Pott fracture (Dupuytren fracture) is a fracture of the lower end of the fibula, often accompanied by a fracture of the medial malleolus or rupture of the deltoid ligament. It is caused by forced eversion of the foot.

Pillion fracture is a T-shaped fracture of the distal femur with displacement of the condyles. It may be caused by a blow to the flexed knee of a person riding pillion on a motorcycle.

Fracture of the fibular neck may cause an injury to the common peroneal nerve, which winds laterally around the neck of the fibula. This injury results in paralysis of all muscles in the anterior and lateral compartments of the leg (dorsiflexors and evertors of the foot), causing foot drop.

III. BONES OF THE ANKLE AND FOOT (Figures 6.2, 6.4, 6.5, and 6.6)

A. Tarsus

- Consists of seven tarsal bones: **talus, calcaneus, navicular bone, cuboid bone**, and **three cuneiform bones.**

1. Talus

- Transmits the weight of the body from the tibia to the foot and is the only tarsal bone without muscle attachments.
- Has a **neck** with a deep groove, the **sulcus tali**, for the **interosseous ligaments** between the talus and the calcaneus.
- Has a **body** with a **groove** on its posterior surface for the **flexor hallucis longus tendon.**
- Has a **head**, which serves as **keystone** of the **medial longitudinal arch** of the foot.

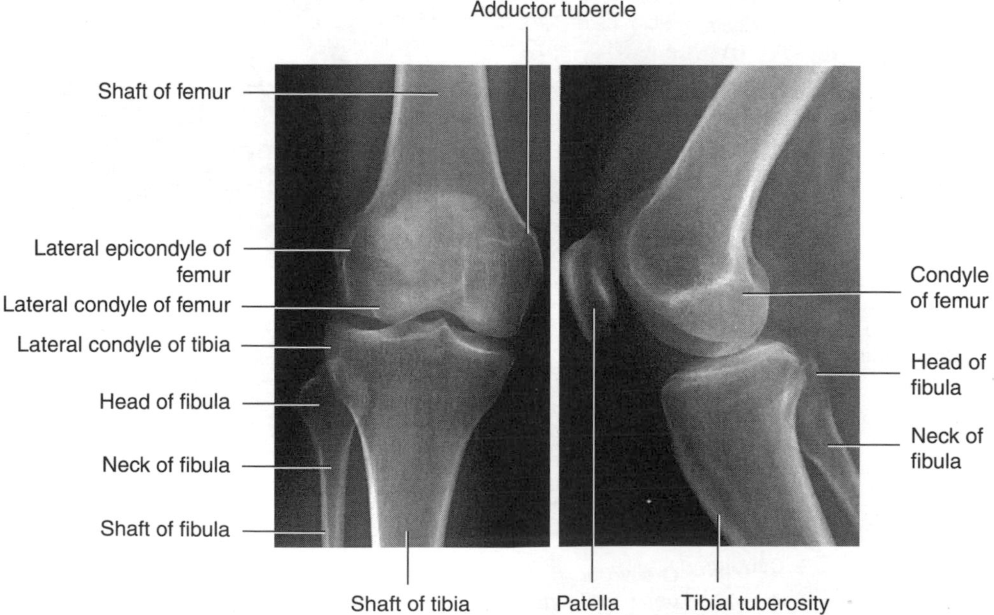

FIGURE 6.4. Anteroposterior and lateral radiographs of the knee.

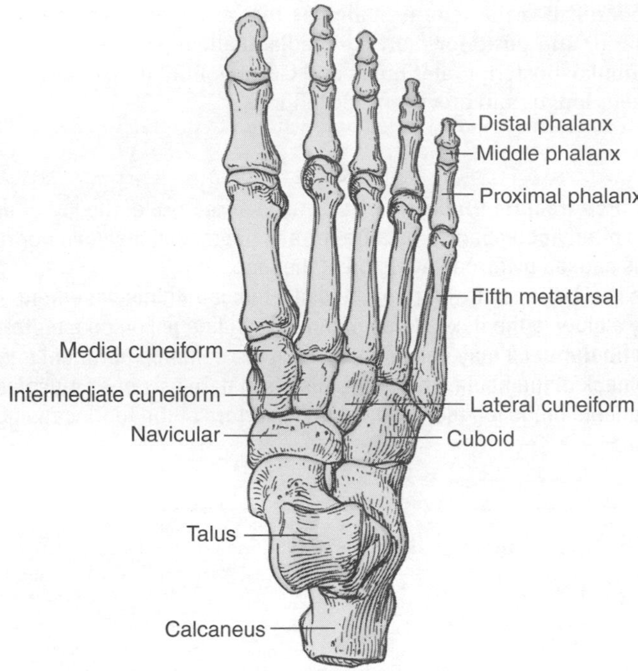

FIGURE 6.5. Bones of the foot.

2. Calcaneus

- Is the largest and strongest bone of the foot and lies below the talus.
- Forms the **heel** of the foot, articulates with the talus superiorly and the cuboid anteriorly, and provides an attachment for the Achilles tendon.
- Has a shelflike medial projection called the **sustentaculum tali**, which **supports** the **head** of the **talus** (with the spring ligament) and has a **groove** on its inferior surface for the **flexor hallucis longus tendon** (which uses the sustentaculum tali as a pulley).

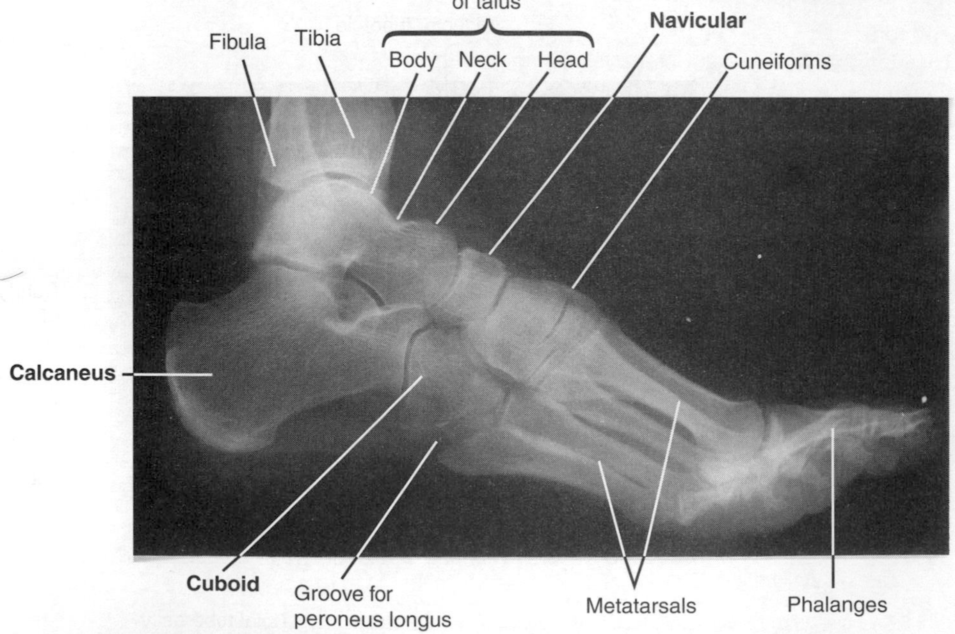

FIGURE 6.6. Radiograph of the ankle and foot.

3. Navicular Bone

- Is a boat-shaped tarsal bone lying between the head of the talus and the three cuneiform bones.

4. Cuboid Bone

- Is the most laterally placed tarsal bone and has a **groove** for the **peroneus longus muscle tendon**.
- Serves as the **keystone** of the **lateral longitudinal arch** of the foot.

5. Cuneiform Bones

- Are three wedge-shaped bones that form a part of the medial longitudinal and proximal transverse arches.
- Articulate with the navicular bone posteriorly and with three metatarsals anteriorly.

B. Metatarsus

- Consists of **five metatarsals** and has prominent medial and lateral sesamoid bones on the first metatarsal.

CLINICAL CORRELATES

March fracture (stress fracture) is a fatigue fracture of one of the metatarsals, which may result from prolonged walking. Metatarsal fractures are also common in female ballet dancers when the dancers lose balance and put their full body weight on the metatarsals.

C. Phalanges

- Consists of 14 bones (two in the first digit and three in each of the others).

JOINTS AND LIGAMENTS OF THE LOWER LIMB

I. HIP (COXAL) JOINT (Figures 6.2, 6.3, and 6.7)

- Is a **multiaxial ball-and-socket synovial joint** between the acetabulum of the hip bone and the head of the femur and allows abduction and adduction, flexion and extension, and circumduction and rotation.
- Is stabilized by the acetabular labrum; the fibrous capsule; and capsular ligaments such as the iliofemoral, ischiofemoral, and pubofemoral ligaments.
- Has a cavity that is deepened by the fibrocartilaginous **acetabular labrum** and is completed below by the **transverse acetabular ligament**, which bridges and converts the **acetabular notch** into a foramen for passage of **nutrient vessels** and nerves.

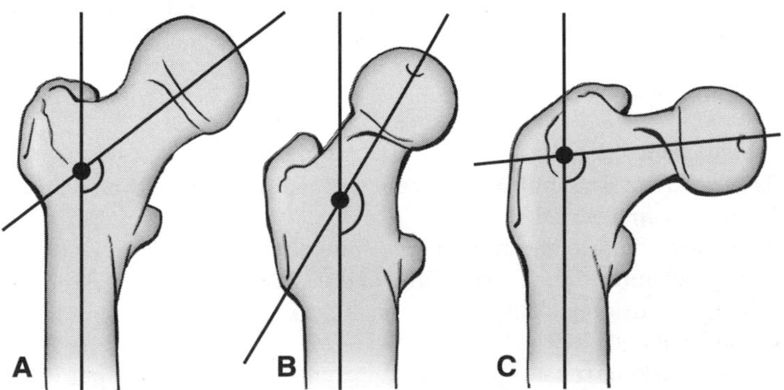

FIGURE 6.7. Angles of the hip joint. **A:** Normal. **B:** Coxa valga (abnormally increased angle of inclination). C: Coxa vara (abnormally decreased angle of inclination).

CLINICAL CORRELATES

Coxa valga is an alteration of the angle made by the axis of the femoral neck to the axis of the femoral shaft so that the angle exceeds 135 degrees and, thus, the femoral neck becomes straighter.

Coxa vara is an alteration of the angle made by the axis of the femoral neck to the axis of the femoral shaft so that the angle is less than 135 degrees and, thus, the femoral neck becomes more horizontal.

- Receives blood from branches of the medial and lateral femoral circumflex, superior and inferior gluteal, and obturator arteries. The posterior branch of the obturator artery gives rise to the artery of the ligamentum teres capitis femoris.
- Is innervated by branches of the femoral, obturator, sciatic and superior gluteal nerves, and by the nerve to the quadratus femoris.

A. Fibrous and Cartilaginous Structures

1. Acetabular Labrum (Figure 6.8)

- Is a complete fibrocartilage rim that deepens the articular socket for the head of the femur and consequently stabilizes the hip joint.

2. Fibrous Capsule

- Is attached proximally to the margin of the acetabulum and to the transverse acetabular ligament.
- Is attached distally to the neck of the femur as follows: anteriorly to the intertrochanteric line and the root of the greater trochanter, and posteriorly to the intertrochanteric crest.
- Encloses part of the head and most of the neck of the femur.
- Is reinforced anteriorly by the **iliofemoral** ligament, posteriorly by the **ischiofemoral** ligament, and inferiorly by the **pubofemoral** ligament.

CLINICAL CORRELATES

Posterior dislocation of the hip joint occurs through a posterior tearing of the joint capsule, accounts for approximately 90% of hip dislocations, and the **fractured femoral head** lies posterior to the acetabulum or the ischium, as occurs in a head-on collision. It results in a probable rupture of both the posterior acetabular labrum and the ligamentum capitis femoris and usually in the injury of the sciatic nerve. It results in the **affected lower limb** being **shortened, flexed, adducted, and medially rotated.**

Anterior dislocation of the hip joint is characterized by the tearing of the joint capsule anteriorly with movement of the femoral head out from the acetabulum; the femoral head is displaced anteroinferior to the acetabulum or the pubic bone. The **affected limb** is slightly flexed, **abducted**, and **laterally rotated.**

Medial (central or intrapelvic) dislocation of the hip joint occurs through a medial tearing of the joint capsule, and the dislocated femoral head lies medial to the pubic bone. This may be accompanied by acetabular fracture and rupture of the bladder.

B. Ligaments

1. Iliofemoral Ligament

- Is the largest and most important ligament that reinforces the fibrous capsule anteriorly and is in the form of an inverted **Y**.
- Is attached proximally to the anterior–inferior iliac spine and the acetabular rim and distally to the intertrochanteric line and the front of the greater trochanter of the femur.
- Resists hyperextension and lateral rotation at the hip joint during standing.

2. Ischiofemoral Ligament

- Reinforces the fibrous capsule posteriorly, extends from the ischial portion of the **acetabular rim** to the neck of the femur medial to the base of the greater trochanter, and limits extension and medial rotation of the thigh.

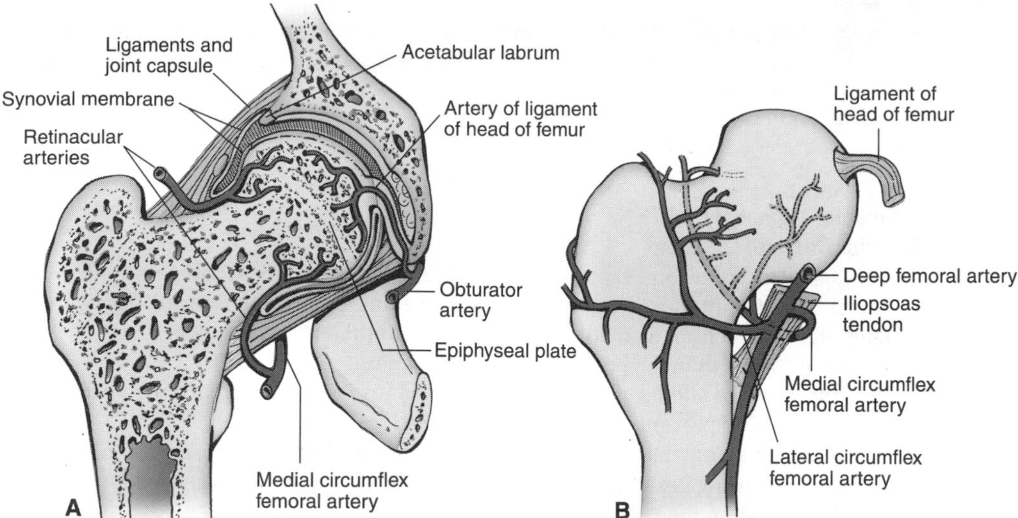

FIGURE 6.8. Blood supply of the head and neck of the femur. **A:** Coronal section. **B:** Anterior view.

3. **Pubofemoral Ligament**
   - Reinforces the fibrous capsule inferiorly, extends from the pubic portion of the acetabular rim and the superior pubic ramus to the lower part of the femoral neck, and limits extension and abduction.
4. **Ligamentum Teres Capitis Femoris (Round Ligament of Head of Femur)**
   - Arises from the floor of the acetabular fossa (more specifically, from the margins of the acetabular notch and from the transverse acetabular ligament) and attaches to the **fovea capitis femoris.**
   - Provides a pathway for the artery of the ligamentum capitis femoris (foveolar artery) from the obturator artery, which is of variable size but represents a significant portion of the blood supply to the femoral head during childhood.
5. **Transverse Acetabular Ligament**
   - Is a fibrous band that bridges the acetabular notch and converts it into a foramen, through which the nutrient vessels enter the joint.

II. KNEE JOINT (Figures 6.9 to 6.10; see also Figure 6.2)

- Is the largest and most complicated joint. Although structurally it resembles a hinge joint, it is a **condylar type of synovial joint** between two condyles of the femur and tibia. In addition, it includes a **saddle joint** between the femur and the patella.
- Is encompassed by a **fibrous capsule** that is rather thin, weak, and incomplete, but it is attached to the margins of the femoral and tibial condyles and to the patella and patellar ligament and surrounds the lateral and posterior aspects of the joint.
- Permits flexion, extension, and some gliding and rotation in the flexed position of the knee; full extension is accompanied by medial rotation of the femur on the tibia, pulling all ligaments taut.
- Is stabilized laterally by the biceps and gastrocnemius (lateral head) tendons, the **iliotibial tract**, and the fibular collateral ligaments.
- Is stabilized medially by the sartorius, gracilis, gastrocnemius (medial head), semitendinosus, and semimembranosus muscles and the tibial collateral ligament.
- Receives blood from the genicular branches (superior medial and lateral, inferior medial and lateral, and middle) of the popliteal artery, a descending branch of the lateral femoral circumflex artery, an articular branch of the descending genicular artery, and the anterior tibial recurrent artery.
- Is innervated by branches of the sciatic, femoral, and obturator nerves.
- Is supported by various ligaments and menisci.

CLINICAL CORRELATES **Hemarthrosis (blood in a joint)** usually causes a rapid swelling of the injured knee joint, whereas inflammatory joint effusion causes a slow swelling of the knee joint.

A. **Ligaments**

1. **Intracapsular Ligaments**

a. **Anterior Cruciate Ligament**

- Lies inside the knee joint capsule but outside the synovial cavity of the joint.
- Arises from the anterior intercondylar area of the tibia and passes upward, backward, and laterally to insert into the medial surface of the **lateral femoral condyle.**
- Is slightly longer than the posterior cruciate ligament.
- **Prevents forward sliding of the tibia on the femur** (or posterior displacement of the femur on the tibia) and prevents hyperextension of the knee joint.
- Is **taut during extension** of the knee and is **lax during flexion**. (The small, more anterior band is taut during flexion.)
- May be torn when the knee is hyperextended.

b. **Posterior Cruciate Ligament**

- Lies outside the synovial cavity but within the fibrous joint capsule.
- Arises from the posterior intercondylar area of the tibia and passes upward, forward, and medially to insert into the lateral surface of the **medial femoral condyle.**
- Is **shorter**, straighter, and **stronger** than the anterior cruciate ligament.
- **Prevents backward sliding of the tibia on the femur** (or anterior displacement of the femur on the tibia) and limits hyperflexion of the knee.
- Is **taut during flexion** of the knee and is **lax during extension**. (The small posterior band is lax during flexion and taut during extension.)

CLINICAL CORRELATES **Drawer sign: anterior drawer sign** is a forward sliding of the tibia on the femur due to a rupture of the **anterior cruciate ligament**, whereas posterior drawer sign is a backward sliding of the tibia on the femur caused by a rupture of the posterior cruciate ligament.

The medial meniscus is more frequently torn in injuries than the lateral meniscus because of its strong attachment to the tibial collateral ligament.

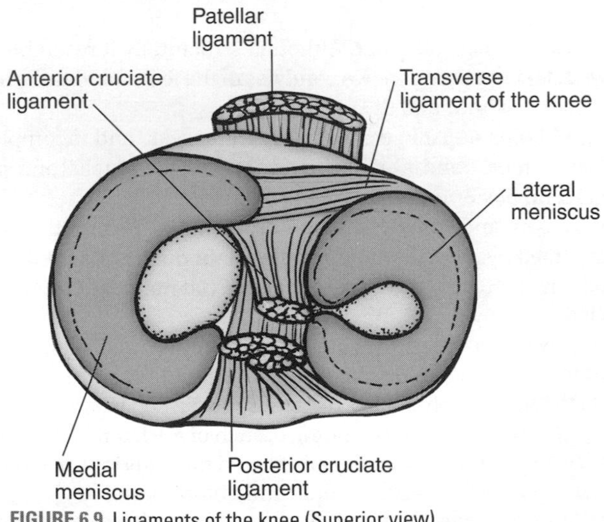

FIGURE 6.9. Ligaments of the knee (Superior view).

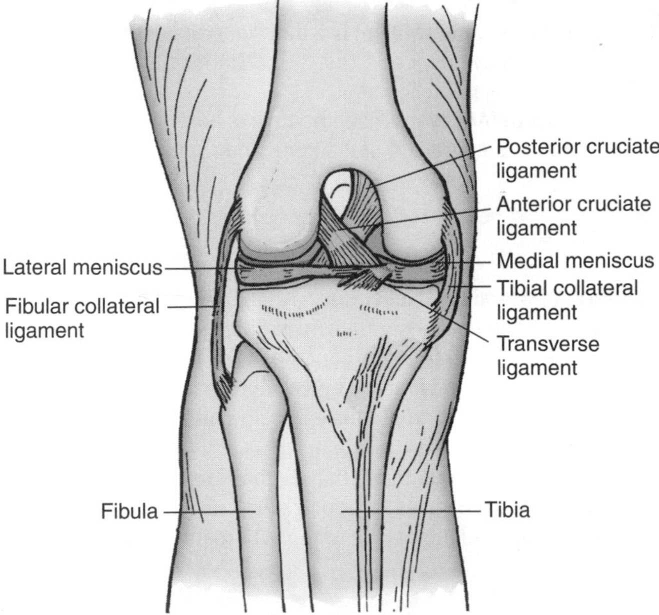

FIGURE 6.10. Ligaments of the knee joint (anterior view).

c. Medial Meniscus

- Lies outside the synovial cavity but within the joint capsule.
- Is **C-shaped** (i.e., forms a semicircle) and is attached to the medial collateral ligament and interarticular area of the tibia.
- Acts as a cushion or shock absorber and lubricates the articular surfaces by distributing synovial fluid in a windshield-wiper manner.

CLINICAL CORRELATES **Unhappy triad or O'Donoghue triad of the knee joint** may occur when a football player's cleated shoe is planted firmly in the turf and the knee is struck from the lateral side. It is indicated by a markedly swollen knee and results in tenderness on application of pressure along the tibial collateral ligament. It is characterized by the (a) rupture of the **tibial collateral ligament**, as a result of excessive abduction; (b) tearing of the **anterior cruciate ligament**, as a result of forward displacement of the tibia; and (c) injury to the **medial meniscus**, as a result of the tibial collateral ligament attachment. However, lateral meniscus injuries are commonly seen among athletes.

d. Lateral Meniscus

- Lies outside the synovial cavity but within the joint capsule.
- Is nearly **circular**, acts as a cushion, and facilitates lubrication.
- Is separated laterally from the fibular (or lateral) collateral ligament by the tendon of the popliteal muscle and aids in forming a more stable base for the articulation of the femoral condyle.

e. Transverse Ligament

- Binds the anterior horns (ends) of the lateral and medial semilunar cartilages (menisci).

2. Extracapsular Ligaments

a. Medial (Tibial) Collateral Ligament

- Is a broad band that extends from the medial femoral epicondyle to the medial tibial condyle.
- Is **firmly attached to the medial meniscus**, and its attachment is of clinical significance because injury to the ligament results in concomitant damage to the medial meniscus.
- **Prevents** medial displacement of the two long bones and thus **abduction** of the leg at the knee.
- Becomes **taut on extension** and thus limits extension and abduction of the leg.

CLINICAL CORRELATES **Knock-knee (genu valgum)** is a deformity in which the tibia is bent or twisted laterally. It may occur as a result of collapse of the lateral compartment of the knee and rupture of the medial collateral ligament.

Bowleg (genu varum) is a deformity in which the tibia is bent medially. It may occur as a result of collapse of the medial compartment of the knee and rupture of the lateral collateral ligament.

b. Lateral (Fibular) Collateral Ligament

- Is a rounded cord that is separated from the lateral meniscus by the tendon of the popliteus muscle and also from the capsule of the joint.
- Extends between the lateral femoral epicondyle and the head of the fibula.
- Becomes **taut on extension** and **limits** extension and **adduction** of the leg.

c. Patellar Ligament (Tendon)

- Is a strong flattened fibrous band that is the continuation of the **quadriceps femoris tendon**. Its portion may be used for repair of the anterior cruciate ligament.
- Extends from the apex of the patella to the tuberosity of the tibia.

CLINICAL CORRELATES **Patellar tendon reflex:** a tap on the patellar tendon elicits extension of the knee joint. Both afferent and efferent limbs of the reflex arc are in the femoral nerve (L2–L4).

A portion of the **patella ligament** may be used for surgical repair of the anterior cruciate ligament of the knee joint. The tendon of the plantaris muscle may be used for tendon autografts to the long flexors of the fingers.

d. Arcuate Popliteal Ligament

- Arises from the head of the fibula, arches superiorly and medially over the tendon of the popliteus muscle on the back of the knee joint, and fuses with the articular capsule.

e. Oblique Popliteal Ligament

- Is an oblique expansion of the **semimembranosus tendon** and passes upward obliquely across the posterior surface of the knee joint from the medial condyle of the tibia.
- Resists hyperextension of the leg and lateral rotation during the final phase of extension.

f. Popliteus Tendon

- Arises as a strong cordlike tendon from the lateral aspect of the lateral femoral condyle and runs between the lateral meniscus and the capsule of the knee joint deep to the fibular collateral ligament.

B. Bursae

1. Suprapatellar Bursa

- Lies deep to the quadriceps femoris muscle and is the major bursa communicating with the knee joint cavity (the semimembranosus bursa also may communicate with it).

2. Prepatellar Bursa

- Lies over the superficial surface of the patella.

3. Infrapatellar Bursa

- Consists of a **subcutaneous infrapatellar bursa** over the patellar ligament and a **deep infrapatellar bursa** deep to the patellar ligament.

4. Anserine Bursa (Known as the Pes Anserinus [Goose Foot])

- Lies between the tibial collateral ligament and the tendons of the sartorius, gracilis, and semitendinosus muscles.

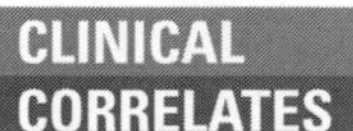

Prepatellar bursitis (housemaid knee) is inflammation and swelling of the prepatellar bursa.

Infrapatellar (superficial) **bursitis** (clergyman knee) is inflammation of the infrapatellar bursa located between the patellar ligament and the skin (the deep bursa lies between the patellar ligament and the tibia).

Popliteal (Baker) cyst is a swelling behind the knee, caused by knee arthritis, meniscus injury, or herniation or tear of the joint capsule. It impairs flexion and extension of the knee joint, and the pain gets worse when the knee is fully extended, such as during prolonged standing or walking. It can be treated by draining and decompressing the cyst.

III. TIBIOFIBULAR JOINTS

A. Proximal Tibiofibular Joint

- Is a plane-type synovial joint between the head of the fibula and the tibia that allows a little gliding movement.

B. Distal Tibiofibular Joint

- Is a fibrous joint between the tibia and the fibula.

IV. ANKLE (TALOCRURAL) JOINT (Figures 6.2 and 6.11)

- Is a **hinge-type (ginglymus) synovial joint** between the tibia and fibula superiorly and the trochlea of the talus inferiorly, permitting dorsiflexion and plantar flexion.

A. Articular Capsule

- Is a thin fibrous capsule that lies both anteriorly and posteriorly, allowing movement.
- Is reinforced medially by the medial (or deltoid) ligament and laterally by the lateral ligament, which prevents anterior and posterior slipping of the tibia and fibula on the talus.

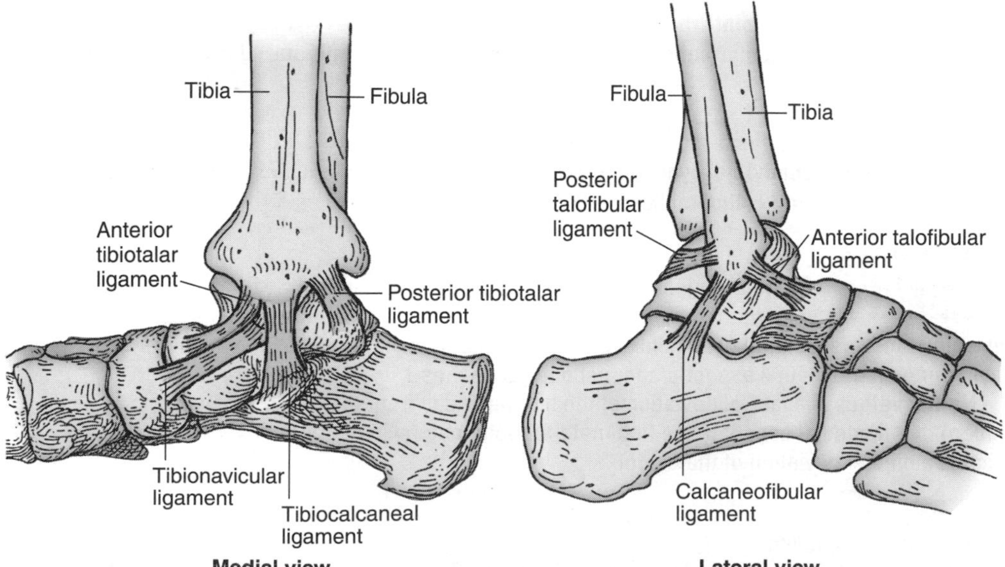

FIGURE 6.11. Ligaments of the ankle joint.

B. Ligaments

1. Medial (Deltoid) Ligament

- Has four parts: the tibionavicular, tibiocalcaneal, anterior tibiotalar, and posterior tibiotalar ligaments.
- Extends from the medial malleolus to the navicular bone, calcaneus, and talus.
- Prevents overeversion of the foot and helps maintain the medial longitudinal arch.

2. Lateral Ligament

- Consists of the anterior talofibular, posterior talofibular, and calcaneofibular (cordlike) ligaments.
- Resists inversion of the foot and may be torn during an **ankle sprain** (inversion injury).

V. TARSAL JOINTS

A. Intertarsal Joints

1. Talocalcaneal (Subtalar) Joint

- Is a plane synovial joint (part of the talocalcaneonavicular joint), and is formed between the talus and calcaneus bones.
- Allows inversion and eversion of the foot.

2. Talocalcaneonavicular Joint

- Is a ball-and-socket joint (part of the transverse tarsal joint), and is formed between the head of the talus (ball) and the calcaneus and navicular bones (socket).
- Is supported by the **spring** (plantar calcaneonavicular) ligament.

3. Calcaneocuboid Joint

- Is part of the transverse tarsal joint and resembles a saddle joint between the calcaneus and the cuboid bones.
- Is supported by the **short plantar** (plantar calcaneocuboid) and **long plantar** ligaments and by the tendon of the peroneus longus muscle.

4. Transverse Tarsal (Midtarsal) Joint

- Is a collective term for the **talonavicular part** of the talocalcaneonavicular joint and the calcaneocuboid joint. The two joints are separated anatomically but act together functionally.
- Is important in inversion and eversion of the foot.

B. Tarsometatarsal Joints

- Are **plane synovial joints** that strengthen the transverse arch.
- Are united by articular capsules and are reinforced by the plantar, dorsal, and interosseous ligaments.

C. Metatarsophalangeal Joints

- Are **ellipsoid (condyloid) synovial joints** that are joined by articular capsules and are reinforced by the plantar and collateral ligaments.

CLINICAL CORRELATES

Bunion is a localized swelling at the medial side of the first metatarsophalangeal joint (or of the first metatarsal head) that is caused by an inflammatory bursa and is unusually associated with hallux valgus. **Bunionectomy** is an excision of an abnormal prominence on the medial aspect of the first metatarsal head.

Hallux valgus is a lateral deviation of the big toe and is frequently accompanied by swelling (bunion) on the medial aspect of the first metatarsophalangeal joint. It contrasts with **hallux varus,** which is a medial deviation of the big toe.

D. Interphalangeal Joints

- Are **hinge-type (ginglymus) synovial joints** that are enclosed by articular capsules and are reinforced by the plantar and collateral ligaments.

CUTANEOUS NERVES, SUPERFICIAL VEINS, AND LYMPHATICS

I. CUTANEOUS NERVES OF THE LOWER LIMB (Figure 6.12)

A. Lateral Femoral Cutaneous Nerve

- Arises from the lumbar plexus (L2–L3), emerges from the lateral border of the psoas major, crosses the iliacus, and passes under the inguinal ligament near the anterior–superior iliac spine.
- Innervates the **skin on the anterior and lateral aspects of the thigh** as far as the knee.

B. Cluneal (Buttock) Nerves

- Innervate the skin of the gluteal region.
- Consist of **superior** (lateral branches of the dorsal rami of the upper three lumbar nerves), **middle** (lateral branches of the dorsal rami of the upper three sacral nerves), and **inferior** (gluteal branches of the posterior femoral cutaneous nerve) nerves.

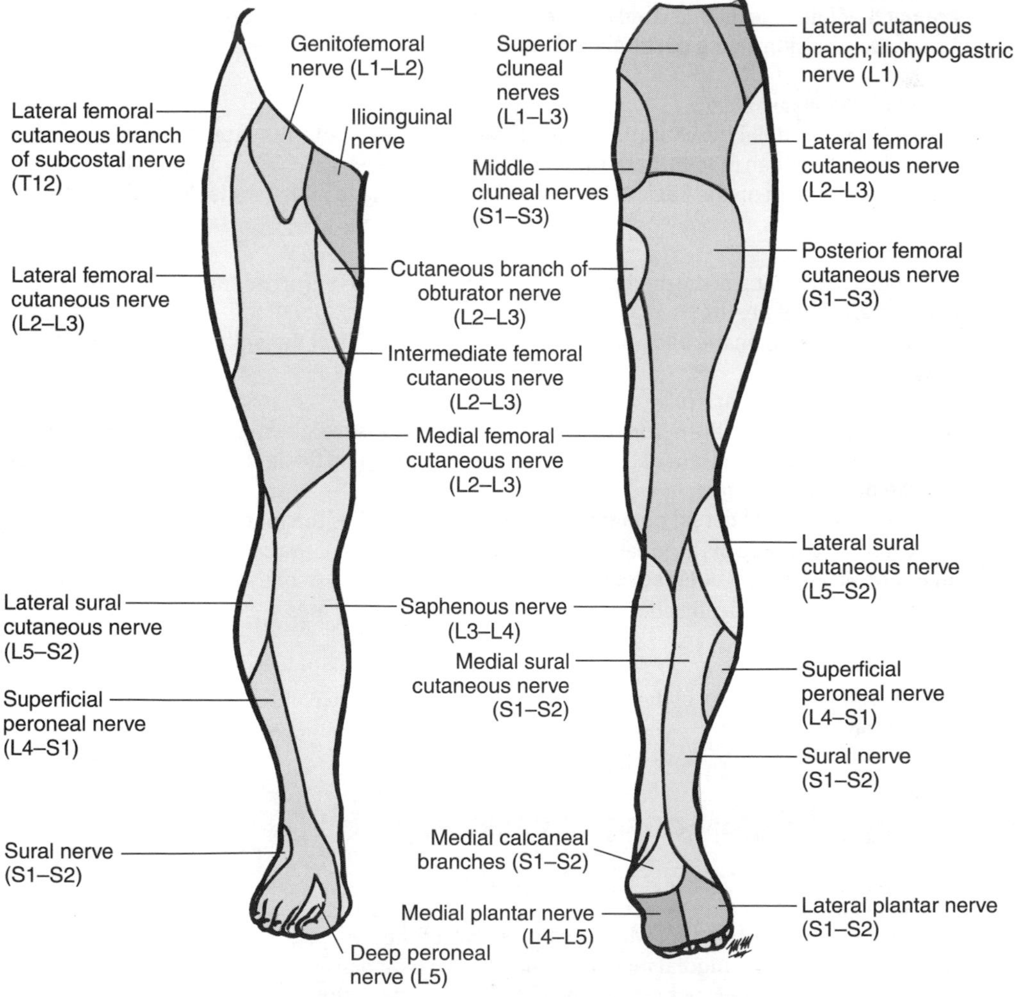

FIGURE 6.12. Cutaneous nerves of the lower limb.

C. Posterior Femoral Cutaneous Nerve

- Arises from the **sacral plexus** (S1–S3), passes through the greater sciatic foramen below the piriformis muscle, runs deep to the gluteus maximus muscle, and emerges from the inferior border of this muscle.
- Descends in the posterior midline of the thigh deep to the fascia lata and pierces the fascia lata near the popliteal fossa.
- Innervates the **skin of the buttock, thigh**, and **calf**.

D. Saphenous Nerve

- Arises from the **femoral nerve** in the **femoral triangle** and descends with the femoral vessels through the femoral triangle and the adductor canal.
- Pierces the fascial covering of the adductor canal at its distal end in company with the saphenous branch of the descending genicular artery.
- Becomes cutaneous between the sartorius and the gracilis and descends behind the condyles of the femur and tibia and medial aspect of the leg in company with the great saphenous vein.
- **Innervates the skin on the medial side of the leg and foot.**
- **Is vulnerable to injury** (proximal portion) during surgery to repair varicose veins.

E. Lateral Sural Cutaneous Nerve

- Arises from the **common peroneal nerve** in the **popliteal fossa** and may have a **communicating branch** that joins the medial sural cutaneous nerve.
- Innervates the **skin on the posterolateral side of the leg**.

F. Medial Sural Cutaneous Nerve

- Arises from the tibial nerve in the popliteal fossa and may join the lateral sural nerve or its communicating branch to form the **sural nerve.**
- Innervates the skin on the **back of the leg** and the **lateral side of the ankle, heel, and foot**.

G. Sural Nerve

- Is formed by the union of the medial sural and lateral sural nerves (or the communicating branch of the lateral sural nerve).
- Innervates the skin on the **back of the leg** and the **lateral side of the ankle, heel, and foot**.

H. Superficial Peroneal (fibular) Nerve

- Passes distally between the peroneus muscles and the extensor digitorum longus and pierces the deep fascia in the lower third of the leg to innervate the **skin on the lateral side of the lower leg and the dorsum of the foot**.
- Divides into a **medial dorsal cutaneous nerve**, which supplies the medial sides of the foot and ankle, the medial side of the great toe, and the adjacent sides of the second and third toes, and an **intermediate dorsal cutaneous nerve**, which supplies the skin of the lateral sides of the foot and ankle and the adjacent sides of the third, fourth, and little toes.

I. Deep Peroneal (fibular) Nerve

- Supplies anterior muscles of the leg and foot and the skin of the contiguous sides of the first and second toes.

II. SUPERFICIAL VEINS OF THE LOWER LIMB

A. Great Saphenous Vein

- Begins at the medial end of the **dorsal venous arch** of the foot.
- Ascends in front of the medial malleolus and along the medial aspect of the tibia along with the saphenous nerve, passes behind the medial condyles of the tibia and femur, and then ascends along the medial side of the femur.
- Passes through the **saphenous opening (fossa ovalis)** in the fascia lata and pierces the femoral sheath to join the femoral vein.

- Receives the external pudendal, superficial epigastric, superficial circumflex ilia, lateral femoral cutaneous, and accessory saphenous veins.
- Is a suitable vessel for use in coronary artery bypass surgery and for venipuncture.

CLINICAL CORRELATES **The great saphenous vein** accompanies the saphenous nerve, which is vulnerable to injury when collected surgically. It is commonly used for **coronary artery bypass** surgery, and the vein should be reversed so its valves do not obstruct blood flow in the graft. This vein and its tributaries become dilated and varicose commonly in the posteromedial parts of the lower limb.

B. Small (Short) Saphenous Vein

- Begins at the lateral end of the **dorsal venous arch** and passes upward along the lateral side of the foot with the sural nerve, behind the lateral malleolus.
- Ascends in company with the sural nerve and passes to the popliteal fossa, where it perforates the deep fascia and terminates in the **popliteal vein**.

CLINICAL CORRELATES **Thrombophlebitis** is a venous inflammation with thrombus formation that occurs in the superficial veins in the lower limb, leading to **pulmonary embolism.** However, most pulmonary emboli originate in deep veins, and the risk of embolism can be reduced by anticoagulant treatment.

Varicose veins develop in the **superficial veins** of the lower limb because of reduced elasticity and incompetent valves in the veins or **thrombophlebitis** of the **deep veins.**

III. LYMPHATICS OF THE LOWER LIMB

A. Lymph Vessels

1. Superficial Lymph Vessels

- Are formed by vessels from the gluteal region, the abdominal wall, and the external genitalia.
- Are divided into a **medial group**, which follows the great saphenous vein to end in the inguinal nodes, and a **lateral group**, which follows the small saphenous vein to end in the popliteal nodes, and their efferents accompany the femoral vessels to end in the inguinal nodes.

2. Deep Lymph Vessels

- Consist of the **anterior tibial**, **posterior tibial**, and **peroneal vessels**, which follow the course of the corresponding blood vessels and enter the **popliteal lymph nodes.** The lymph vessels from the popliteal nodes accompany the femoral vessels to the inguinal nodes, which enter the external iliac nodes and ultimately drain into the lumbar (aortic) nodes and vessels.

B. Lymph Nodes

1. Superficial Inguinal Group of Lymph Nodes

- Is located subcutaneously near the **saphenofemoral junction** and drains the superficial thigh region.
- Receives lymph from the anterolateral abdominal wall below the umbilicus, gluteal region, lower parts of the vagina and anus, and external genitalia except the glans, and drains into the **external iliac nodes.**

2. Deep Inguinal Group of Lymph Nodes

- Lies deep to the fascia lata on the medial side of the femoral vein.
- Receives lymph from deep lymph vessels (i.e., efferents of the popliteal nodes) that accompany the femoral vessels and from the glans penis or glans clitoris, and drains into the external iliac nodes through the femoral canal.

MUSCLES OF THE LOWER LIMB

I. MUSCLES OF THE GLUTEAL REGION (Table 6.1)

A. Sacrotuberous Ligament

- Extends from the ischial tuberosity to the posterior iliac spines, lower sacrum, and coccyx.
- Converts, with the sacrospinous ligament, the lesser sciatic notch into the lesser sciatic foramen.

B. Sacrospinous Ligament

- Extends from the ischial spine to the lower sacrum and coccyx.
- Converts the greater sciatic notch into the greater sciatic foramen.

C. Sciatic Foramina

1. Greater Sciatic Foramen

- Provides a pathway for the piriformis muscle, superior and inferior gluteal vessels and nerves, internal pudendal vessels and pudendal nerve, sciatic nerve, posterior femoral cutaneous nerve, and the nerves to the obturator internus and quadratus femoris muscles.

2. Lesser Sciatic Foramen

- Provides a pathway for the tendon of the obturator internus, the nerve to the obturator internus, and the internal pudendal vessels and pudendal nerve.

3. Structures That Pass through Both the Greater and the Lesser Sciatic Foramina

- Include the pudendal nerve, the internal pudendal vessels, and the nerve to the obturator internus.

D. Iliotibial Tract

- Is a thick lateral portion of the **fascia lata**.
- Provides insertion for the gluteus maximus and tensor fasciae latae muscles.
- Helps form the **fibrous capsule of the knee joint** and is important in maintaining posture and locomotion.

table 6.1 Muscles of the Gluteal Region

Muscle	Origin	Insertion	Nerve	Action
Gluteus maximus	Ilium, sacrum, coccyx, sacrotuberous ligament	Gluteal tuberosity, iliotibial tract	Inferior gluteal	Extends and rotates thigh laterally
Gluteus medius	Ilium between iliac crest, and anterior and posterior gluteal lines	Greater trochanter	Superior gluteal	Abducts and rotates thigh medially, stabilizes pelvis
Gluteus minimus	Ilium between anterior and inferior gluteal lines	Greater trochanter	Superior gluteal	Abducts and rotates thigh medially
Tensor fasciae latae	Iliac crest, anterior–superior iliac spine	Iliotibial tract	Superior gluteal	Flexes, abducts, and rotates thigh medially
Piriformis	Pelvic surface of sacrum, sacrotuberous ligament	Upper end of greater trochanter	Sacral (S1–S2)	Rotates thigh laterally
Obturator internus	Ischiopubic rami, obturator membrane	Greater trochanter	Nerve to obturator internus	Abducts and rotates thigh laterally
Superior gemellus	Ischial spine	Obturator internus tendon	Nerve to obturator internus	Rotates thigh laterally
Interior gemellus	Ischial tuberosity	Obturator internus tendon	Nerve to quadratus femoris	Rotates thigh laterally
Quadratus femoris	Ischial tuberosity	Intertrochanteric crest	Nerve to quadratus femoris	Rotates thigh laterally

E. **Fascia Lata**

- Is a membranous, deep fascia covering muscles of the thigh and forms the **lateral and medial intermuscular septa** by its inward extension to the femur.
- Is attached to the pubic symphysis, pubic crest, pubic rami, ischial tuberosity, inguinal and sacrotuberous ligaments, and the sacrum and coccyx.

CLINICAL CORRELATES

Gluteal gait (gluteus medius limp) is a waddling gait characterized by the pelvis falling (or drooping) toward the unaffected side when the opposite leg is raised at each step. It results from paralysis of the gluteus medius muscle, which normally functions to stabilize the pelvis when the opposite foot is off the ground.

The **common site for intramuscular injection of medications** is in the **superior lateral quadrant** of the gluteal region to avoid injury to the underlying sciatic nerve and other neurovascular structures.

II. POSTERIOR MUSCLES OF THE THIGH (Table 6.2)

CLINICAL CORRELATES

Piriformis syndrome is a condition in which the piriformis muscle irritates and places pressure on the sciatic nerve, causing pain in the buttocks and referring pain along the course of the sciatic nerve. This referred pain, called "**sciatica**," in the lower back and hip radiates down the back of the thigh and into the lower back. (The pain initially was attributed to sciatic nerve dysfunction but now is known to be due to herniation of a lower lumbar intervertebral disk compromising nerve roots.) It can be treated with progressive piriformis stretching. If this fails, then a corticosteroid may be administered into the piriformis muscle. Finally, surgery may be opted as a last resort.

CLINICAL CORRELATES

Positive Trendelenburg sign is seen in a fracture of the femoral neck, dislocated hip joint (head of femur), or weakness and paralysis of the gluteus medius (abductor). If the right gluteus medius muscle is paralyzed, the left side (**sound side**) of **the pelvis falls** (sags) instead of rising; normally, the pelvis rises.

CLINICAL CORRELATES

Hamstring injuries or strains (pulled or torn hamstrings) are very painful and common in persons who are involved in running, jumping, and quick-start sports. **Avulsion of the ischial tuberosity** (the origin of the hamstrings) may result from forcible flexion of the hip with the knee extended.

table 6.2 Posterior Muscles of the Thigh*

Muscle	Origin	Insertion	Nerve	Action
Semitendinosus	Ischial tuberosity	Medial surface of upper part of tibia	Tibial portion of sciatic nerve	Extends thigh, flexes and rotates leg medially
Semimembranosus	Ischial tuberosity	Medical condyle of tibia	Tibial portion of sciatic nerve	Extends thigh, flexes and rotates leg medially
Biceps femoris	Long head from ischial tuberosity, short head from linea aspera and upper supracondylar line	Head of fibula	Tibial (long head) and common peroneal (short head) divisions of sciatic nerve	Extends thigh, flexes and rotates leg laterally

* All posterior thigh muscles are hamstrings except the short head of the biceps femoris. Hamstrings cross two joints and are innervated by the tibial portion of the sciatic nerve.

III. MUSCLES OF THE ANTERIOR AND MEDIAL THIGH (Tables 6.3 to 6.4)

A. Femoral Triangle

- Is bounded by the inguinal ligament superiorly, the sartorius muscle laterally, and the adductor longus muscle medially.
- Has the **floor**, which is formed by the iliopsoas, pectineus, and adductor longus muscles. Its **roof** is formed by the fascia lata and the cribriform fascia.
- Contains the femoral **n**erve, **a**rtery, **v**ein, and **l**ymphatics (in the canal). A mnemonic NAVeL is used to remember the order of the structures, and the mnemonic NAVY is used to remember

table 6.3 Anterior Muscles of the Thigh

Muscle	Origin	Insertion	Nerve	Action
Iliacus	Iliac fossa, ala of sacrum	Lesser trochanter	Femoral	Flexes thigh (with psoas major)
Sartorius	Anterior–superior iliac spine	Upper medial side of tibia	Femoral	Flexes and rotates thigh laterally, flexes and rotates leg medially
Rectus femoris	Anterior–inferior iliac spine, posterior–superior rim of acetabulum	Base of patella, tibial tuberosity	Femoral	Flexes thigh, extends leg
Vastus medialis	Intertrochanteric line, linea aspera, medial intermuscular septum	Medial side of patella, tibial tuberosity	Femoral	Extends leg
Vastus lateralis	Intertrochanteric line, greater trochanter, linea aspera, gluteal tuberosity, lateral intermuscular septum	Lateral side of patella, tibial tuberosity	Femoral	Extends leg
Vastus intermedius	Upper shaft of femur, lower lateral intermuscular septum	Upper border of patella, tibial tuberosity	Femoral	Extends leg

table 6.4 Medial Muscles of the Thigh

Muscle	Origin	Insertion	Nerve	Action
Adductor longus	Body of pubis below its crest	Middle third of linea aspera	Obturator	Adducts and flexes thigh
Adductor brevis	Body and inferior pubic ramus	Pectineal line, upper part of linea aspera	Obturator	Adducts and flexes thigh
Adductor magnus	Ischiopubic ramus, ischial tuberosity	Linea aspera, medial supracondylar line, adductor tubercle	Obturator and sciatic (tibial part)	Adducts, flexes, and extends thigh
Pectineus	Pectineal line of pubis	Pectineal line of femur	Obturator and femoral	Adducts and flexes thigh
Gracilis	Body and inferior pubic ramus	Medial surface of upper quarter of tibia	Obturator	Adducts and flexes thigh, flexes and rotates leg medially
Obturator externus	Margin of obturator foramen and obturator membrane	Intertrochanteric fossa of femur	Obturator	Rotates thigh laterally

the structures from lateral to medial (**n**erve, **a**rtery, **v**ein, **y**ahoo!!!). The pulsation of the femoral artery may be felt just inferior to the midpoint of the inguinal ligament.

B. Femoral Ring

- Is the abdominal opening of the femoral canal.
- Is bounded by the inguinal ligament anteriorly, the femoral vein laterally, the lacunar ligament medially, and the pectineal ligament posteriorly.

C. Femoral Canal

- Lies medial to the femoral vein in the femoral sheath.
- Contains fat, areolar connective tissue, and lymph nodes and vessels.
- Transmits **lymphatics** from the lower limb and perineum to the peritoneal cavity.
- Is a potential weak area and a site of **femoral herniation**, which occurs most frequently in women because of the greater width of the superior pubic ramus of the female pelvis.

CLINICAL CORRELATES

Femoral hernia is more common in women than in men, passes through the femoral ring and canal, and lies lateral and inferior to the pubic tubercle and deep and inferior to the inguinal ligament; its sac is formed by the parietal peritoneum. Strangulation of a femoral hernia may occur because of the sharp, stiff boundaries of the femoral ring, and the strangulation interferes with the blood supply to the herniated intestine, resulting in death of the tissues.

D. Femoral Sheath

- Is formed by a prolongation of the **transversalis** and **iliac fasciae** in the thigh.
- Contains the femoral artery and vein, the femoral branch of the genitofemoral nerve, and the femoral canal. (The femoral nerve lies outside the femoral sheath, lateral to the femoral artery.)
- Reaches the level of the proximal end of the saphenous opening with its distal end.

E. Adductor Canal

- Begins at the apex of the femoral triangle and ends at the **adductor hiatus** (hiatus tendineus).
- Lies between the adductor magnus and longus muscles and the vastus medialis muscle, and is covered by the sartorius muscle and fascia.
- Contains the femoral vessels, the saphenous nerve, the nerve to the vastus medialis, and the descending genicular artery.

F. Adductor Hiatus (Hiatus Tendineus)

- Is the aperture in the tendon of insertion of the adductor magnus.
- Allows the passage of the femoral vessels into the popliteal fossa.

G. Saphenous Opening (Saphenous Hiatus) or Fossa Ovalis

- Is an oval gap in the fascia lata below the inguinal ligament that is covered by the **cribriform fascia**, which is a part of the superficial fascia of the thigh.
- Provides a pathway for the greater saphenous vein.

CLINICAL CORRELATES

Groin injury or pulled groin is a strain, stretching, or tearing of the origin of the flexor and adductor of the thigh and often occurs in sports that require quick starts such as a 100-m dash and football.

The gracilis is a relatively weak member of the adductor group of muscles, and thus surgeons often transplant this muscle or part of it, with nerve and blood vessels, to replace a damaged muscle in the hand. The proximal muscle attachments are in the inguinal region or groin.

Muscle strains of the adductor longus may occur in horseback riders and produce pain because the riders adduct their thighs to keep from falling from the animal.

IV. ANTERIOR AND LATERAL MUSCLES OF THE LEG (Table 6.5)

A. Popliteal Fossa

- Is bounded superomedially by the semitendinosus and semimembranosus muscles, superolaterally by the biceps muscle, inferolaterally by the lateral head of the gastrocnemius and plantaris muscles, and inferomedially by the medial head of the gastrocnemius muscle.
- Has a floor that is composed of the femur, the oblique popliteal ligament, and the popliteus muscle.
- Contains the popliteal vessels, the common peroneal and tibial nerves, and the small saphenous vein.

B. Pes Anserinus

- Is the combined tendinous expansions of the sartorius, gracilis, and semitendinosus muscles at the medial border of the tuberosity of the tibia. It may be used for surgical repair of the anterior cruciate ligament of the knee joint.

CLINICAL CORRELATES

Anterior tibial compartment syndrome is an ischemic necrosis of the muscles of the anterior compartment of the leg, resulting from compression of the anterior tibial artery and its branches by swollen muscles following excessive exertion. It is accompanied by extreme tenderness and pain on the anterolateral aspect of the leg.

Shin splint is a painful condition caused by swollen muscles in the anterior compartment of the leg along the shin bone (tibia), particularly the tibialis anterior muscle, following athletic overexertion. It may be a mild form of the anterior compartment syndrome.

Muscle cramp ("charley horse") is a sudden, involuntary, painful contraction of muscles of the lower limb. It is caused by muscle fatigue from prolonged sitting, overexertion, dehydration, and depletion or imbalance of salt and minerals (electrolytes) as well as a poor blood supply to leg muscles. It occurs most commonly in the calf muscle, hamstrings, and quadriceps. The cramp goes away within a few minutes, or it can be treated by a gentle stretch and massage of the cramped muscle, pain relievers, and muscle relaxers.

Intermittent claudication is a condition of limping caused by ischemia of the muscles in the lower limbs, chiefly the calf muscles, and is seen in occlusive peripheral arterial diseases particularly in the popliteal artery and its branches. The main symptom is leg pain that occurs during walking and intensifies until walking is impossible, but the pain is relieved by rest.

table 6.5 Anterior and Lateral Muscles of the Leg

Muscle	Origin	Insertion	Nerve	Action
Tibialis anterior	Lateral tibial condyle, interosseous membrane	First cuneiform, first metatarsal	Deep peroneal (fibular)	Dorsiflexes and inverts foot
Extensor hallucis longus	Middle half of anterior surface of fibula, interosseous membrane	Base of distal phalanx of big toe	Deep peroneal (fibular)	Extends big toe, dorsiflexes and inverts foot
Extensor digitorum longus	Lateral tibial condyle, upper two-thirds of fibula, interosseous membrane	Bases of middle and distal phalanges	Deep peroneal (fibular)	Extends toes, dorsiflexes and everts foot
Peroneus (fibularis) tertius	Distal one-third of fibula, interosseous membrane	Base of fifth metatarsal	Deep peroneal (fibular)	Dorsiflexes and everts foot
Lateral				
Peroneus (fibularis) longus	Lateral tibial condyle, head and upper lateral side of fibula	Base of first metatarsal, medial cuneiform	Superficial peroneal (fibular)	Everts and plantar flexes foot
Peroneus (fibularis) brevis	Lower lateral side of fibula, intermuscular septa	Base of fifth metatarsal	Superficial peroneal (fibular)	Everts and plantar flexes foot

V. POSTERIOR MUSCLES OF THE LEG (Table 6.6)

CLINICAL CORRELATES **Restless legs syndrome** is a sense of restless unpleasant discomfort inside the legs when sitting or lying down, accompanied by an irresistible urge to move the legs. Movement like walking brings temporary relief, but it is worse at rest and in the evening or at night. Its cause is unknown (idiopathic).

Knee-jerk (patellar) reflex occurs when the patellar ligament is tapped, resulting in a sudden contraction of the quadriceps femoris. It **tests** the **L2 to L4 spinal (femoral) nerves** by activating muscle spindle in the quadriceps. Both afferent and efferent impulses are transmitted in the femoral nerve.

Ankle-jerk (Achilles) reflex is a reflex twitch of the triceps surae (i.e., the medial and lateral heads of the gastrocnemius and the soleus muscles) induced by tapping the tendo calcaneus. It causes plantar flexion of the foot and tests its reflex center in the L5 to S1 or S1 to S2 segments of the spinal cord. Both afferent and efferent limbs of the reflex arc are carried in the tibial nerve.

VI. MUSCLES OF THE FOOT (Table 6.7)

A. Superior Extensor Retinaculum

- Is a **broad band of deep fascia** extending between the tibia and fibula above the ankle.

B. Inferior Extensor Retinaculum

- Is a **Y-shaped band of deep fascia** that forms a loop for the tendons of the extensor digitorum longus and the peroneus tertius and then divides into an upper band, which attaches to the medial malleolus, and a **lower band**, which attaches to the deep fascia of the foot and the plantar aponeurosis.

table 6.6 Posterior Muscles of the Leg

Muscle	Origin	Insertion	Nerve	Action
Superficial group				
Gastrocnemius	Lateral (lateral head) and medial (medial head) femoral condyles	Posterior aspect of calcaneus via tendo calcaneus	Tibial	Flexes knee, plantar flexes foot
Soleus	Upper fibula head, soleal line on tibia	Posterior aspect of calcaneus via tendo calcaneus	Tibial	Plantar flexes foot
Plantaris	Lower lateral supracondylar line	Posterior surface of calcaneus	Tibial	Flexes leg, plantar flexes foot
Deep group				
Popliteus	Lateral condyle of femur, popliteal ligament	Upper posterior side of tibia	Tibial	Flexes by unlocking knee and rotates leg medially
Flexor hallucis longus	Lower two-thirds of fibula, interosseous membrane, intermuscular septa	Base of distal phalanx of big toe	Tibial	Plantar flexes foot, flexes distal phalanx of big toe
Flexor digitorum longus	Middle posterior aspect of tibia	Distal phalanges of lateral four toes	Tibial	Flexes lateral four toes, plantar flexes foot
Tibialis posterior	Interosseous membrane, upper parts of tibia and fibula	Tuberosity of navicular, sustentacula tali, three cuneiforms, cuboid, bases of metatarsals 2–4	Tibial	Plantar flexes and inverts foot

table 6.7 Muscles of the Foot

Muscle	Origin	Insertion	Nerve	Action
Dorsum of foot				
Extensor digitorum brevis	Dorsal surface of calcaneus	Tendons of extensor digitorum longus	Deep peroneal	Extends toes
Extensor hallucis brevis	Dorsal surface of calcaneus	Base of proximal phalanx of big toe	Deep peroneal	Extends big toe
Sole of foot				
First layer				
Abductor hallucis	Medical tubercle of calcaneus	Base of proximal phalanx of big toe	Medial plantar	Abducts big toe
Flexor digitorum brevis	Medial tubercle of calcaneus	Middle phalanges of lateral four toes	Medial plantar	Flexes middle phalanges of lateral four toes
Abductor digiti minimi	Medial and lateral tubercles of calcaneus	Proximal phalanx of little toe	Lateral plantar	Abducts little toe
Second layer				
Quadratus plantae	Medial and lateral side of calcaneus	Tendons of flexor digitorum longus	Lateral plantar	Aids in flexing toes
Lumbricals (4)	Tendons of flexor digitorum longus	Proximal phalanges, extensor expansion	First by medial plantar, lateral three by lateral plantar	Flex metatarsophalangeal joints and extend interphalangeal joints
Third layer				
Flexor hallucis brevis	Cuboid, third cuneiform	Proximal phalanx of big toe	Medial plantar	Flexes big toe
Adductor hallucis				
Oblique head	Bases of metatarsals 2–4	Proximal phalanx of big toe	Lateral plantar	Adducts big toe
Transverse head	Capsule of lateral four metatarsophalangeal joints			
Flexor digiti minimi brevis	Base of metatarsal 5	Proximal phalanx of little toe	Lateral plantar	Flexes little toe
Fourth layer				
Plantar interossei (3)	Medial sides of metatarsals 3–5	Medial sides of base of proximal phalanges 3–5	Lateral plantar	Adduct toes, flex proximal, and extend distal phalanges
Dorsal interossei (4)	Adjacent shafts of metatarsals	Proximal phalanges of second toe (medial and lateral sides), and third and fourth toes (lateral sides)	Lateral plantar	Abduct toes, flex proximal, and extend distal phalanges

C. Flexor Retinaculum

- Is a deep fascial band that passes between the medial malleolus and the medial surface of the calcaneus and forms the **tarsal tunnel** with tarsal bones for the tibial nerve, posterior tibial vessels, and flexor tendons.
- Holds three tendons and blood vessels and a nerve in place deep to it (from anterior to posterior): the **t**ibialis posterior, flexor **d**igitorum longus, posterior tibial **a**rtery and **v**ein, tibial **n**erve, and flexor **h**allucis longus (mnemonic device: **T**om, **D**ick **AN**d **H**arry or **T**om **D**rives **A** **V**ery **N**ervous **H**orse).
- Provides a pathway for the tibial nerve and posterior tibial artery beneath it.

CLINICAL CORRELATES **Tarsal tunnel syndrome** is a complex symptom resulting from compression of the tibial nerve or its medial and lateral plantar branches in the **tarsal tunnel**, with pain, numbness, and tingling sensations on the ankle, heel, and sole of the foot. It may be caused by repetitive stress with activities, flat feet, or excess weight.

D. Tendo Calcaneus (Achilles Tendon)

- Is the tendon of insertion of the **triceps surae** (gastrocnemius and soleus) into the tuberosity of the calcaneus.

CLINICAL CORRELATES **Avulsion or rupture of the Achilles tendon** disables the triceps surae (gastrocnemius and soleus) muscles; thus, the patient is unable to plantar flex the foot.

Forced eversion of the foot avulses the medial malleolus or ruptures the deltoid ligament, whereas **forced inversion** avulses the lateral malleolus or tears the lateral collateral (anterior and posterior talofibular and calcaneofibular) ligament.

Ankle sprain (inversion injury) results from rupture of calcaneofibular and talofibular ligaments and a fracture of the lateral malleolus caused by forced inversion of the foot.

E. Plantar Aponeurosis

- Is a thick fascia investing the plantar muscles.
- Radiates from the **calcaneal tuberosity** (tuber calcanei) toward the toes and provides attachment to the short flexor muscles of the toes.

F. Arches of the Foot (Figure 6.13)

1. Medial Longitudinal Arch

- Is formed and maintained by the interlocking of the talus, calcaneus, navicular, cuneiform, and three medial metatarsal bones.
- Has, as its **keystone**, the **head of the talus**, which is located at the summit between the sustentaculum tali and the navicular bone.
- Is supported by the spring ligament and the tendon of the flexor hallucis longus.

CLINICAL CORRELATES **Flat foot (pes planus or talipes planus)** is a condition of disappearance or **collapse of the medial longitudinal arch** with eversion and abduction of the forefoot and causes greater wear on the inner border of the soles and heels of shoes than on the outer border. It causes pain as a result of stretching of the plantar muscles and straining of the spring ligament and the long and short plantar ligaments. **Pes cavus** exhibits an exaggerated height of the medial longitudinal arch of the foot.

2. Lateral Longitudinal Arch

- Is formed by the calcaneus, the cuboid bone, and the lateral two metatarsal bones. The **keystone** is the **cuboid bone**.
- Is supported by the peroneus longus tendon and the long and short plantar ligaments.
- Supports the body in the erect position and acts as a spring in locomotion.

3. Transverse Arch

a. Proximal (metatarsal) Arch

- Is formed by the navicular bone, the three cuneiform bones, the cuboid bone, and the bases of the five metatarsal bones of the foot.
- Is supported by the tendon of the **peroneus longus**.

b. Distal Arch

- Is formed by the heads of five metatarsal bones.
- Is maintained by the **transverse head** of the **adductor hallucis**.

G. Ligaments (Figure 6.13)

1. Long Plantar (Plantar Calcaneocuboid) Ligament

- Extends from the plantar aspect of the calcaneus in front of its tuberosity to the tuberosity of the cuboid bone and the base of the metatarsals and forms a canal for the tendon of the peroneus longus.
- Supports the lateral side of the longitudinal arch of the foot.

2. Short Plantar (Plantar Calcaneocuboid) Ligament

- Extends from the front of the plantar surface of the calcaneus to the plantar surface of the cuboid bone.
- Lies deep to the long plantar ligament and supports the lateral longitudinal arch.

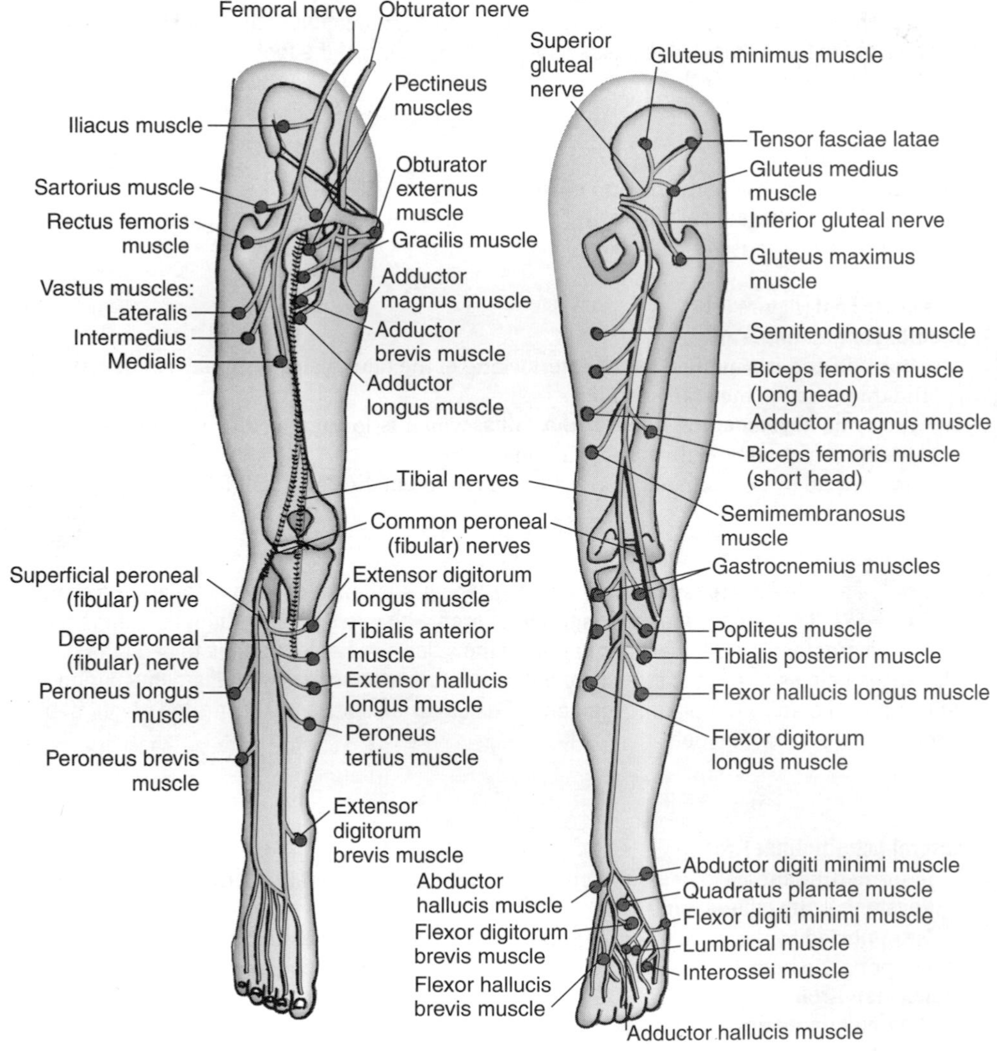

FIGURE 6.13. Distribution of the nerves of the lower limb.

3. **Spring (Plantar Calcaneonavicular) Ligament**
   - Passes from the sustentaculum tali of the calcaneus to the navicular bone.
   - Supports the **head of the talus** and the medial longitudinal arch.
   - Is called the spring ligament because it contains considerable numbers of elastic fibers to give elasticity to the arch and spring to the foot.
   - Is supported by the tendon of the tibialis posterior.

CLINICAL CORRELATES **Clubfoot (talipes equinovarus)** is a congenital deformity of the foot in which the foot is plantar-flexed, inverted, and adducted. It may involve a deformity in which the **heel is elevated** (the longitudinal arch is abnormally high) and **turns medially** (equinovarus) or laterally (euinovalgus).

NERVES OF THE LOWER LIMB

I. BRANCHES OF THE LUMBAR AND SACRAL PLEXUSES (Figure 6.14)

A. Obturator Nerve (L2–L4)

- Arises from the **lumbar plexus** and enters the thigh through the obturator foramen.
- Divides into anterior and posterior branches.

1. **Anterior Branch**
   - Descends between the adductor longus and adductor brevis muscles.
   - Innervates the adductor longus, adductor brevis, gracilis, and pectineus muscles.
2. **Posterior Branch**
   - Descends between the adductor brevis and adductor magnus muscles.

CLINICAL CORRELATES **Damage to the obturator nerve** causes a weakness of adduction and a lateral swinging of the limb during walking because of the unopposed abductors.

B. Femoral Nerve (L2–L4)

- Arises from the **lumbar plexus** within the substance of the psoas major, emerges between the iliacus and psoas major muscles, and enters the thigh by passing deep to the inguinal ligament and lateral to the femoral sheath.
- Gives rise to **muscular branches; articular branches** to the hip and knee joints; and **cutaneous branches**, including the anterior femoral cutaneous nerve and the saphenous nerve, which descends through the femoral triangle and accompanies the femoral vessels in the adductor canal.

CLINICAL CORRELATES **Damage to the femoral nerve** causes impaired flexion of the hip and impaired extension of the leg resulting from paralysis of the quadriceps femoris.

C. Superior Gluteal Nerve (L4–S1)

- Arises from the **sacral plexus** and enters the buttock through the greater sciatic foramen above the piriformis.
- Passes between the gluteus medius and minimus muscles and divides into numerous branches.
- Innervates the gluteus medius and minimus, the tensor fasciae latae, and the hip joint.

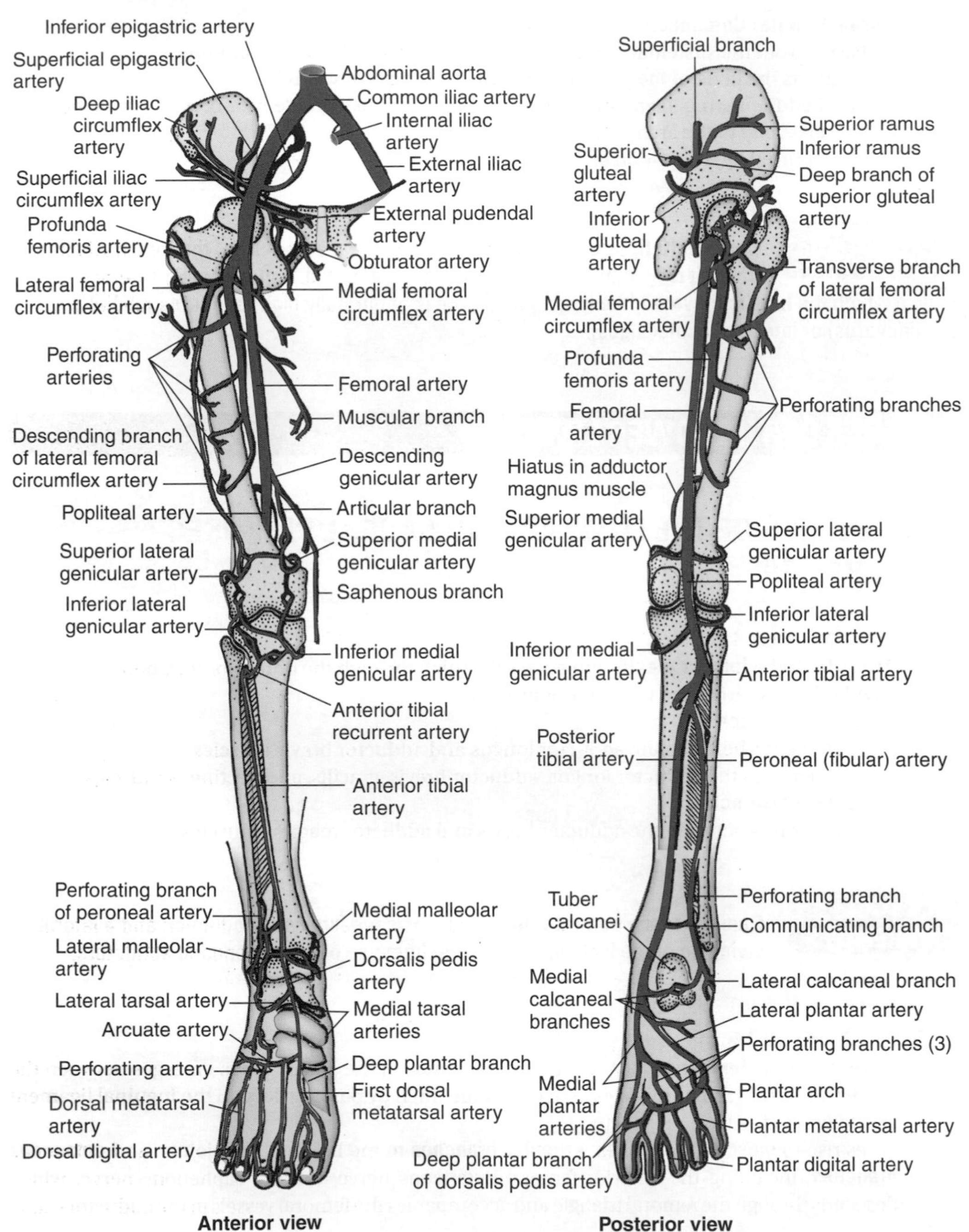

FIGURE 6.14. Blood supply to the lower limb.

CLINICAL CORRELATES

Injury to the superior gluteal nerve causes a characteristic motor loss, resulting in weakened abduction of the thigh by the gluteus medius, a disabling gluteus medius limp, and gluteal gait.

D. Inferior Gluteal Nerve (L5–S2)

- Arises from the **sacral plexus** and enters the buttock through the greater sciatic foramen below the piriformis.
- Divides into numerous branches.
- Innervates the overlying gluteus maximus.

E. Posterior Femoral Cutaneous Nerve (S1–S3)

- Arises from the **sacral plexus** and enters the buttock through the greater sciatic foramen below the piriformis.
- Runs deep to the gluteus maximus and emerges from the inferior border of this muscle.
- Descends on the posterior thigh.
- Innervates the skin of the buttock, thigh, and calf, as well as scrotum or labium majus.

F. Sciatic Nerve (L4–S3)

- Arises from the **sacral plexus** and is the **largest nerve in the body**.
- Divides at the superior border of the popliteal fossa into the **tibial nerve**, which runs through the fossa to disappear deep to the gastrocnemius, and the **common peroneal nerve**, which runs along the medial border of the biceps femoris and superficial to the lateral head of the gastrocnemius.
- Enters the buttock through the greater sciatic foramen below the piriformis.
- Descends over the obturator internus gemelli and quadratus femoris muscles between the ischial tuberosity and the greater trochanter.
- **Innervates the hamstring muscles** by its tibial division, except for the short head of the biceps femoris, which is innervated by its common peroneal division.
- Provides articular branches to the hip and knee joints.

CLINICAL CORRELATES

Damage to the sciatic nerve causes impaired extension at the hip and impaired flexion at the knee, loss of dorsiflexion and plantar flexion at the ankle, inversion and eversion of the foot, and peculiar gait because of increased flexion at the hip to lift the dropped foot off the ground.

1. Common Peroneal (Fibular) Nerve (L4–S2)

- Arises as the smaller terminal portion of the sciatic nerve at the apex of the popliteal fossa, descends through the fossa, and superficially crosses the lateral head of the gastrocnemius muscle.
- Passes behind the head of the fibula, then winds laterally around the neck of the fibula, and pierces the peroneus longus, where it divides into the deep peroneal and superficial peroneal nerves.
- **Is vulnerable to injury as it winds around the neck of the fibula**, where it also can be palpated.
- Gives rise to the **lateral sural cutaneous nerve**, which supplies the skin on the lateral part of the back of the leg, and the **recurrent articular branch** to the knee joint.

CLINICAL CORRELATES

Phantom limb pain is intermittent or continuous pain perceived as originating in an absent (amputated) limb.

CLINICAL CORRELATES

Damage to the common peroneal (fibular) nerve may occur as a result of fracture of the head or neck of the fibula because it passes behind the head of the fibula and then winds laterally around the neck of the fibula. The nerve damage results in **foot drop** (loss of dorsiflexion) and loss of sensation on the dorsum of the foot and lateral aspect of the leg and causes paralysis of all muscles in the anterior and lateral compartments of the leg (dorsiflexor and evertor muscles of the foot).

a. Superficial Peroneal (Fibular) Nerve (See Cutaneous Nerves, Superficial Veins, and Lymphatics: I. H.)

- Arises from the common peroneal (fibular) nerve in the substance of the peroneus longus on the lateral side of the neck of the fibula; thus, it is **less vulnerable** to injury than the common peroneal nerve.
- Innervates the peroneus longus and brevis muscles and then emerges between the peroneus longus and brevis muscles by piercing the deep fascia at the lower third of the leg to become subcutaneous.
- Descends in the lateral compartment and innervates the skin on the lateral side of the lower leg and the dorsum of the foot.

CLINICAL CORRELATES **Damage to the superficial peroneal (fibular) nerve** causes no foot drop but does cause loss of eversion of the foot.

Damage to the deep peroneal (fibular) nerve results in **foot drop** (loss of dorsiflexion) and hence a characteristic high-stepping gait.

b. Deep Peroneal (Fibular) Nerve

- Arises from the common peroneal (fibular) nerve in the substance of the peroneus longus on the lateral side of the neck of the fibula (where it is vulnerable to injury but less vulnerable than the common peroneal nerve).
- Enters the anterior compartment by passing through the extensor digitorum longus muscle.
- Descends on the **interosseous membrane** between the extensor digitorum longus and the tibialis anterior and then between the extensor digitorum longus and the extensor hallucis longus muscles.
- Innervates the anterior muscles of the leg and then divides into a **lateral branch**, which supplies the extensor hallucis brevis and extensor digitorum brevis, and a **medial branch**, which accompanies the dorsalis pedis artery to supply the skin on the adjacent sides of the first and second toes.

2. Tibial Nerve (L4–S3)

- Descends through the popliteal fossa and then lies on the popliteus muscle.
- Gives rise to **three articular branches**, which accompany the medial superior genicular, middle genicular, and medial inferior genicular arteries to the knee joint.
- Gives rise to **muscular branches** to the posterior muscles of the leg.
- Gives rise to the medial sural cutaneous nerve, the medial calcaneal branch to the skin of the heel and sole, and the articular branches to the ankle joint.
- Terminates beneath the flexor retinaculum by dividing into the **medial** and **lateral plantar nerves.**

CLINICAL CORRELATES **Damage to the tibial nerve** causes **loss of plantar flexion** of the foot and impaired inversion resulting from paralysis of the tibialis posterior and causes a difficulty in getting the heel off the ground and a shuffling of the gait. It results in a characteristic clawing of the toes and sensory loss on the sole of the foot, affecting posture and locomotion.

a. Medial Plantar Nerve

- Arises beneath the flexor retinaculum, deep to the posterior portion of the abductor hallucis muscle, as the larger terminal branch from the tibial nerve.
- Passes distally between the abductor hallucis and flexor digitorum brevis muscles and innervates them.
- Gives rise to **common digital branches** that divide into proper digital branches, which supply the flexor hallucis brevis and the first lumbrical and the skin of the medial three and one-half toes.

b. Lateral Plantar Nerve

- Is the smaller terminal branch of the tibial nerve.
- Runs distally and laterally between the quadratus plantae and the flexor digitorum brevis, innervating the quadratus plantae and the abductor digiti minimi muscles.
- Divides into a **superficial branch**, which innervates the flexor digiti minimi brevis, and a **deep branch**, which innervates the plantar and dorsal interossei, the lateral three lumbricals, and the adductor hallucis.

BLOOD VESSELS OF THE LOWER LIMB

I. ARTERIES OF THE LOWER LIMB (Figures 6.15 to 6.16)

A. Superior Gluteal Artery

- Arises from the **internal iliac artery**, passes between the lumbosacral trunk and the first sacral nerve, and enters the buttock through the greater sciatic foramen above the piriformis muscle.

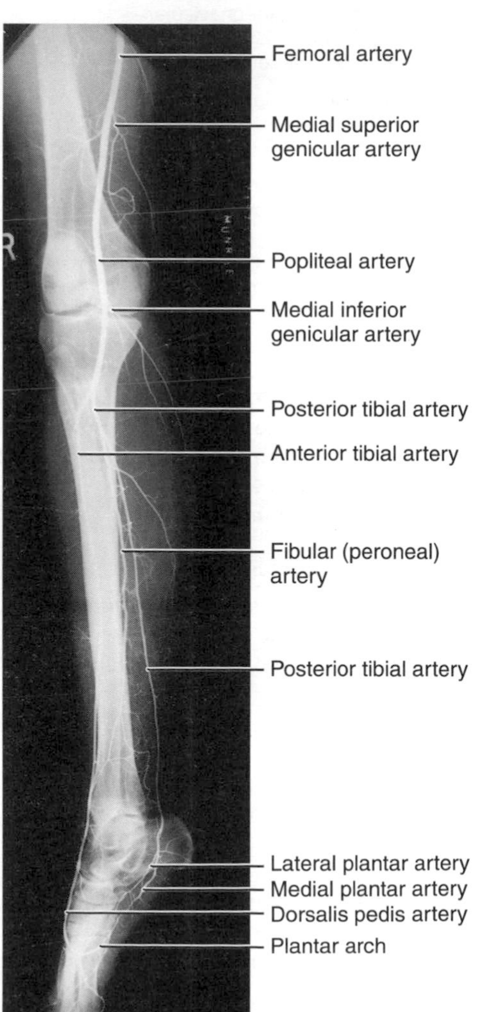

FIGURE 6.15. Arteriograph of the lower limb, oblique view.

(Reprinted with permission from Agur AMR, Lee JL. *Grant's Atlas of Anatomy.* 10th ed. Philadelphia, PA: Lippincott Williams & Wilkins; 1999:379.)

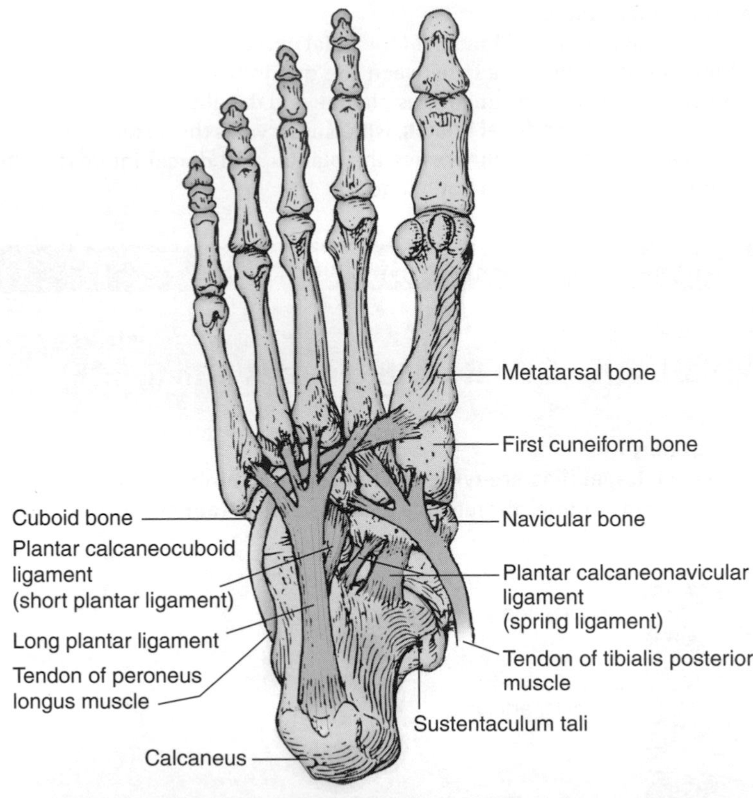

FIGURE 6.16. Plantar ligaments (plantar view).

- Runs deep to the gluteus maximus muscle and divides into a **superficial branch**, which forms numerous branches to supply the gluteus maximus and anastomoses with the inferior gluteal and lateral sacral arteries, and a **deep branch**, which runs between the gluteus medius and minimus muscles and supplies these muscles and the tensor fasciae latae.
- Anastomoses with the lateral and medial circumflex and inferior gluteal arteries.

B. Inferior Gluteal Artery

- Arises from the **internal iliac artery**, usually passes between the first and second sacral nerves, and enters the buttock through the greater sciatic foramen below the piriformis.
- Enters the deep surface of the gluteus maximus and descends on the medial side of the sciatic nerve, in company with the posterior femoral cutaneous nerve.
- Supplies the gluteus maximus, the lateral rotators of the hips, the hamstrings (upper part), and the hip joint.
- Enters the **cruciate anastomosis** and also anastomoses with the superior gluteal, internal pudendal, and obturator arteries.

C. Obturator Artery

- Arises from the **internal iliac artery** in the pelvis and passes through the obturator foramen, where it divides into **anterior and posterior branches**.
- May arise from the external iliac or inferior epigastric artery, which may pass toward the pelvic brim along the medial margin of the femoral ring.

1. Anterior Branch

- Descends in front of the adductor brevis muscle and gives rise to muscular branches.

2. Posterior Branch

- Descends behind the adductor brevis muscle to supply the adductor muscles.
- Gives rise to the **acetabular branch**, which enters the hip joint through the acetabular notch, ramifies in the acetabular fossa, and sends an **artery to the head of the femur**, which is an important source of blood to the femoral head in children. It may or may not persist in adults, or it may be insufficient to sustain the viability of the femoral head; thus, ischemic necrosis gradually takes place.

CLINICAL CORRELATES

Corona mortis (crown of death) is defined as the vascular anastomoses between the obturator and external iliac systems. A vascular anastomosis between pubic branches of the obturator artery and of the external iliac (or inferior epigastric) artery is called the corona mortis because these vessels in the retropubic area are hard to distinguish and can be injured in groin or pubic surgery, leading to massive uncontrolled bleeding. Since a venous connection is more probable than an arterial one, surgeons dealing with inguinal and femoral hernias should avoid venous bleeding and need to be aware of these anastomoses and their proximity to the femoral ring. An **aberrant obturator artery** may arise from the external iliac or inferior epigastric artery and is vulnerable during surgical repair of a femoral hernia.

D. Femoral Artery

- Begins as the continuation of the **external iliac artery** distal to the inguinal ligament, descends through the femoral triangle, and enters the adductor canal.
- Has a **palpable pulsation**, which may be felt just inferior to the midpoint of the inguinal ligament.
- Is **vulnerable to injury** because of its relatively superficial position in the femoral triangle.
- Includes several branches:

1. Superficial Epigastric Artery

- Runs subcutaneously upward toward the umbilicus.

2. Superficial Circumflex Iliac Artery

- Runs laterally almost parallel with the inguinal ligament.

3. Superficial External Pudendal Artery

- Emerges through the saphenous ring, runs medially over the spermatic cord (or the round ligament of the uterus), and sends inguinal branches and anterior scrotal (or labial) branches.

4. Deep External Pudendal Artery

- Passes medially across the pectineus and adductor longus and is distributed to the skin of the perineum, scrotum, or labium majus.

5. Profunda Femoris (Deep Femoral) Artery

- Arises from the **femoral artery** within the femoral triangle.
- Descends in front of the pectineus, adductor brevis, and adductor magnus muscles but behind the adductor longus muscle.
- Gives rise to the medial and lateral femoral circumflex and muscular branches.
- Provides, in the adductor canal, **four perforating arteries** that perforate and supply the adductor magnus and hamstring muscles. The **first perforating artery sends** an ascending branch, which joins the **cruciate anastomosis** of the buttock.

6. Medial Femoral Circumflex Artery

- Arises from the **femoral or profunda femoris artery** in the femoral triangle.
- Runs between the pectineus and iliopsoas muscles, continues between the obturator externus and adductor brevis muscles, and enters the gluteal region between the adductor magnus and quadratus femoris muscles.
- Gives rise to **muscular branches** and an **acetabular branch** to the hip joint and then divides into an **ascending branch**, which anastomoses with branches of the superior and inferior gluteal arteries, and a **transverse branch**, which joins the **cruciate anastomosis**.

CLINICAL CORRELATES **The medial femoral circumflex artery** is clinically important because its branches run through the neck to reach the head, and it **supplies most of the blood to the neck and head of the femur** except for the small proximal part that receives blood from a branch of the obturator artery.

The cruciate anastomosis of the buttock is formed by an ascending branch of the **first perforating** artery, the **inferior gluteal** artery, and the transverse branches of the **medial** and **lateral femoral circumflex** arteries. The cruciate anastomosis bypasses an obstruction of the external iliac or femoral artery.

7. **Lateral Femoral Circumflex Artery**
   - Arises from the **femoral or profunda femoris artery** and passes laterally deep to the sartorius and rectus femoris muscles.
   - Divides into three branches: an **ascending branch**, which forms a vascular circle with branches of the medial femoral circumflex artery around the femoral neck and also anastomoses with the superior gluteal artery; a **transverse branch**, which joins the **cruciate anastomosis**; and a **descending branch**, which anastomoses with the superior lateral genicular branch of the popliteal artery.
8. **Descending Genicular Artery**
   - Arises from the **femoral artery** in the adductor canal just before it passes through the adductor hiatus.
   - Divides into the **articular branch**, which enters the anastomosis around the knee, and the **saphenous branch**, which supplies the superficial tissue and skin on the medial side of the knee.

CLINICAL CORRELATES **The femoral artery** is easily exposed and cannulated at the base of the femoral triangle just inferior to the midpoint of the inguinal ligament. The superficial position of the femoral artery in the femoral triangle makes it **vulnerable to injury** by laceration and gunshot wounds. When it is necessary to ligate the femoral artery, the cruciate anastomosis supplies blood to the thigh and leg.

E. **Popliteal Artery**
- Is a continuation of the **femoral artery** at the adductor hiatus and runs through the popliteal fossa.
- Terminates at the lower border of the popliteus muscle by dividing into the anterior and posterior tibial arteries.
- May be felt by gentle palpation in the depth of the popliteal fossa.
- Is vulnerable to injury from fracture of the femur and dislocation of the knee joint.
- Gives rise to five genicular arteries:
  1. **Superior lateral genicular artery**, which passes deep to the biceps femoris tendon.
  2. **Superior medial genicular artery**, which passes deep to the semimembranosus and semitendinosus muscles and enters the substance of the vastus medialis.
  3. **Inferior lateral genicular artery**, which passes laterally above the head of the fibula and then deep to the fibular collateral ligament.
  4. **Inferior medial genicular artery**, which passes medially along the upper border of the popliteus muscle, deep to the popliteus fascia.
  5. **Middle genicular artery**, which pierces the oblique popliteal ligament and enters the knee joint.

CLINICAL CORRELATES **A popliteal aneurysm** usually results in edema and pain in the popliteal fossa. If it is necessary to ligate the femoral artery for surgical repair, blood can bypass the occlusion through the genicular anastomoses and reach the popliteal artery distal to the ligation.

F. Posterior Tibial Artery

- Arises from the popliteal artery at the lower border of the popliteus, between the tibia and the fibula.
- Is accompanied by two venae comitantes and the tibial nerve on the posterior surface of the tibialis posterior muscle. Its **pulsation** is often palpable between the medial malleolus and the calcaneal tendon.
- Gives rise to the **peroneal (fibular) artery**, which descends between the tibialis posterior and the flexor hallucis longus muscles and supplies the lateral muscles in the posterior compartment. The peroneal artery passes behind the lateral malleolus, gives rise to the **posterior lateral malleolar branch**, and ends in branches to the ankle and heel.
- Gives rise also to the posterior medial malleolar, perforating, and muscular branches and terminates by dividing into the **medial** and **lateral plantar arteries**.

1. Medial Plantar Artery

- Is the smaller terminal branch of the posterior tibial artery.
- Runs between the abductor hallucis and the flexor digitorum brevis muscles.
- Gives rise to a **superficial branch**, which supplies the big toe, and a **deep branch**, which forms three superficial digital branches.

2. Lateral Plantar Artery

- Is the larger terminal branch of the posterior tibial artery.
- Runs forward laterally in company with the lateral plantar nerve between the quadratus plantae and the flexor digitorum brevis muscles and then between the flexor digitorum brevis and the adductor digiti minimi muscles.
- Forms the **plantar arch** by joining the deep plantar branch of the dorsalis pedis artery. The plantar arch gives rise to four plantar metatarsal arteries.

G. Anterior Tibial Artery

- Arises from the **popliteal artery** and enters the anterior compartment by passing through the **gap between the tibia and fibula (neck)** at the upper end of the interosseous membrane.
- Descends along with the deep peroneal vessels on the interosseous membrane between the tibialis anterior and extensor digitorum longus muscles. Its **pulsation** may be felt between the two malleoli and lateral to the extensor hallucis longus tendon.
- Gives rise to the **anterior tibial recurrent artery**, which ascends to the knee joint, and the **anterior medial** and **lateral malleolar arteries** at the ankle.
- Runs distally and ends at the ankle midway between the lateral and medial malleoli, where it becomes the dorsalis pedis artery.

H. Dorsalis Pedis Artery

- Begins anterior to the ankle joint midway between the two malleoli as the continuation of the **anterior tibial artery**.
- Descends on the dorsum of the foot between the tendons of the extensor hallucis longus and extensor digitorum longus muscles, where its **pulsation** can be felt.
- Gives rise to the **medial tarsal, lateral tarsal, arcuate**, and **first dorsal metatarsal arteries**. The **arcuate artery** gives rise to the second, third, and fourth dorsal metatarsal arteries.
- Terminates as the **deep plantar artery**, which enters the sole of the foot by passing between the two heads of the first dorsal interosseous muscle and joins the lateral plantar artery to form the **plantar arch**.
- Exhibits a pulsation that may be felt on the navicular and cuneiform bones lateral to the tendon of the flexor hallucis longus.

II. DEEP VEINS OF THE LOWER LIMB

A. Deep Veins of the Leg

- Are the venae comitantes to the anterior and posterior tibial arteries.

B. Popliteal Vein

- Ascends through the popliteal fossa behind the popliteal artery.
- Receives the small saphenous vein and those veins corresponding to the branches of the popliteal artery.

C. Femoral Vein

- Accompanies the femoral artery as a continuation of the popliteal vein through the upper two-thirds of the thigh.
- Has valves, receives tributaries corresponding to branches of the femoral artery, and is joined by the great saphenous vein, which passes through the saphenous opening.

III. DEVELOPMENT OF THE LOWER LIMB

- Is similar to development of the upper limb, except that the lower limb is somewhat behind in development due to cephalocaudal development of the embryo.
- The limb skeletons develop from **lateral plate somatic mesoderm**, while the musculature develops from ventral and dorsal condensations of somatic mesoderm **(myotomic portions of somites)**. All appendicular musculature is innervated by branches of ventral primary rami of the spinal nerves.
- The lower limb rotates along its longitudinal axis 90 degrees medially; in contrast, the upper limb rotates laterally 90 degrees. The limb rotations result in the knee facing anterior with a medial big toe versus the elbow facing posterior and the thumb on the lateral aspect of the upper limb.
- Separation of the digits occurs via apoptosis and is complete by 8 weeks in the lower limb.
- Limb joints form between developing bones in an area called the interzone. Cells in this zone will form articular cartilage and the joint capsule, while cavitation of the innermost cells forms the joint cavity.

HIGH-YIELD TOPICS

- **Pelvic girdle**—bony ring formed by the **hip bones** (ilium, ischium, and pubis) and the **sacrum** that provides a strong connection between the trunk and the lower limb.
- The **iliofemoral ligament** (that forms an inverted **Y shape**) is the strongest ligament of the hip joint and **limits hyperextension**.
- The **femoral triangle** is bounded by the **inguinal ligament**, the **sartorius**, and the **adductor longus**. Its floor is formed by the iliopsoas, pectineus and adductor longus, and the roof is formed by the fascia lata and cribriform fascia. The contents from lateral to medial are the femoral nerve, then the **femoral sheath** that contains the **femoral artery**, **vein**, and **deep lymphatics**.
- The **popliteal fossa** is bounded by the semimembranosus and semitendinosus, biceps femoris, medial and lateral heads of the gastrocnemius, and the plantaris. It contains the popliteal vessels, the common peroneal and tibial nerves, and the small saphenous vein.
- The **pes anserinus** (Latin for **"goose foot"**) is the combined tendinous expansions of the **sartorius**, **gracilis**, and **semitendinosus**, and attaches these muscles to the medial tibial condyle. The semitendinosus tendon may be used for surgical reconstruction of the anterior cruciate ligament.
- The **anterior cruciate ligament** prevents excessive **anterior translation (sliding)** of the tibia in relation to the femur and **prevents hyperextension** of the knee joint. It is taut during extension of the knee and is lax during flexion. The **posterior cruciate ligament** prevents **posterior translation** of the tibia and **limits hyperflexion** of the knee. It is taut during flexion of the knee and is lax during extension. The **patellar ligament** may be used for surgical repair of the anterior cruciate ligament, and the plantaris tendon may be used for tendon autografts to the long flexors of the fingers.
- The **medial (deltoid) ligament** of the ankle **prevents overeversion** of the foot, whereas the lateral ligament (anterior and posterior talofibular and calcaneofibular ligaments) **resists inversion** of the foot.
- The **long and short plantar** (plantar calcaneocuboid) ligaments **support the lateral** side of the **longitudinal arch** of the foot, whereas the **spring** (plantar calcaneonavicular) ligament **supports the**

head of the talus and the **medial longitudinal arch**. The spring ligament is fairly elastic, hence its name.

- **Gluteal gait** (gluteus medius limp) is a waddling gait characterized by the **pelvis falling** (or drooping) **toward the unaffected side** when the opposite leg is raised. It results from **paralysis of the gluteus medius** muscle.
- The common site for **intramuscular injection** of medications is in the **superior lateral quadrant of the gluteal region** to avoid injury to the underlying sciatic nerve and other neurovascular structures.
- **Piriformis syndrome** is a condition in which the **piriformis muscle irritates and places pressure on the sciatic nerve**, causing pain in the lower back, buttocks, and referring pain along the course of the sciatic nerve. This referred pain is called **sciatica**.
- **Positive Trendelenburg sign** is seen in the **fracture of the femoral neck**, **hip dislocation** (head of femur), or weakness **and paralysis of the gluteus medius** (abductor). If the right gluteus medius muscle is paralyzed, the left side **(sound side) of the pelvis falls (sags)** instead of rising; normally, the pelvis rises on the unsupported side.
- **Hamstring injuries** or strains (**pulled or torn hamstrings**) are very painful and common in persons who are involved in running, jumping, and quick-start sports. **Avulsion of the ischial tuberosity** (the origin of the hamstrings) may result from forcible flexion of the hip with the knee extended.
- **Femoral hernia** passes through the femoral ring and canal, and lies lateral and inferior to the pubic tubercle and deep and inferior to the inguinal ligament; its sac is formed by the parietal peritoneum. **Strangulation** of a femoral hernia may interfere with the blood supply to the herniated intestine, resulting in **death of the tissues**.
- **Groin injury** or pulled groin is a strain, stretching, or **tearing of the origin of the flexor and adductor** of the thigh and often occurs in sports that require quick starts such as a 100-m dash and football. Muscle strains of the **adductor longus** may occur in horseback riders and produce pain because the riders adduct their thighs to keep from falling from the animal.
- The **gluteus maximus** is the **strongest extensor** of the thigh at the hip and especially important when walking uphill, climbing stairs, or rising from a sitting position.
- The **iliopsoas muscle** is a **powerful flexor** of the thigh and attaches to the lesser trochanter.
- The **tensor fascia lata** and **rectus femoris** muscles can **flex the thigh at the hip joint and extend the leg at the knee**.
- The **hamstring muscles** include the **semitendinosus, semimembranosus**, and **long head of the biceps** femoris, which **extend the thigh at the hip and flex the leg at the knee**.
- The **dorsal interossei abduct** toes and flex metacarpophalangeal (MP) joints, whereas the **plantar interossei adduct** toes and flex MP joints.
- **Anterior tibial compartment syndrome** is an **ischemic necrosis** of the muscles of the **anterior compartment** of the leg, resulting from **compression of the anterior tibial artery** and its branches by swollen muscles following excessive exertion. It is accompanied by extreme tenderness and pain on the anterolateral aspect of the leg.
- **Knock-knee** (genu valgum) is a condition in which the tibia is bent or twisted laterally and the **knees are abnormally close** together. Genu valgum is normal in early childhood, but can occur with **damage to the medial collateral ligament** in adults. **Bowleg** (genu varum) is a condition in which the tibia is bent medially, resulting from **collapse of lateral collateral ligament**.
- **Shin splint** is a **painful condition** caused by swollen muscles in **the anterior compartment** of the leg **along the shin bone** (tibia), particularly the tibialis anterior muscle, following athletic overexertion. It may be a mild form of the anterior compartment syndrome.
- **Muscle cramp** is a sudden, involuntary, painful contraction of muscles. It is caused by muscle fatigue from prolonged sitting, overexertion, dehydration, and depletion or imbalance of salt and minerals (electrolytes) as well as a **poor blood supply** to leg muscles. It occurs commonly **in the calf muscle**, **hamstrings**, and **quadriceps**.
- **Patellar (knee-jerk) reflex** occurs when the **patellar ligament is tapped**, resulting in a sudden contraction of the quadriceps femoris. Its afferent and efferent impulses are transmitted in the femoral nerve (L2–L4).
- **Ankle-jerk (Achilles) reflex** is a reflex twitch of the **triceps surae** (i.e., the medial and lateral heads of the gastrocnemius and the soleus muscles) induced by **tapping the tendo calcaneus**. It causes plantar flexion of the foot. Both afferent and efferent limbs of the reflex arc are carried in the tibial nerve.

- **Damage to the obturator nerve** causes a weakness of adduction and a lateral swinging of the limb during walking because of the unopposed abductors.
- **Damage to the femoral nerve** causes impaired flexion of the hip and impaired extension of the leg resulting from **paralysis of the quadriceps femoris.**
- **Injury to the superior gluteal nerve** causes a characteristic motor loss, resulting in weakened abduction of the thigh by the gluteus medius, a disabling gluteus medius limp, and **gluteal gait.**
- **Damage to the sciatic nerve** causes impaired extension at the hip and impaired flexion at the knee, loss of dorsiflexion (foot drop) and plantar flexion at the ankle, inversion and eversion of the foot, and high-stepping gait (increased flexion) at the hip to lift the dropped foot off the ground.
- **Phantom limb pain** is intermittent or continuous pain perceived as originating in an absent **(amputated) limb.**
- **Damage to the common peroneal** (fibular) nerve may occur as a result of fracture of the head or neck of the fibula. The nerve damage results in foot drop (loss of dorsiflexion), loss of foot eversion, and loss of sensation on the dorsum of the foot and lateral aspect of the leg.
- **Damage to the superficial peroneal** (fibular) nerve results in loss of foot eversion, while damage to the deep peroneal (fibular) nerve results in foot drop (loss of dorsiflexion).
- **Damage to the tibial nerve** causes loss of plantar flexion of the foot and impaired inversion resulting from paralysis of the tibialis posterior. It results in sensory loss on the sole of the foot and can cause clawing of the toes.
- **Tarsal tunnel syndrome** results from **compression of the tibial nerve** or its medial and lateral plantar branches in the tarsal tunnel, with pain, numbness, and tingling sensations on the ankle, heel, and sole of the foot. It may be caused by repetitive stress, flat feet, or excess weight.
- The **greater saphenous vein** drains venous blood from the dorsal venous arch, ascends along the medial side of the lower limb, passes through the saphenous opening (fossa ovalis) in the fascia lata, and **joins the femoral vein**, whereas the **small saphenous vein** drains blood from the lateral dorsal venous arch, ascends the lateral leg, and **enters into the popliteal vein.**
- **Thrombophlebitis** is a venous inflammation with thrombus formation, especially **in the deep veins of the lower limb**, and can lead to **pulmonary embolism.**
- **Varicose veins** develop in the **superficial veins of the lower limb** because of reduced elasticity and incompetent valves in the veins.
- The **major blood supply to the femoral head** comes from the medial and lateral femoral circumflex arteries, and the acetabular branch of the posterior obturator artery, which runs in the round ligament of the femoral head.
- The **femoral artery** reaches the popliteal fossa, passing **through the adductor hiatus** (an aperture in the insertion tendon of the adductor magnus) to become the **popliteal artery.** The femoral artery is easily exposed and cannulated at the base of the femoral triangle.
- The **popliteal artery** gives rise to the anterior and posterior tibial arteries, and the later provides a fibular branch.
- The **sole of the foot** receives blood from the medial and lateral plantar arteries derived from the **posterior tibial artery.**
- The **medial femoral circumflex artery** is clinically important because its branches supply most of the blood **to the neck and head of the femur** except for the small proximal part that receives blood from a branch of the obturator artery.
- The **cruciate anastomosis** of the buttock is formed by a branch of **the first perforating artery**, the **inferior gluteal artery**, and the transverse branches of the **medial** and **lateral femoral circumflex arteries.** The cruciate anastomosis allows blood to bypass an obstruction of the external iliac or femoral artery.
- A **popliteal aneurysm** usually results in edema and pain in the popliteal fossa. If it is necessary to ligate the femoral artery for surgical repair, blood can bypass the occlusion through the **genicular anastomoses** and reach the popliteal artery distal to the ligation.
- The **femoral artery pulse** can be felt at the midpoint along the inguinal ligament; the **popliteal artery pulse** can sometimes be felt in the depths of the popliteal fossa; the **posterior tibial artery pulse** can be felt behind the medial malleolus and between the flexor digitorum longus and flexor hallucis longus tendons; and the **dorsalis pedis artery pulse** can be felt between the extensor hallucis longus and extensor digitorum longus tendons midway between the medial and lateral malleoli of the ankle.

- The **superficial lymph vessels** are divided into a medial group, which follows the greater saphenous vein to drain into superficial inguinal nodes, and a lateral group, which follows the small saphenous vein to the popliteal nodes. The **deep lymph vessels** follow vasculature in the muscle compartments; the leg drains via the anterior tibial, posterior tibial, and peroneal vessels to popliteal nodes, while the thigh drains to deep inguinal nodes.
- The **weight-bearing bone** of the leg is the **tibia**. The fibula is largely a bone for muscle attachment. The most common fracture in long bones is fracture of the tibial shaft.
- **The most important tarsal bones are the calcaneus** (heel bone) and the talus (which articulates with the leg bones at the ankle joint).
- **The most fractured tarsal bone is the calcaneus.**
- The weight of the body is transferred to the foot through the talus (ankle bone).
- **Fracture of the femoral head** is caused by **posterior hip dislocation** in advanced age (osteoporosis) and requires hip replacement. It presents as a shortened lower limb with medial rotation.
- **Fracture of the femoral neck** can result in **ischemic necrosis of the neck and head**. The affected lower limb is shortened with lateral rotation.
- **Pertrochanteric fracture** is a femoral fracture through the trochanters and is a form of extracapsular hip fracture, producing shortening and lateral rotation of the leg.
- A **dislocated knee or fractured distal femur** may injure the **popliteal artery** because of its deep position adjacent to the femur and the knee joint capsule.
- **Pott fracture (Dupuytren fracture)** is a **fracture of the lower end of the fibula** often accompanied by fracture of the medial malleolus or rupture of the deltoid ligament. It is caused by forced eversion of the foot.
- **Pillion fracture** is a **T-shaped fracture of the distal femur** with displacement of the condyles. It may be caused by a blow to the flexed knee of a person riding pillion on a motorcycle.
- **Fracture of the fibular neck** may cause an injury to **the common peroneal nerve**, which winds laterally around the neck of the fibula. This injury results in paralysis of all muscles in the anterior and lateral compartments of the leg (dorsiflexors and evertors of the foot), causing foot drop.
- The **talar neck fracture** causes avascular necrosis of the body of the talus, because most of the blood supply to the talus passes through the talar neck.
- **March fracture** (stress fracture) is a fatigue fracture of one of the **metatarsals**, which may result from prolonged walking. Metatarsal fractures are also **common in female ballet dancers** when the dancers lose balance and put their full body weight on the metatarsals.
- **Unhappy (O'Donoghue) triad** is the injury to the **anterior cruciate ligament**, **tibial collateral ligament**, and **medial meniscus**. However, **lateral meniscus injuries** are commonly seen among athletes.
- Drawer sign: **anterior drawer sign is a forward sliding of the tibia on the femur** due to a rupture of the **anterior cruciate ligament**, whereas **posterior drawer sign is a backward sliding of the tibia** on the femur caused by a rupture of the **posterior cruciate ligament**. The anterior cruciate ligament is injured more than the posterior cruciate ligament.
- **Prepatellar bursitis (housemaid knee)** is inflammation and swelling of the prepatellar bursa.
- Avulsion **or rupture of the Achilles tendon** disables the triceps surae (gastrocnemius and soleus) muscles; thus, the patient is **unable to plantar flex the foot**.
- **Forced eversion** of the foot avulses the **medial malleolus or ruptures the deltoid ligament**, whereas **forced inversion** avulses the lateral malleolus or **tears the lateral collateral** (anterior and posterior talofibular and calcaneofibular) ligament.
- **Ankle sprain** is stretching (or tearing) of the ankle ligaments. The weaker lateral ligament is sprained more often.
- **Flat foot** (pes planus or talipes planus) results from collapse of the **medial longitudinal arch** with eversion and abduction of the forefoot, causing greater wear on the inner border of the soles and heels of shoes. **Pes cavus** is an abnormally **high medial longitudinal arch**.
- **Club foot** (talipes equinovarus) is a condition in which the foot is plantar-flexed, inverted, and adducted. **The heel is elevated and turned medially**.
- **Bunion** is a swelling at the **medial side of the first metatarsal head** that is caused by an inflamed bursa or a bony projection and is unusually associated with hallux valgus.
- **Hallux valgus** is a **deviation of the big toe toward the lateral side** of the foot. **Hallux varus** is a **deviation of the big toe toward the medial side** of the foot.

- **Claudication** (intermittent) is **limping** caused by ischemia of the muscles, **chiefly in the calf muscles.**
- **Gout** is a joint inflammation from **deposition of urate in a synovial cavity**, resulting from abnormalities of purine metabolism. The most common location for gout is the **metatarsophalangeal joint** of the great toe.
- **Foot drop** is weakened dorsiflexion due to **common or deep peroneal nerve lesion.**
- The **lower limb rotates in utero medially 90 degree**, while the **upper limb** rotates **laterally** 90 degree. Thus, the limbs are 180 degree out of phase with one another (knee anterior and big toe medial versus elbow posterior and thumb lateral).

Summary

MUSCLE ACTIONS OF THE LOWER LIMB

Movements at the Hip Joint (Ball-and-Socket Joint)

Flexion—iliopsoas, tensor fasciae latae, rectus femoris, adductors, sartorius, pectineus, gracilis

Extension—hamstrings, gluteus maximus, adductor magnus

Adduction—adductor magnus, adductor longus, adductor brevis, pectineus, gracilis

Abduction—gluteus medius, gluteus minimus

Medial rotation—tensor fasciae latae, gluteus medius, gluteus minimus

Lateral rotation—obturator internus, obturator externus, gemelli, piriformis, quadratus femoris, gluteus maximus

Movements at the Knee Joint (Hinge Joint)

Flexion—hamstrings, gracilis, sartorius, gastrocnemius, popliteus

Extension—quadriceps femoris

Medial rotation—semitendinosus, semimembranosus, popliteus

Lateral rotation—biceps femoris

Movements at the Ankle Joint (Hinge Joint)

Dorsiflexion—anterior tibialis, extensor digitorum longus, extensor hallucis longus, peroneus tertius

Plantar flexion—triceps surae, plantaris, posterior tibialis, peroneus longus and brevis, flexor digitorum longus, flexor hallucis longus (when the knee is fully flexed)

Movements at the Intertarsal Joint (Talocalcaneal, Transverse Tarsal Joint)

Inversion—tibialis posterior, tibialis anterior, triceps surae, extensor hallucis longus

Eversion—peroneus longus, brevis, and tertius, extensor digitorum longus

Movements at the Metatarsophalangeal Joint (Ellipsoid Joint)

Flexion—lumbricals, interossei, flexor hallucis brevis, flexor digiti minimi brevis

Extension—extensor digitorum longus and brevis, extensor hallucis longus

Movements at the Interphalangeal Joint (Hinge Joint)

Flexion—flexor digitorum longus and brevis, flexor hallucis longus

Extension—extensor digitorum longus and brevis, extensor hallucis longus

MUSCLE INNERVATIONS OF THE LOWER LIMB

Muscles of the Gluteal Region

Gluteus maximus (inferior gluteal nerve)

Gluteus medius (superior gluteal nerve)

Gluteus minimus (superior gluteal nerve)

Tensor fasciae latae (superior gluteal nerve)

Piriformis (nerve to piriformis)

Obturator internus (nerve to obturator internus)

Superior gemellus (nerve to obturator internus)
Inferior gemellus (nerve to quadratus femoris)
Quadratus femoris (nerve to quadratus femoris)

Muscles of the Thigh

Muscles of the Anterior Compartment: Femoral Nerve

Sartorius, quadriceps femoris, rectus femoris, vastus medialis, vastus intermedius, vastus lateralis

Muscles of the Medial Compartment: Obturator Nerve

Adductor longus, adductor brevis, adductor magnus (obturator and tibial nerves),* gracilis, obturator externus, pectineus (femoral and obturator nerves)*

Muscles of the Posterior Compartment: Tibial Part of Sciatic Nerve

Semitendinosus; semimembranosus; biceps femoris, long head; biceps femoris, short head (common peroneal part of sciatic nerve)*; adductor magnus (tibial part of sciatic and obturator nerve)*

Muscles of the Leg

Muscles of the Anterior Compartment: Deep Peroneal Nerve

Tibialis anterior, extensor digitorum longus, extensor hallucis longus, peroneus tertius

Muscles of the Lateral Compartment: Superficial Peroneal Nerve

Peroneus longus, peroneus brevis

Muscles of the Posterior Compartment: Tibial Nerve

Superficial layer—gastrocnemius, soleus, plantaris

Deep layer—popliteus, tibialis posterior, flexor digitorum longus, flexor hallucis longus

Muscles of the Foot

Muscles of the Anterior Compartment (Dorsum): Deep Peroneal Nerve

Extensor digitorum brevis, extensor hallucis brevis

Muscles of the Plantar Compartment (Sole): Medial and Lateral Plantar Nerves

Flexor digitorum brevis, abductor hallucis, flexor hallucis brevis, first lumbrical (medial plantar nerve)

Quadratus plantae, abductor digiti minimi, lateral three lumbricals, adductor hallucis, flexor digiti minimi brevis, plantar interossei, dorsal interossei (lateral plantar nerve)

*Indicates exception.

Review Test

Directions: Each of the numbered items or incomplete statements in this section is followed by answers or by completions of the statement. Select the **one**-lettered answer or completion that is **best** in each case.

1. A 27-year-old patient exhibits a loss of skin sensation and paralysis of muscles on the plantar aspect of the medial side of the foot. Which of the following nerves is most likely damaged?

(A) Common peroneal
(B) Tibial
(C) Superficial peroneal
(D) Deep peroneal
(E) Sural

2. A patient with a deep knife wound in the buttock walks with a waddling gait that is characterized by the pelvis falling toward one side at each step. Which of the following nerves is damaged?

(A) Obturator nerve
(B) Nerve to obturator internus
(C) Superior gluteal nerve
(D) Inferior gluteal nerve
(E) Femoral nerve

3. A patient is unable to prevent anterior displacement of the femur on the tibia when the knee is flexed. Which of the following ligaments is most likely damaged?

(A) Anterior cruciate
(B) Fibular collateral
(C) Patellar
(D) Posterior cruciate
(E) Tibial collateral

4. A 41-year-old man was involved in a fight and felt weakness in extending the knee joint. On examination, he was diagnosed with a lesion of the femoral nerve. Which of the following symptoms would be a result of this nerve damage?

(A) Paralysis of the psoas major muscle
(B) Loss of skin sensation on the lateral side of the foot
(C) Loss of skin sensation over the greater trochanter
(D) Paralysis of the vastus lateralis muscle
(E) Paralysis of the tensor fasciae latae

5. A 47-year-old woman is unable to invert her foot after she stumbled on her driveway. Which of the following nerves are most likely injured?

(A) Superficial and deep peroneal
(B) Deep peroneal and tibial
(C) Superficial peroneal and tibial
(D) Medial and lateral plantar
(E) Obturator and tibial

6. A 22-year-old patient is unable to "unlock" the knee joint to permit flexion of the leg. Which of the following muscles is most likely damaged?

(A) Rectus femoris
(B) Semimembranosus
(C) Popliteus
(D) Gastrocnemius
(E) Biceps femoris

7. A patient presents with sensory loss on adjacent sides of the great and second toes and impaired dorsiflexion of the foot. These signs probably indicate damage to which of the following nerves?

(A) Superficial peroneal
(B) Lateral plantar
(C) Deep peroneal
(D) Sural
(E) Tibial

8. A motorcyclist falls from his bike in an accident and gets a deep gash that severs the superficial peroneal nerve near its origin. Which of the following muscles is paralyzed?

(A) Peroneus longus
(B) Extensor hallucis longus
(C) Extensor digitorum longus
(D) Peroneus tertius
(E) Extensor digitorum brevis

9. A 67-year-old patient has been given a course of antibiotics by gluteal intramuscular injections after a major abdominal surgery. To avoid damaging the sciatic nerve during an injection, the needle should be inserted into which of the following areas?

(A) Over the sacrospinous ligament
(B) Midway between the ischial tuberosity and the lesser trochanter
(C) Midpoint of the gemelli muscles
(D) Upper lateral quadrant of the gluteal region
(E) Lower medial quadrant of the gluteal region

10. A 20-year-old patient cannot flex and medially rotate the thigh while running and climbing. Which of the following muscles is most likely damaged?

(A) Semimembranosus
(B) Sartorius
(C) Rectus femoris
(D) Vastus intermedius
(E) Tensor fasciae latae

11. A 21-year-old man was involved in a motorcycle accident, resulting in destruction of the groove in the lower surface of the cuboid bone. Which of the following muscle tendons is most likely damaged?

(A) Flexor hallucis longus
(B) Peroneus brevis
(C) Peroneus longus
(D) Tibialis anterior
(E) Tibialis posterior

12. A construction worker falls feet first from a roof. He sustains a fracture of the groove on the undersurface of the sustentaculum tali of the calcaneus bone. Which of the following muscle tendons is most likely torn?

(A) Flexor digitorum brevis
(B) Flexor digitorum longus
(C) Flexor hallucis brevis
(D) Flexor hallucis longus
(E) Tibialis posterior

13. A thoracic surgeon is going to collect a portion of the greater saphenous vein for coronary bypass surgery. He has observed that this vein runs

(A) Posterior to the medial malleolus
(B) Into the popliteal vein
(C) Anterior to the medial condyles of the tibia and femur
(D) Superficial to the fascia lata of the thigh
(E) Along with the femoral artery

14. A 52-year-old woman slipped and fell and now complains of being unable to extend her leg at the knee joint. Which of the following muscles was paralyzed as a result of this accident?

(A) Semitendinosus
(B) Sartorius
(C) Gracilis
(D) Quadriceps femoris
(E) Biceps femoris

15. A patient experiences weakness in dorsiflexing and inverting the foot. Which of the following muscles is damaged?

(A) Peroneus longus
(B) Peroneus brevis
(C) Tibialis anterior
(D) Extensor digitorum longus
(E) Peroneus tertius

Questions 16 to 20: A 62-year-old woman slips and falls on the bathroom floor. As a result, she has a posterior dislocation of the hip joint and a fracture of the neck of the femur.

16. Rupture of the ligamentum teres capitis femoris may lead to damage to a branch of which of the following arteries?

(A) Medial circumflex femoral
(B) Lateral circumflex femoral
(C) Obturator
(D) Superior gluteal
(E) Inferior gluteal

17. Fracture of the neck of the femur results in avascular necrosis of the femoral head, probably resulting from lack of blood supply from which of the following arteries?

(A) Obturator
(B) Superior gluteal
(C) Inferior gluteal
(D) Medial femoral circumflex
(E) Lateral femoral circumflex

18. If the acetabulum is fractured at its posterosuperior margin by dislocation of the hip joint, which of the following bones could be involved?

(A) Pubis
(B) Ischium
(C) Ilium
(D) Sacrum
(E) Head of the femur

19. The woman experiences weakness when abducting and medially rotating the thigh after this accident. Which of the following muscles is most likely damaged?

(A) Piriformis
(B) Obturator internus
(C) Quadratus femoris
(D) Gluteus maximus
(E) Gluteus minimus

20. The woman undergoes hip surgery. If all of the arteries that are part of the cruciate anastomosis of the upper thigh are ligated, which of the following arteries maintains blood flow?

(A) Medial femoral circumflex
(B) Lateral femoral circumflex
(C) Superior gluteal
(D) Inferior gluteal
(E) First perforating

21. A 34-year-old woman sustains a deep cut on the dorsum of the foot just distal to her ankle joint by a falling kitchen knife. A physician in the emergency department has ligated the dorsalis pedis artery proximal to the injured area. Which of the following conditions most likely occurs as a result of the injury?

(A) Ischemia in the peroneus longus muscle
(B) Aneurysm in the plantar arterial arch
(C) Reduction of blood flow in the medial tarsal artery
(D) Low blood pressure in the anterior tibial artery
(E) High blood pressure in the arcuate artery

22. A patient experiences paralysis of the muscle that originates from the femur and contributes directly to the stability of the knee joint. Which of the following muscles is involved?

(A) Vastus lateralis
(B) Semimembranosus
(C) Sartorius
(D) Biceps femoris (long head)
(E) Rectus femoris

23. A patient is involved in a motorcycle wreck that results in avulsion of the skin over the anterolateral leg and ankle. Which of the following structures is most likely destroyed with this type of injury?

(A) Deep peroneal nerve
(B) Extensor digitorum longus muscle tendon
(C) Dorsalis pedis artery
(D) Great saphenous vein
(E) Superficial peroneal nerve

24. A knife wound penetrates the superficial vein that terminates in the popliteal vein. Bleeding occurs from which of the following vessels?

(A) Posterior tibial vein
(B) Anterior tibial vein
(C) Peroneal vein
(D) Great saphenous vein
(E) Lesser saphenous vein

25. A 10-year-old boy falls from a tree house. The resultant heavy compression of the sole of his foot against the ground caused a fracture of the head of the talus. Which of the following structures is unable to function normally?

(A) Transverse arch
(B) Medial longitudinal arch
(C) Lateral longitudinal arch
(D) Tendon of the peroneus longus
(E) Long plantar ligament

26. A 24-year-old woman complains of weakness when she extends her thigh and rotates it laterally. Which of the following muscles is paralyzed?

(A) Obturator externus
(B) Sartorius
(C) Tensor fasciae latae
(D) Gluteus maximus
(E) Semitendinosus

27. A patient with hereditary blood clotting problems presents with pain in the back of her knee. An arteriograph reveals a blood clot in the popliteal artery at its proximal end. Which of the following arteries will allow blood to reach the foot?

(A) Anterior tibial
(B) Posterior tibial
(C) Peroneal
(D) Lateral circumflex femoral
(E) Superior medial genicular

28. A 72-year-old woman complains of a cramplike pain in her thigh and leg. She was diagnosed as having a severe intermittent claudication. Following surgery, an infection was found in the adductor canal, damaging the enclosed structures. Which of the following structures remains intact?

(A) Femoral artery
(B) Femoral vein
(C) Saphenous nerve
(D) Great saphenous vein
(E) Nerve to the vastus medialis

29. A basketball player was hit in the thigh by an opponent's knee. Which of the following arteries is likely to compress and cause ischemia because of the bruise and damage to the extensor muscles of the leg?

(A) Popliteal
(B) Deep femoral
(C) Anterior tibial
(D) Posterior tibial
(E) Peroneal

30. An elderly woman fell at home and fractured the greater trochanter of her femur. Which of the following muscles would continue to function normally?

(A) Piriformis
(B) Obturator internus
(C) Gluteus medius
(D) Gluteus maximus
(E) Gluteus minimus

Questions 31 to 35: A 20-year-old college student receives a severe blow on the inferolateral side of the left knee joint while playing football. Radiographic examination reveals a fracture of the head and neck of the fibula.

31. Which of the following nerves is damaged?

(A) Sciatic
(B) Tibial
(C) Common peroneal
(D) Deep peroneal
(E) Superficial peroneal

32. After injury to this nerve, which of the following muscles could be paralyzed?

(A) Gastrocnemius
(B) Popliteus
(C) Extensor hallucis longus
(D) Flexor digitorum longus
(E) Tibialis posterior

33. If the lateral (fibular) collateral ligament is torn by this fracture, which of the following conditions may occur?

(A) Abnormal passive abduction of the extended leg
(B) Abnormal passive adduction of the extended leg
(C) Anterior displacement of the femur on the tibia
(D) Posterior displacement of the femur on the tibia
(E) Maximal flexion of the leg

34. Which of the following arteries could also be damaged by this fracture?

(A) Popliteal
(B) Posterior tibial
(C) Anterior tibial
(D) Peroneal
(E) Lateral inferior genicular

35. Which of the following conditions would occur from this fracture?

(A) Ischemia in the gastrocnemius
(B) Loss of plantar flexion
(C) Trendelenburg sign
(D) Anterior tibial compartment syndrome
(E) Flat foot

36. A construction worker is hit on the leg with a concrete block and is subsequently unable to plantar flex and invert his foot. Which of the following muscles is most likely damaged?

(A) Extensor digitorum longus
(B) Tibialis anterior
(C) Tibialis posterior
(D) Peroneus longus
(E) Peroneus brevis

37. The obturator nerve and the sciatic (tibial portion) nerve of a 15-year-old boy are transected as a result of a motorcycle accident. This injury would result in complete paralysis of which of the following muscles?

(A) Rectus femoris
(B) Biceps femoris, short head
(C) Pectineus
(D) Adductor magnus
(E) Sartorius

38. A 24-year-old woman presents to her physician with weakness in flexing the hip joint and extending the knee joint. Which muscle is most likely involved in this scenario?

(A) Sartorius
(B) Gracilis
(C) Rectus femoris
(D) Vastus medialis
(E) Semimembranosus

39. A 17-year-old boy was stabbed during a gang fight, resulting in the transection of the obturator nerve. Which of the following muscles is completely paralyzed?

(A) Pectineus
(B) Adductor magnus
(C) Adductor longus
(D) Biceps femoris
(E) Semimembranosus

40. A 32-year-old carpenter fell from the roof. The lateral longitudinal arch of his foot was flattened from fracture and displacement of the keystone for the arch. Which of the following bones is damaged?

(A) Calcaneus
(B) Cuboid bone
(C) Head of the talus
(D) Medial cuneiform
(E) Navicular bone

41. While playing football, a 19-year-old college student receives a twisting injury to his knee when being tackled from the lateral side. Which of the following conditions most likely has occurred?

(A) Tear of the medial meniscus
(B) Ruptured fibular collateral ligament
(C) Tenderness on pressure along the fibular collateral ligament
(D) Injury of the posterior cruciate ligament
(E) Swelling on the back of the knee joint

42. A patient has weakness when flexing both her thigh and leg. Which of the following muscles is most likely injured?

(A) Rectus femoris
(B) Semitendinosus
(C) Biceps femoris
(D) Sartorius
(E) Adductor longus

43. A 35-year-old man has difficulty in dorsiflexing the foot. Which of the following muscles is most likely damaged?

(A) Tibialis posterior
(B) Flexor digitorum longus
(C) Tibialis anterior
(D) Peroneus longus
(E) Peroneus brevis

44. An injury to the leg of a golfer results in loss of the ability to invert the foot. Which of the following muscles is most likely paralyzed?

(A) Tibialis posterior
(B) Peroneus longus
(C) Peroneus brevis
(D) Peroneus tertius
(E) Extensor digitorum longus

45. An orthopedic surgeon ligates the posterior tibial artery at its origin. Which of the following arteries has no blood flow immediately after the ligation?

(A) Peroneal
(B) Dorsalis pedis
(C) Superior medial genicular
(D) Anterior tibial
(E) Descending genicular

46. Before knee surgery, a surgeon ligates arteries participating in the anastomosis around the knee joint. Which of the following arteries is most likely spared?

(A) Lateral superior genicular
(B) Medial inferior genicular
(C) Descending branch of the lateral femoral circumflex
(D) Saphenous branch of the descending genicular
(E) Anterior tibial recurrent

47. A 25-year-old gladiator sustains a penetrating injury that severs the superficial peroneal nerve. This will most likely cause paralysis of which of the following muscles?

(A) Peroneus tertius
(B) Peroneus brevis
(C) Flexor hallucis longus
(D) Tibialis anterior
(E) Tibialis posterior

48. A patient presents with a thrombosis in the popliteal vein. This thrombosis most likely causes reduction of blood flow in which of the following veins?

(A) Greater saphenous
(B) Lesser saphenous
(C) Femoral
(D) Posterior tibial
(E) Anterior tibial

49. A 21-year-old tennis player comes to an emergency room and complains of pain in the knee joint. On examination, he has an infection inside the knee joint capsule but outside the synovial cavity. Which of the following structures is preserved from this infection?

(A) Anterior cruciate ligament
(B) Posterior cruciate ligament
(C) Lateral meniscus
(D) Lateral collateral ligament
(E) Medial meniscus

50. A 14-year-old gymnastic silver medalist falls from the parallel bar and complains of pains from the knee and ankle joints. On physical examination, her physician found that the muscle responsible for flexing the leg at the knee joint and plantar flexing the foot is severely weakened. Which of the following muscles involved in both movements was most likely damaged in this accident?

(A) Tibialis posterior
(B) Gastrocnemius
(C) Soleus
(D) Peroneus longus
(E) Flexor digitorum longus

51. A 28-year-old basketball player falls while rebounding and is unable to run and jump. On physical examination, he has pain and weakness when extending his thigh and flexing his leg. Which muscle involved in both movements is most likely injured?

(A) Short head of biceps femoris
(B) Adductor magnus
(C) Semitendinosus
(D) Sartorius
(E) Gracilis

52. A 52-year-old woman comes to an orthopedic surgeon complaining of an uncomfortable feeling in her knee and ankle joints. After a thorough examination, she is diagnosed as having arthritis with mild discomfort with passive movements. The muscles acting at the ankle joint appear normal with good strength. Which muscle can both dorsiflex and invert her foot?

(A) Peroneus longus
(B) Peroneus brevis
(C) Peroneus tertius
(D) Extensor hallucis longus
(E) Extensor digitorum longus

Questions 53 to 56: Choose the appropriate lettered site or structure in the following radiographs of the knee joint (see Figure below) to match the following descriptions.

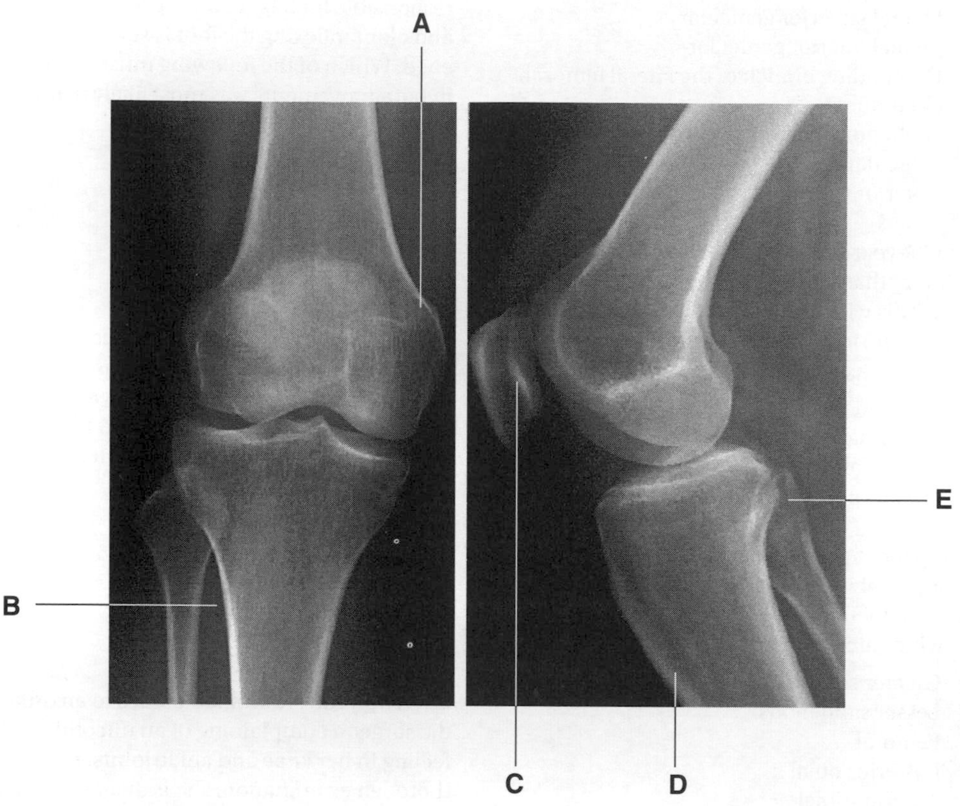

53. Rupture of the tendon superior to this structure would most likely cause an inability to extend the knee joint.

54. Fracture of this structure would most likely cause weakness in adduction, flexion, and extension of the thigh.

55. A knife penetrating through this point would most likely cause muscle ischemia in the anterior compartment of the leg.

56. Fracture of this structure would most likely cause a lesion of the common peroneal nerve, resulting in paralysis of the muscles in the anterior and lateral compartments of the leg.

Questions 57 to 60: Choose the appropriate lettered site or structure in the radiograph of the hip and pelvis (see Figure below) to match the following descriptions.

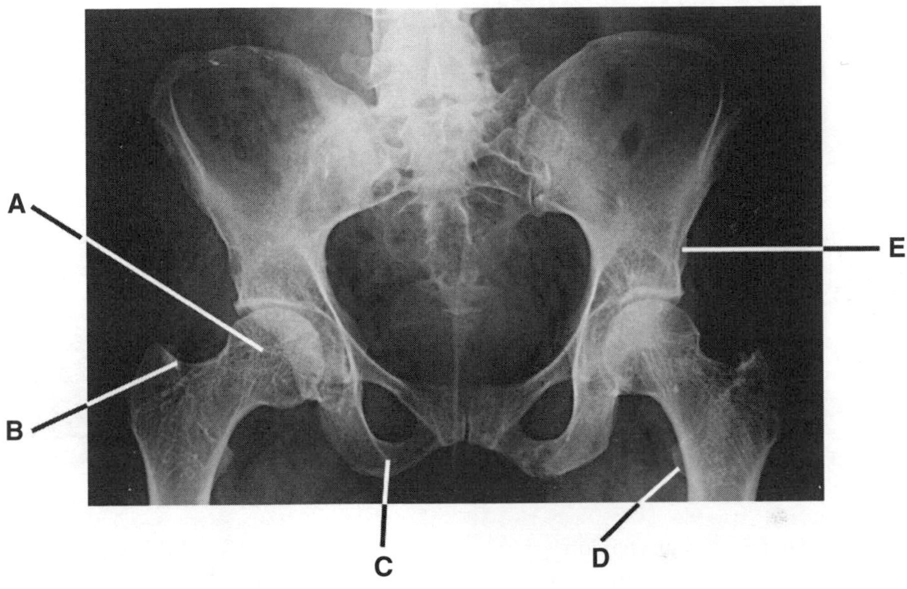

57. Which structure in this radiograph may be fractured, resulting in loss of the chief flexor of the thigh?

58. Fracture of which structure may destroy the site of insertion of the muscle that can rotate the thigh laterally and its tendon that passes through the lesser sciatic foramen?

59. Which fractured structure is likely to cause paralysis of the adductor magnus?

60. Which structure becomes necrotic after the medial femoral circumflex artery is severed?

Questions 61 to 64: Choose the appropriate lettered site or structure in the following radiograph of the ankle and foot (see Figure below) to match the following descriptions.

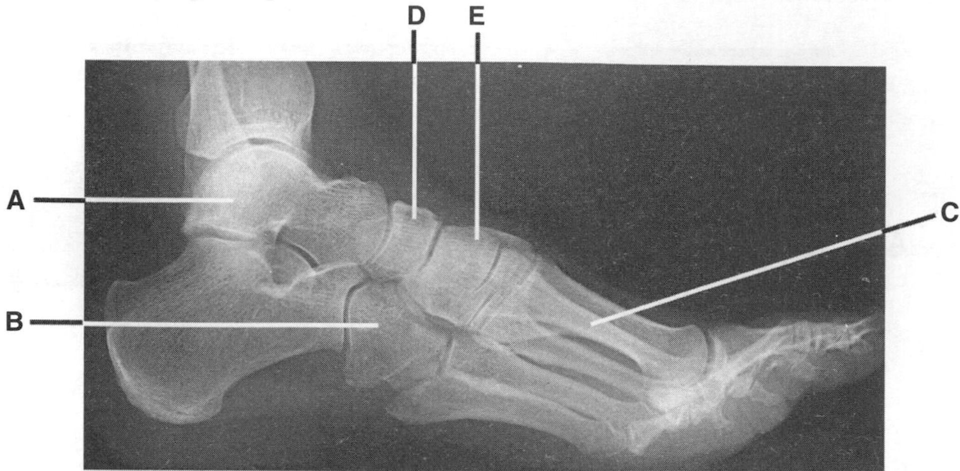

61. The flexor hallucis longus tendon is damaged in a groove on the posterior surface of a tarsal bone. Which bone in the radiograph is likely fractured?

62. The tibialis anterior and peroneus longus muscles are weakened. Which bone in the radiograph is most likely fractured?

63. The medial longitudinal arch of the foot is flattened because the spring ligament is torn. Which bone in the radiograph is most likely fractured?

64. The peroneus longus muscle tendon is damaged in a groove of a tarsal bone by fracture. Which bone in the radiograph is most likely fractured?

Answers and Explanations

1. **The Answer is B.** The common peroneal nerve divides into the deep peroneal nerve, which innervates the anterior muscles of the leg and supplies the adjacent skin of the first and second toes, and the superficial peroneal nerve, which innervates the lateral muscles of the leg and supplies the skin on the side of the lower leg and the dorsum of the ankle and foot. The sural nerve supplies the lateral aspect of the foot and the little toe.

2. **The Answer is C.** The superior gluteal nerve innervates the gluteus medius muscle. Paralysis of this muscle causes gluteal gait, a waddling gait characterized by a falling of the pelvis toward the unaffected side at each step. The gluteus medius muscle normally functions to stabilize the pelvis when the opposite foot is off the ground. The inferior gluteal nerve innervates the gluteus maximus, and the nerve to the obturator internus supplies the obturator internus and superior gemellus muscles. The obturator nerve innervates the adductor muscles of the thigh, and the femoral nerve supplies the flexors of the thigh.

3. **The Answer is D.** The posterior cruciate ligament is important because it prevents forward displacement of the femur on the tibia when the knee is flexed. The anterior cruciate ligament prevents backward displacement of the femur on the tibia.

4. **The answer is D.** The femoral nerve innervates the quadratus femoris, sartorius, and vastus muscles. Therefore, damage to this nerve results in paralysis of these muscles. The second and third lumbar nerves innervate the psoas major muscle, the sural nerve innervates the skin on the lateral side of the foot, the iliohypogastric nerve and superior cluneal nerves supply the skin over the greater trochanter, and the superior gluteal nerve innervates the tensor fasciae latae.

5. **The Answer is B.** The deep peroneal and tibial nerves innervate the chief evertors of the foot, which are the tibialis anterior, tibialis posterior, triceps surae, and extensor hallucis longus muscles. The tibialis anterior and extensor hallucis longus muscles are innervated by the deep peroneal nerve, and the tibialis posterior and triceps surae are innervated by the tibial nerve.

6. **The Answer is C.** The popliteus muscle rotates the femur laterally ("unlocks" the knee) or rotates the tibia medially, depending on which bone is fixed. This action results in unlocking of the knee joint to initiate flexion of the leg at the joint. The rectus femoris flexes the thigh and extends the knee. The gastrocnemius flexes the knee and plantar flexes the foot. The semimembranosus extends the thigh and flexes and rotates the leg medially. The biceps femoris extends the thigh and flexes and rotates the leg laterally.

7. **The Answer is C.** The deep peroneal nerve supplies the anterior muscles of the leg, including the tibialis anterior, extensor hallucis longus, extensor digitorum longus, and peroneus tertius muscles, which dorsiflex the foot. The medial branch of the deep peroneal nerve supplies the skin of adjacent sides of the great and second toes, whereas the lateral branch supplies the extensor digitorum brevis and extensor hallucis brevis. The superficial peroneal nerve innervates the peroneus longus and brevis, which plantar flexes the foot, and supplies the skin on the side of the lower leg and the dorsum of the ankle and foot. The tibial nerve innervates the muscles of the posterior compartment that plantar flexes and supplies the skin on the heel and plantar aspect of the foot. The lateral plantar nerve innervates muscles and skin of the lateral plantar aspect of the foot. The sural nerve supplies the skin on the posterolateral aspect of the leg and the lateral aspect of the foot and the little toe.

8. **The Answer is A.** The superficial peroneal nerve supplies the peroneus longus and brevis muscles. Other muscles are innervated by the deep peroneal nerve.

9. **The Answer is D.** To avoid damaging the sciatic nerve during an intramuscular injection, the clinician should insert the needle in the upper lateral quadrant of the gluteal region.

The inserted needle in the lower medial quadrant may damage the pudendal and sciatic nerves. The inserted needle midway between the ischial tuberosity and the lesser trochanter may damage the sciatic and posterior femoral cutaneous nerves on the quadratus femoris. The inserted needle over the sacrospinous ligament may damage the pudendal nerve and vessels.

10. **The Answer is E.** The tensor fasciae latae can flex and medially rotate the thigh, so this is the muscle most likely damaged. The hamstring muscles (semitendinosus, semimembranosus, and biceps femoris) can extend the thigh and flex the leg. The sartorius can flex the thigh and leg. The rectus femoris can flex the thigh and extend the leg. The vastus intermedius can extend the leg.

11. **The Answer is C.** The groove in the lower surface of the cuboid bone is occupied by the tendon of the peroneus longus muscle. The flexor hallucis longus tendon occupies a groove on the posterior surface of the body of the talus and a groove on the inferior surface of the calcaneus during its course. The tibialis posterior muscle tendon occupies the medial malleolar groove of the tibia. Other muscle tendons are not in the groove of the tarsal bones.

12. **The Answer is D.** The tendon of the flexor hallucis longus muscle occupies first the groove on the posterior surface of the talus and then the groove on the undersurface of the sustentaculum tali. None of the other tendons would have been affected in such an injury.

13. **The Answer is D.** The greater saphenous vein ascends superficial to the fascia lata. It courses anterior to the medial malleolus and posterior to the medial condyles of the tibia and femur and terminates in the femoral vein by passing through the saphenous opening. The small saphenous vein drains into the popliteal vein. The greater saphenous vein does not run along with the femoral artery.

14. **The Answer is D.** The quadriceps femoris muscle includes the rectus femoris muscle and the vastus medialis, intermedialis, and lateralis muscles. They extend the leg at the knee joint. The semitendinosus, semimembranosus, and biceps femoris muscles (the hamstrings) extend the thigh and flex the leg. The sartorius and gracilis muscles can flex the thigh and the leg.

15. **The Answer is C.** The tibialis anterior can dorsiflex and invert the foot. The peroneus longus and brevis muscles can plantar flex and evert the foot, the peroneus tertius can dorsiflex and evert the foot, and the extensor digitorum longus can dorsiflex the foot and extend the toes.

16. **The Answer is C.** The obturator artery gives rise to an acetabular branch that runs in the round ligament of the head of the femur.

17. **The Answer is D.** In adults, the chief arterial supply to the head of the femur is from the branches of the medial femoral circumflex artery. The lateral femoral circumflex artery may supply the femoral head by anastomosing with the medial femoral circumflex artery. The posterior branch of the obturator artery gives rise to the artery of the head of the femur, which runs in the round ligament of the femoral head and is usually insufficient to supply the head of the femur in adults but is an important source of blood to the femoral head in children. The superior and inferior gluteal arteries do not supply the head of the femur.

18. **The Answer is C.** The acetabulum is a cup-shaped cavity on the lateral side of the hip bone and is formed superiorly by the ilium, posteroinferiorly by the ischium, and anteromedially by the pubis. The sacrum and the head of the femur do not participate in the formation of the acetabulum.

19. **The Answer is E.** The gluteus medius or minimus abducts and rotates the thigh medially. The piriformis, obturator internus, quadratus femoris, and gluteus maximus muscles can rotate the thigh laterally.

20. **The Answer is C.** The superior gluteal artery does not participate in the cruciate anastomosis of the thigh. The inferior gluteal artery, transverse branches of the medial and lateral femoral circumflex arteries, and an ascending branch of the first perforating artery form the cruciate anastomosis of the thigh.

21. **The Answer is C.** Reduction of blood flow in the medial tarsal artery occurs because it is a branch of the dorsalis pedis artery, which begins at the ankle joint as the continuation of the anterior tibial artery. The anterior tibial and peroneal arteries supply the peroneus longus muscle. The deep plantar arterial arch is formed mainly by the lateral plantar artery. Blood pressure in the anterior tibial artery should be higher than normal. The arcuate artery should have a low blood pressure because it is a terminal branch of the dorsalis pedis artery.

22. **The Answer is A.** The vastus lateralis muscles arise from the femur and all the other muscles originate from the hip (coxal) bone. The biceps femoris inserts on the fibula, and other muscles insert on the tibia; thus, all of them contribute to the stability of the knee joint.

23. **The Answer is E.** The superficial peroneal nerve emerges between the peroneus longus and peroneus brevis muscles and descends superficial to the extensor retinaculum of the ankle on the anterolateral side of the leg and ankle, innervating the skin of the lower leg and foot. The great saphenous vein begins at the medial end of the dorsal venous arch of the foot and ascends in front of the medial malleolus and along the medial side of the tibia along with the saphenous nerve. Other structures pass deep to the extensor retinaculum.

24. **The Answer is E.** The lesser (small) saphenous vein ascends on the back of the leg in company with the sural nerve and terminates in the popliteal vein. The peroneal vein empties into the posterior tibial vein. The anterior and posterior tibial veins are deep veins and join to form the popliteal vein. The great saphenous vein drains into the femoral vein.

25. **The Answer is B.** The keystone of the medial longitudinal arch of the foot is the head of the talus, which is located at the summit between the sustentaculum tali and the navicular bone. The medial longitudinal arch is supported by the spring ligament and the tendon of the flexor hallucis longus muscle. The cuboid bone serves as the keystone of the lateral longitudinal arch, which is supported by the peroneus longus tendon and the long and short plantar ligaments. The transverse arch is formed by the navicular, the three cuneiform, the cuboid, and the five metatarsal bones and is supported by the peroneus longus tendon and the transverse head of the adductor hallucis.

26. **The Answer is D.** The gluteus maximus can extend and rotate the thigh laterally. The obturator externus rotates the thigh laterally. The sartorius can flex both the hip and knee joints. The tensor fasciae latae can flex and medially rotate the thigh. The semitendinosus can extend the thigh and medially rotate the leg.

27. **The Answer is D.** If the proximal end of the popliteal artery is blocked, blood may reach the foot by way of the descending branch of the lateral circumflex femoral artery, which participates in the anastomosis around the knee joint. Other blood vessels are direct or indirect branches of the popliteal artery.

28. **The Answer is D.** The great saphenous nerve remains intact because it is not in the adductor canal. The adductor canal contains the femoral vessels, the saphenous nerve, and the nerve to the vastus medialis.

29. **The Answer is C.** A muscular spasm or hypertrophy of the extensor muscles of the leg may compress the anterior tibial artery, causing ischemia. The popliteal artery supplies muscles of the popliteal fossa. The deep femoral artery supplies deep muscles of the thigh. The posterior tibial and peroneal arteries supply muscles of the posterior and lateral compartments of the leg.

30. **The Answer is D.** The gluteus maximus is inserted into the gluteal tuberosity of the femur and the iliotibial tract. All of the other muscles insert on the greater trochanter of the femur, and their functions are impaired.

31. **The Answer is C.** The common peroneal nerve is vulnerable to injury as it passes behind the head of the fibula and then winds around the neck of the fibula and pierces the peroneus longus muscle, where it divides into the deep and superficial peroneal nerves. In addition, the deep and superficial peroneal nerves pass superficial to the neck of the fibula in the substance of the peroneus longus muscle and are less susceptible to injury than the common peroneal nerve. Other nerves are not closely associated with the head and neck of the fibula.

32. **The Answer is C.** The extensor hallucis longus is innervated by the deep peroneal nerve, whereas other muscles are innervated by the posterior tibial nerve.

33. **The Answer is B.** The lateral (fibular) collateral ligament prevents adduction at the knee. Therefore, a torn lateral collateral ligament can be recognized by abnormal passive adduction of the extended leg. Abnormal passive abduction of the extended leg may occur when the medial (tibial) collateral ligament is torn. The anterior cruciate ligament prevents posterior displacement of the femur on the tibia; the posterior cruciate ligament prevents anterior displacement of the femur on the tibia. In addition, the posterior cruciate ligament is taut when the knee is fully flexed.

34. **The Answer is C.** The anterior tibial artery, which arises from the popliteal artery, enters the anterior compartment by passing through the gap between the fibula and tibia at the upper end of the interosseous membrane. The other arteries would not be affected because they are not closely associated with the head and neck of the fibula.

35. **The Answer is D.** Anterior tibial compartment syndrome is characterized by ischemic necrosis of the muscles of the anterior tibial compartment of the leg resulting from damage to the anterior tibial artery. The gastrocnemius receives blood from sural branches of the popliteal artery. Loss of plantar flexion is due to necrosis of the posterior muscles of the leg, which are supplied by the posterior tibial and peroneal arteries. Trendelenburg sign is caused by weakness or paralysis of the gluteus medius and minimus muscles. Flat foot results from the collapse of the medial longitudinal arch of the foot.

36. **The Answer is C.** The tibialis posterior can plantar flex and invert the foot. The extensor digitorum longus can dorsiflex and evert the foot, the tibialis anterior can dorsiflex and invert the foot, and the peroneus longus and brevis can plantar flex and evert the foot.

37. **The Answer is D.** The adductor magnus is innervated by both the obturator and sciatic (tibial portion) nerves. Hence, a lesion here could cause paralysis. The rectus femoris and sartorius are innervated by the femoral nerve. The biceps femoris long head is innervated by the tibial portion of the sciatic nerve, whereas the short head is innervated by the common peroneal portion of the sciatic nerve. The pectineus is innervated by both the femoral and obturator nerves.

38. **The Answer is C.** The rectus femoris flexes the thigh and extends the leg. The sartorius can flex both the hip and knee joints. The gracilis adducts and flexes the thigh and flexes the leg, the vastus medialis extends the knee joint, and the semimembranosus extends the hip joint and flexes the knee joint.

39. **The Answer is C.** The adductor longus is innervated by only the obturator nerve. Thus, injury here could completely paralyze the adductor longus. The pectineus is innervated by both the obturator and femoral nerves. The adductor magnus is innervated by both the obturator nerve and tibial part of the sciatic nerve. The biceps femoris is innervated by the tibial portion (long head) and common peroneal portion (short head) of the sciatic nerve. The semimembranosus is innervated by the tibial portion of the sciatic nerve.

40. **The Answer is B.** The keystone for the lateral longitudinal arch is the cuboid bone, whereas the keystone for the medial longitudinal arch is the head of the talus. The calcaneus, navicular, and medial cuneiform bones form a part of the medial longitudinal arch, but they are not keystones. The calcaneus also forms a part of the lateral longitudinal arch.

41. **The Answer is A.** The "unhappy triad" of the knee joint is characterized by tear of the medial meniscus, rupture of the tibial collateral ligament, and rupture of the anterior cruciate ligament. This injury may occur when a cleated shoe, as worn by football players, is planted firmly in the turf and the knee is struck from the lateral side. Tenderness along the medial collateral ligament and over the medial meniscus and swelling on the front of the joint are due to excessive production of synovial fluid, which fills the joint cavity and the suprapatellar bursa.

42. **The Answer is D.** The sartorius can flex and rotate the thigh laterally, and flex and rotate the leg medially. The rectus femoris flexes the thigh and extends the leg. The semimembranosus extends the thigh and flexes and rotates the leg medially. The biceps femoris extends the thigh and flexes and rotates the leg laterally. The adductor longus adducts and flexes the thigh.

43. **The Answer is C.** The tibialis anterior muscle can dorsiflex the foot, whereas all other muscles are able to plantar flex the foot.

44. **The Answer is A.** The tibialis posterior inverts the foot. The peroneus longus, brevis, and tertius and extensor digitorum longus can evert the foot.

45. **The Answer is A.** The peroneal artery is a branch of the posterior tibial artery. The dorsalis pedis artery begins anterior to the ankle as the continuation of the anterior tibial artery. The superior medial genicular artery is a branch of the popliteal artery, and the descending genicular artery arises from the femoral artery.

46. **The Answer is D.** The descending genicular artery gives off the articular branch, which enters the anastomosis around the knee joint, and the saphenous branch, which is not involved in the anastomosis but supplies the superficial tissue and skin on the medial side of the knee. Other arteries are involved in the anastomosis around the knee joint.

47. **The Answer is B.** The peroneus brevis muscle is innervated by the superficial peroneal nerve. The peroneus tertius and tibialis anterior muscles are innervated by the deep peroneal nerve. The flexor hallucis longus and tibialis posterior muscles are innervated by the tibial nerve.

48. **The Answer is C.** The popliteal vein drains blood into the femoral vein; thus, blood flow in the femoral vein is reduced. The great saphenous vein drains into the upper part of the femoral vein. Other veins empty into the popliteal vein.

49. **The Answer is D.** The lateral (fibular) collateral ligament extends between the lateral femoral epicondyle and the head of the fibula and is not attached to the lateral meniscus. All other ligaments lie outside the synovial cavity but within the joint capsule.

50. **The Answer is B.** The gastrocnemius can flex the knee joint and also plantar flex the foot. The tibialis posterior can plantar flex and invert the foot. The soleus can plantar flex the foot. The peroneus longus can plantar flex and evert the foot. The flexor digitorum longus can plantar flex the foot and flex the lateral four toes.

51. **The Answer is C.** The semitendinosus extends the thigh and flexes the leg. The short head of the biceps femoris flexes the leg. The adductor magnus adducts, flexes, and extends the thigh. The sartorius and gracilis can flex the thigh and leg.

52. **The Answer is D.** The extensor hallucis longus can dorsiflex and invert the foot. The peroneus longus, peroneus tertius, and extensor digitorum longus can dorsiflex and evert foot. The peroneus brevis can plantar flex and evert the foot.

53. **The Answer is C.** The quadriceps tendon is ruptured. The quadriceps muscle is a powerful knee extensor used in climbing, running, jumping, and rising from a seated position.

54. **The Answer is A.** The adductor tubercle is fractured. The adductor magnus inserts on the adductor tubercle on the femur and functions to adduct, flex, and extend the thigh.

55. **The Answer is B.** The anterior tibial artery enters the anterior compartment by passing through a gap between the neck of the fibula and tibia. Therefore, a knife wound through the gap may cause an injury to the anterior tibial artery, resulting in muscle ischemia in the anterior compartment of the leg.

56. **The Answer is E.** The common peroneal nerve is vulnerable to injury as it passes behind the head of the fibula and then winds laterally around the neck of the fibula. Fracture of the fibular head causes a lesion of the common peroneal nerve, resulting in paralysis of the muscles in the anterior and lateral compartments of the leg.

57. **The Answer is D.** The iliopsoas muscle is the chief flexor of the thigh and inserts on the lesser trochanter.

58. **The Answer is B.** The greater trochanter is the site for insertion of the obturator internus muscle tendon, which leaves the pelvis through the lesser sciatic foramen.

59. **The Answer is C.** The ischiopubic ramus and ischial tuberosity provide attachment for the adductor magnus.

60. **The Answer is A.** The distal part of the femoral head receives blood mainly from the medial femoral circumflex artery, whereas the proximal part is supplied by a branch from the posterior division of the obturator artery.

61. **The Answer is A.** The body of the talus has a groove on its posterior surface for the flexor hallucis longus tendon. This tendon also occupies the groove on the undersurface of the sustentaculum tali.

62. **The Answer is E.** The first or medial cuneiform bone provides insertions for the tibialis anterior, tibialis posterior, and peroneus longus muscles.

63. **The Answer is D.** The spring (plantar calcaneonavicular) ligament extends from the sustentaculum tali of the calcaneus to the navicular bone.

64. **The Answer is B.** The cuboid bone has a groove for the peroneus longus muscle tendon.

chapter 7 Upper Limb

BONES AND JOINTS OF THE UPPER LIMB

I. BONES OF THE SHOULDER GIRDLE (Figure 7.1)

A. Clavicle (Collarbone)

- Is a **commonly fractured bone** that forms the **pectoral (shoulder) girdle** with the **scapula**, which connects the upper limb to the sternum (axial skeleton), by articulating with the sternum at the sternoclavicular joint and with the acromion of the scapula at the acromioclavicular joint.
- Is **the first bone to begin ossification** during fetal development, but it is **the last one to complete ossification**, at approximately 21 years of age.
- Is the only long bone to be **ossified intramembranously** and forms from somatic lateral plate mesoderm.

CLINICAL CORRELATES

Fracture of the clavicle may result from a fall on the shoulder or outstretched hand or may be caused during delivery through the birth canal of a baby who is breech presentation. Its fracture occurs most commonly at the junction of its middle and lateral thirds, resulting in upward displacement of the proximal fragment and downward displacement of the distal fragment. It may cause injury to the brachial plexus (lower trunk), fatal hemorrhage from the subclavian artery, and thrombosis of the subclavian vein, leading to pulmonary embolism.

B. Scapula (Shoulder Blade)

1. Spine of the Scapula

- Is a triangular-shaped process that continues laterally as the **acromion**.
- Divides the posterior scapula into the upper **supraspinous** and lower **infraspinous fossae**, and also provides an origin for the deltoid and an insertion for the trapezius.

2. Acromion

- Is the lateral end of the spine and articulates with the clavicle.
- Provides an origin for the deltoid and an insertion for the trapezius.

3. Coracoid Process

- Provides the origin of the coracobrachialis and short head of biceps brachii, the insertion of the pectoralis minor, and the attachment site for the coracoclavicular, coracohumeral, and coracoacromial ligaments and the costocoracoid membrane.

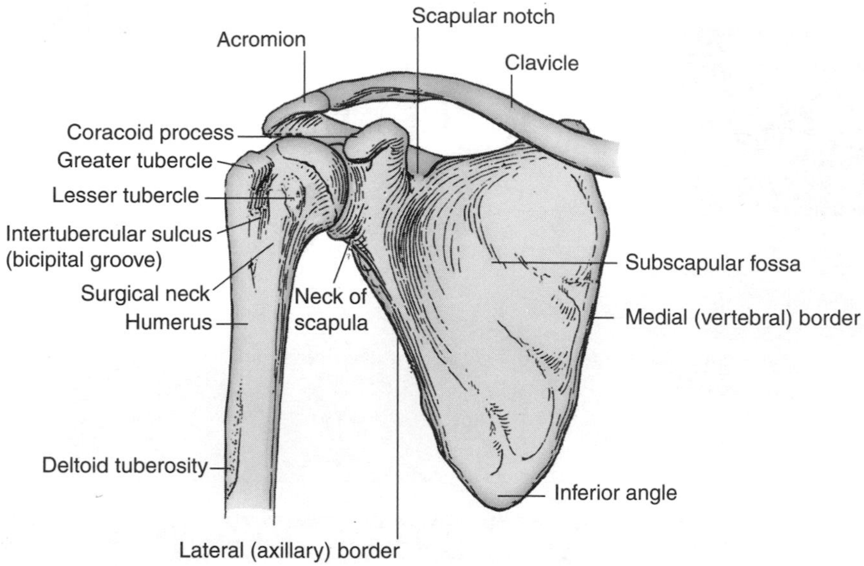

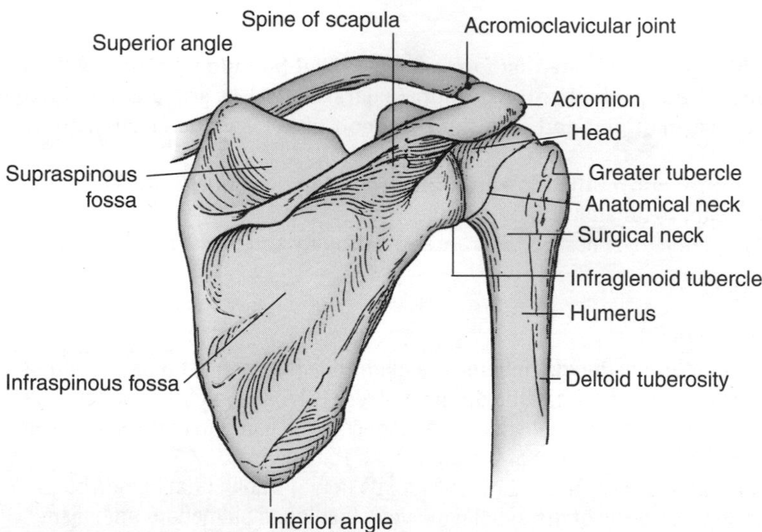

FIGURE 7.1. Pectoral girdle and humerus (anterior and posterior views).

4. Scapular Notch

- Is bridged by the superior transverse scapular ligament and converted into a foramen that transmits the **suprascapular nerve**.

CLINICAL CORRELATES **Calcification of the superior transverse scapular ligament** may trap or compress the suprascapular nerve as it passes through the scapular notch under the superior transverse scapular ligament, affecting functions of the supraspinatus and infraspinatus muscles.

5. **Glenoid Cavity**
   - Is deepened by the **glenoid labrum** for the head of the **humerus**.
6. **Supraglenoid and Infraglenoid Tubercles**
   - Provide origins for the tendons of the long heads of the biceps brachii and triceps brachii muscles, respectively.

II. BONES OF THE ARM AND FOREARM

A. Humerus (See Figure 7.1)

1. **Head**
   - Articulates with the scapula at the **glenohumeral joint**.
2. **Anatomic Neck**
   - Is an indentation distal to the head and provides an attachment for the fibrous joint capsule.
3. **Greater Tubercle**
   - Lies just lateral and distal to the anatomic neck and provides attachments for the supraspinatus, infraspinatus, and teres minor muscles.

CLINICAL CORRELATES **Fracture of the greater tuberosity** commonly occurs by direct trauma or by violent contractions of the supraspinatus muscle. The bone fragment has the attachments of the supraspinatus, infraspinatus, and teres minor muscles, whose tendons form parts of the rotator cuff.

Fracture of the lesser tuberosity accompanies posterior dislocation of the shoulder joint, and the bone fragment has the insertion of the subscapularis tendon.

Fracture of the surgical neck may injure the axillary nerve and the posterior humeral circumflex artery as they pass through the quadrangular space.

4. **Lesser Tubercle**
   - Lies on the anterior medial side of the humerus, just distal to the anatomic neck, and provides an insertion for the subscapularis muscle.
5. **Intertubercular (Bicipital) Groove**
   - Lies between the greater and lesser tubercles, lodges the tendon of the long head of the biceps brachii muscle, and is bridged by the **transverse humeral ligament**.
   - Provides insertions for the pectoralis major on its **lateral lip**, the teres major on its **medial lip**, and the latissimus dorsi on its **floor**.
6. **Surgical Neck**
   - Is a narrow area distal to the tubercles that is a **common site of fracture** and is in contact with the axillary nerve and the posterior humeral circumflex artery.
7. **Deltoid Tuberosity**
   - Is a rough triangular elevation on the lateral aspect of the midshaft that marks the insertion of the deltoid muscle.
8. **Spiral Groove**
   - Contains the radial nerve, separating the origin of the lateral head of the triceps above and the origin of the medial head below.

CLINICAL CORRELATES **Fracture of the shaft** of the humerus may injure the radial nerve and deep brachial artery in the spiral groove.

Supracondylar fracture is a fracture of the distal end of the humerus; it is common in children and occurs when the child falls on the outstretched hand with the elbow partially flexed and may injure the median nerve.

Fracture of the medial epicondyle may damage the ulnar nerve. This nerve may be compressed in a groove behind the medial epicondyle "funny bone," causing numbness.

9. Trochlea

- Is a spool-shaped medial articular surface and articulates with the **trochlear notch of the ulna**.

10. Capitulum

- Is the lateral articular surface, globular in shape, and articulates with the **head of the radius**.

11. Olecranon Fossa

- Is a posterior depression above the trochlea of the humerus that houses the **olecranon** of the ulna on full extension of the forearm.

12. Coronoid Fossa

- Is an anterior depression above the trochlea of the humerus that accommodates the **coronoid process** of the ulna on flexion of the elbow.

13. Radial Fossa

- Is an anterior depression above the capitulum that is occupied by the **head of the radius** during full flexion of the elbow joint.

14. Lateral Epicondyle

- Projects from the capitulum and provides the origin of the supinator and extensor muscles of the forearm. It is an attachment site for the radial collateral ligament.

15. Medial Epicondyle

- Projects from the trochlea and has a groove on the back for the ulnar nerve and superior ulnar collateral artery.
- Provides attachment sites for the ulnar collateral ligament, the pronator teres, and the common tendon of the forearm flexor muscles.

B. Radius (Figure 7.2)

- Is shorter than the ulna and is situated lateral to the ulna.

1. Head (Proximal End)

- Articulates with the **capitulum** of the humerus and the **radial notch** of the ulna and is surrounded by the **annular ligament**.

2. Neck

- Is enclosed by the lower margin of the annular ligament, and the neck and head are free from capsular attachment and thus can rotate freely within the socket.

3. Distal End

- Articulates with the **proximal row of carpal bones**, including the scaphoid, lunate, and triquetral bones but excludes the pisiform bone.

4. Radial Tuberosity

- Is an oblong prominence just distal to the neck and provides an attachment site for the biceps brachii tendon.

5. Styloid Process

- Is located on the distal end of the radius and is approximately 1 cm distal to that of the ulna and provides insertion of the brachioradialis muscle.
- Can be palpated in the proximal part of the anatomic snuffbox between the extensor pollicis longus and brevis tendons.

CLINICAL CORRELATES

Colles fracture of the wrist is a **distal radius fracture** in which the distal fragment is displaced (tilted) posteriorly, producing a characteristic bump described as **dinner (silver) fork deformity** because the forearm and wrist resemble the shape of a dinner fork. If the distal fragment is displaced anteriorly, it is called a **reverse Colles fracture (Smith fracture)**. This fracture may show styloid processes of the radius and ulna lineup on a radiograph.

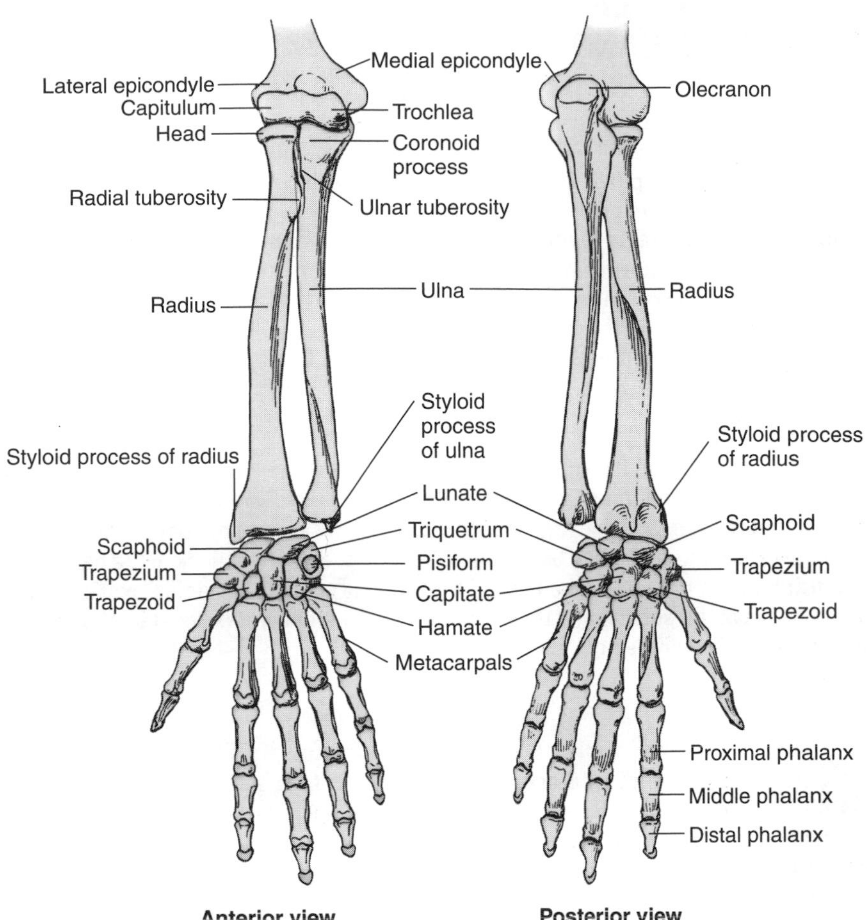

FIGURE 7.2. Bones of the forearm and hand (anterior and posterior views).

C. Ulna (See Figure 7.2)

1. Olecranon

- Is the curved projection on the back of the elbow that provides an attachment site for the triceps tendon.

2. Coronoid Process

- Is located below the trochlear notch and provides an attachment site for the brachialis.

3. Trochlear Notch

- Receives the trochlea of the humerus.

4. Ulnar Tuberosity

- Is a roughened prominence distal to the coronoid process that provides an attachment site for the brachialis.

5. Radial Notch

- Accommodates the head of the radius at the proximal radioulnar joint.

6. Head (Distal End)

- Articulates with the articular disk of the **distal radioulnar joint** and has a styloid process.

III. BONES OF THE HAND

A. Carpal Bones (See Figure 7.2)

- Are arranged in two rows of four (lateral to medial): scaphoid, lunate, triquetrum, pisiform, trapezium, trapezoid, capitate, and hamate (mnemonic device: **S**andra **L**ikes **T**o **P**at **T**om's **T**wo **C**old **H**ands). (Trapezium precedes trapezoid alphabetically.)

1. Proximal Row (Lateral to Medial): Scaphoid, Lunate, Triquetrum, and Pisiform

- Except for the pisiform, articulates with the radius and the articular disk (the ulna has no contact with the carpal bones). The pisiform is said to be a sesamoid bone contained in the flexor carpi ulnaris tendon.

2. Distal Row (Lateral to Medial): Trapezium, Trapezoid, Capitate, and Hamate

CLINICAL CORRELATES **Fracture of the scaphoid** occurs on a fall on the outstretched hand, shows a deep tenderness in anatomical snuffbox, and damages the radial artery and can cause avascular necrosis of the bone and degenerative joint disease of the wrist. **Fracture of the hamate** may injure the ulnar nerve and artery because they are near the hook of the hamate.

Bennett fracture is a fracture of the base of the metacarpal of the thumb. **Boxer's fracture** is a fracture of the necks of the second and third metacarpals, seen in professional boxers, and typically of the fifth metacarpal in unskilled boxers.

CLINICAL CORRELATES **Guyon canal syndrome** is an entrapment of the ulnar nerve in the Guyon canal, which causes pain, numbness, and tingling in the ring and little fingers, followed by loss of sensation and motor weakness. It can be treated by surgical decompression of the nerve. **Guyon canal (ulnar tunnel)** is formed by the pisiform, hook of the hamate, and pisohamate ligament, deep to the palmaris brevis and palmar carpal ligament and transmits the ulnar nerve and artery.

B. Metacarpals

- Are miniature long bones consisting of **bases** (proximal ends), **shafts** (bodies), and **heads** (distal ends). Heads form the knuckles of the fist.

C. Phalanges

- Are miniature long bones consisting of **bases, shafts, and heads**. The heads of the proximal and middle phalanges form the knuckles.
- Occur in fingers (three each) and thumb (two).

IV. JOINTS AND LIGAMENTS OF THE UPPER LIMB (See Figures 7.1 to 7.3)

A. Acromioclavicular Joint

- Is a synovial **plane joint** that allows a gliding movement when the scapula rotates and is reinforced by the **coracoclavicular ligament**, which consists of the conoid and trapezoid ligaments.

B. Sternoclavicular Joint

- Is a double synovial **plane (gliding) joint** united by the fibrous capsule.
- Is reinforced by the anterior and posterior sternoclavicular, interclavicular, and costoclavicular ligaments.
- Allows elevation and depression, protraction and retraction, and circumduction of the shoulder.

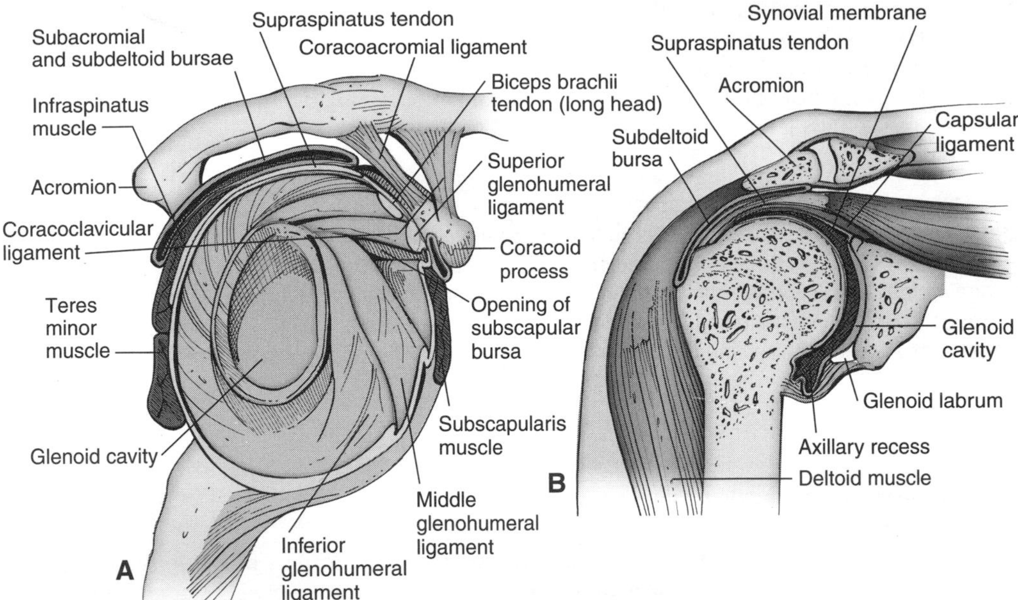

FIGURE 7.3. Shoulder joint with bursae and rotator cuff. **A:** Anterior view. **B:** Coronal section.

CLINICAL CORRELATES

Dislocation of the acromioclavicular joint can result from a fall on the shoulder with the impact taken by the acromion or from a fall on the outstretched arm. It is called a shoulder separation because the **shoulder is separated** from the clavicle when the joint dislocation with rupture of the coracoclavicular ligament occurs.

C. Shoulder (Glenohumeral) Joint

- Is a synovial **ball-and-socket joint** between the glenoid cavity of the scapula and the head of the humerus. Both articular surfaces are covered with hyaline cartilage.
- Is surrounded by the **fibrous capsule** that is attached superiorly to the margin of the glenoid cavity and inferiorly to the **anatomic neck** of the humerus. The capsule is reinforced by the **rotator cuff**, the **glenohumeral ligaments**, and the **coracohumeral ligaments**.
- Has a cavity that is deepened by the fibrocartilaginous **glenoid labrum**; communicates with the subscapular bursa; and allows abduction and adduction, flexion and extension, and circumduction and rotation.
- Is innervated by the axillary, suprascapular, and lateral pectoral nerves.
- Receives blood from branches of the suprascapular, anterior and posterior humeral circumflex, and scapular circumflex arteries.
- May be subject to inferior or anterior **dislocation**, which stretches the fibrous capsule, avulses the glenoid labrum, and may injure the axillary nerve.

CLINICAL CORRELATES

Dislocation (subluxation) of the shoulder joint occurs usually in the anteroinferior direction because of the lack of support by tendons of the rotator cuff. It may damage the axillary nerve and the posterior humeral circumflex vessels.

Referred pain to the shoulder most probably indicates involvement of the phrenic nerve (or diaphragm). The supraclavicular nerve (C3–C4), which supplies sensory fibers over the shoulder, has the same origin as the phrenic nerve (C3–C5), which supplies the diaphragm. Examples of referred pain are gallbladder pain radiating to right shoulder and splenic pain radiating to left shoulder.

1. **Rotator (Musculotendinous) Cuff (See** Figure 7.3
   - Is formed by the tendons of the **s**upraspinatus, **i**nfraspinatus, **t**eres minor, and **s**ubscapularis (SITS); fuses with the joint capsule; and provides mobility.
   - Keeps the head of the humerus in the glenoid fossa during movements and thus stabilizes the shoulder joint.

CLINICAL CORRELATES **Rupture of rotator cuff** may occur by a chronic wear and tear or an acute fall on the outstretched arm and is manifested by severe limitation of shoulder joint motion, chiefly abduction. A rupture of the rotator cuff, most frequently attrition of the supraspinatus tendon by friction among middle-aged persons may cause degenerative inflammatory changes (degenerative **tendonitis**) of the rotator cuff, resulting in a painful abduction of the arm or a **painful shoulder**.

2. **Ligaments of the shoulder joint**
   - **(a) Glenohumeral Ligaments**
     - Extend from the **supraglenoid tubercle** to the upper part of the lesser tubercle of the humerus **(superior glenohumeral ligament)**, to the lower anatomic neck of the humerus **(middle glenohumeral ligament)**, and to the lower part of the lesser tubercle of the humerus **(inferior glenohumeral ligament)**.
   - **(b) Transverse Humeral Ligament**
     - Extends between the greater and lesser tubercles and holds the tendon of the long head of the biceps in the intertubercular groove.
   - **(c) Coracohumeral Ligament**
     - Extends from the coracoid process to the greater tubercle.
   - **(d) Coracoacromial Ligament**
     - Extends from the coracoid process to the acromion.
   - **(e) Coracoclavicular Ligament**
     - Extends from the coracoid process to the clavicle and consists of the trapezoid and conoid ligaments.
3. **Bursae around the Shoulder**
   - Form a **lubricating mechanism** between the rotator cuff and the coracoacromial arch during movement of the shoulder joint.
   - **(a) Subacromial Bursa**
     - Lies between the coracoacromial arch and the supraspinatus muscle, usually communicates with the subdeltoid bursa, and protects the supraspinatus tendon against friction with the acromion.
   - **(b) Subdeltoid Bursa**
     - Lies between the deltoid muscle and the shoulder joint capsule, usually communicates with the subacromial bursa, and facilitates the movement of the deltoid muscle over the joint capsule and the supraspinatus tendon.
   - **(c) Subscapular Bursa**
     - Lies between the subscapularis tendon and the neck of the scapula and communicates with the synovial cavity of the shoulder joint.

D. Elbow Joint

- Forms a synovial **hinge joint**, consisting of the **humeroradial** and **humeroulnar joints**, and allows flexion and extension. It also includes the **proximal radioulnar (pivot) joint**, within a common articular capsule.

- Is innervated by the musculocutaneous, median, radial, and ulnar nerves.
- Receives blood from the anastomosis formed by branches of the brachial artery and recurrent branches of the radial and ulnar arteries.
- Is reinforced by the following ligaments:

1. **Annular Ligament**
   - Is a fibrous band that is attached to the anterior and posterior margins of the radial notch of the ulna and forms nearly four-fifths of a circle around the head of the radius; the **radial notch** forms the remainder.
   - Encircles the head of the radius and holds it in position and fuses with the radial collateral ligament and the articular capsule.
2. **Radial Collateral Ligament**
   - Extends from the lateral epicondyle to the anterior and posterior margins of the radial notch of the ulna and the annular ligament of the radius.
3. **Ulnar Collateral Ligament**
   - Is **triangular** and is composed of anterior, posterior, and oblique bands.
   - Extends from the medial epicondyle to the coronoid process and the olecranon of the ulna.

E. Proximal Radioulnar Joint

- Forms a synovial **pivot joint** in which the head of the radius articulates with the radial notch of the ulna and allows **pronation** and **supination** by permitting the head of radius to rotate within the encircling annular ligament.

F. Distal Radioulnar Joint

- Forms a synovial **pivot joint** between the head of the ulna and the ulnar notch of the radius and allows **pronation** and **supination**.

G. Wrist (Radiocarpal) Joint

- Is a synovial **condylar joint** formed superiorly by the radius and the articular disk and inferiorly by the proximal row of carpal bones (scaphoid, lunate, and rarely triquetrum).
- Its capsule is strengthened by radial and ulnar collateral ligaments and dorsal and palmar radiocarpal ligaments, and it allows flexion and extension, abduction and adduction, and circumduction.

H. Midcarpal Joint

- Forms a synovial **plane joint** between the proximal and distal rows of carpal bones and allows gliding and sliding movements.

I. Carpometacarpal Joints

- Form synovial **saddle (sellar) joints** between the carpal bone (trapezium) and the first metacarpal bone, allowing flexion and extension, abduction and adduction, and circumduction.
- Also form **plane joints** between the carpal bones and the medial four metacarpal bones, allowing a simple gliding movement.

J. Metacarpophalangeal Joints

- Are **condyloid joints** that allow flexion and extension, and abduction and adduction.

K. Interphalangeal Joints

- Are **hinge joints** that allow flexion and extension.

CUTANEOUS NERVES, SUPERFICIAL VEINS, AND LYMPHATICS

I. CUTANEOUS NERVES OF THE UPPER LIMB (Figure 7.4)

A. Supraclavicular Nerve

- Arises from the cervical plexus (C3, C4) and innervates the skin over the upper pectoral, deltoid, and outer trapezius areas.

B. Medial Brachial Cutaneous Nerve

- Arises from the medial cord of the brachial plexus and innervates the medial side of the arm.

C. Medial Antebrachial Cutaneous Nerve

- Arises from the medial cord of the brachial plexus and innervates the medial side of the forearm.

D. Lateral Brachial Cutaneous Nerve

- Arises from the axillary nerve and innervates the lateral side of the arm.

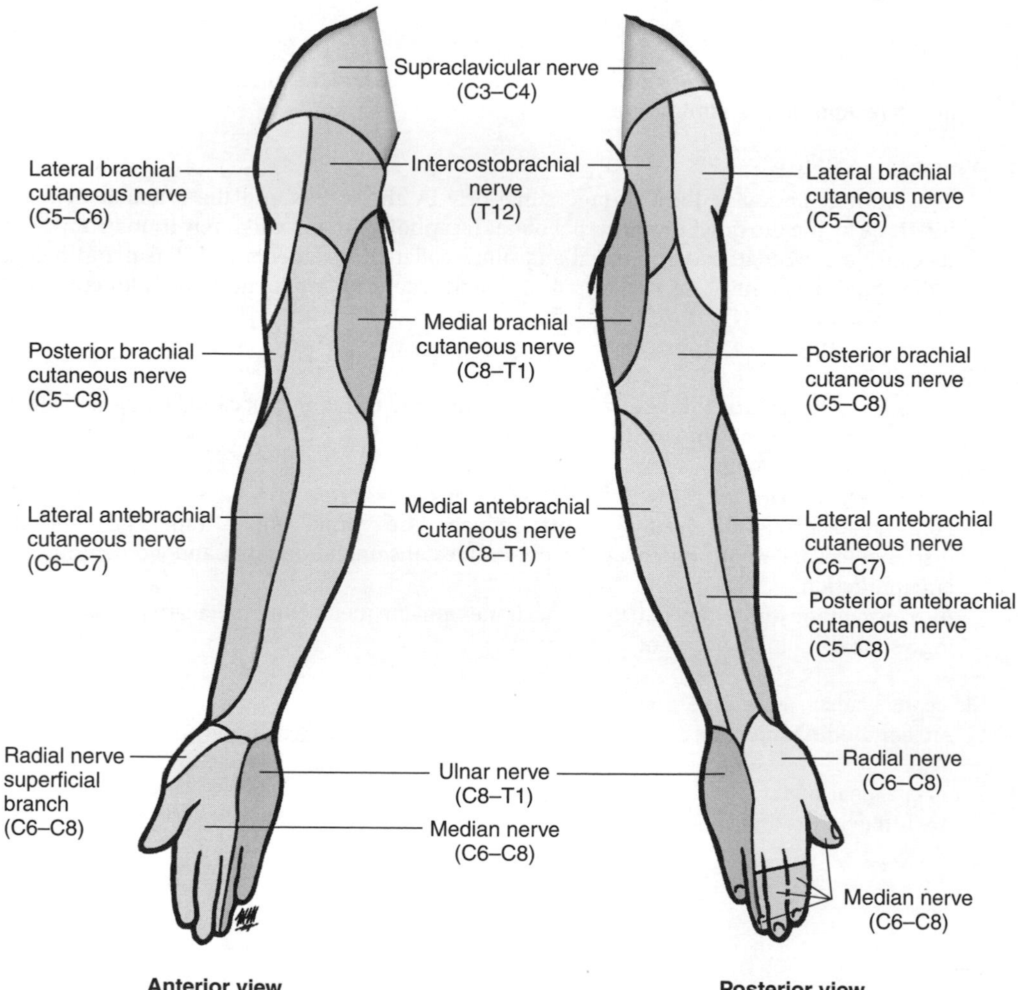

FIGURE 7.4. Cutaneous nerves of the upper limb (anterior and posterior views).

E. Lateral Antebrachial Cutaneous Nerve

- Arises from the musculocutaneous nerve and innervates the lateral side of the forearm.

F. Posterior Brachial and Antebrachial Cutaneous Nerves

- Arise from the radial nerve and innervate the posterior sides of the arm and forearm, respectively.

G. Intercostobrachial Nerve

- Is the lateral cutaneous branch of the second intercostal nerve emerging from the second intercostal space and may communicate with the medial brachial cutaneous nerve.

II. SUPERFICIAL VEINS OF THE UPPER LIMB (Figure 7.5)

A. Cephalic Vein

- Begins as a radial continuation of the dorsal venous network, runs on the lateral side, and is often connected with the basilic vein by the **median cubital vein** in front of the elbow.
- Ascends along the lateral surface of the biceps, pierces the brachial fascia, and lies in the deltopectoral triangle with the deltoid branch of the thoracoacromial trunk.
- Pierces the costocoracoid membrane of the clavipectoral fascia and ends in the axillary vein.

B. Basilic Vein

- Arises from the dorsal venous arch of the hand and accompanies the medial antebrachial cutaneous nerve along the ulnar border of the forearm and passes anterior to the medial epicondyle.
- Pierces the deep fascia of the arm and joins the brachial veins (the **venae comitantes** of the brachial artery) to form the **axillary vein** at the lower border of the teres major muscle.

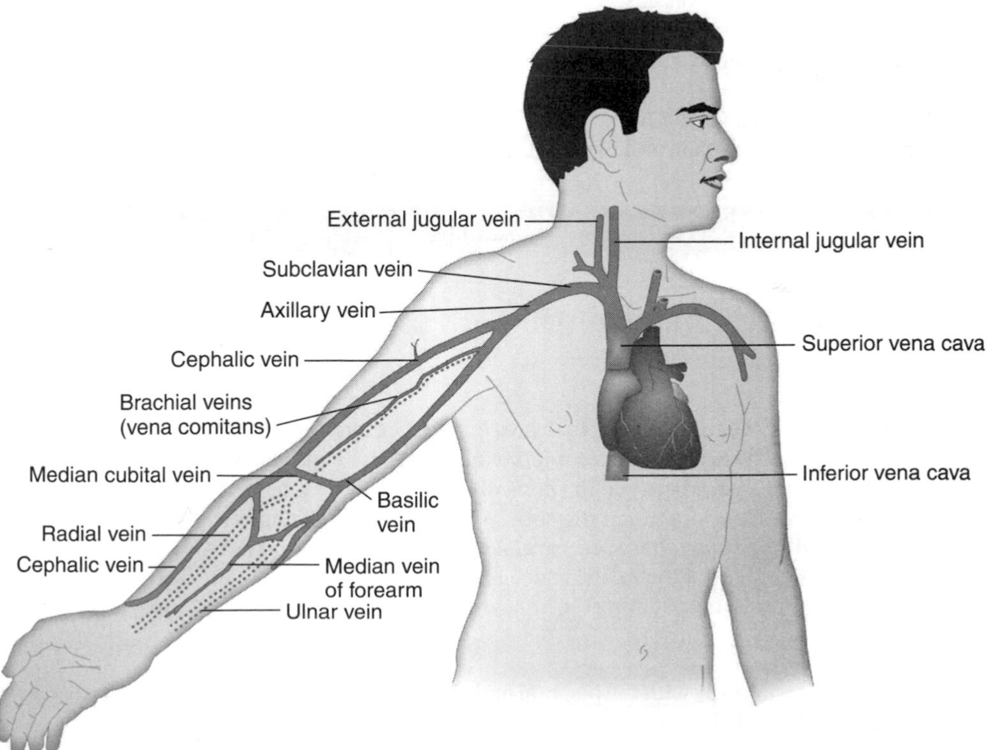

FIGURE 7.5. Venous drainage of the upper limb.

C. Median Cubital Vein

- Connects the cephalic vein to the basilic vein over the cubital fossa.
- Lies superficial to the **bicipital aponeurosis**, and thus separates it from the brachial artery, which is vulnerable to being punctured during intravenous injections and blood transfusions. The median nerve on the medial side of the artery is also vulnerable to an incorrectly placed needle.

D. Median Antebrachial Vein

- Arises in the palmar venous network, ascends on the front of the forearm, and terminates in the median cubital or the basilic vein.

E. Dorsal Venous Network

- Is a network of veins formed by the dorsal metacarpal veins that receive dorsal digital veins and continues proximally as the **cephalic vein** and the **basilic vein**.

III. SUPERFICIAL LYMPHATICS OF THE UPPER LIMB

A. Lymphatics of the Finger

- Drain into the plexuses on the dorsum and palm of the hand, which form the medial and lateral lymph vessels.

B. Medial Group of Lymphatic Vessels

- Accompanies the basilic vein; passes through the cubital or supratrochlear nodes; and ascends to enter the **lateral axillary nodes**, which drain first into the **central axillary nodes** and then into the **apical axillary nodes**.

C. Lateral Group of Lymphatic Vessels

- Accompanies the cephalic vein and drains into the **lateral axillary nodes** and also into the **deltopectoral** (infraclavicular) node, which then drain into the **apical nodes**.

D. Axillary Lymph Nodes (Figure 7.6

- Lie in the axilla (see Axilla and Breast: II. C).

AXILLA AND BREAST

I. FASCIAE OF THE AXILLA AND PECTORAL REGIONS

A. Clavipectoral Fascia

- Extends between the coracoid process, clavicle, and the thoracic wall and envelops the subclavius and pectoralis minor muscles. Its components are (1) the **costocoracoid ligament**, which is a thickening of the fascia between the coracoid process and the first rib; (2) the **costocoracoid membrane**, which lies between the subclavius and pectoralis minor muscles and is pierced by the **cephalic vein**, the **thoracoacromial artery**, and the **lateral pectoral nerve**; and (3) the **suspensory ligament of the axilla**, which is the inferior extension of the fascia and is attached to the axillary fascia, maintaining the hollow of the armpit.

B. Axillary Fascia

- Is contiguous anteriorly with the pectoral and clavipectoral fasciae (suspensory ligament of the axilla), laterally with the brachial fascia, and posteromedially with the fascia over the latissimus dorsi.

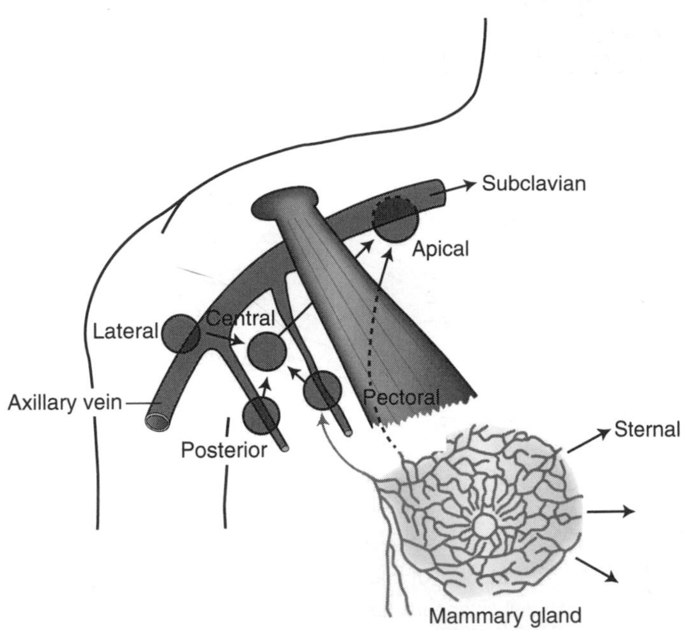

FIGURE 7.6. Lymphatic drainage of the breast and axillary lymph nodes.

- Forms the floor of the axilla and is attached to the suspensory ligament of the axilla that forms the hollow of the armpit by traction when the arm is abducted.

C. Axillary Sheath

- Is a tubular fascial prolongation of the prevertebral layer of the deep cervical fascia into the axilla, enclosing the axillary vessels and the brachial plexus.

II. AXILLA (ARMPIT)

- Is a pyramid-shaped space between the upper thoracic wall and the arm.

A. Boundaries of the Axilla

- Include **medial wall**: upper ribs and their intercostal muscles and serratus anterior muscle; **lateral wall**: intertubercular groove of the humerus; **posterior wall**: subscapularis, teres major, and latissimus dorsi muscles; **anterior wall**: pectoralis major and pectoralis minor muscles and clavipectoral fascia; **base**: axillary fascia and skin; and **apex**: interval between the clavicle, first rib, and upper border of the scapula.

B. Contents of the Axilla (Figures 7.7 to 7.9)

- **Brachial plexus** and its branches (see Figure 7.7).
- **Axillary artery** has many branches, including the superior thoracic, thoracoacromial, lateral thoracic, thoracodorsal, and circumflex humeral (anterior and posterior) arteries.
- **Axillary vein** is formed by the union of the brachial veins (venae comitantes of the brachial artery) and the basilic vein, receives the cephalic vein and veins that correspond to the branches of the axillary artery, and drains into the subclavian vein.
- **Lymph nodes** and areolar tissue are present.
- **Axillary tail** (tail of Spence) is a superolateral extension of the mammary gland.

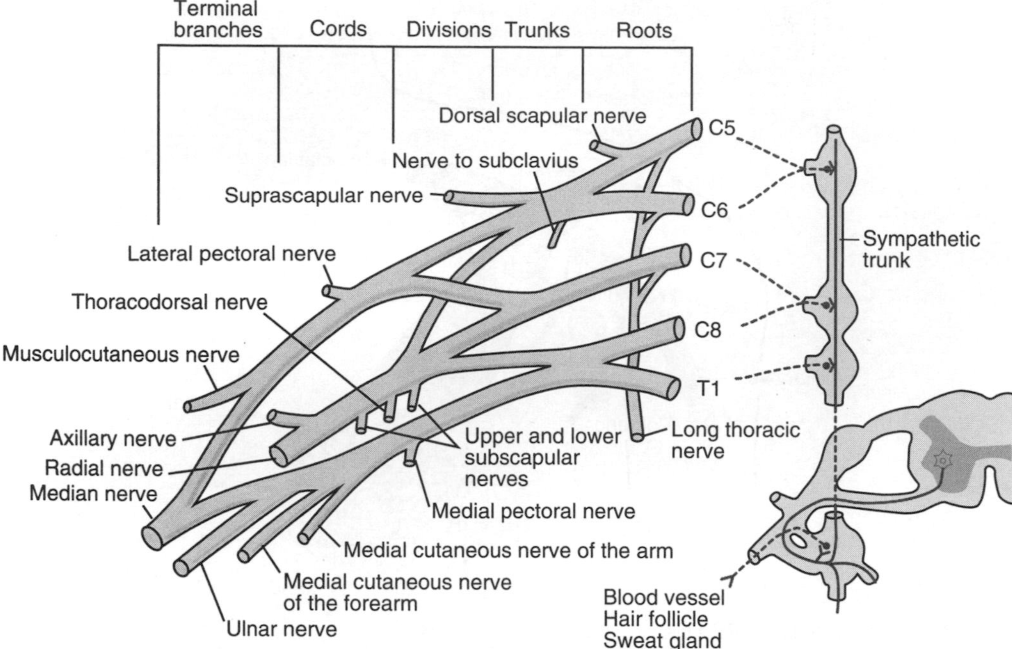

FIGURE 7.7. Brachial plexus.

C. Axillary Lymph Nodes (Figure 7.6)

1. Central Nodes

- Lie near the base of the axilla between the lateral thoracic and subscapular veins; receive lymph from the lateral, anterior, and posterior groups of nodes; and drain into the apical nodes.

2. Brachial (Lateral) Nodes

- Lie posteromedial to the axillary veins, receive lymph from the upper limb, and drain into the central nodes.

3. Subscapular (Posterior) Nodes

- Lie along the subscapular vein, receive lymph from the posterior thoracic wall and the posterior aspect of the shoulder, and drain into the central nodes.

4. Pectoral (Anterior) Nodes

- Lie along the inferolateral border of the pectoralis minor muscle; receive lymph from the anterior and lateral thoracic walls, including the breast; and drain into the central nodes.

5. Apical (Medial or Subclavicular) Nodes

- Lie at the apex of the axilla medial to the axillary vein and above the upper border of the pectoralis minor muscle, receive lymph from all of the other axillary nodes (and occasionally from the breast), and drain into the subclavian trunks, which usually empty into the junction of the subclavian and internal jugular veins.

III. BREAST AND MAMMARY GLAND (Figure 7.10)

A. Breast

- Consists of mammary gland tissue, fibrous and fatty tissue, blood and lymph vessels, and nerves.
- Extends from the second to sixth ribs and from the sternum to the midaxillary line and is divided into the upper and lower lateral and medial quadrants.
- Has mammary glands, which lie in the **superficial fascia**.

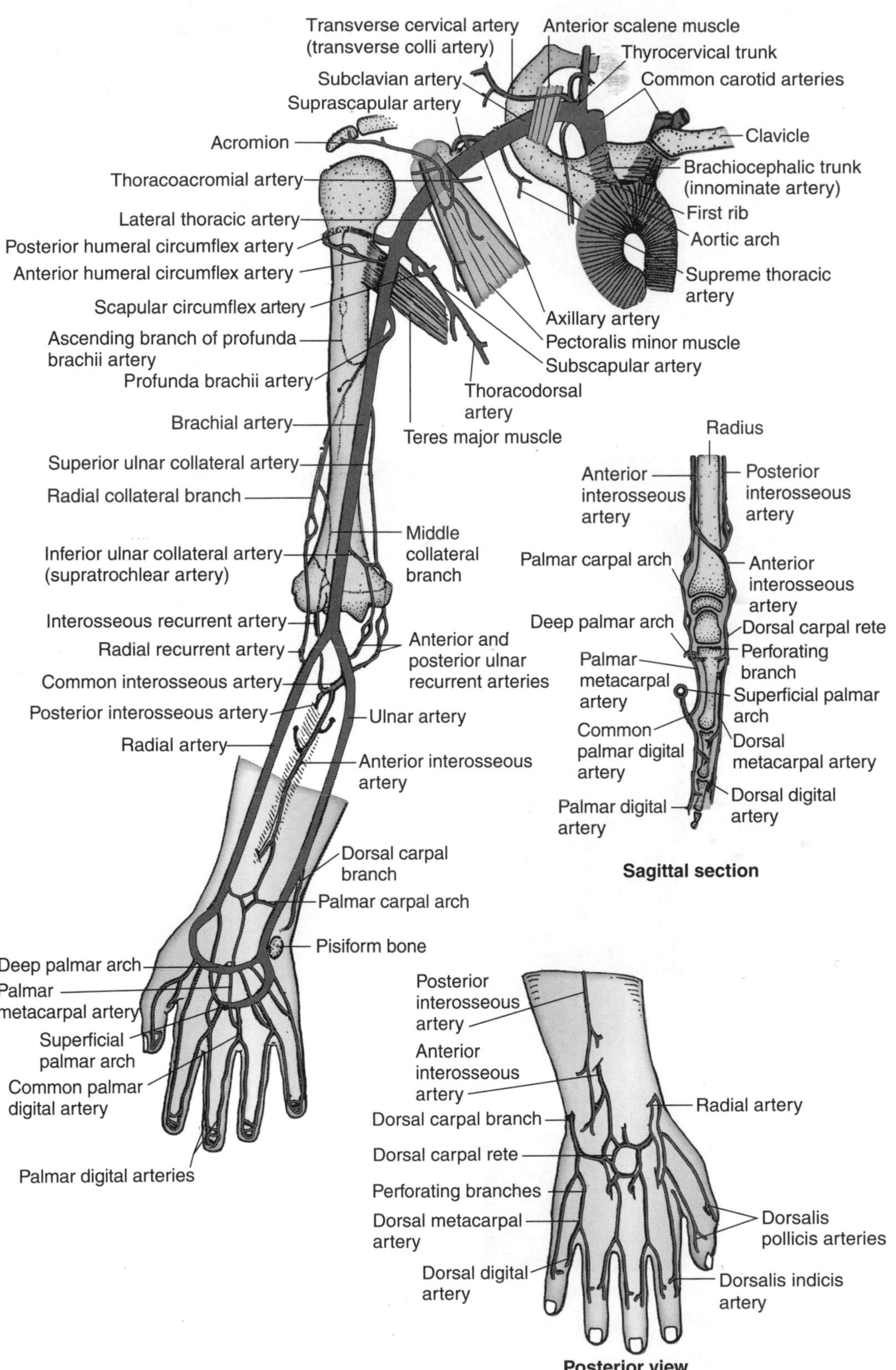

FIGURE 7.8. Blood supply to the upper limb.

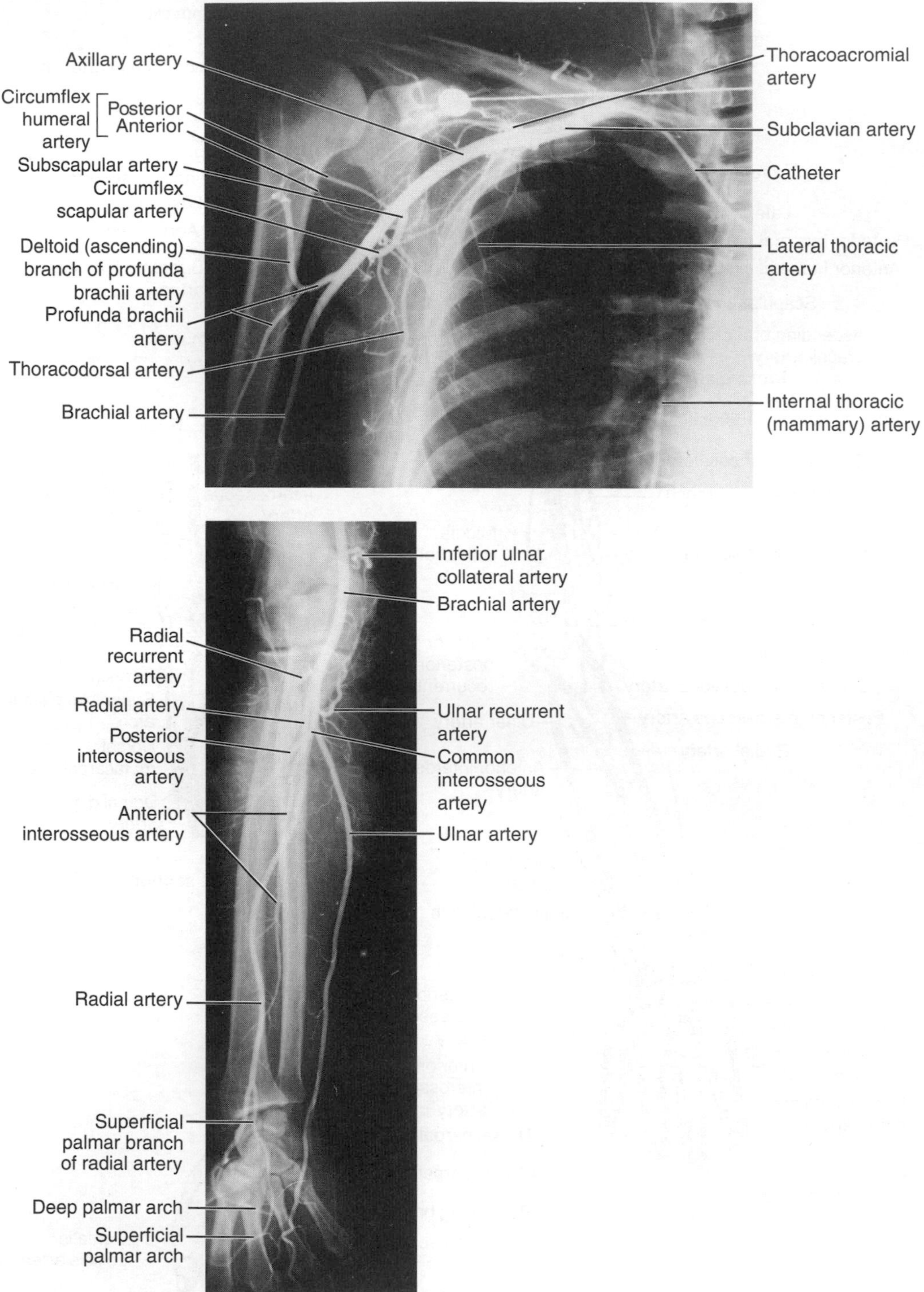

FIGURE 7.9. Arteriographs of the axillary, brachial, radial, and ulnar arteries.

(Reprinted with permission from Augur AMR, Lee MJ. *Grant's Atlas of Anatomy*. 10th ed. Philadelphia, PA: Lippincott Williams & Wilkins; 1999:435, 473.)

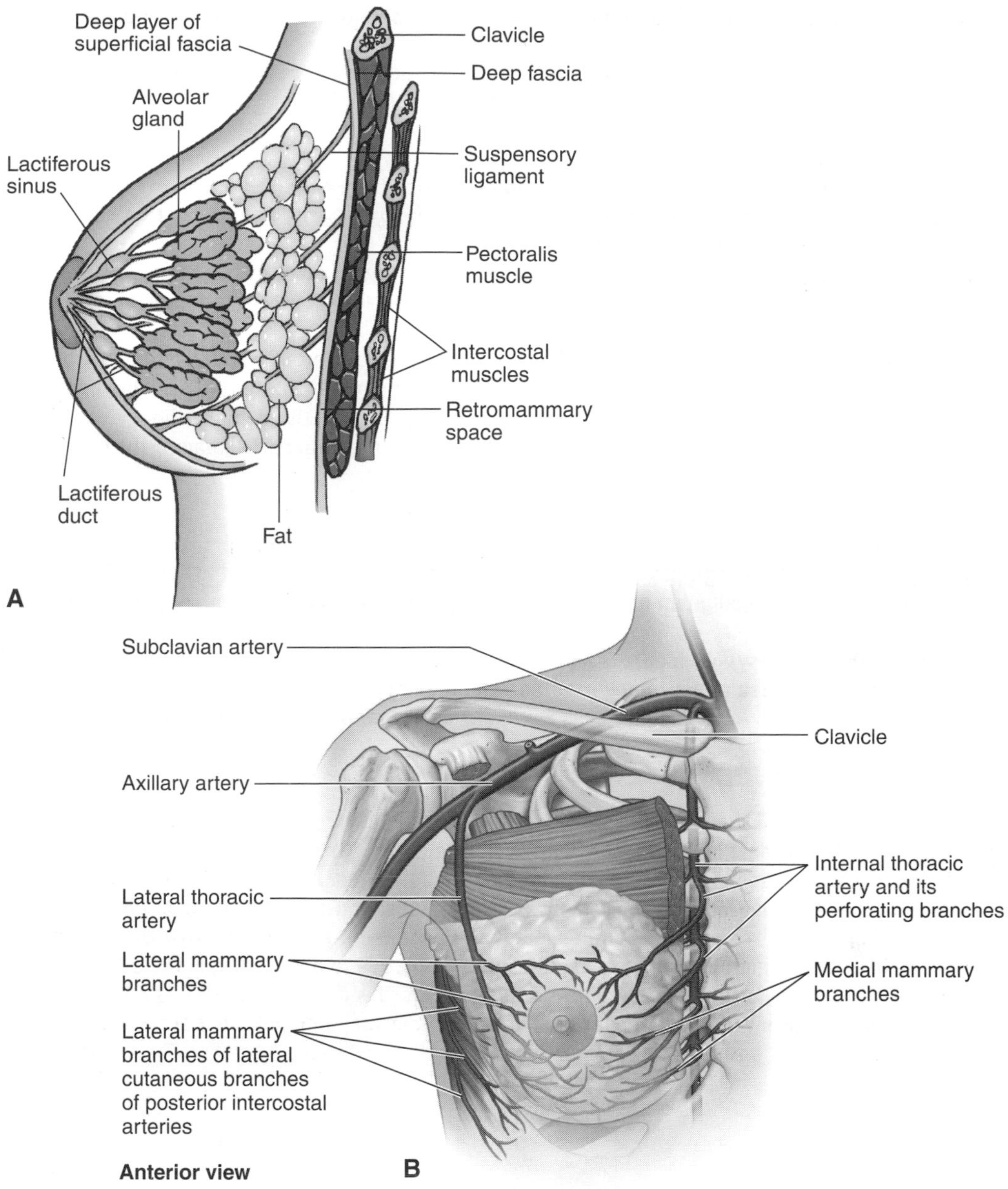

FIGURE 7.10. **A:** Female breast structures. **B:** Arterial supply of the breast.

- Is supported by the **suspensory ligaments (of Cooper)**, strong fibrous processes, that run from the dermis of the skin to the deep layer of the superficial fascia through the breast.
- **Nipple** usually lies at the level of the fourth intercostal space and contain smooth muscle fibers that contract on tactile stimulation inducing firmness and prominence.
- **Areola** is a ring of pigmented skin around the nipple.
- Receives blood from the **medial mammary** branches of the anterior perforating branches of the internal thoracic artery, the **lateral mammary** branches of the lateral thoracic artery, the **pectoral** branches of the thoracoacromial trunk, and the lateral cutaneous branches of the posterior intercostal arteries.

- Is innervated by the anterior and lateral cutaneous branches of the second to the sixth intercostal nerves.
- May have more than one pair of breasts (polymastia), more than one pair of nipples (polythelia), absence of breasts (amastia), and absence of nipples (athelia).

B. Mammary Gland

- Is a **modified sweat gland** located in the fatty superficial fascia.
- Has the **axillary tail**, a small part of the mammary gland that extends superolaterally sometimes through the deep fascia to lie in the axilla.
- Is separated from the deep fascia covering the underlying muscles by an area of loose areolar tissue known as the **retromammary space**, which allows the breast some degree of movement over the pectoralis major muscle.
- Has 15 to 20 lobes of glandular tissue, which are separated by fibrous septa that radiate from the nipple. Each lobe opens by a **lactiferous duct** onto the tip of the nipple, and each duct enlarges to form a **lactiferous sinus**, which serves as a reservoir for milk during lactation.
- Usually warrants radial incisions to avoid spreading any infection and damaging the lactiferous ducts.

CLINICAL CORRELATES

Mammography is a radiographic examination of the breast to screen for benign and malignant tumors and cysts. It plays a central part in early detection of breast cancers.

Sentinel node (biopsy) procedure is a surgical procedure to determine the extent of spread or the stage of cancer by use of an isotope injected into the tumor region. The **sentinel lymph node** is the first lymph node(s) to which cancer cells are likely to spread from the primary tumor.

CLINICAL CORRELATES

Breast cancer occurs in the **upper lateral quadrant** (approximately 60% of cases) and forms a palpable mass in advanced stages. It enlarges, attaches to Cooper ligaments, and produces shortening of the ligaments, causing depression or **dimpling** of the overlying **skin**. Advanced sign of **inflammatory breast cancer,peau d'orange** (texture of an orange peel), is the edematous swollen and pitted breast skin due to obstruction of the subcutaneous lymphatics. Cancer may also attach to and shorten the lactiferous ducts, resulting in a retracted or **inverted nipple**. It may invade the deep fascia of the pectoralis major muscle so that the contraction of the muscle produces a sudden upward movement of the entire breast.

CLINICAL CORRELATES

Radical mastectomy is the extensive surgical removal of the breast and its related structures, including the pectoralis major and minor muscles, axillary lymph nodes and fascia, and part of the thoracic wall. It may injure the **long thoracic** and **thoracodorsal nerves** and may cause postoperative swelling (edema) of the upper limb as a result of lymphatic obstruction caused by the removal of most of the lymphatic channels that drain the arm or by venous obstruction caused by thrombosis of the axillary vein.

Modified radical mastectomy involves excision of the entire breast and axillary lymph nodes, with preservation of the pectoralis major and minor muscles. (The pectoralis minor muscle is usually retracted or severed near its insertion into the coracoid process.)

Lumpectomy (tylectomy) is the surgical excision of only the palpable mass in carcinoma of the breast.

C. Lymphatic Drainage of the Breast (See Figure 7.6)

- Is of great importance in view of the frequent development of cancer and subsequent dissemination of cancer cells through the lymphatic stream.

- Removes lymphatic fluid from the lateral quadrants into the axillary nodes and the medial quadrants into the parasternal (internal thoracic) nodes.
- Drains primarily (75%) to the **axillary** nodes, more specifically to the **pectoral (anterior)** nodes (including drainage of the nipple).
- Follows the perforating vessels through the pectoralis major muscle and the thoracic wall to enter the **parasternal (internal thoracic) nodes**, which lie along the internal thoracic artery.
- Also drains to the apical nodes and may connect to lymphatics draining the opposite breast and to lymphatics draining the anterior abdominal wall.

MUSCLES OF THE UPPER LIMB

I. MUSCLES OF THE PECTORAL REGION AND AXILLA (Figure 7.11; Table 7.1)

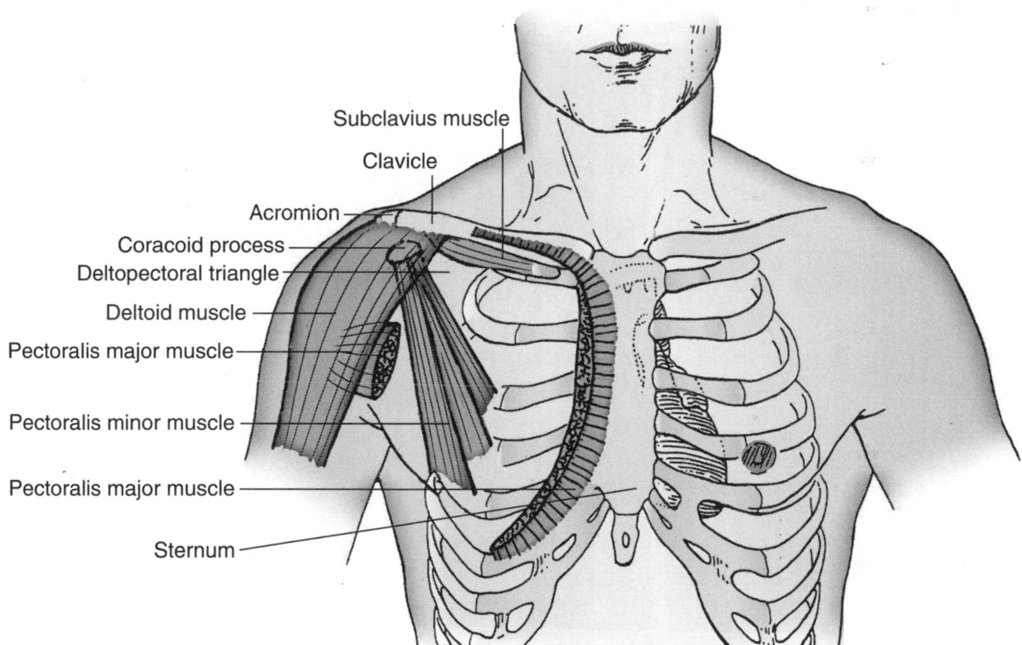

FIGURE 7.11. Muscles of the pectoral region.

table 7.1 Muscles of the Pectoral Region and Axilla

Muscle	Origin	Insertion	Nerve	Action
Pectoralis major	Medial half of clavicle; manubrium and body of sternum; upper six costal cartilages	Lateral lip of intertubercular groove of humerus	Lateral and medial pectoral	Flexes, adducts, and medially rotates arm
Pectoralis minor	Third, fourth, and fifth ribs	Coracoid process of scapula	Medial (and lateral) pectoral	Depresses scapula; elevates ribs
Subclavius	Junction of first rib and costal cartilage	Inferior surface of clavicle	Nerve to subclavius	Depresses lateral part of clavicle
Serratus anterior	Upper eight ribs	Medial border of scapula	Long thoracic	Rotates scapula upward; abducts scapula with arm and elevates it above the horizontal

II. MUSCLES OF THE SHOULDER REGION (See Figure 7.12; Table 7.2)

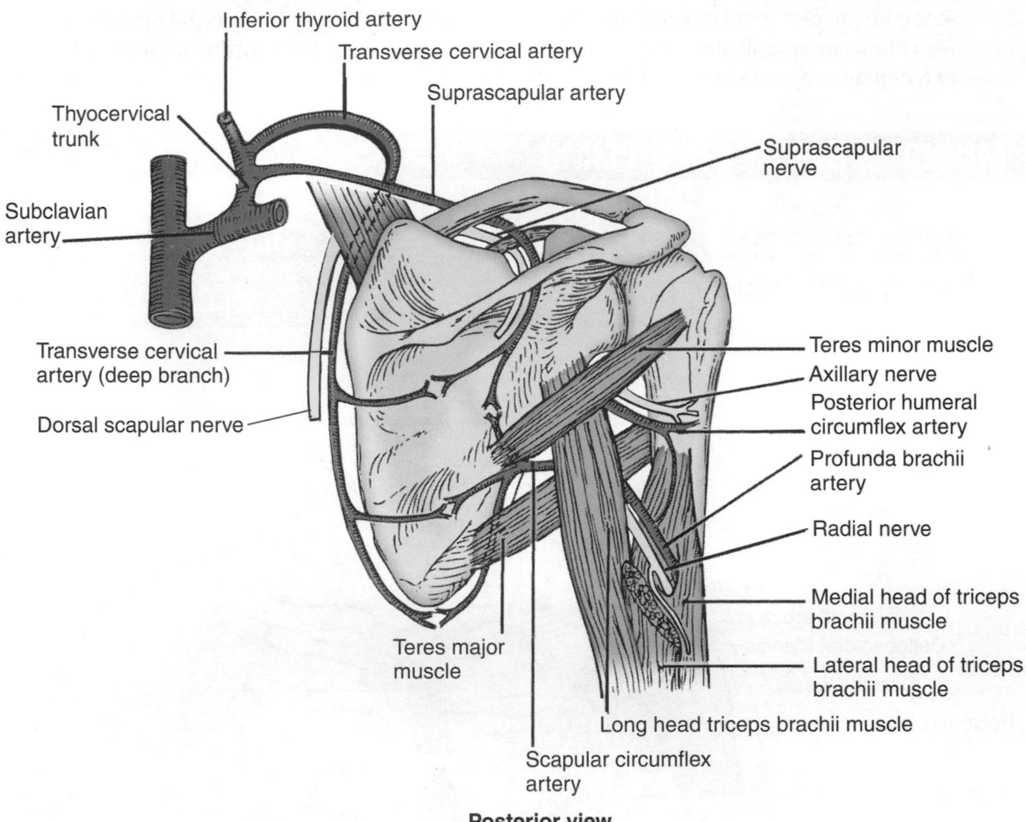

FIGURE 7.12. Structures of the shoulder region (posterior view).

table 7.2 Muscles of the Shoulder

Muscle	Origin	Insertion	Nerve	Action
Deltoid	Lateral third of clavicle, acromion, and spine of scapula	Deltoid tuberosity of humerus	Axillary	Abducts, adducts, flexes, extends, and rotates arm medially and laterally
Supraspinatus	Supraspinous fossa of scapula	Superior facet of greater tubercle of humerus	Suprascapular	Abducts arm
Infraspinatus	Infraspinous fossa	Middle facet of greater tubercle of humerus	Suprascapular	Rotates arm laterally
Subscapularis	Subscapular fossa	Lesser tubercle of humerus	Upper and lower subscapular	Adducts and rotates arm medially
Teres major	Dorsal surface of inferior angle of scapula	Medial lip of intertubercular groove of humerus	Lower subscapular	Adducts and rotates arm medially
Teres minor	Upper portion of lateral border of scapula	Lower facet of greater tubercle of humerus	Axillary	Rotates arm laterally
Latissimus dorsi	Spines of T7–T12 thoracolumbar fascia, iliac crest, ribs 9–12	Floor of bicipital groove of humerus	Thoracodorsal	Adducts, extends, and rotates arm medially

A. Rotator (Musculotendinous) Cuff (See Figure 7.3)

- Is formed by the tendons of supraspinatus, infraspinatus, teres minor, and subscapularis (SITS).; fuses with the joint capsule; and provides mobility.
- Keeps the head of the humerus in the glenoid fossa during movements and thus stabilizes the shoulder joint.

B. Quadrangular Space (Figures 7.11 and 7.13)

- Is bounded superiorly by the teres minor and subscapularis muscles, inferiorly by the teres major muscle, medially by the long head of the triceps, and laterally by the surgical neck of the humerus.
- Transmits the **axillary nerve** and the **posterior humeral circumflex vessels**.

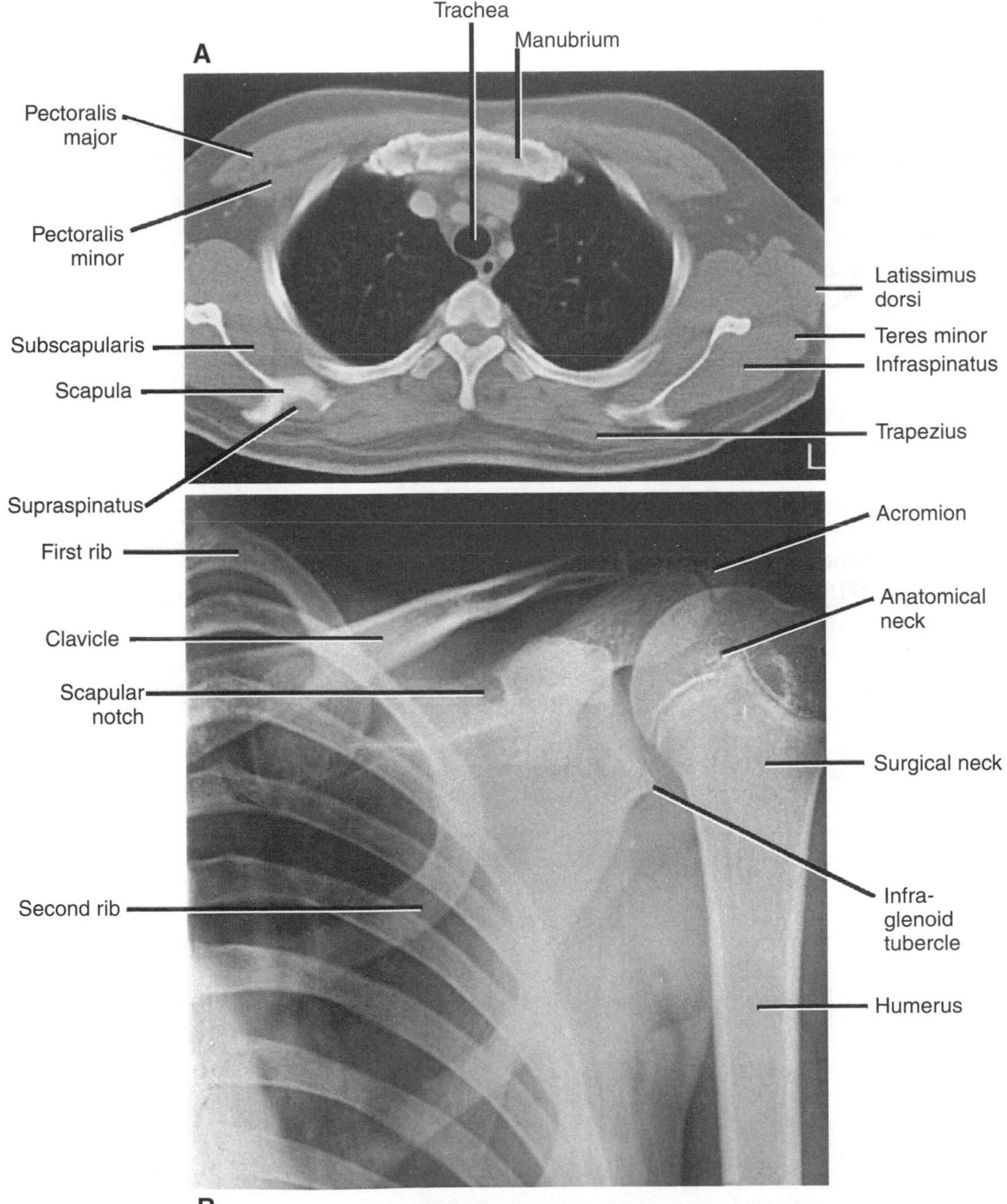

FIGURE 7.13. Views of the shoulder region. **A:** Transverse computed tomography image through the shoulders and upper thorax. **B:** Radiograph of the shoulder region in a 11-year-old boy.

C. Triangular Space (Upper)

- Is bounded superiorly by the teres minor muscle, inferiorly by the teres major muscle, and laterally by the long head of the triceps.
- Contains the **circumflex scapular vessels**.

D. Triangular Space (Lower)

- Is formed superiorly by the teres major muscle, medially by the long head of the triceps, and laterally by the medial head of the triceps.
- Contains the **radial nerve** and the **profunda brachii (deep brachial) artery**.

E. Triangle of Auscultation

- Is bounded by the upper border of the latissimus dorsi muscle, the lateral border of the trapezius muscle, and the medial border of the scapula; its floor is formed by the rhomboid major muscle.
- Is the site at which **breathing sounds** are heard most clearly.

III. MUSCLES OF THE ARM AND FOREARM (Tables 7.3 to 7.5)

A. Brachial Intermuscular Septa

- Extend from the brachial fascia, a portion of the deep fascia, enclosing the arm.
- Consist of medial and lateral intermuscular septa, which divide the arm into the anterior compartment (**flexor compartment**) and the posterior compartment (**extensor compartment**).

B. Cubital Fossa

- Is a V-shaped interval on the anterior aspect of the elbow that is bounded laterally by the **brachioradialis** muscle, medially by the **pronator teres** muscle, and superiorly by an imaginary horizontal line connecting the epicondyles of the humerus with a floor formed by the brachialis and supinator muscles.
- At its lower end, the brachial artery divides into the radial and ulnar arteries, with a fascial roof strengthened by the bicipital aponeurosis.
- Contains (from lateral to medial) the **r**adial nerve, **b**iceps tendon, **b**rachial artery, and **m**edian nerve (mnemonic device: **R**on **B**eats **B**ad **M**an).

table 7.3 Muscles of the Arm

Muscle	Origin	Insertion	Nerve	Action
Coracobrachialis	Coracoid process	Middle third of medial surface of humerus	Musculocutaneous	Flexes and adducts arm
Biceps brachii	Long head, supraglenoid tubercle; short head, coracoid process	Radial tuberosity of radius	Musculocutaneous	Flexes arm and forearm, supinates forearm
Brachialis	Lower anterior surface of humerus	Coronoid process of ulna and ulnar tuberosity	Musculocutaneous	Flexes forearm
Triceps	Long head, infraglenoid tubercle; lateral head, superior to radial groove of humerus; medial head, inferior to radial groove	Posterior surface of olecranon process of ulna	Radial	Extends forearm
Anconeus	Lateral epicondyle of humerus	Olecranon and upper posterior surface of ulna	Radial	Extends forearm

table 7.4 Muscles of the Anterior Forearm

Muscle	Origin	Insertion	Nerve	Action
Pronator teres	Medial epicondyle and coronoid process of ulna	Middle of lateral side of radius	Median	Pronates and flexes forearm
Flexor carpi radialis	Medial epicondyle of humerus	Bases of second and third metacarpals	Median	Flexes forearm, flexes and abducts hand
Palmaris longus	Medial epicondyle of humerus	Flexor retinaculum, palmar aponeurosis	Median	Flexes forearm and hand
Flexor carpi ulnaris	Medial epicondyle (humeral head); medial olecranon, and posterior border of ulna (ulnar head)	Pisiform, hook of hamate, and base of fifth metacarpal	Ulnar	Flexes forearm; flexes and adducts hand
Flexor digitorum superficialis	Medial epicondyle, coronoid process, oblique line of radius	Middle phalanges of finger	Median	Flexes proximal interphalangeal joints, flexes hand and forearm
Flexor digitorum profundus	Anteromedial surface of ulna, interosseous membrane	Bases of distal phalanges of fingers	Ulnar and median	Flexes distal interphalangeal joints and hand
Flexor pollicis longus	Anterior surface of radius, interosseous membrane, and coronoid process	Base of distal phalanx of thumb	Median	Flexes thumb
Pronator quadratus	Anterior surface of distal ulna	Anterior surface of distal radius	Median	Pronates forearm

table 7.5 Muscles of the Posterior Forearm

Muscle	Origin	Insertion	Nerve	Action
Brachioradialis	Lateral supracondylar ridge of humerus	Base of radial styloid process	Radial	Flexes forearm
Extensor carpi radialis longus	Lateral supracondylar ridge of humerus	Dorsum of base of second metacarpal	Radial	Extends and abducts hand
Extensor carpi radialis brevis	Lateral epicondyle of humerus	Posterior base of third metacarpal	Radial	Extends and abducts hands
Extensor digitorum	Lateral epicondyle of humerus	Extensor expansion, base of middle and digital phalanges	Radial	Extends fingers and hand
Extensor digiti minimi	Common extensor tendon and interosseous membrane	Extensor expansion, base of middle and distal phalanges	Radial	Extends little finger
Extensor carpi ulnaris	Lateral epicondyle and posterior surface of ulna	Base of fifth metacarpal	Radial	Extends and adducts hand
Supinator	Lateral epicondyle, radial collateral and annular ligaments, supinator fossa and crest of ulna	Lateral side of upper part of radius	Radial	Supinates forearm
Abductor pollicis longus	Interosseous membrane, middle third of posterior surfaces of radius and ulna	Lateral surface of base of first metacarpal	Radial	Abducts thumb and hand
Extensor pollicis longus	Interosseous membrane and middle third of posterior surface of ulna	Base of distal phalanx of thumb	Radial	Extends distal phalanx of thumb and abducts hand
Extensor pollicis brevis	Interosseous membrane and posterior surface of middle third of radius	Base of proximal phalanx of thumb	Radial	Extends proximal phalanx of thumb and abducts hand
Extensor indicis	Posterior surface of ulna and interosseous membrane	Extensor expansion of index finger	Radial	Extends index finger

C. Bicipital Aponeurosis

- Originates from the medial border of the biceps tendon, **lies on the brachial artery and the median nerve**, and blends with the deep fascia of the forearm.

D. Interosseous Membrane of the Forearm

- Is a **dense connective tissue** sheet between the radius and the ulna. Its proximal border forms a gap through which the posterior interosseous vessels pass, and it is pierced (distally) by the anterior interosseous vessels.
- Provides attachments for the deep extrinsic flexor, extensor, and abductor muscles of the hand.

E. Characteristics of the Arm and Forearm

1. Carrying Angle

- Is formed laterally by the axis of the arm and forearm when the elbow is extended, because the medial edge of the trochlea projects more inferiorly than its lateral edge. The forearm deviated (5–15 degrees) laterally from a straight line of the arm.
- Is wider in women than in men and disappears when the forearm is flexed or pronated.

2. Pronation and Supination

- Occur at the **proximal** and **distal radioulnar joints** and have unequal strengths, with supination being stronger.

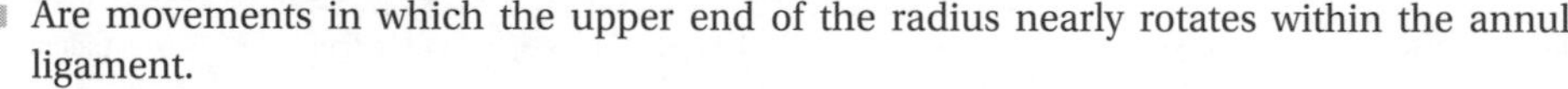

- Are movements in which the upper end of the radius nearly rotates within the annular ligament.
- **Supination:** palm faces forward (lateral rotation); **pronation:** the radius rotates over the ulna, and thus, the palm faces backward (medial rotation, in which case the shafts of the radius and ulna cross each other).

CLINICAL CORRELATES

Tennis elbow (lateral epicondylitis) is caused by a chronic inflammation or irritation of the origin (tendon) of the extensor muscles of the forearm from the lateral epicondyle of the humerus as a result of repetitive strain. It is a painful condition and common in tennis players and violinists.

Golfer's elbow (medial epicondylitis) is a painful condition caused by a small tear or an inflammation or irritation in the origin of the flexor muscles of the forearm from the medial epicondyle. Treatment may include injection of glucocorticoids into the inflamed area or avoidance of repetitive bending (flexing) of the forearm in order to not compress the ulnar nerve.

Nursemaid's elbow or pulled elbow is a radial head subluxation and occurs in toddlers when the child is lifted by the wrist. It is caused by a partial tear (or loose) of the annular ligament and thus the radial head to slip out of position.

CLINICAL CORRELATES

Cubital tunnel syndrome results from compression on the ulnar nerve in the cubital tunnel behind the medial epicondyle (**funny bone**), causing numbness and tingling in the ring and little fingers. The tunnel is formed by the medial epicondyle, ulnar collateral ligament, and two heads of the flexor carpi ulnaris muscle and transmits the ulnar nerve and superior ulnar collateral or posterior ulnar recurrent artery.

IV. MUSCLES OF THE HAND (Figures 7.14 and 7.16; Table 7.6)

A. Extensor Retinaculum (Figures 7.15 and 7.16)

- Is a thickening of the antebrachial fascia on the back of the wrist, is subdivided into compartments, and places the extensor tendons beneath it.

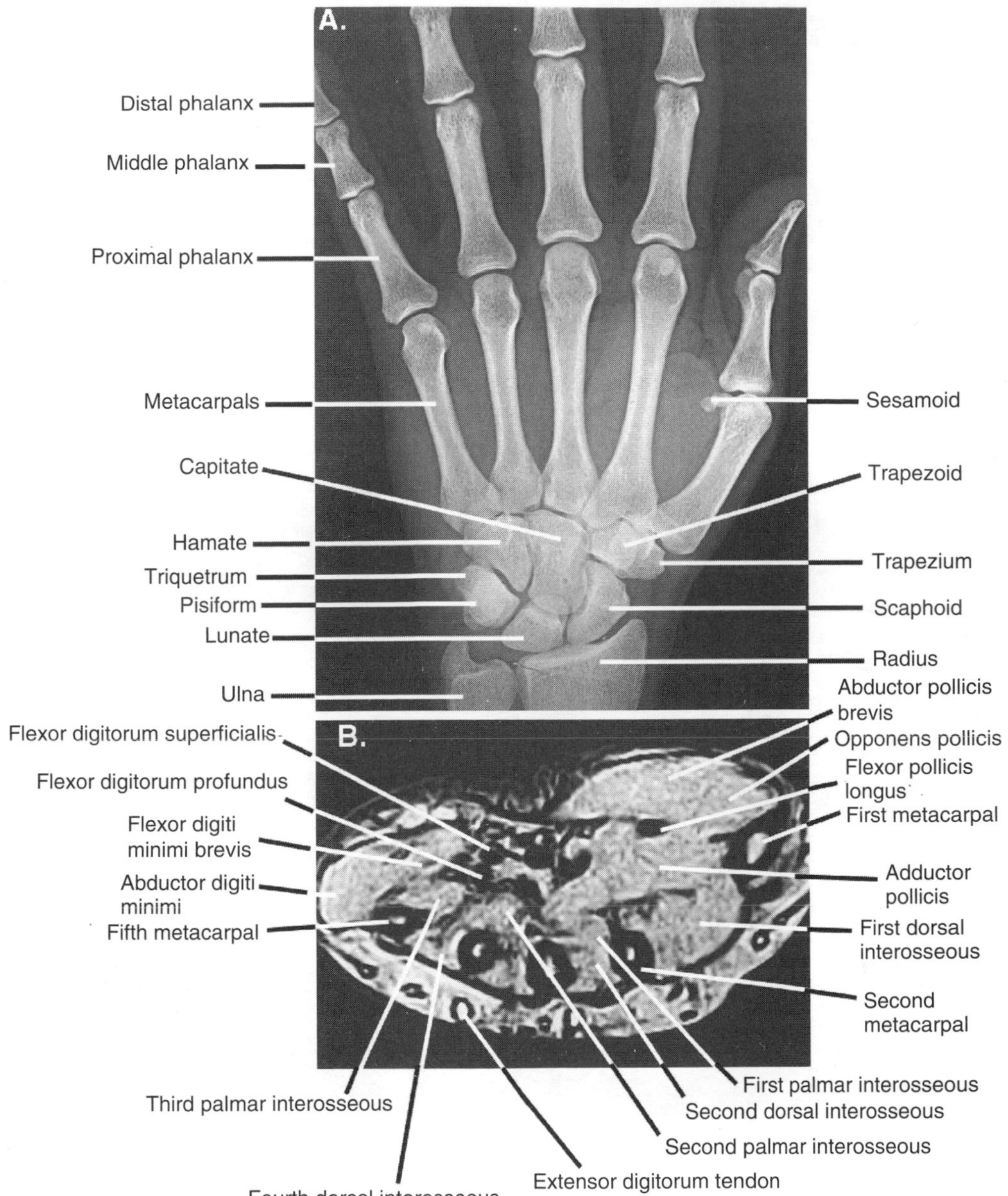

FIGURE 7.14. Bones and muscles of the hand. **A:** Radiograph of the wrist and hand. **B:** Transverse magnetic resonance image of the palm of the hand.

- Extends from the lateral margin of the radius to the styloid process of the ulna, the pisiform, and the triquetrum and is crossed superficially by the superficial branch of the radial nerve.

B. Palmar Aponeurosis

- Is a triangular fibrous layer overlying the tendons in the palm and is continuous with the palmaris longus tendon, the thenar and hypothenar fasciae, the flexor retinaculum, and the palmar carpal ligament.
- Protects the superficial palmar arterial arch, the palmar digital nerves, and the long flexor tendons.

C. Palmar Carpal Ligament

- Is a thickening of deep antebrachial fascia at the wrist, covering the tendons of the flexor muscles, median nerve, and ulnar artery and nerve, except palmar branches of the median and ulnar nerves.

table 7.6 Muscles of the Hand

Muscle	Origin	Insertion	Nerve	Action
Abductor pollicis brevis	Flexor retinaculum, scaphoid, trapezium	Lateral side of base of proximal phalanx of thumb	Median	Abducts thumb
Flexor pollicis brevis	Flexor retinaculum and trapezium	Base of proximal phalanx of thumb	Median	Flexes thumb
Opponens pollicis	Flexor retinaculum and trapezium	Lateral side of first metacarpal	Median	Opposes thumb to other digits
Adductor pollicis	Capitate and bases of second and third metacarpals (oblique head); palmar surface of third metacarpal (transverse head)	Medial side of base of proximal phalanx of the thumb	Ulnar	Adducts thumb
Palmaris brevis	Medial side of flexor retinaculum, palmar aponeurosis	Skin of medial side of palm	Ulnar	Wrinkles skin on medial side of palm
Abductor digiti minimi	Pisiform and tendon of flexor carpi ulnaris	Medial side of base of proximal phalanx of little finger	Ulnar	Abducts little finger
Flexor digiti minimi brevis	Flexor retinaculum and hook of hamate	Medial side of base of proximal phalanx of little finger	Ulnar	Flexes proximal phalanx of little finger
Opponens digiti minimi	Flexor retinaculum and hook of hamate	Medial side of fifth metacarpal	Ulnar	Opposes little finger
Lumbricals (4)	Lateral side of tendons of flexor digitorum profundus	Lateral side of extensor expansion	Median (two lateral) and ulnar (two medial)	Flex metacarpophalangeal joints and extend interphalangeal joints
Dorsal interossei (4) (bipennate)	Adjacent sides of metacarpal bones	Lateral sides of bases of proximal phalanges, extensor expansion	Ulnar	Abduct fingers, flex metacarpophalangeal joints, extend interphalangeal joints
Palmar interossei (3) (unipennate)	Medial side of second metacarpal; lateral sides of fourth and fifth metacarpals	Bases of proximal phalanges in same sides as their origins, extensor expansion	Ulnar	Adduct fingers, flex metacarpophalangeal joints, extend interphalangeal joints

CLINICAL CORRELATES **Dupuytren contracture** is a progressive thickening, shortening, and **fibrosis of the palmar fascia**, especially the palmar aponeurosis, producing a flexion deformity of fingers in which the fingers are pulled toward the palm (inability to fully extend fingers), especially the third and fourth fingers.

Volkmann contracture is an ischemic muscular contracture (flexion deformity) of the fingers and sometimes of the wrist, resulting from **ischemic necrosis of the forearm flexor muscles**, caused by a pressure injury, such as compartment syndrome, or a tight cast. The muscles are replaced by fibrous tissue, which contracts, producing the flexion deformity.

D. Flexor Retinaculum (See Figure 7.15)

- Serves as an origin for muscles of the thenar eminence.
- Forms the **carpal (osteofascial) tunnel** on the anterior aspect of the wrist.
- Is attached medially to the triquetrum, the pisiform, and the hook of the hamate and laterally to the tubercles of the scaphoid and trapezium.
- Is crossed superficially by the **ulnar nerve**, **ulnar artery**, **palmaris longus tendon**, and **palmar cutaneous branch of the median nerve**.

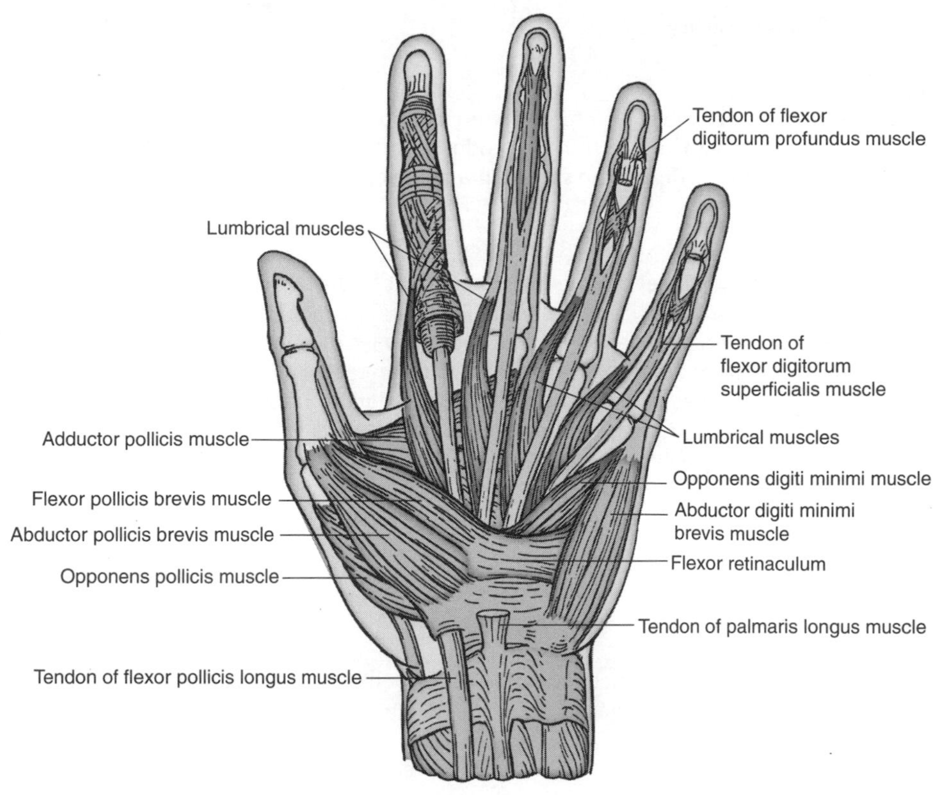

FIGURE 7.15. Superficial muscles of the hand (anterior view).

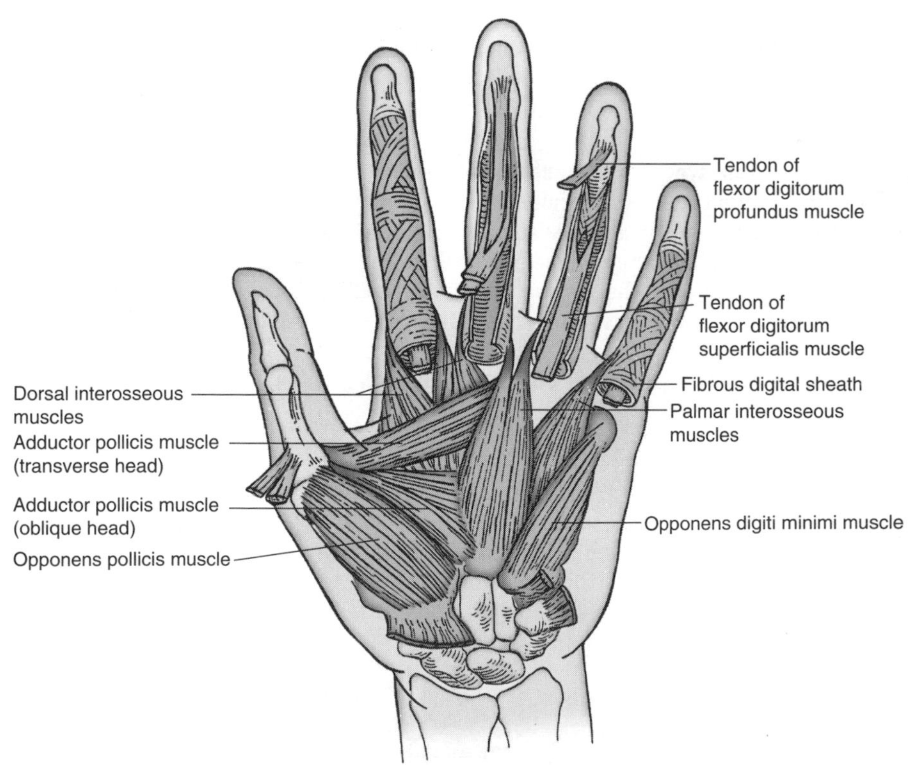

FIGURE 7.16. Deep muscles of the hand (anterior view).

E. Carpal Tunnel

- Is formed anteriorly by the flexor retinaculum and posteriorly by the carpal bones.
- Transmits the **median nerve** and the tendons of **flexor pollicis longus**, **flexor digitorum profundus**, and **flexor digitorum superficialis muscles**.

CLINICAL CORRELATES

Carpal tunnel syndrome is caused by compression of the median nerve due to the reduced size of the osseofibrous carpal tunnel, resulting from inflammation of the flexor retinaculum, arthritic changes in the carpal bones, or inflammation or thickening of the synovial sheaths of the flexor tendons. It leads to **pain** and **paresthesia** (tingling, burning, and numbness) in the hand in the area supplied by the median nerve and may also cause **atrophy of the thenar muscles** in cases of severe compression. However, no paresthesia occurs over the thenar eminence of skin because this area is supplied by the palmar cutaneous branch of the median nerve.

F. Fascial Spaces of the Palm

- Are fascial spaces deep to the palmar aponeurosis and divided by a midpalmar (oblique) septum into the **thenar space** and the **midpalmar space**.

1. Thenar Space

- Is the lateral space that contains the flexor pollicis longus tendon and the other flexor tendons of the index finger.

2. Midpalmar Space

- Is the medial space that contains the flexor tendons of the medial three digits.

G. Synovial Flexor Sheaths

1. Common Synovial Flexor Sheath (Ulnar Bursa)

- Envelops or contains the tendons of both the flexor digitorum superficialis and profundus muscles.

2. Synovial Sheath for Flexor Pollicis Longus (Radial Bursa)

- Envelops the tendon of the flexor pollicis longus muscle.

CLINICAL CORRELATES

Tenosynovitis is an **inflammation of the tendon and synovial sheath**, and puncture injuries cause infection of the synovial sheaths of the digits. The tendons of the second, third, and fourth digits have separate synovial sheaths so that the infection is confined to the infected digit, but rupture of the proximal ends of these sheaths allows the infection to spread to the **midpalmar space**. The synovial sheath of the little finger is usually continuous with the common synovial sheath (**ulnar bursa**), and thus, infection may spread to the common sheath and thus through the palm and carpal tunnel to the forearm. Likewise, infection in the thumb may spread through the synovial sheath of the flexor pollicis longus (**radial bursa**).

CLINICAL CORRELATES

Trigger finger results from stenosing tenosynovitis or occurs when the flexor tendon develops a nodule or swelling that interferes with its gliding through the pulley, causing an audible clicking or snapping. Symptoms are pain at the joints and a clicking when extending or flexing the joints. This condition may be caused by rheumatoid arthritis, repetitive trauma, and wear and tear of aging of the tendon. It can be treated by immobilization by a splint, an injection of corticosteroid into the flexor tendon sheath to shrink the nodule, or surgical incision of the thickened area.

Mallet finger (hammer or baseball finger) is a finger with permanent flexion of the distal phalanx due to an avulsion of the lateral bands of the extensor tendon to the distal phalanx. **Boutonniere deformity** is a finger with abnormal flexion of the middle phalanx and hyperextension of the distal phalanx due to an avulsion of the central band of the extensor tendon to the middle phalanx or rheumatoid arthritis.

H. Tendons of the Flexor and Extensor Digitorum Muscles

- The **flexor digitorum superficialis** tendon splits into two medial and lateral bands and inserts on the base of the middle phalanx, whereas the **flexor digitorum profundus** tendon inserts on the base of the distal phalanx as a single tendon. On the dorsum of the hand, a single central band of the extensor digitorum tendon inserts on the base of the middle phalanx, whereas two lateral bands of the extensor digitorum tendon join to form a single band to insert on the base of the distal phalanx.

I. Extensor Expansion (Figure 7.17)

- Is the expansion of the extensor tendon over the metacarpophalangeal joint and is referred to by clinicians as the **extensor hood**.
- Provides the insertion of the lumbrical and interosseous muscles and the extensor indicis and extensor digiti minimi muscles.

J. Anatomic Snuffbox

- **Is a triangular interval** bounded medially by the tendon of the extensor pollicis longus muscle and laterally by the tendons of the extensor pollicis brevis and abductor pollicis longus muscles.
- Is limited proximally by the styloid process of the radius.
- Has a floor formed by the scaphoid and trapezium bones and crossed by the **radial artery**.

K. Fingernails

- Are keratinized plates on the dorsum of the tips of the fingers that consist of the proximal hidden part or **root**, the exposed part or **body**, and the distal **freeborder**. Parts of the nail include the following:

1. Nail bed

- The skin underneath the nail is the **nail bed** in which sensory nerve endings and blood vessels are abundant. The **matrix** or proximal part of the nail bed produces hard keratin and is responsible for nail growth.

2. Other structures

- The root is partially covered by a fold of skin known as the **nail fold**. The narrow band of epidermis prolonged from the proximal nail fold onto the nail is termed the **eponychium**. The half-moon, or **lunula,** is distal to the eponychium. The **hyponychium** represents the thickened epidermis deep to the distal end of the nail.

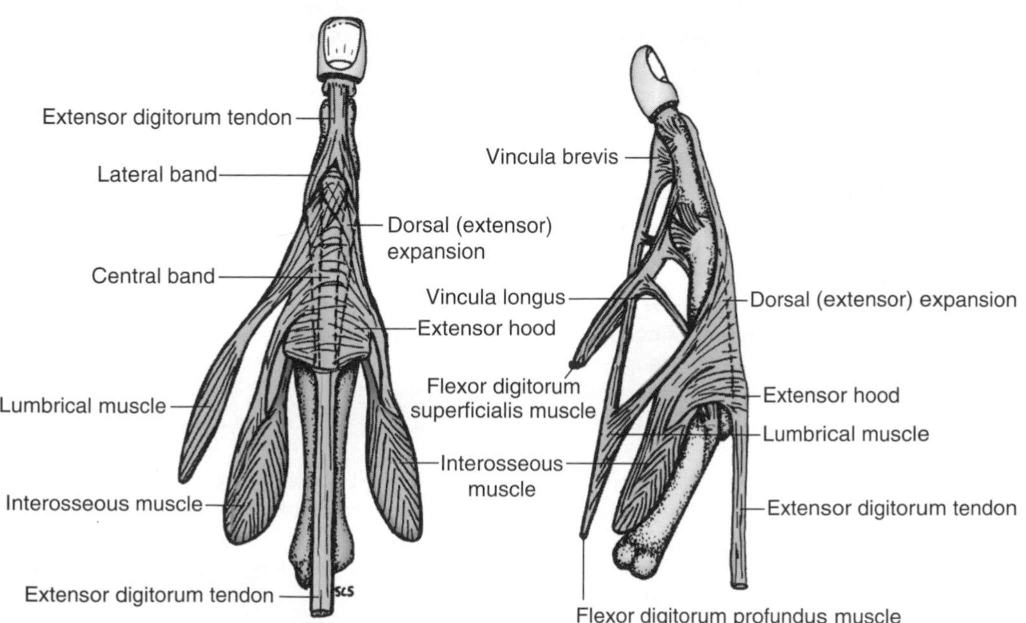

FIGURE 7.17. Dorsal (extensor) expansion of the middle finger.

NERVES OF THE UPPER LIMB

I BRACHIAL PLEXUS (See Figure 7.7)

- Is formed by the ventral primary rami of the lower four cervical nerves and the first thoracic nerve (C5–T1).
- Has roots that pass between the scalenus anterior and medius muscles.
- Is enclosed with the axillary artery and vein in the **axillary sheath**, which is formed by a prolongation of the prevertebral fascia.
- Has the following subdivisions:

A. Branches from the Roots

1. Dorsal Scapular Nerve (C5)

- Pierces the scalenus medius muscle to reach the posterior cervical triangle and descends deep to the levator scapulae and the rhomboid minor and major muscles.
- Innervates the rhomboids and frequently the levator scapulae muscles.

2. Long Thoracic Nerve (C5–C7)

- Descends behind the brachial plexus and runs on the external surface of the serratus anterior muscle, which it supplies.

CLINICAL CORRELATES **Injury to the long thoracic nerve** is commonly caused by a stab wound or during radical mastectomy or thoracic surgery. It results in paralysis of the serratus anterior muscle and inability to elevate the arm above the horizontal. It produces a **winged scapula** in which the vertebral (medial) border of the scapula protrudes away from the thorax.

B. Branches from the Upper Trunk

1. Suprascapular Nerve (C5–C6)

- Runs laterally across the posterior cervical triangle.
- Passes through the scapular notch under the superior transverse scapular ligament, whereas the suprascapular artery passes over the ligament. (Thus, it can be said that the army [**artery**] runs over the bridge [**ligament**], and the navy [**nerve**] runs under the bridge.)
- Supplies the supraspinatus muscle and the shoulder joint and then descends through the notch of the scapular neck to innervate the infraspinatus muscle.

2. Nerve to Subclavius (C5)

- Descends in front of the brachial plexus and the subclavian artery and behind the clavicle to reach the subclavius muscle.
- Also innervates the sternoclavicular joint.
- Usually branches to the **accessory phrenic nerve (C5)**, which enters the thorax to join the phrenic nerve.

C. Branches from the Lateral Cord

1. Lateral Pectoral Nerve (C5–C7)

- Innervates the **pectoralis major muscle** primarily and also supplies the **pectoralis minor muscle** by way of a nerve loop.
- Sends a branch over the first part of the axillary artery to the medial pectoral nerve and forms a nerve loop through which the lateral pectoral nerve conveys motor fibers to the pectoralis minor muscle.
- Pierces the costocoracoid membrane of the clavipectoral fascia.
- Is accompanied by the pectoral branch of the thoracoacromial artery.

2. Musculocutaneous Nerve (C5–C7)

- Pierces the coracobrachialis muscle, descends between the biceps brachii and brachialis muscles, and innervates these three muscles.

D. Branches from the Medial Cord

1. Medial Pectoral Nerve (C8–T1)

- Passes forward between the axillary artery and vein and forms a loop in front of the axillary artery with the lateral pectoral nerve.
- Enters and supplies the pectoralis minor muscle and reaches the overlying pectoralis major muscle.

2. Medial Brachial Cutaneous Nerve (C8–T1)

- Runs along the medial side of the axillary vein.
- Innervates the skin on the medial side of the arm.
- May communicate with the **intercostobrachial nerve**, which arises as a lateral branch of the second intercostal nerve.

3. Medial Antebrachial Cutaneous Nerve (C8–T1)

- Runs between the axillary artery and vein and then runs medial to the brachial artery.
- Innervates the skin on the medial side of the forearm.

4. Ulnar Nerve (C7–T1)

- Runs down the medial aspect of the arm but does not branch in the brachium.

E. Branches from the Medial and Lateral Cords: Median Nerve (C5–T1)

- Is formed by heads from both the medial and lateral cords.
- Runs down the anteromedial aspect of the arm but does not branch in the brachium.

F. Branches from the Posterior Cord

1. Upper Subscapular Nerve (C5–C6)

- Innervates the upper portion of the subscapularis muscle.

2. Thoracodorsal Nerve (C7–C8)

- Runs behind the axillary artery and accompanies the thoracodorsal artery to enter the latissimus dorsi muscle.

CLINICAL CORRELATES

Injury to the posterior cord is caused by the pressure of the crosspiece of a crutch, resulting in the paralysis of the arm called **crutch palsy**. It results in the loss in function of the extensors of the arm, forearm, and hand and produces a **wrist drop**.

3. Lower Subscapular Nerve (C5–C6)

- Innervates the lower part of the subscapularis and teres major muscles.
- Runs downward behind the subscapular vessels to the teres major muscle.

4. Axillary Nerve (C5–C6)

- Innervates the deltoid and teres minor muscles and gives rise to the **lateral brachial cutaneous nerve**.
- Passes posteriorly through the quadrangular space accompanied by the posterior circumflex humeral artery and winds around the surgical neck of the humerus (may be injured when this part of the bone is fractured).

CLINICAL CORRELATES

Injury to the axillary nerve is commonly caused by a fracture of the surgical neck of the humerus or inferior dislocation of the humerus. It results in weakness of lateral rotation and abduction of the arm (the supraspinatus can abduct the arm but not to a horizontal level).

5. Radial Nerve (C5–T1)

- Is the largest branch of the brachial plexus and occupies the musculospiral groove on the back of the humerus with the profunda brachii artery.

CLINICAL CORRELATES **Injury to the radial nerve** is commonly caused by a fracture of the midshaft of the humerus. It results in loss of function in the extensors of the forearm, hand, metacarpals, and phalanges. It also results in the loss of wrist extension, leading to **wrist drop**, and produces a weakness of abduction and adduction of the hand.

II. NERVES OF THE ARM, FOREARM, AND HAND (Figures 7.18 to 7.19)

A. Musculocutaneous Nerve (C5–C7)

- Pierces the coracobrachialis muscle and descends between the biceps and brachialis muscles.
- Innervates all of the flexor muscles in the anterior compartment of the arm, such as the coracobrachialis, biceps, and brachialis muscles.
- Continues into the forearm as the **lateral antebrachial cutaneous nerve**.

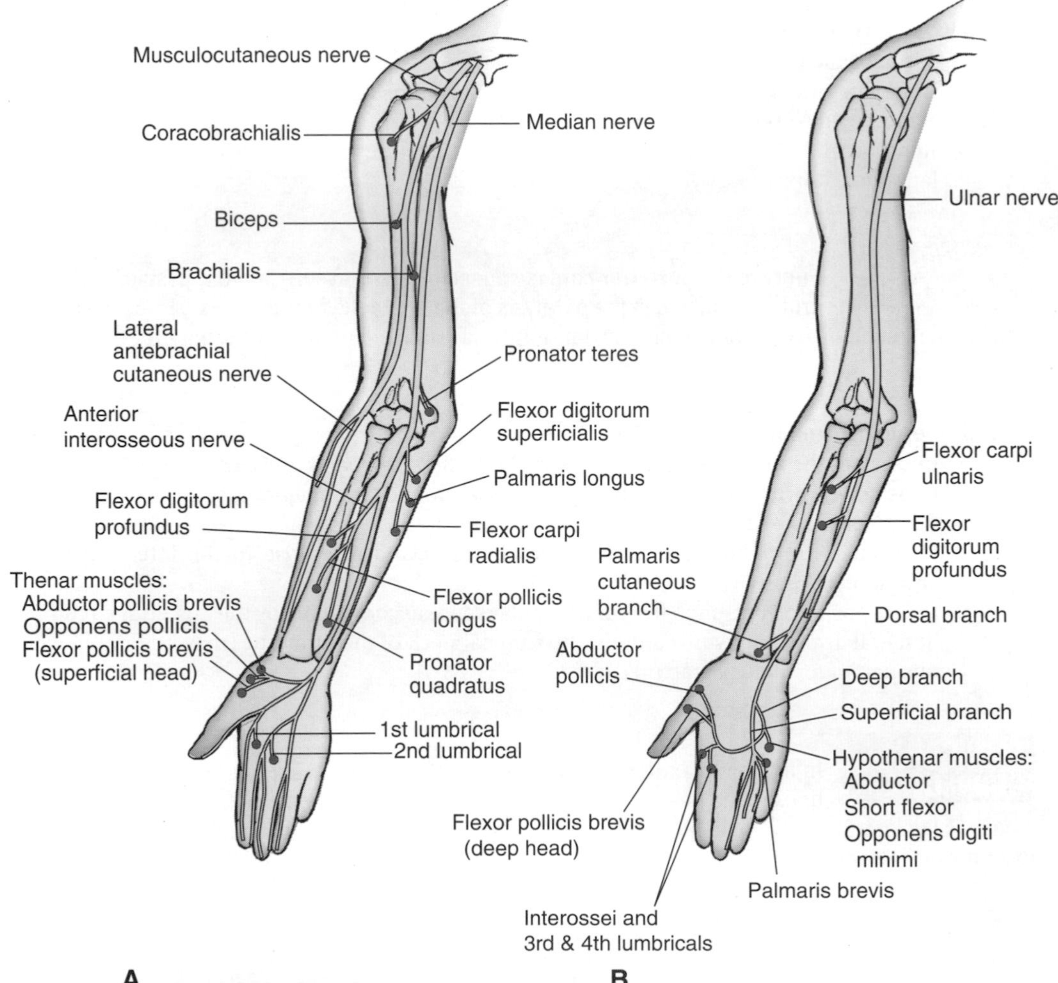

FIGURE 7.18. Distribution of the musculocutaneous, median, and ulnar nerves **A:** Distribution of musculocutaneous and median nerves. **B:** Distribution of ulnar nerve.

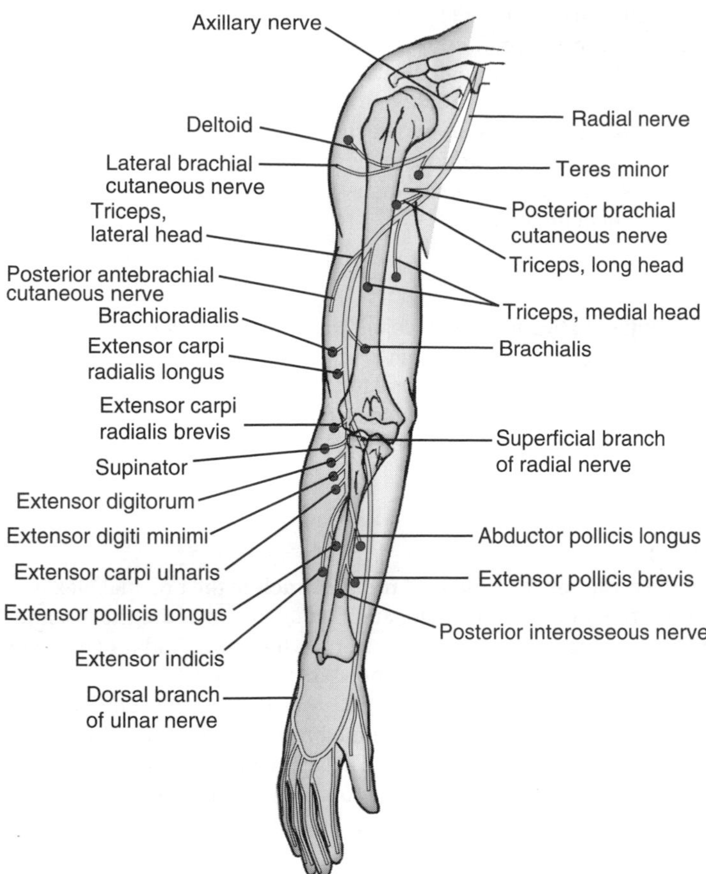

FIGURE 7.19. Distribution of the axillary and radial nerves.

CLINICAL CORRELATES

Injury to the musculocutaneous nerve results in weakness of supination (biceps) and flexion (biceps and brachialis) of forearm and loss of sensation on the lateral side of forearm.

B. Median Nerve (C5–T1)

- Runs down the anteromedial aspect of the arm, and at the elbow, it lies medial to the brachial artery on the brachialis muscle (has no muscular branches in the arm).
- Passes through the cubital fossa, deep to the bicipital aponeurosis, and medial to the brachial artery.
- Enters the forearm between the humeral and ulnar heads of the pronator teres muscle, passes between the flexor digitorum superficialis and the flexor digitorum profundus muscles, and then becomes superficial by passing between the tendons of the flexor digitorum superficialis and flexor carpi radialis near the wrist.
- In the cubital fossa, it gives rise to the **anterior interosseous nerve**, which descends on the interosseous membrane between the flexor digitorum profundus and the flexor pollicis longus; passes behind the pronator quadratus, supplying these three muscles; and then ends in sensory "twigs" to the wrist joint.

- Innervates all of the anterior muscles of the forearm except the flexor carpi ulnaris and the ulnar half of the flexor digitorum profundus.
- Enters the palm of the hand through the carpal tunnel deep to the flexor retinaculum; gives off a muscular branch (**recurrent branch**) to the thenar muscles; and terminates by dividing into three **common palmar digital nerves**, which then divide into the palmar digital branches.
- Innervates also the lateral two lumbricals, the skin of the lateral side of the palm, and the palmar side of the lateral three and one-half fingers and the dorsal side of the index finger, middle finger, and one-half of the ring finger.

CLINICAL CORRELATES

Injury to the median nerve may be caused by a supracondylar fracture of the humerus or a compression in the carpal tunnel. It results in the loss of pronation, opposition of the thumb, and flexion of the lateral two interphalangeal joints and impairment of the medial two interphalangeal joints. It also produces a characteristic flattening of the thenar eminence, often referred to as the **ape hand**.

C. Radial Nerve (C5–T1)

- Arises from the posterior cord and the **largest branch** of the brachial plexus.
- Descends posteriorly between the long and medial heads of the triceps, after which it passes inferolaterally with the profunda brachii artery in the spiral (radial) groove on the back of the humerus between the medial and lateral heads of the triceps.
- Pierces the lateral intermuscular septum to enter the anterior compartment and descends anterior to the lateral epicondyle between the brachialis and brachioradialis muscles to enter the cubital fossa, where it divides into superficial and deep branches.
- Gives rise to muscular branches (which supply the brachioradialis and extensor carpi radialis longus), articular branches, and posterior brachial and posterior antebrachial cutaneous branches.

1. Deep Branch

- Enters the supinator muscle, winds laterally around the radius in the substance of the muscle, and supplies the extensor carpi radialis brevis and supinator muscles.
- Emerges from the supinator as the **posterior interosseous nerve** and continues with the posterior interosseous artery and innervates the extensor muscles of the forearm.

2. Superficial Branch

- Descends in the forearm under cover of the brachioradialis muscle and then passes dorsally around the radius under the tendon of the brachioradialis.
- Runs distally to the dorsum of the hand to innervate the skin of the radial side of the hand and the radial two and one-half digits over the proximal phalanx. This nerve does not supply the skin of the distal phalanges.

D. Ulnar Nerve (C7–T1)

- Arises from the medial cord of the brachial plexus, runs down the medial aspect of the arm, pierces the medial intermuscular septum at the middle of the arm, and descends together with the superior ulnar collateral branch of the brachial artery.
- Descends behind the medial epicondyle in a groove or tunnel (cubital tunnel), where it is readily palpated and most commonly injured. It may be damaged by a fracture of the medial epicondyle and produce **funny bone** symptoms.
- Enters the forearm by passing between the two heads of the flexor carpi ulnaris and descends between and innervates the flexor carpi ulnaris and flexor digitorum profundus muscles.
- Enters the hand superficial to the flexor retinaculum and lateral to the pisiform bone, where it is vulnerable to damage from cuts or stab wounds.
- Terminates by dividing into superficial and deep branches at the root of the hypothenar eminence.

CLINICAL CORRELATES **Injury to the ulnar nerve** is commonly caused by a fracture of the medial epicondyle and results in a **claw hand**, in which the ring and little fingers are hyperextended at the metacarpophalangeal joints and flexed at the interphalangeal joints. It results in loss of abduction and adduction of the fingers and flexion of the metacarpophalangeal joints because of the paralysis of the palmar and dorsal interossei muscles and the medial two lumbricals. It also produces wasting of the hypothenar eminence and palm and also leads to loss of adduction of the thumb because of the paralysis of the adductor pollicis muscle.

1. **Superficial Branch**
   - Innervates the palmaris brevis and the skin over the palmar and dorsal surfaces of the medial one-third of the hand, including the hypothenar eminence.
   - Terminates in the palm by dividing into **threepalmar digital branches**, which supply the skin of the little finger and the medial side of the ring finger.
2. **Deep Branch**
   - Arises at and travels through the Guyon canal, and then passes between the pisiform and the hook of the hamate, and then deep to the opponens digiti minimi.
   - Curves medial to the hook of the hamate, and then turns laterally to follow the course of the deep palmar arterial arch across the interossei, and then runs between two heads of the adductor pollicis.
   - Innervates the hypothenar muscles, the medial two lumbricals, all of the interossei, the adductor pollicis, and usually the deep head of the flexor pollicis brevis.

III. FUNCTIONAL COMPONENTS OF THE PERIPHERAL NERVES

A. Somatic Motor Nerves

- Include radial, axillary, median, musculocutaneous, and ulnar nerves and ventral or dorsal primary rami and other nerves.
- Contain nerve fibers with cell bodies that are located in the following structures:
  1. **Dorsal root ganglia for general somatic afferent (GSA) and general visceral afferent (GVA) fibers.**
  2. **Anterior horn of the spinal cord for general somatic efferent (GSE) fibers.**
  3. **Sympathetic chain ganglia for sympathetic postganglionic general visceral efferent (GVE) fibers.**

B. Cutaneous Nerves

- Include medial brachial, medial antebrachial, lateral antebrachial, and other cutaneous nerves.
- Contain nerve fibers with cell bodies that are located in the following structures:
  1. **Dorsal root ganglia for GSA and GVA fibers.**
  2. **Sympathetic chain ganglia for sympathetic postganglionic GVE fibers.**

CLINICAL CORRELATES **Upper trunk injury (Erb–Duchenne paralysis or Erb palsy)** is caused by a birth injury during a breech delivery or a violent displacement of the head from the shoulder such as might result from a fall from a motorcycle or horse. It results in a loss of abduction, flexion, and lateral rotation of the arm, producing a **waiter's tip hand**, in which the arm tends to lie in medial rotation resulting from paralysis of lateral rotator muscles.

Lower trunk injury (Klumpke paralysis) may be caused during a difficult breech delivery (birth palsy or obstetric paralysis), by a cervical rib (cervical rib syndrome), or by abnormal insertion or spasm of the anterior and middle scalene muscles (scalene syndrome). The injury causes a **claw hand**.

Thoracic outlet syndrome is a syndrome involving the **compression of neurovascular structures** such as brachial plexus (lower trunk or C8 and T1 nerve roots) and subclavian vessels in the **thoracic outlet** (a space between the clavicle and the first rib) between the base of the neck and axilla. It is caused by (1) **abnormal insertion** or spasm of the anterior and middle scalene muscles, causing ischemic muscle pain in the arm; (2) a **cervical rib** (cartilaginous elongation of the transverse process of the seventh cervical vertebra), compressing the subclavian artery, causing impaired circulation; (3) a **fractured clavicle**, causing subclavian venous bleeding and thrombosis, leading to **pulmonary embolism**; or (4) physical trauma and repetitive strain injury. Symptoms include pain, numbness, tingling, and weakness in the upper limb. Its treatment involves physical measures, medications, and surgery.

BLOOD VESSELS OF THE UPPER LIMB

I. BRANCHES OF THE SUBCLAVIAN ARTERY (Figure 7.8)

A. Suprascapular Artery

- Is a branch of the thyrocervical trunk.
- Passes over the superior transverse scapular ligament (whereas the suprascapular nerve passes under the ligament).
- Anastomoses with the deep branch of the transverse cervical artery (**dorsal scapular artery**) and the circumflex scapular artery around the scapula, providing a collateral circulation.
- Supplies the supraspinatus and infraspinatus muscles and the shoulder and acromioclavicular joints.

B. Dorsal Scapular or Descending Scapular Artery

- Arises from the subclavian artery but may be a deep branch of the transverse cervical artery.
- Accompanies the dorsal scapular nerve.
- Supplies the levator scapulae, rhomboids, and serratus anterior muscles.

C. Arterial Anastomoses around Scapular

- Occur between three groups of arteries: (a) suprascapular, descending scapular, and circumflex scapular arteries; (b) acromial and posterior humeral circumflex arteries; and (c) descending scapular and posterior intercostal arteries.

II. AXILLARY ARTERY (See Figures 7.8 to 7.9)

- Is considered to be the central structure of the axilla.
- Extends from the outer border of the first rib to the inferior border of the teres major muscle, where it becomes the **brachial artery**. The axillary artery is bordered on its medial side by the axillary vein.
- Is divided into three parts by the pectoralis minor muscle.

A. Superior or Supreme Thoracic Artery

- Supplies the intercostal muscles in the first and second anterior intercostal spaces and adjacent muscles.

B. Thoracoacromial Artery

- Is a short trunk from the first or second part of the axillary artery and has pectoral, clavicular, acromial, and deltoid branches.
- Pierces the costocoracoid membrane (or clavipectoral fascia).

C. Lateral Thoracic Artery

- Runs along the lateral border of the pectoralis minor muscle.
- Supplies the pectoralis major, pectoralis minor, and serratus anterior muscles and the axillary lymph nodes and gives rise to **lateral mammary branches**.

D. Subscapular Artery

- Is the largest branch of the axillary artery, arises at the lower border of the subscapularis muscle, and descends along the axillary border of the scapula.
- Divides into the thoracodorsal and circumflex scapular arteries.

1. Thoracodorsal Artery

- Accompanies the thoracodorsal nerve and supplies the latissimus dorsi muscle and the lateral thoracic wall.

2. Circumflex Scapular Artery

- Passes posteriorly into the triangular space bounded by the subscapularis muscle and the teres minor muscle above, the teres major muscle below, and the long head of the triceps brachii laterally.
- Ramifies in the infraspinous fossa and anastomoses with branches of the dorsal scapular and suprascapular arteries.

E. Anterior Humeral Circumflex Artery

- Passes anteriorly around the surgical neck of the humerus.
- Anastomoses with the posterior humeral circumflex artery.

F. Posterior Humeral Circumflex Artery

- Runs posteriorly with the axillary nerve through the quadrangular space bounded by the teres minor and teres major muscles, the long head of the triceps brachii, and the humerus.
- Anastomoses with the anterior humeral circumflex artery and an ascending branch of the profunda brachii artery and also sends a branch to the acromial rete.

CLINICAL CORRELATES If the **axillary artery** is ligated between the thyrocervical trunk and the subscapular artery, then blood from **anastomoses in the scapular region** arrives at the subscapular artery in which the blood flow is reversed to reach the axillary artery distal to the ligature. The axillary artery may be compressed or felt for the pulse in front of the teres major or against the humerus in the lateral wall of the axilla.

III. BRACHIAL ARTERY (See Figures 7.8 to 7.9)

- Extends from the inferior border of the teres major muscle to its bifurcation in the cubital fossa.
- Lies on the triceps brachii and then on the brachialis muscles medial to the coracobrachialis and biceps brachii and is accompanied by the basilic vein in the middle of the arm.
- Lies in the center of the cubital fossa, medial to the biceps tendon, lateral to the median nerve, and deep to the bicipital aponeurosis. The stethoscope should be placed in this place when taking **blood pressure** and listening to the **arterial pulse**.
- Provides muscular branches and terminates by dividing into the radial and ulnar arteries at the level of the radial neck, approximately 1 cm below the bend of the elbow, in the cubital fossa.

A. Profunda Brachii (Deep Brachial) Artery

- Descends posteriorly with the radial nerve and gives off an **ascending branch**, which anastomoses with the descending branch of the posterior humeral circumflex artery.
- Divides into the **middle collateral artery**, which anastomoses with the interosseous recurrent artery, and the **radial collateral artery**, which follows the radial nerve through the lateral

intermuscular septum and ends in front of the lateral epicondyle by anastomosing with the radial recurrent artery of the radial artery.

B. Superior Ulnar Collateral Artery

- Pierces the medial intermuscular septum and accompanies the ulnar nerve behind the septum and medial epicondyle.
- Anastomoses with the posterior ulnar recurrent branch of the ulnar artery.

C. Inferior Ulnar Collateral Artery

- Arises just above the elbow and descends in front of the medial epicondyle.
- Anastomoses with the anterior ulnar recurrent branch of the ulnar artery.

CLINICAL CORRELATES If the **brachial artery** is tied off distal to the inferior ulnar collateral artery, sufficient blood reaches the ulnar and radial arteries via the existing **anastomoses around the elbow**. The brachial artery may be compressed or felt for the **pulse** on the brachialis against the humerus but medial to the biceps and its tendon and can be used for taking blood pressure.

IV. RADIAL ARTERY (See Figures 7.8, 7.9, and 7.20)

- Arises as the smaller lateral branch of the brachial artery in the cubital fossa and descends laterally under cover of the brachioradialis muscle, with the superficial radial nerve on its lateral side, on the supinator and flexor pollicis longus muscles.
- Curves over the radial side of the carpal bones beneath the tendons of the abductor pollicis longus muscle, the extensor pollicis longus and brevis muscles, and over the surface of the scaphoid and trapezium bones.
- Runs through the anatomic snuffbox, enters the palm by passing between the two heads of the first dorsal interosseous muscle and then between the heads of the adductor pollicis muscle, and divides into the **princeps pollicis artery** and the **deep palmar arch**.
- Accounts for the **radial pulse**, which can be felt proximal to the wrist between the tendons of the brachioradialis and flexor carpi radialis muscles. The radial pulse may also be palpated in the anatomic snuffbox between the tendons of the extensor pollicis longus and brevis muscles.
- Gives rise to the following branches:

A. Radial Recurrent Artery

- Arises from the radial artery just below its origin and ascends on the supinator and then between the brachioradialis and brachialis muscles.
- Anastomoses with the radial collateral branch of the profunda brachii artery.

B. Palmar Carpal Branch

- Joins the palmar carpal branch of the ulnar artery and forms the palmar carpal arch.

C. Superficial Palmar Branch

- Passes through the thenar muscles and anastomoses with the superficial branch of the ulnar artery to complete the superficial palmar arterial arch.

D. Dorsal Carpal Branch

- Joins the dorsal carpal branch of the ulnar artery and the dorsal terminal branch of the anterior interosseous artery to form the **dorsal carpal rete**.

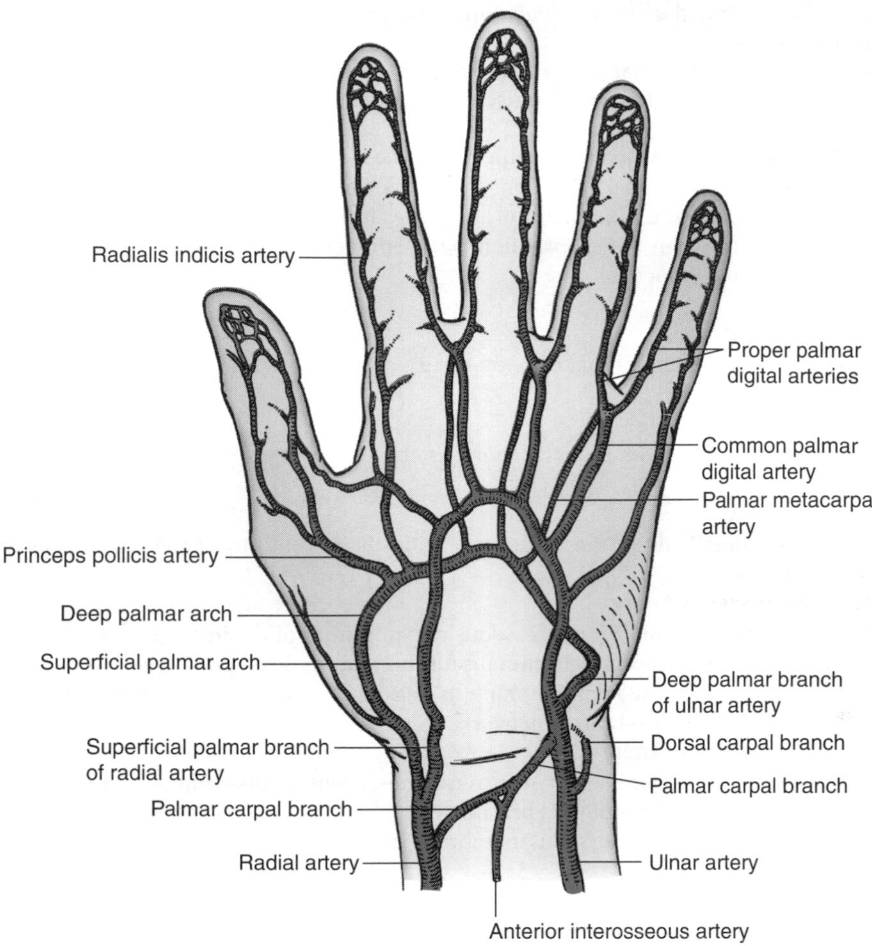

FIGURE 7.20. Blood supply to the hand.

E. Princeps Pollicis Artery

- Descends along the ulnar border of the first metacarpal bone under the flexor pollicis longus tendon.
- Divides into two **proper digital arteries** for each side of the thumb.

F. Radialis Indicis Artery

- Also may arise from the deep palmar arch or the princeps pollicis artery.

G. Deep Palmar Arch

- Is formed by the main termination of the radial artery and usually is completed by the deep palmar branch of the ulnar artery.
- Passes between the transverse and oblique heads of the adductor pollicis muscle.
- Gives rise to **threepalmar metacarpal arteries**, which descend on the interossei and join the common palmar digital arteries from the superficial palmar arch.

V. ULNAR ARTERY (See Figures 7.8, 7.9, and 7.20)

- Is the **larger medial branch of the brachial artery** in the cubital fossa.
- Descends behind the ulnar head of the pronator teres muscle and lies between the flexor digitorum superficialis and profundus muscles.

- Enters the hand anterior to the flexor retinaculum, lateral to the pisiform bone, and medial to the hook of the hamate bone.
- Divides into the superficial palmar arch and the deep palmar branch, which passes between the abductor and flexor digiti minimi brevis muscles and runs medially to join the radial artery to complete the deep palmar arch.
- Accounts for the **ulnar pulse**, which is palpable just to the radial side of the insertion of the flexor carpi ulnaris into the pisiform bone. If the ulnar artery arises high from the brachial artery and runs invariably superficial to the flexor muscles, the artery may be mistaken for a vein for certain drugs, resulting in disastrous gangrene with subsequent partial or total loss of the hand.
- Gives rise to the following branches:

A. Anterior Ulnar Recurrent Artery

- Anastomoses with the inferior ulnar collateral artery.

B. Posterior Ulnar Recurrent Artery

- Anastomoses with the superior ulnar collateral artery.

C. Common Interosseous Artery

- Arises from the lateral side of the ulnar artery and divides into the anterior and posterior interosseous arteries.

1. Anterior Interosseous Artery

- Descends with the anterior interosseous nerve in front of the interosseous membrane, located between the flexor digitorum profundus and the flexor pollicis longus muscles.
- Perforates the interosseous membrane to anastomose with the posterior interosseous artery and join the dorsal carpal network.

2. Posterior Interosseous Artery

- Gives rise to the interosseous recurrent artery, which anastomoses with a middle collateral branch of the profunda brachii artery.
- Descends behind the interosseous membrane in company with the posterior interosseous nerve.
- Anastomoses with the dorsal carpal branch of the anterior interosseous artery.

CLINICAL CORRELATES If the **ulnar artery** arises high from the brachial artery and runs invariably superficial to the flexor muscles, then when injecting, the artery may be mistaken for a vein for certain drugs, resulting in disastrous gangrene with subsequent partial or total loss of the hand. The ulnar artery may be compressed or felt for the **pulse** on the anterior aspect of the flexor retinaculum on the lateral side of the pisiform bone.

D. Palmar Carpal Branch

- Joins the palmar carpal branch of the radial artery to form the palmar carpal arch.

E. Dorsal Carpal Branch

- Passes around the ulnar side of the wrist and joins the dorsal carpal rete.

F. Superficial Palmar Arterial Arch

- Is the main termination of the ulnar artery, usually completed by anastomosis with the superficial palmar branch of the radial artery.
- Lies immediately under the palmar aponeurosis.
- Gives rise to three **common palmar digital arteries**, each of which bifurcates into proper palmar digital arteries, which run distally to supply the adjacent sides of the fingers.

G. Deep Palmar Branch

- Accompanies the deep branch of the ulnar nerve through the hypothenar muscles and anastomoses with the radial artery, thereby completing the **deep palmar arch**.
- Gives rise to the palmar metacarpal arteries, which join the common palmar digital arteries.

CLINICAL CORRELATES The **Allen test** is a test for occlusion of the radial or ulnar artery; either the radial or ulnar artery is digitally compressed by the examiner after blood has been forced out of the hand by making a tight fist; failure of the blood to return to the palm and fingers on opening indicates that the uncompressed artery is occluded.

VI. VEINS OF THE UPPER LIMB (See Figure 7.4)

A. Deep and Superficial Venous Arches

- Are formed by a pair of venae comitantes, which accompany each of the deep and superficial palmar arterial arches.

B. Deep Veins of the Arm and Forearm

- Follow the course of the arteries, accompanying them as their venae comitantes. (The radial veins receive the dorsal metacarpal veins. The ulnar veins receive tributaries from the deep palmar venous arches. The brachial veins are the vena comitantes of the brachial artery and are joined by the basilic vein to form the axillary vein.)

C. Axillary Vein

- Is formed at the lower border of the teres major muscle by the union of the brachial veins (venae comitantes of the brachial artery) and the basilic vein and ascends along the medial side of the axillary artery.
- Continues as the subclavian vein at the inferior margin of the first rib.
- Commonly receives the thoracoepigastric veins directly or indirectly and thus provides a collateral circulation if the inferior vena cava becomes obstructed.
- Has tributaries that include the cephalic vein, brachial veins (venae comitantes of the brachial artery that join the basilic vein to form the axillary vein), and veins that correspond to the branches of the axillary artery.

CLINICAL CORRELATES **Venipuncture of the upper limb** is performed on veins by applying a tourniquet to the arm, when the venous return is occluded and the veins are distended and are visible and palpable. Venipuncture may be performed on the axillary vein to locate the central line, on the median cubital vein for drawing blood, and on the dorsal venous network or the cephalic and basilic veins at their origin for long-term introduction of fluids or intravenous feeding.

VII. DEVELOPMENT OF THE LIMBS

- Begins with the activation of mesenchymal cells in the **lateral plate somatic mesoderm**.

A. Appendicular Skeleton

- Develops from mesenchyme derived from the somatic mesoderm in the limb buds.

1. Limb Buds

- Consist of a **mesenchymal core** covered with ectoderm and capped by an **apical ectodermal ridge** that induces limb growth and development.
- Arise in somatic mesoderm at week 4. The upper limb buds arise first, and the lower limb buds soon follow.
  - (a) **Upper limb** buds rotate laterally through 90 degrees, whereas the lower limb buds rotate medially through almost 90 degrees. The upper limb buds become elongated by week 5, and soon after, they are subdivided into the precursors of the arm, forearm, and hand.

(b) The hand and foot are subdivided into digits by week 6, and individual fingers and toes are visible by week 8.

2. **Bones of Limbs**
- Are derived from the **lateral plate somatic mesoderm** and develop by endochondral ossification except the clavicle, which develops by intramembranous ossification. (**Endochondral ossification** involves development of hyaline cartilage models that are replaced by bone, except at epiphyseal plates and articular cartilages, whereas **intramembranous ossification** involves direct ossification of mesenchyme and lacks a cartilaginous precursor.) Epimysium, perimysium, and tendons develop from the lateral plate somatic mesoderm.
- Continue to grow after birth due to activity of the epiphyseal plates. (At birth, the diaphysis of the bone is ossified but the epiphyses are still cartilaginous.)

3. **Muscles of Limbs**
- Develop exclusively from the myotomic portions of the **somites** and also from ventral (flexor) and dorsal (extensor) condensations of somitic mesoderm.

B. Limb Abnormalities
- Include congenital absence of a limb (amelia); partial absence of a limb (meromelia), in which hands and feet are attached to the trunk by a small irregular bone; fusion of digits (syndactyly); and extra digits (polydactyly).

HIGH-YIELD TOPICS

- **Pectoral (shoulder) girdle**—formed by the **clavicle** and **scapula**, attaches the upper limb (appendicular skeleton) to the sternum (axial skeleton). The clavicle is a commonly fractured bone, the first bone to begin ossification but the last bone to complete ossification, and the only long bone to be ossified intramembranously (other bones of the upper limb develop by endochondral ossification).
- The **quadrangular space** is bounded by the teres minor (with subscapularis), teres major, triceps (long head), and the humerus and transmits the **axillary nerve** and the posterior humeral circumflex vessels. The **auscultation triangle** is bounded by the trapezius, latissimus dorsi, and scapula and is the most audible site for breath sounds.
- **Rotator cuff**—is formed by the tendons of the **s**upraspinatus, **i**nfraspinatus, **t**eres minor, and **s**ubscapularis (**SITS**). **Rupture of rotator cuff** occurs most frequently by **attrition of the supraspinatus tendon** by friction, resulting in degenerative **tendonitis**,a **painful shoulder**, and **subacromial bursitis**.
- **Breast**—is supported by the **suspensory ligaments of Cooper**. The **mammary gland**, which lies in the superficial fascia, has 15 to 20 lobes and has an **axillary tail** that extends superolaterally into the axilla. Each lobe opens by a **lactiferous duct** onto the tip of the nipple, and each duct enlarges to form a **lactiferous sinus** for milk storage during lactation. The chief **lymphatic drainage** is to the axillary nodes, more specifically to the pectoral nodes.
- **Breast Cancer**: commonly occurs in the upper lateral quadrant, produces a **dimpling of the skin** due to cancer on the suspensory ligament of Cooper and a retracted or **inverted nipple** due to cancer on the lactiferous ducts. An advanced sign of inflammatory breast cancer, **peau d'orange** (texture of an orange peel) is the edematous (swollen) and pitted breast skin due to obstruction of the subcutaneous lymphatics.
- **Sentinel node** is the first lymph node(s) to which cancer cells are likely to spread from the primary tumor.
- The **biceps brachii muscle** flexes the arm at the elbow and is a powerful supinator.
- **Palmar aponeurosis** is a triangular fibrous layer overlying the tendons in the palm and protects the superficial palmar arterial arch and palmar digital nerves. The **flexor retinaculum** forms the **carpal tunnel** through which the median nerve and tendons of the long flexor muscles are transmitted. The **extensor expansion** provides the insertion of the lumbrical, interosseous, and extensor muscles of the hand and fingers.

- The **flexor digitorum superficialis** tendon splits into medial and lateral bands, which pass around the flexor digitorum profundus tendon and insert on the base of the middle phalanx, while the **flexor digitorum profundus** tendon inserts on the base of the distal phalanx as a single tendon. On the dorsum of the hand, a single central band of the **extensor digitorum** tendon inserts on the base of the middle phalanx, whereas two lateral bands of the extensor digitorum tendon join to form a single terminal band to insert on the base of the distal phalanx.
- **Fracture of the clavicle** may cause injury to the **brachial plexus** (lower trunk), fatal hemorrhage from the s**ubclavian vein**, or **pulmonary embolism**.
- **Fracture of the lower end of the radius** (**Colles fracture**) causes the distal fragment of the radius to be displaced posteriorly, producing the **dinner (silver) fork deformity**.
- **Smith facture** is sometimes called a reverse Colles fracture. It is also a fracture of the distal radius, but the fracture fragment displaces anteriorly, resulting in a **garden spade deformity**.
- The **scaphoid bone** lies deep to the anatomical snuffbox and is f**requently fractured** by falls on an outstretched hand, causing damage to the radial artery. **Fracture of the hamate** may injure the **ulnar nerve** and artery. **Bennett fracture** is a fracture of the base of the **metacarpal of the thumb**. **Boxer's fracture** is the fracture of the **metacarpal neck**.
- **Tennis elbow** (lateral epicondylitis) is caused by a chronic **inflammation or irritation of the origin (tendon) of the extensor muscles** of the forearm from the lateral epicondyle of the humerus as a result of repetitive strain.
- **Golfer's elbow** (medial epicondylitis) is caused by a chronic **inflammation or irritation of the tendon (origin) of the flexor muscles** of the forearm from the medial epicondyle of the humerus.
- **Nursemaid's elbow** is a radial head subluxation, which occurs when the child is lifted by the wrist. It is caused by a partial tear (or loosening) of the annular ligament and causes the radial head to slip out of position.
- **Cubital tunnel syndrome** results from **compression on the ulnar nerve** in the cubital tunnel behind the medial epicondyle (funny bone), causing numbness and tingling in the ring and little fingers. The **cubital tunnel** is formed by the medial epicondyle, ulnar collateral ligament, and two heads of the flexor carpi ulnaris, and **transmits the ulnar nerve** and superior ulnar collateral artery.
- The **anatomic snuffbox** is bounded medially by the extensor pollicis tendon and laterally by the extensor pollicis brevis and abductor pollicis longus tendons. Its floor is formed by the scaphoid and trapezium bones and is crossed by the radial artery.
- **Guyon canal syndrome** is an **entrapment of the ulnar nerve** in the Guyon canal, which is formed by the pisiform, hook of hamate, and pisohamate ligament.
- The **carpal tunnel** is an osteofascial tunnel consisting of the **carpal arch** and overlying **flexor retinaculum**, and contains nine muscle tendons and the **median nerve**. **Carpal tunnel syndrome** is caused by **compression of the median nerve**, resulting in **pain** and **paresthesia** (tingling, burning, and numbness) and **atrophy of the thenar muscles**.
- **Dupuytren contracture** is a progressive thickening, shortening, and **fibrosis of the palmar fascia**, producing a **fixed flexion contracture of the hand**, in which the fingers bend toward the palm and cannot be fully extended (commonly fourth and fifth fingers). **Volkmann contracture** is an ischemic contracture (flexion deformity) resulting from necrosis of the forearm flexor muscles.
- **Tenosynovitis** is an **infection of the synovial sheath and tendon** (the long flexor tendon), causing pain, swelling, and difficulty moving a joint. **Rupture** of the tendon sheath (puncture injury of the palm) may cause the **spread** of infection to the **midpalmar space** and to the carpal tunnel. Likewise, tenosynovitis in the thumb may spread to the **radial bursa** and in the little finger to the **ulnar bursa**.
- **Trigger finger** occurs when the **long flexor tendon develops a nodule** or swelling that **interferes with its gliding** through the pulley, causing **pain at the joint** and an **audible clicking** or snapping. The condition is caused by rheumatoid arthritis, repetitive trauma, and wear and tear of aging of the tendon.
- **Mallet finger** (hammer finger or baseball finger) is a finger with **permanent flexion of the distal phalanx** due to an **avulsion of the lateral bands of the extensor tendon** to the distal phalanx.
- **Boutonniere deformity** is a finger with **abnormal flexion of the middle phalanx** and hyperextension of the distal phalanx due to a **rupture of the central band of the extensor tendon** to the middle phalanx.

- **Brachial plexopathy** is pain, decreased sensation, or muscular deficits due to a nerve problem in the upper limb.
- **Upper trunk injury** (Erb–Duchenne paralysis or Erb palsy) is caused by a difficult delivery in infants or a fall onto the shoulder in adults. It results in a loss of abduction, flexion, and lateral rotation of the arm, producing a **Waiter's tip hand**, in which the arm tends to lie in medial rotation and the forearm pronated.
- **Lower trunk injury** (Klumpke paralysis) may be caused by excessive traction on the upper limb as seen in a breech delivery (**birth palsy**), a cervical rib, or abnormal insertion or spasm of the anterior and middle scalene muscles (**scalene syndrome**). It results in a **claw hand deformity** due to nonfunctioning intrinsic hand muscles.
- **A Pancoast tumor** in the apex of the lung can result in the lower trunk injury and occasionally **Horner syndrome** due to sympathetic ganglion compression (ptosis, anhidrosis, pupillary constriction). It can also cause thoracic outlet syndrome.
- **Injury to the long thoracic nerve** results in paralysis of the serratus anterior muscle, causing a **winged scapula** (the medial border of the scapula moves or protrudes posteriorly away from the thoracic wall) when pushing against resistance. It may also cause difficulty in raising the arm above the head.
- **Injury to the suprascapular nerve** is characterized by atrophy of the supraspinatus and infraspinatus muscles. Deficits will include difficulty in initiation of arm abduction and weakness in external rotation of the arm.
- **Injury to the posterior cord** of the brachial plexus results in the weakness of shoulder abduction (axillary), **extensors** of the forearm, wrist, and metacarpophalangeal joint (radial), and produces a **wrist drop**.
- **Injury to the axillary nerve** caused by a **fracture of the surgical neck** of the humerus or **inferior dislocation** of the humerus results in the **weakness of lateral rotation and abduction** of the arm.
- **Injury to the radial nerve** caused by a **fracture of the midshaft of the humerus**, results in **loss of function in the extensors** of the forearm, hand, metacarpals, and phalanges. It also results in **wrist drop** and produces a weakness of abduction and adduction of the hand.
- **Injury to the musculocutaneous nerve** results in **weakness of supination (biceps) and flexion** (biceps, brachialis, and coracobrachialis) of the forearm and loss of sensation on the lateral side of the forearm.
- **Injury to the median nerve** may be caused by a **supracondylar fracture** of the humerus or a **compression in the carpal tunnel**, resulting in loss of pronation, opposition, and abduction of the thumb, flexion of the lateral two interphalangeal joints, and impairment of the medial two interphalangeal joints. It also produces the **ape hand deformity** (thenar eminence wasting and inability to abduct the thumb).
- **Pronator syndrome** is caused by entrapment of the **median nerve** between the heads of the pronator teres muscle. Pain and weakness result when pronating against resistance.
- **Injury to the ulnar nerve** is caused by a **fracture of the medial epicondyle** or fracture dislocation of the elbow joint, resulting in loss of sensation in the fourth and fifth digits and a **claw hand deformity**. It also results in **loss of abduction and adduction of the fingers**, **flexion of the metacarpophalangeal joints**, and **adduction of the thumb**, and produces a **wasted hypothenar eminence** and palm.
- **Thoracic outlet syndrome** is the compression of a neurovascular bundle in the thoracic outlet between the clavicle and the first rib. It can be caused by the abnormal insertion of scalene muscles, by a cervical rib, or by a fractured clavicle.
- **Anastomosis around the scapula** is formed by the dorsal scapular (also called deep branch of the transverse cervical), suprascapular, and subscapular (circumflex scapular branch) arteries.
- **Axillary artery** pulse is felt in front of the teres major, **the brachial artery** on the brachialis but medial to the biceps tendon, **the radial artery** in front of the distal end of the radius between the tendons of the brachioradialis and flexor carpi radialis, and the **ulnar artery** anterior to the flexor retinaculum on the lateral side of the pisiform bone.
- The **ulnar artery** is the major contribution to the **superficial palmar arterial arch**, whereas the **radial artery** is the major contribution to the **deep palmar arch**.
- The **cephalic vein** drains the lateral aspect of the forearm and arm and then drains into the axillary vein.

- The **basilic vein** runs along the ulnar border of the forearm and pierces the deep fascia of the arm and joins the brachial veins (the venae comitantes of the brachial artery) to **form the axillary vein**.
- The **median cubital vein connects the cephalic and basilica veins in the cubital fossa and** is commonly used for **venipuncture** and **blood transfusion**.

Summary

MUSCLE ACTIONS OF THE UPPER LIMB

Movement of the Scapula

Elevation—trapezius (upper part), levator scapulae
Depression—trapezius (lower part), serratus anterior, pectoralis minor
Protrusion (forward or lateral movement; abduction)—serratus anterior
Retraction (backward or medial movement; adduction)—trapezius, rhomboids
Anterior or inferior rotation of the glenoid fossa—rhomboid major
Posterior or superior rotation of the glenoid fossa—serratus anterior, trapezius

Movement at the Shoulder Joint (Ball-and-Socket Joint)

Adduction—pectoralis major, latissimus dorsi, deltoid (posterior part)
Abduction—deltoid, supraspinatus
Flexion—pectoralis major (clavicular part), deltoid (anterior part), coracobrachialis, biceps
Extension—latissimus dorsi, deltoid (posterior part)
Medial rotation—subscapularis, pectoralis major, deltoid (anterior part), latissimus dorsi, teres major
Lateral rotation—infraspinatus, teres minor, deltoid (posterior part)

Movement at the Elbow Joint (Hinge Joint)

Flexion—brachialis, biceps, brachioradialis, pronator teres
Extension—triceps, anconeus

Movement at the Radioulnar Joints (Pivot Joints)

Pronation—pronator quadratus, pronator teres
Supination—supinator, biceps brachii

Movement at the Wrist (Radiocarpal) Joint (Condylar or Ellipsoidal Joint)

Adduction—flexor carpi ulnaris, extensor carpi ulnaris
Abduction—flexor carpi radialis, extensor carpi radialis longus and brevis
Flexion—flexor carpi radialis, flexor carpi ulnaris, palmaris longus, abductor pollicis longus
Extension—extensor carpi radialis longus and brevis, extensor carpi ulnaris

Movement at the Metacarpophalangeal Joint (Condyloid Joint)

Adduction—palmar interossei (palmer adducts or PAD)
Abduction—dorsal interossei (dorsal abducts or DAB)
Flexion—lumbricals and interossei
Extension—extensor digitorum

Movement at the Interphalangeal Joint (Hinge Joint)

Flexion—flexor digitorum superficialis (proximal interphalangeal joint), flexor digitorum profundus (distal interphalangeal joint)
Extension—lumbricals and interossei (when metacarpophalangeal joint is extended by extensor digitorum)
Extension—extensor digitorum (when metacarpophalangeal joint is flexed by lumbricals and interossei)

MUSCLE INNERVATIONS OF THE UPPER LIMB

Muscles of the Anterior Compartment of the Arm: Musculocutaneous Nerve

Biceps brachii
Coracobrachialis
Brachialis

Muscles of the Posterior Compartment of the Arm: Radial Nerve

Triceps

Anconeus

Muscles of the Posterior Compartment of the Forearm: Radial Nerve

Superficial layer—brachioradialis, extensor carpi radialis longus, extensor carpi radialis brevis, extensor carpi ulnaris, extensor digitorum communis, extensor digiti minimi

Deep layer—supinator, abductor pollicis longus, extensor pollicis longus, extensor pollicis brevis, extensor indicis

Muscles of the Anterior Compartment of the Forearm: Median Nerve

Superficial layer—pronator teres, flexor carpi radialis, palmaris longus, flexor carpi ulnaris (ulnar nerve)*

Middle layer—flexor digitorum superficialis

Deep layer—flexor digitorum profundus (median nerve and ulnar nerve)*, flexor pollicis longus, pronator quadratus

Thenar Muscles: Median Nerve

Abductor pollicis brevis

Opponens pollicis

Flexor pollicis brevis (median and ulnar nerves)*

Adductor Pollicis Muscle: Ulnar Nerve

Hypothenar Muscles: Ulnar Nerve

Abductor digiti minimi

Opponens digiti minimi

Flexor digiti minimi

Interossei (Dorsal and Palmar) Muscles: Ulnar Nerve

Lumbrical Muscles (Medial Two): Ulnar Nerve

Lumbrical Muscles (Lateral Two): Median Nerve

*Indicates exception or dual innervation.

Review Test

Directions: Each of the numbered items or incomplete statements in this section is followed by answers or by completions of the statement. Select the **one**-lettered answer or completion that is **best** in each case.

1. A 21-year-old patient has a lesion of the upper trunk of the brachial plexus (Erb–Duchenne paralysis). Which of the following is the most likely diagnosis?

(A) Paralysis of the rhomboid major
(B) Inability to elevate the arm above the horizontal
(C) Arm tending to lie in medial rotation
(D) Loss of sensation on the medial side of the arm
(E) Inability to adduct the thumb

2. A patient comes in with a gunshot wound and requires surgery in which his thoracoacromial trunk needs to be ligated. Which of the following arterial branches would maintain normal blood flow?

(A) Acromial
(B) Pectoral
(C) Clavicular
(D) Deltoid
(E) Superior thoracic

3. A 29-year-old man comes in with a stab wound, cannot raise his arm above horizontal, and exhibits a condition known as "winged scapula." Which of the following structures of the brachial plexus would most likely be damaged?

(A) Medial cord
(B) Posterior cord
(C) Lower trunk
(D) Roots
(E) Upper trunk

4. A 16-year-old patient has weakness flexing the metacarpophalangeal joint of the ring finger and is unable to adduct the same finger. Which of the following muscles is most likely paralyzed?

(A) Flexor digitorum profundus
(B) Extensor digitorum
(C) Lumbrical
(D) Dorsal interosseous
(E) Palmar interosseous

5. A 27-year-old patient presents with an inability to draw the scapula forward and downward because of paralysis of the pectoralis minor. Which of the following would most likely be a cause of his condition?

(A) Fracture of the clavicle
(B) Injury to the posterior cord of the brachial plexus
(C) Fracture of the coracoid process
(D) Axillary nerve injury
(E) Defects in the posterior wall of the axilla

6. A 22-year-old patient received a stab wound in the chest that injured the intercostobrachial nerve. Which of the following conditions results from the described lesion of the nerve?

(A) Inability to move the ribs
(B) Loss of tactile sensation on the lateral aspect of the arm
(C) Absence of sweating on the posterior aspect of the arm
(D) Loss of sensory fibers from the second intercostal nerve
(E) Damage to the sympathetic preganglionic fibers

7. A 16-year-old boy fell from a motorcycle, and his radial nerve was severely damaged because of a fracture of the midshaft of the humerus. Which of the following conditions would most likely result from this accident?

(A) Loss of wrist extension leading to wrist drop
(B) Weakness in pronating the forearm
(C) Sensory loss over the ventral aspect of the base of the thumb
(D) Inability to oppose the thumb
(E) Inability to abduct the fingers

8. A patient comes in complaining that she cannot flex her proximal interphalangeal joints. Which of the following muscles appear(s) to be paralyzed on further examination of her finger?

(A) Palmar interossei
(B) Dorsal interossei
(C) Flexor digitorum profundus
(D) Flexor digitorum superficialis
(E) Lumbricals

9. A 21-year-old woman walks in with a shoulder and arm injury after falling during horseback riding. Examination indicates that she cannot adduct her arm because of paralysis of which of the following muscles?

(A) Teres minor
(B) Supraspinatus
(C) Latissimus dorsi
(D) Infraspinatus
(E) Serratus anterior

10. A 35-year-old man walks in with a stab wound to the most medial side of the proximal portion of the cubital fossa. Which of the following structures would most likely be damaged?

(A) Biceps brachii tendon
(B) Radial nerve
(C) Brachial artery
(D) Radial recurrent artery
(E) Median nerve

11. The police bring in a murder suspect who has been in a gunfight with a police officer. The suspect was struck by a bullet in the arm; his median nerve has been damaged. Which of the following symptoms is likely produced by this nerve damage?

(A) Waiter's tip hand
(B) Claw hand
(C) Wrist drop
(D) Ape hand
(E) Flattening of the hypothenar eminence

12. An automobile body shop worker has his middle finger crushed while working on a transmission. Which of the following muscles is most likely to retain function?

(A) Extensor digitorum
(B) Flexor digitorum profundus
(C) Palmar interosseous
(D) Dorsal interosseous
(E) Lumbrical

13. A 14-year-old boy falls on his outstretched hand and has a fracture of the scaphoid bone. The fracture is most likely accompanied by a rupture of which of the following arteries?

(A) Brachial artery
(B) Ulnar artery
(C) Deep palmar arterial arch
(D) Radial artery
(E) Princeps pollicis artery

14. A 12-year-old boy walks in; he fell out of a tree and fractured the upper portion of his humerus. Which of the following nerves are intimately related to the humerus and are most likely to be injured by such a fracture?

(A) Axillary and musculocutaneous
(B) Radial and ulnar
(C) Radial and axillary
(D) Median and musculocutaneous
(E) Median and ulnar

15. A man injures his wrist on broken glass. Which of the following structures entering the palm superficial to the flexor retinaculum may be damaged?

(A) Ulnar nerve and median nerve
(B) Median nerve and flexor digitorum profundus
(C) Median nerve and flexor pollicis longus
(D) Ulnar artery and ulnar nerve
(E) Ulnar nerve and flexor digitorum superficialis

16. A patient with Bennett fracture (a fracture of the base of the first metacarpal bone) experiences an impaired thumb movement. Which of the following intrinsic muscles of the thumb is most likely injured?

(A) Abductor pollicis brevis
(B) Flexor pollicis brevis (superficial head)
(C) Opponens pollicis
(D) Adductor pollicis
(E) Flexor pollicis brevis (deep head)

17. A 27-year-old pianist with a known carpal tunnel syndrome experiences difficulty in finger movements. Which of the following intrinsic muscles of her hand is paralyzed?

(A) Palmar interossei and adductor pollicis
(B) Dorsal interossei and lateral two lumbricals
(C) Lateral two lumbricals and opponens pollicis

(D) Abductor pollicis brevis and palmar interossei
(E) Medial two and lateral two lumbricals

18. A 31-year-old roofer walks in with tenosynovitis resulting from a deep penetrated wound in the palm by a big nail. Examination indicates that he has an infection in the ulnar bursa. This infection most likely resulted in necrosis of which of the following tendons?

(A) Tendon of the flexor carpi ulnaris
(B) Tendon of the flexor pollicis longus
(C) Tendon of the flexor digitorum profundus
(D) Tendon of the flexor carpi radialis
(E) Tendon of the palmaris longus

19. An 18-year-old boy involved in an automobile accident presents with an arm that cannot abduct. His paralysis is caused by damage to which of the following nerves?

(A) Suprascapular and axillary
(B) Thoracodorsal and upper subscapular
(C) Axillary and musculocutaneous
(D) Radial and lower subscapular
(E) Suprascapular and dorsal scapular

20. A 17-year-old boy with a stab wound received multiple injuries on the upper part of the arm and required surgery. If the brachial artery were ligated at its origin, which of the following arteries would supply blood to the profunda brachii artery?

(A) Lateral thoracic
(B) Subscapular
(C) Posterior humeral circumflex
(D) Superior ulnar collateral
(E) Radial recurrent

21. A 23-year-old woman who receives a deep cut to her ring finger by a kitchen knife is unable to move the metacarpophalangeal joint. Which of the following pairs of nerves was damaged?

(A) Median and ulnar
(B) Radial and median
(C) Musculocutaneous and ulnar
(D) Ulnar and radial
(E) Radial and axillary

22. A 27-year-old baseball player is hit on his forearm by a high-speed ball during the World Series, and the muscles that form the floor of the cubital fossa appear to be torn. Which of the following groups of muscles have lost their functions?

(A) Brachioradialis and supinator
(B) Brachialis and supinator
(C) Pronator teres and supinator
(D) Supinator and pronator quadratus
(E) Brachialis and pronator teres

23. A 23-year-old man complains of numbness on the medial side of the arm following a stab wound in the axilla. On examination, he is diagnosed with an injury of his medial brachial cutaneous nerve. In which of the following structures are the cell bodies of the damaged nerve involved in numbness located?

(A) Sympathetic chain ganglion
(B) Dorsal root ganglion
(C) Anterior horn of the spinal cord
(D) Lateral horn of the spinal cord
(E) Posterior horn of the spinal cord

24. A 38-year-old homebuilder was involved in an accident and is unable to supinate his forearm. Which of the following nerves are most likely damaged?

(A) Suprascapular and axillary
(B) Musculocutaneous and median
(C) Axillary and radial
(D) Radial and musculocutaneous
(E) Median and ulnar

25. A 31-year-old patient complains of sensory loss over the anterior and posterior surfaces of the medial third of the hand and the medial one and one-half fingers. He is diagnosed by a physician as having "funny bone" symptoms. Which of the following nerves is injured?

(A) Axillary
(B) Radial
(C) Median
(D) Ulnar
(E) Musculocutaneous

26. A patient with a deep stab wound in the middle of the forearm has impaired movement of the thumb. Examination indicates a lesion of the anterior interosseous nerve. Which of the following muscles is paralyzed?

(A) Flexor pollicis longus and brevis
(B) Flexor pollicis longus and opponens pollicis
(C) Flexor digitorum profundus and pronator quadratus

(D) Flexor digitorum profundus and superficialis
(E) Flexor pollicis brevis and pronator quadratus

27. A 29-year-old patient comes in; he cannot flex the distal interphalangeal (DIP) joint of the index finger. His physician determines that he has nerve damage from a supracondylar fracture. Which of the following conditions is also a symptom of this nerve damage?

(A) Inability to flex the DIP joint of the ring finger
(B) Atrophy of the hypothenar eminence
(C) Loss of sensation over the distal part of the second digit
(D) Paralysis of all the thumb muscles
(E) Loss of supination

28. A 27-year-old man with cubital tunnel syndrome complains of numbness and tingling in the ring and little finger and back and sides of his hand because of damage to a nerve in the tunnel at the elbow. Which of the following muscles is most likely to be paralyzed?

(A) Flexor digitorum superficialis
(B) Opponens pollicis
(C) Two medial lumbricals
(D) Pronator teres
(E) Supinator

29. A secretary comes in to your office complaining of pain in her wrists from typing all day. You determine that she likely has carpal tunnel syndrome. Which of the following conditions would help you determine the diagnosis?

(A) Inability to adduct the little finger
(B) Inability to flex the DIP joint of the ring finger
(C) Flattened thenar eminence
(D) Loss of skin sensation of the medial one and one-half fingers
(E) Atrophied adductor pollicis muscle

30. A man is unable to hold typing paper between his index and middle fingers. Which of the following nerves was likely injured?

(A) Radial nerve
(B) Median nerve
(C) Ulnar nerve
(D) Musculocutaneous nerve
(E) Axillary nerve

31. The victim of an automobile accident has a destructive injury of the proximal row of carpal bones. Which of the following bones is most likely damaged?

(A) Capitate
(B) Hamate
(C) Trapezium
(D) Triquetrum
(E) Trapezoid

32. A patient has a torn rotator cuff of the shoulder joint as the result of an automobile accident. Which of the following muscle tendons is intact and has normal function?

(A) Supraspinatus
(B) Subscapularis
(C) Teres major
(D) Teres minor
(E) Infraspinatus

33. A patient complains of having pain with repeated movements of his thumb (claudication). His physician performs the Allen test and finds an insufficiency of the radial artery. Which of the following conditions would be a result of the radial artery stenosis?

(A) A marked decrease in the blood flow in the superficial palmar arterial arch
(B) Decreased pulsation in the artery passing superficial to the flexor retinaculum
(C) Ischemia of the entire extensor muscles of the forearm
(D) A marked decrease in the blood flow in the princeps pollicis artery
(E) A low blood pressure in the anterior interosseous artery

34. A patient bleeding from the shoulder secondary to a knife wound is in fair condition because there is vascular anastomosis around the shoulder. Which of the following arteries is most likely a direct branch of the subclavian artery that is involved in the anastomosis?

(A) Dorsal scapular artery
(B) Thoracoacromial artery
(C) Circumflex scapular artery
(D) Transverse cervical artery
(E) Suprascapular artery

35. During a breast examination of a 56-year-old woman, the physician found a palpable mass in her breast. Which of the following characteristics of breast cancer and its diagnosis is correct?

(A) Elevated nipple
(B) Polymastia
(C) Shortening of the clavipectoral fascia
(D) Dimpling of the overlying skin
(E) Enlargement of the breast

36. A patient with a stab wound receives a laceration of the musculocutaneous nerve. Which of the following conditions is most likely to have occurred?

(A) Lack of sweating on the lateral side of the forearm
(B) Inability to extend the forearm
(C) Paralysis of brachioradialis muscle
(D) Loss of tactile sensation on the arm
(E) Constriction of blood vessels on the hand

37. A 20-year-old man fell from the parallel bar during the Olympic trial. A neurologic examination reveals that he has a lesion of the lateral cord of the brachial plexus. Which of the following muscles is most likely weakened by this injury?

(A) Subscapularis
(B) Teres major
(C) Latissimus dorsi
(D) Teres minor
(E) Pectoralis major

38. A 24-year-old carpenter suffers a crush injury of his entire little finger. Which of the following muscles is most likely to be spared?

(A) Flexor digitorum profundus
(B) Extensor digitorum
(C) Palmar interossei
(D) Dorsal interossei
(E) Lumbricals

39. A 7-year-old boy falls from a tree house and is brought to the emergency department of a local hospital. On examination, he has weakness in rotating his arm laterally because of an injury of a nerve. Which of the following conditions is most likely to cause a loss of this nerve function?

(A) Injury to the lateral cord of the brachial plexus
(B) Fracture of the anatomic neck of the humerus
(C) Knife wound on the teres major muscle
(D) Inferior dislocation of the head of the humerus
(E) A tumor in the triangular space in the shoulder region

40. A 49-year-old woman is diagnosed as having a large lump in her right breast. Lymph from the cancerous breast drains primarily into which of the following nodes?

(A) Apical nodes
(B) Anterior (pectoral) nodes
(C) Parasternal (internal thoracic) nodes
(D) Supraclavicular nodes
(E) Nodes of the anterior abdominal wall

41. A 17-year-old boy fell from his motorcycle and complains of numbness of the lateral part of the arm. Examination reveals that the axillary nerve is severed. Which of the following types of axons is most likely spared?

(A) Postganglionic sympathetic axons
(B) Somatic afferent axons
(C) Preganglionic sympathetic axons
(D) General somatic efferent axons
(E) General visceral afferent axons

42. A construction worker suffers a destructive injury of the structures related to the anatomic snuffbox. Which of the following structures would most likely be damaged?

(A) Triquetral bone
(B) Trapezoid bone
(C) Extensor indicis tendon
(D) Abductor pollicis brevis tendon
(E) Radial artery

43. A rock climber falls on his shoulder, resulting in a chipping off of the lesser tubercle of the humerus. Which of the following structures would most likely have structural and functional damage?

(A) Supraspinatus muscle
(B) Infraspinatus muscle
(C) Subscapularis muscle
(D) Teres minor muscle
(E) Coracohumeral ligament

44. A 22-year-old female Macarena dancer fell from the stage and complains of elbow pain and inability to supinate her forearm. Which of the following nerves are most likely injured from this accident?

(A) Median and ulnar nerves
(B) Axillary and radial nerves
(C) Radial and musculocutaneous nerves
(D) Ulnar and axillary nerves
(E) Musculocutaneous and median nerves

Questions 45 to 47: A 37-year-old female patient has a fracture of the clavicle. The junction of the middle and lateral thirds of the bone exhibits overriding of the medial and lateral fragments. The arm is rotated medially, but it is not rotated laterally.

45. The lateral portion of the fractured clavicle is displaced downward by which of the following?

(A) Deltoid and trapezius muscles
(B) Pectoralis major and deltoid muscles
(C) Pectoralis minor muscle and gravity
(D) Trapezius and pectoralis minor muscles
(E) Deltoid muscle and gravity

46. Which of the following muscles causes upward displacement of the medial fragment?

(A) Pectoralis major
(B) Deltoid
(C) Trapezius
(D) Sternocleidomastoid
(E) Scalenus anterior

47. Which of the following conditions is most likely to occur secondary to the fractured clavicle?

(A) A fatal hemorrhage from the brachiocephalic vein
(B) Thrombosis of the subclavian vein, causing a pulmonary embolism
(C) Thrombosis of the subclavian artery, causing an embolism in the ascending aorta
(D) Damage to the upper trunk of the brachial plexus
(E) Damage to the long thoracic nerve, causing the winged scapula

Questions 48 to 50: A 21-year-old man injures his right arm in an automobile accident. Radiographic examination reveals a fracture of the medial epicondyle of the humerus.

48. Which of the following nerves is most likely injured as a result of this accident?

(A) Axillary
(B) Musculocutaneous
(C) Radial
(D) Median
(E) Ulnar

49. Which of the following muscles is most likely paralyzed as a result of this accident?

(A) Extensor pollicis brevis
(B) Abductor pollicis longus
(C) Abductor pollicis brevis
(D) Adductor pollicis
(E) Opponens pollicis

50. After this injury, the patient is unable to do which of the following?

(A) Flex the proximal interphalangeal joint of his ring finger
(B) Flex the DIP joint of his index finger
(C) Feel sensation on his middle finger
(D) Abduct his thumb
(E) Adduct his index finger

Questions 51 to 55: A 10-year-old boy falls off his bike, has difficulty in moving his shoulder, and is brought to the emergency department. His radiograph and angiograph reveal fracture of the surgical neck of his humerus and bleeding from the point of the fracture.

51. Which of the following nerves is most likely injured as a result of this accident?

(A) Musculocutaneous
(B) Axillary
(C) Radial
(D) Median
(E) Ulnar

52. Following this accident, the damaged nerve causes difficulty in abduction, extension, and lateral rotation of his arm. Cell bodies of the injured nerve involved in movement of his arm are located in which of the following structures?

(A) Dorsal root ganglion
(B) Sympathetic chain ganglion
(C) Anterior horn of the spinal cord
(D) Lateral horn of the spinal cord
(E) Posterior horn of the spinal cord

53. The damaged nerve causes numbness of the lateral side of the arm. Cell bodies of the injured nerve fibers involved in sensory loss are located in which of the following structures?

(A) Anterior horn of the spinal cord
(B) Posterior horn of the spinal cord
(C) Lateral horn of the spinal cord
(D) Dorsal root ganglia
(E) Sympathetic chain ganglia

54. This accident most likely leads to the damage of which of the following arteries?

(A) Axillary
(B) Deep brachial
(C) Posterior humeral circumflex
(D) Superior ulnar collateral
(E) Scapular circumflex

55. Following this accident, the boy has weakness in rotating his arm laterally. Which of the following muscles are paralyzed?

(A) Teres major and teres minor
(B) Teres minor and deltoid
(C) Infraspinatus and deltoid
(D) Supraspinatus and subscapularis
(E) Teres minor and infraspinatus

Questions 56 to 57: A 64-year-old man with a history of liver cirrhosis has been examined for hepatitis A, B, and C viruses. In an attempt to obtain a blood sample from the patient's median cubital vein, a registered nurse inadvertently procures arterial blood.

56. The blood most likely comes from which of the following arteries?

(A) Brachial
(B) Radial
(C) Ulnar
(D) Common interosseous
(E) Superior ulnar collateral

57. During the procedure, the needle hits a nerve medial to the artery. Which of the following nerves is most likely damaged?

(A) Radial
(B) Median
(C) Ulnar
(D) Lateral antebrachial
(E) Medial antebrachial

Questions 58 to 62: A 17-year-old boy is injured in an automobile accident. He has a fracture of the shaft of the humerus.

58. Which of the following nerves is most likely damaged?

(A) Axillary nerve
(B) Radial nerve
(C) Musculocutaneous nerve
(D) Median nerve
(E) Ulnar nerve

59. As a result of this fracture, the patient shows lack of sweating on the back of the arm and forearm. Cell bodies of the damaged nerve fibers involved in sweating are located in which of the following structures?

(A) Anterior horn of the spinal cord
(B) Posterior horn of the spinal cord
(C) Lateral horn of the spinal cord
(D) Sympathetic chain ganglion
(E) Dorsal root ganglion

60. Following this accident, the patient has no cutaneous sensation in which of the following areas?

(A) Medial aspect of the arm
(B) Lateral aspect of the forearm
(C) Palmar aspect of the second and third digits
(D) Area of the anatomic snuffbox
(E) Medial one and one-half fingers

61. Which of the following arteries may be damaged?

(A) Brachial artery
(B) Posterior humeral circumflex artery
(C) Profunda brachii artery
(D) Radial artery
(E) Radial recurrent artery

62. After this accident, supination is still possible through contraction of which of the following muscles?

(A) Supinator
(B) Pronator teres
(C) Brachioradialis
(D) Biceps brachii
(E) Supraspinatus

63. A cyclist is thrown over his handle bars and breaks his clavicle as he hits the ground on his shoulder. Which of the following is correct regarding the development of the clavicle?

(A) It develops through intramembranous ossification
(B) It is the last upper limb bone to begin ossification
(C) The clavicle forms from somitic mesoderm
(D) It is the first limb bone to complete ossification
(E) Associated muscles form from somatic lateral plate mesoderm

64. A patient presents with pain in the neck, numbness and tingling in the fingers, and a week grip. This presentation suggests thoracic outlet syndrome. Which of the following causes has an embryological etiology?

(A) Traumatic injury
(B) Cardiovascular disease
(C) Cervical rib
(D) Pancoast tumor
(E) Scalene muscle inflammation

Questions 65 to 66: A 11-year-old boy falls down the stairs. A physician examines the radiograph of the boy's shoulder region (see Figure below).

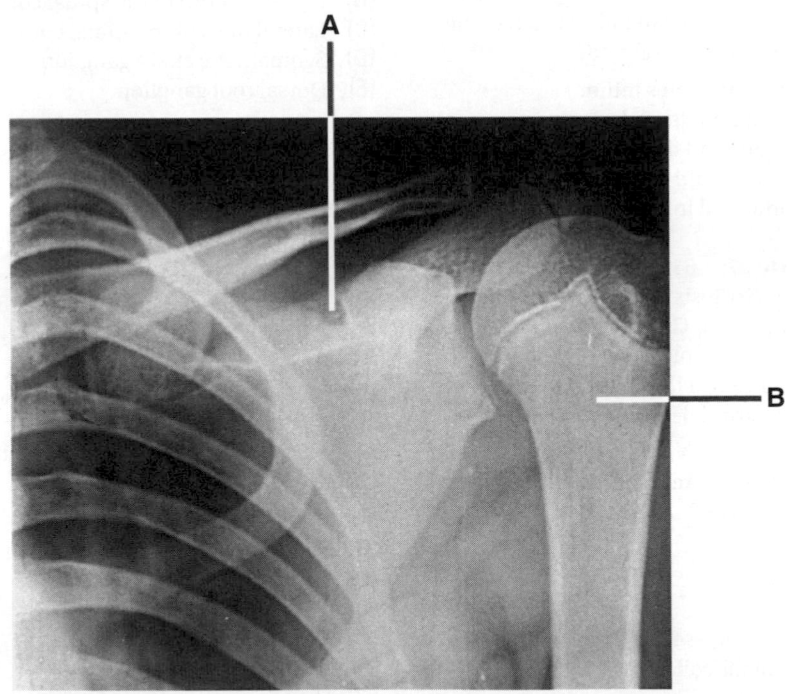

65. If the structure indicated by the letter **A** is calcified, which of the following muscles is most likely paralyzed?

(A) Deltoid
(B) Teres major
(C) Teres minor
(D) Infraspinatus
(E) Subscapularis

66. If the structure indicated by the letter **B** is fractured, which of the following structures is most likely injured?

(A) Musculocutaneous nerve
(B) Radial nerve
(C) Deep brachial artery
(D) Posterior humeral circumflex artery
(E) Scapular circumflex artery

Questions 67 to 69: Choose the appropriate lettered site or structure in the radiograph of the elbow joint (see Figure below) and its associated structures to match the following descriptions.

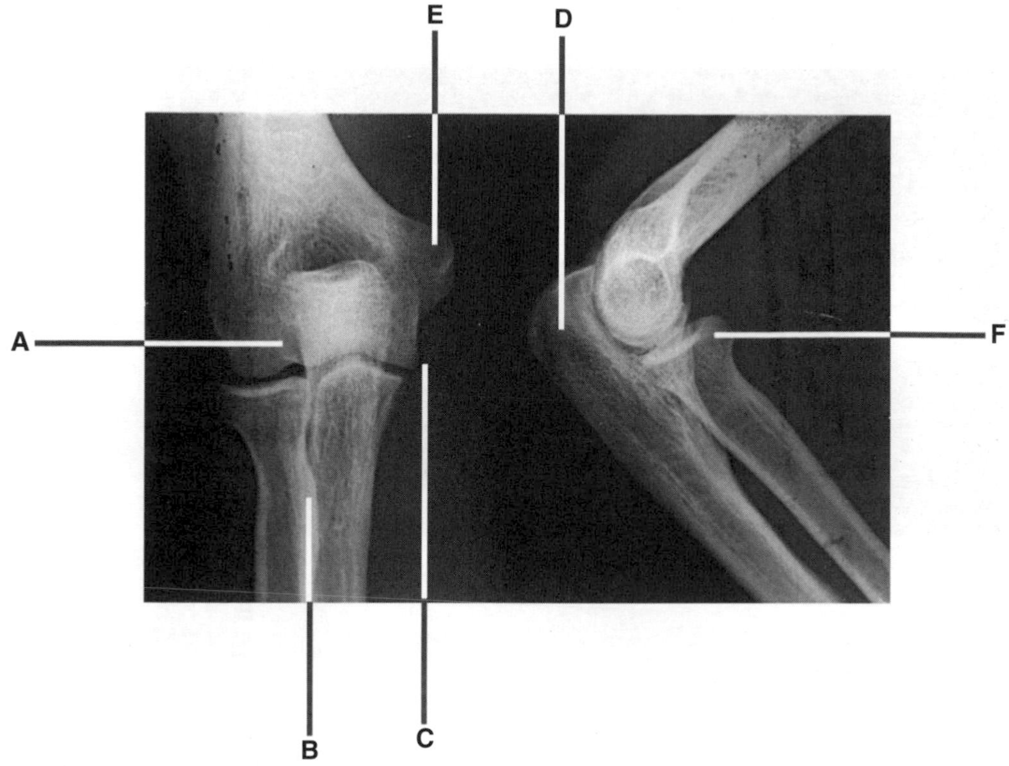

67. Destruction of this area would most likely cause weakness of supination and flexion of the forearm.

68. Destruction of this area would most likely cause weakness of pronation of the forearm and flexion of the wrist joints.

69. A lesion of the radial nerve would most likely cause paralysis of muscles that are attached to this area.

Questions 70 to 71: Choose the appropriate lettered site or structure in the following radiograph of the wrist and hand (see Figure below).

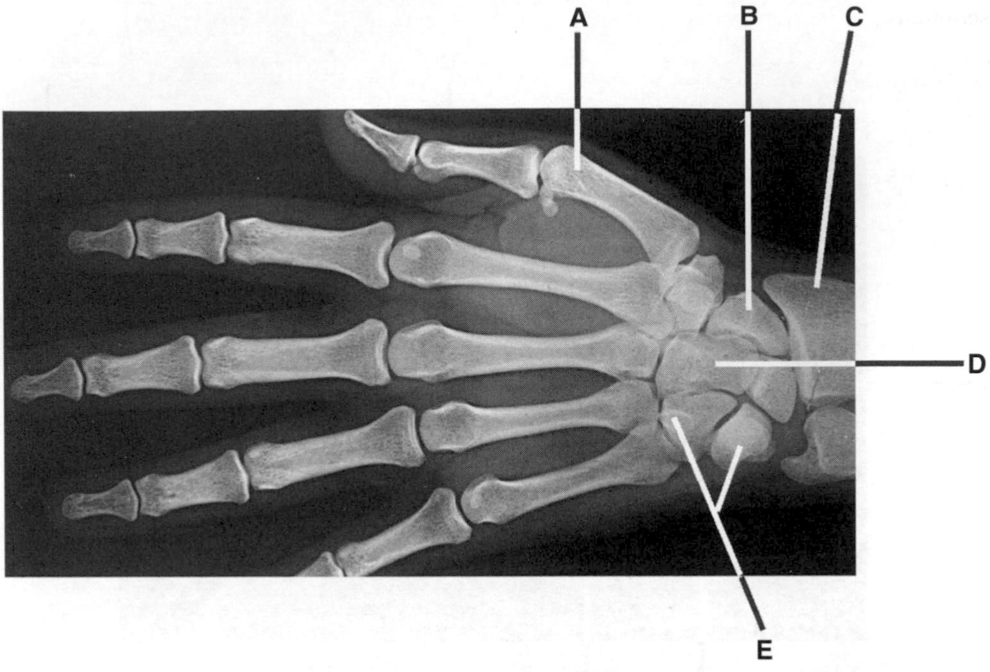

70. Destruction of the structure indicated by the letter **E** most likely causes weakness of which of the following muscles?

(A) Flexor carpi radialis
(B) Palmaris longus
(C) Flexor carpi ulnaris
(D) Brachioradialis
(E) Flexor digitorum superficialis

71. If the floor of the anatomic snuffbox and origin of the abductor pollicis brevis are damaged, which of the following bones is most likely to be involved?

(A) A
(B) B
(C) C
(D) D
(E) E

Questions 72 to 75: Choose the appropriate lettered site or structure in this transverse magnetic resonance imaging through the middle of the palm of a woman's right hand (see Figure below) that matches the following descriptions.

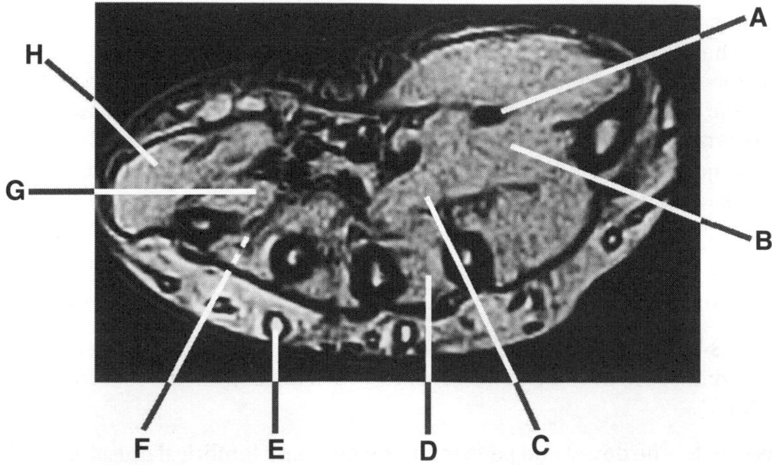

72. The patient is unable to abduct her middle finger because of paralysis of this structure.

73. A lesion of the median nerve causes paralysis of this structure.

74. The patient is unable to adduct her little finger because of paralysis of this structure.

75. Atrophy of this structure impairs extension of both the metacarpophalangeal and interphalangeal joints.

Answers and Explanations

1. **The answer is C.** A lesion of the upper trunk of the brachial plexus results in a condition called "waiter's tip hand," in which the arm tends to lie in medial rotation because of paralysis of lateral rotators and abductors of the arm. The long thoracic nerve, which arises from the root (C5–C7) of the brachial plexus, innervates the serratus anterior muscle that can elevate the arm above the horizontal. The dorsal scapular nerve, which arises from the root (C5), innervates the rhomboid major. The medial side of the arm receives cutaneous innervation from the medial brachial cutaneous nerve of the medial cord. The adductor pollicis is innervated by the ulnar nerve.

2. **The answer is E.** The superior thoracic artery is a direct branch of the axillary artery. The thoracoacromial trunk has four branches: the pectoral, clavicular, acromial, and deltoid.

3. **The answer is D.** Winged scapula is caused by paralysis of the serratus anterior muscle that results from damage to the long thoracic nerve, which arises from the roots of the brachial plexus (C5–C7).

4. **The answer is E.** The dorsal and palmar interosseous and lumbrical muscles can flex the metacarpophalangeal joints and extend the interphalangeal joints. The palmar interosseous muscles adduct the fingers, while the dorsal interosseous muscles abduct the fingers. The flexor digitorum profundus flexes the distal interphalangeal (DIP) joints.

5. **The answer is C.** The pectoralis minor inserts on the coracoid process, originates from the second to the fifth ribs, and is innervated by the medial and lateral pectoral nerves that arise from the medial and lateral cords of the brachial plexus. It depresses the shoulder and forms the anterior wall of the axilla. The pectoralis minor has no attachment on the clavicle.

6. **The answer is D.** The intercostobrachial nerve arises from the lateral cutaneous branch of the second intercostal nerve and pierces the intercostal and serratus anterior muscles. It may communicate with the medial brachial cutaneous nerve, and it supplies skin on the medial side of the arm. It contains no skeletal motor fibers but does contain sympathetic postganglionic fibers, which supply sweat glands.

7. **The answer is A.** Injury to the radial nerve results in loss of wrist extension, leading to wrist drop. The median nerve innervates the pronator teres, pronator quadratus, and opponens pollicis muscles and the skin over the ventral aspect of the thumb. The ulnar nerve innervates the dorsal interosseous muscles, which act to abduct the fingers.

8. **The answer is D.** The flexor digitorum superficialis muscle flexes the proximal interphalangeal joints. The flexor digitorum profundus muscle flexes the DIP joints. The palmar and dorsal interossei and lumbricals can flex metacarpophalangeal joints and extend the interphalangeal joints. The palmar interossei adduct the fingers, and the dorsal interossei abduct the fingers.

9. **The answer is C.** The latissimus dorsi adducts the arm, and the supraspinatus muscle abducts the arm. The infraspinatus and the teres minor rotate the arm laterally. The serratus anterior rotates the glenoid cavity of the scapula upward, abducts the arm, and elevates it above a horizontal position.

10. **The answer is E.** The contents of the cubital fossa from medial to lateral side are the median nerve, the brachial artery, the biceps brachii tendon, and the radial nerve. Thus, the median nerve is damaged. The radial recurrent artery ascends medial to the radial nerve.

11. **The answer is D.** Injury to the median nerve produces the ape hand (a hand with the thumb permanently extended). Injury to the radial nerve results in loss of wrist extension, leading to wrist drop. Damage to the upper trunk of the brachial plexus produces waiter's tip hand. A claw

hand and flattening of the hypothenar eminence or atrophy of the hypothenar muscles result from damage to the ulnar nerve.

12. **The answer is C.** The extensor digitorum, flexor digitorum profundus, dorsal interosseous, and lumbrical muscles are attached to the middle digit, but no palmar interosseous muscle is attached to the middle digit.

13. **The answer is D.** The scaphoid bone forms the floor of the anatomic snuffbox, through which the radial artery passes to enter the palm. The radial artery divides into the princeps pollicis artery and the deep palmar arch.

14. **The answer is C.** The axillary nerve passes posteriorly around the surgical neck of the humerus, and the radial nerve lies in the radial groove of the middle of the shaft of the humerus. The ulnar nerve passes behind the medial epicondyle, and the median nerve is vulnerable to injury by supracondylar fracture of the humerus, but these nerves lie close to or in contact with the lower portion of the humerus. The musculocutaneous nerve is not in direct contact with the humerus.

15. **The answer is D.** Structures entering the palm superficial to the flexor retinaculum include the ulnar nerve, ulnar artery, palmaris longus tendon, and palmar cutaneous branch of the median nerve. The median nerve, the flexor pollicis longus, and the flexor digitorum superficialis and profundus run deep to the flexor retinaculum.

16. **The answer is C.** The opponens pollicis inserts on the first metacarpal. All other intrinsic muscles of the thumb, including the abductor pollicis brevis, the flexor pollicis brevis, and the adductor pollicis muscles, insert on the proximal phalanges.

17. **The answer is C.** The median nerve innervates the abductor pollicis brevis, opponens pollicis, and two lateral lumbricals. The ulnar nerve innervates all interossei (palmar and dorsal), the adductor pollicis, and the two medial lumbricals.

18. **The answer is C.** The ulnar bursa, or common synovial flexor sheath, contains the tendons of both the flexor digitorum superficialis and profundus muscles. The radial bursa envelops the tendon of the flexor pollicis longus. The tendons of the flexor carpi ulnaris and the palmaris longus are not contained in the ulnar bursa.

19. **The answer is A.** The abductors of the arm are the deltoid and supraspinatus muscles, which are innervated by the axillary and suprascapular nerves, respectively. The thoracodorsal nerve supplies the latissimus dorsi, which can adduct, extend, and rotate the arm medially. The upper and lower subscapular nerves supply the subscapularis, and the lower subscapular nerve also supplies the teres major; both of these structures can adduct and rotate the arm medially. The musculocutaneous nerve supplies the flexors of the arm, and the radial nerve supplies the extensors of the arm. The dorsal scapular nerve supplies the levator scapulae and rhomboid muscles; these muscles elevate and adduct the scapula, respectively.

20. **The answer is C.** The posterior humeral circumflex artery anastomoses with an ascending branch of the profunda brachii artery, whereas the lateral thoracic and subscapular arteries do not. The superior ulnar collateral and radial recurrent arteries arise inferior to the origin of the profunda brachii artery.

21. **The answer is D.** The metacarpophalangeal joint of the ring finger is flexed by the lumbrical, palmar, and dorsal interosseous muscles, which are innervated by the ulnar nerve. The extensor digitorum, which is innervated by the radial nerve, extends this joint. The musculocutaneous and axillary nerves do not supply muscles of the hand. The median nerve supplies the lateral two lumbricals, which can flex metacarpophalangeal joints of the index and middle fingers.

22. **The answer is B.** The brachialis and supinator muscles form the floor of the cubital fossa. The brachioradialis and pronator teres muscles form the lateral and medial boundaries, respectively. The pronator quadratus is attached to the distal ends of the radius and the ulna.

23. **The answer is B.** The medial brachial cutaneous nerve contains sensory (general somatic afferent [GSA]) fibers that have cell bodies in the dorsal root ganglia, and an injury of these GSA fibers causes numbness of the medial side of the arm. It also contains sympathetic

postganglionic fibers that have cell bodies in the sympathetic chain ganglia. The anterior horn of the spinal cord contains cell bodies of skeletal motor (general somatic efferent [GSE]) fibers, and the lateral horn contains cell bodies of sympathetic preganglionic fibers. The posterior horn contains cell bodies of interneurons.

24. **The answer is D.** The supinator and biceps brachii muscles, which are innervated by the radial and musculocutaneous nerves, respectively, produce supination of the forearm. This is a question of two muscles that can supinate the forearm.

25. **The answer is D.** The ulnar nerve supplies sensory fibers to the skin over the palmar and dorsal surfaces of the medial third of the hand and the medial one and one-half fingers. The median nerve innervates the skin of the lateral side of the palm; the palmar side of the lateral three and one-half fingers; and the dorsal side of the index finger, the middle finger, and one-half of the ring finger. The radial nerve innervates the skin of the radial side of the hand and the radial two and one-half digits over the proximal phalanx.

26. **The answer is C.** The anterior interosseous nerve is a branch of the median nerve and supplies the flexor pollicis longus, half of the flexor digitorum profundus, and the pronator quadratus. The median nerve supplies the pronator teres, flexor digitorum superficialis, palmaris longus, and flexor carpi radialis muscles. A muscular branch (the recurrent branch) of the median nerve innervates the thenar muscles.

27. **The answer is C.** The flexor digitorum profundus muscle flexes the DIP joints of the index and middle fingers and is innervated by the median nerve, which also supplies sensation over the distal part of the second digit. The same muscle flexes the DIP joints of the ring and little fingers but receives innervation from the ulnar nerve, which also innervates the hypothenar muscles. The median nerve innervates the thenar muscles. The radial nerve innervates the supinator, abductor pollicis longus, and extensor pollicis longus and brevis muscles. The ulnar nerve innervates the adductor pollicis. The musculocutaneous nerve supplies the biceps brachii that can supinate the arm.

28. **The answer is C.** The ulnar nerve innervates the two medial lumbricals. However, the median nerve innervates the two lateral lumbricals, the flexor digitorum superficialis, the opponens pollicis, and the pronator teres muscles.

29. **The answer is C.** The carpal tunnel contains the median nerve and the tendons of flexor pollicis longus, flexor digitorum profundus, and flexor digitorum superficialis muscles. Carpal tunnel syndrome results from injury to the median nerve, which supplies the thenar muscle. Thus, injury to this nerve causes the flattened thenar eminence. The middle finger has no attachment for the adductors. The ulnar nerve innervates the medial half of the flexor digitorum profundus muscle, which allows flexion of the DIP joints of the ring and little fingers. The ulnar nerve supplies the skin over the medial one and one-half fingers and adductor pollicis muscle.

30. **The answer is C.** To hold a typing paper, the index finger is adducted by the palmar interosseous muscle, and the middle finger is abducted by the dorsal interosseous muscle. Both muscles are innervated by the ulnar nerve.

31. **The answer is D.** The proximal row of carpal bones consists of the scaphoid, lunate, triquetrum, and pisiform bones, whereas the distal row consists of the trapezium, trapezoid, capitate, and hamate bones.

32. **The answer is C.** The rotator cuff consists of the tendons of the supraspinatus, infraspinatus, subscapularis, and teres minor muscles. It stabilizes the shoulder joint by holding the head of the humerus in the glenoid cavity during movement. The teres major inserts on the medial lip of the intertubercular groove of the humerus.

33. **The answer is D.** The radial artery divides into the princeps pollicis artery and the deep palmar arterial arch. Thus, stenosis of the radial artery results in a decreased blood flow in the princeps pollicis artery. The superficial palmar arterial arch is formed primarily by the ulnar artery, which passes superficial to the flexor retinaculum. The extensor compartment of the forearm receives blood from the posterior interosseous artery, which arises from the common

interosseous branch of the ulnar artery. However, the radial and radial recurrent arteries supply the brachioradialis and the extensor carpi radialis longus and brevis.

34. **The answer is A.** The dorsal scapular artery arises directly from the third part of the subclavian artery and replaces the deep (descending) branch of the transverse cervical artery. The suprascapular and transverse cervical arteries are branches of the thyrocervical trunk of the subclavian artery. The thoracoacromial artery is a short trunk from the first or second part of the axillary artery and has pectoral, clavicular, acromial, and deltoid branches.

35. **The answer is D.** Breast cancer may cause dimpling of the overlying skin because of shortening of the suspensory (Cooper) ligaments and inverted or retracted nipple because of pulling on the lactiferous ducts. Polymastia is a condition in which more than two breasts are present.

36. **The answer is A.** The musculocutaneous nerve contains sympathetic postganglionic fibers that supply sweat glands and blood vessels on the lateral side of the forearm as the lateral antebrachial cutaneous nerve. The musculocutaneous nerve does not supply the extensors of the forearm and the brachioradialis. This nerve also supplies tactile sensation on the lateral side of the forearm but not the arm and supplies blood vessels on the lateral side of the forearm but not the hand.

37. **The answer is E.** The pectoralis major is innervated by the lateral and medial pectoral nerves originating from the lateral and medial cords of the brachial plexus, respectively. The subscapularis, teres major, latissimus dorsi, and teres minor muscles are innervated by nerves originating from the posterior cord of the brachial plexus.

38. **The answer is D.** The dorsal interossei are abductors of the fingers. The little finger has no attachment for the dorsal interosseous muscle because it has its own abductor. Therefore, the dorsal interosseous muscle is not affected. Other muscles are attached to the little finger; thus, they are injured.

39. **The answer is D.** Inferior dislocation of the head of the humerus may damage the axillary nerve, which arises from the posterior cord of the brachial plexus, runs through the quadrangular space accompanied by the posterior humeral circumflex vessels around the surgical neck of the humerus, and supplies the deltoid and teres minor, which are lateral rotators of the arm.

40. **The answer is B.** Lymph from the breast drains mainly (75%) to the axillary nodes, more specifically to the anterior (pectoral) nodes.

41. **The answer is C.** The axillary nerve contains no preganglionic sympathetic general visceral efferent (GVE) fibers, but it contains postganglionic sympathetic GVE fibers. The axillary nerve also contains GSA, GSE, and general visceral afferent (GVA) fibers.

42. **The answer is E.** The radial artery lies on the floor of the anatomic snuffbox. Other structures are not related to the snuffbox. The tendons of the extensor pollicis longus, extensor pollicis brevis, and abductor pollicis longus muscles form the boundaries of the anatomic snuffbox. The scaphoid and trapezium bones form its floor.

43. **The answer is C.** The subscapularis muscle inserts on the lesser tubercle of the humerus. The supraspinatus, infraspinatus, and teres minor muscles insert on the greater tubercle of the humerus. The coracohumeral ligament attaches to the greater tubercle.

44. **The answer is C.** The supinator and biceps brachii muscles supinate the forearm. The supinator is innervated by the radial nerve, and the biceps brachii is innervated by the musculocutaneous nerve.

45. **The answer is E.** The lateral fragment of the clavicle is displaced downward by the pull of the deltoid muscle and gravity. The medial fragment is displaced upward by the pull of the sternocleidomastoid muscle. None of the other muscles are involved.

46. **The answer is D.** The sternocleidomastoid muscle is attached to the superior border of the medial third of the clavicle, and the medial fragment of a fractured clavicle is displaced upward by the pull of the muscle.

47. **The answer is B.** The fractured clavicle may damage the subclavian vein, resulting in a pulmonary embolism; cause thrombosis of the subclavian artery, resulting in embolism of the brachial artery; or damage the lower trunk of the brachial plexus.

48. **The answer is E.** The ulnar nerve runs down the medial aspect of the arm and behind the medial epicondyle in a groove, where it is vulnerable to damage by fracture of the medial epicondyle. Other nerves are not in contact with the medial epicondyle.

49. **The answer is D.** The ulnar nerve innervates the adductor pollicis muscle. The radial nerve innervates the abductor pollicis longus and extensor pollicis brevis muscles, whereas the median nerve innervates the abductor pollicis brevis and opponens pollicis muscles.

50. **The answer is E.** The fingers are adducted by the palmar interosseous muscles; abduction is performed by the dorsal interosseous muscles. The palmar and dorsal interosseous muscles are innervated by the ulnar nerve. The proximal interphalangeal joints are flexed by the flexor digitorum superficialis, which is innervated by the median nerve. However, the DIP joints of the index and middle fingers are flexed by the flexor digitorum profundus, which is innervated by the median nerve (except the medial half of the muscle, which is innervated by the ulnar nerve). The median nerve supplies sensory innervation on the palmar aspect of the middle finger. The abductor pollicis brevis is innervated by the median nerve; the abductor pollicis longus is innervated by the radial nerve.

51. **The answer is B.** The axillary nerve runs posteriorly around the surgical neck of the humerus and is vulnerable to injury such as fracture of the surgical neck of the humerus or inferior dislocation of the humerus. The other nerves listed are not in contact with the surgical neck of the humerus.

52. **The answer is C.** The (injured) axillary nerve contains GSE fibers whose cell bodies are located in the anterior horn of the spinal cord, and these GSE fibers supply the deltoid and teres minor muscles. The axillary nerve also contains GSA and GVA fibers, whose cell bodies are located in the dorsal root ganglia, and sympathetic postganglionic fibers, whose cell bodies are located in sympathetic chain ganglia. The lateral horn of the spinal cord between T1 and L2 contains cell bodies of sympathetic preganglionic fibers. The posterior horn of the spinal cord contains cell bodies of interneurons.

53. **The answer is D.** Axillary nerve contains GSE, GSA, GVA, and sympathetic postganglionic GVE fibers. Cell bodies of GSA and GVA fibers are located in the dorsal root ganglia. Cell bodies of GSE fibers are located in the anterior horn of the spinal cord. Cell bodies of sympathetic postganglionic GVE fibers are located in the sympathetic chain ganglia, but cell bodies of sympathetic preganglionic GVE fibers lie in the lateral horn of the spinal cord.

54. **The answer is C.** The posterior humeral circumflex artery accompanies the axillary nerve that passes around the surgical neck of the humerus. None of the other arteries are involved.

55. **The answer is B.** The lateral rotators of the arm include the teres minor, deltoid, and infraspinatus muscles, but the infraspinatus muscle is innervated by the suprascapular nerve.

56. **The answer is A.** The median cubital vein lies superficial to the bicipital aponeurosis and thus separates it from the brachial artery, which can be punctured during intravenous injections and blood transfusions.

57. **The answer is B.** The median nerve is damaged because it lies medial to the brachial artery. The bicipital aponeurosis lies on the brachial artery and the median nerve. The V-shaped cubital fossa contains (from medial to lateral) the median nerve, brachial artery, biceps tendon, and radial nerve. The ulnar nerve runs behind the medial epicondyle; the lateral and medial antebrachial cutaneous nerves are not closely related to the brachial artery.

58. **The answer is B.** The radial nerve runs in the radial groove on the back of the shaft of the humerus with the profunda brachii artery. The axillary nerve passes around the surgical neck of the humerus. The ulnar nerve passes the back of the medial epicondyle. The musculocutaneous

and median nerves are not in contact with the bone, but the median nerve can be damaged by supracondylar fracture.

59. **The answer is D.** The (damaged) radial nerve contains sympathetic postganglionic nerve fibers whose cell bodies are located in the sympathetic chain ganglion. Sympathetic postganglionic fibers supply sweat glands, blood vessels, and hair follicles (arrector pili muscles). The radial nerve also contains GSE fibers whose cell bodies are located in the anterior horn of the spinal cord, and GSA and GVA fibers whose cell bodies are located in the dorsal root ganglion. The lateral horn of the spinal cord between T1 and L2 contains cell bodies of sympathetic preganglionic nerve fibers.

60. **The answer is D.** The superficial branch of the radial nerve runs distally to the dorsum of the hand to innervate the radial side of the hand, including the area of the anatomic snuffbox and the radial two and one-half digits over the proximal phalanx. The medial aspect of the arm is innervated by the medial brachial cutaneous nerve; the lateral aspect of the forearm is innervated by the lateral antebrachial cutaneous nerve of the musculocutaneous nerve; the palmar aspect of the second and third digits is innervated by the median nerve; and the medial one and one-half fingers are innervated by the ulnar nerve.

61. **The answer is C.** The radial nerve accompanies the profunda brachii artery in the radial groove on the posterior aspect of the shaft of the humerus. The posterior humeral circumflex artery accompanies the axillary nerve around the surgical neck of the humerus. Other arteries are not associated with the radial groove of the humerus.

62. **The answer is D.** A lesion of the radial nerve causes paralysis of the supinator and brachioradialis. The biceps brachii muscle is a flexor of the elbow and also a strong supinator; thus, supination is still possible through action of the biceps brachii muscle. Other muscles cannot supinate the forearm.

63. **The answer is A.** The clavicle is the only upper limb bone to develop through intramembranous ossification. It is the first upper limb bone to begin ossification and is the last bone to complete ossification. The clavicle forms from somatic lateral plate mesoderm and the associated muscles develop from somitic mesoderm (from somites).

64. **The answer is C.** A cervical rib is a congenital abnormality that can cause thoracic outlet syndrome because the space that transmits the neurovasculature to the arm is reduced. Other causes listed are not a result of embryological development.

65. **The answer is D.** The scapular notch transmits the suprascapular nerve below the superior transverse ligament, whereas the suprascapular artery and vein run over the ligament. The suprascapular nerve supplies the supraspinatus and infraspinatus muscles. The axillary nerve innervates the deltoid and teres minor muscles. The subscapular nerves innervate the teres major and subscapularis muscles.

66. **The answer is D.** Fracture of the surgical neck of the humerus occurs commonly and damages the axillary nerve and the posterior humeral circumflex artery.

67. **The answer is B.** The radial tuberosity is the site for tendinous attachment of the biceps brachii muscle, which supinates and flexes the forearm. When the tuberosity is destroyed, the biceps brachii is paralyzed.

68. **The answer is E.** The medial epicondyle is the site of origin for the common flexor tendon and pronator teres. The common flexors include the flexor carpi radialis and ulnaris and palmaris longus muscles, which can flex the elbow and wrist joints. Thus, destruction of this area causes weakness of pronation because the pronator teres is paralyzed but the pronator quadratus is normal. Similarly, destruction of this area causes paralysis of the flexors of the wrist. However, it can be weakly flexed by the flexor pollicis longus, flexor digitorum superficialis, and profundus muscles.

69. **The answer is D.** The olecranon is the site for insertion of the triceps brachii, which is innervated by the radial nerve. When the olecranon is destroyed, the triceps brachii is paralyzed.

70. The answer is C. The hook of hamate and the pisiform provide insertion for the flexor carpi ulnaris.

71. The answer is B. The scaphoid forms the floor of the anatomic snuffbox and provides a site for origin of the abductor pollicis brevis.

72. The answer is D. This is the second dorsal interosseous muscle, which abducts the middle finger.

73. The answer is A. This is the flexor pollicis longus, which is innervated by the median nerve.

74. The answer is G. This is the third palmar interosseous muscle, which adducts the little finger.

75. The answer is E. The extensor digitorum extends both the metacarpophalangeal and interphalangeal joints.

chapter 8

Head and Neck

STRUCTURES OF THE NECK

I. MAJOR DIVISIONS AND BONES (Figure 8.1)

A. Posterior Triangle

- Is bounded by the posterior border of the **sternocleidomastoid** muscle, the anterior border of the **trapezius** muscle, and the superior border of the **clavicle**.
- Has a roof formed by the **platysma** and the investing (superficial) layer of the **deep cervical fascia**.
- Has a floor formed by the splenius capitis and levator scapulae muscles and the anterior, middle, and posterior scalene muscles.

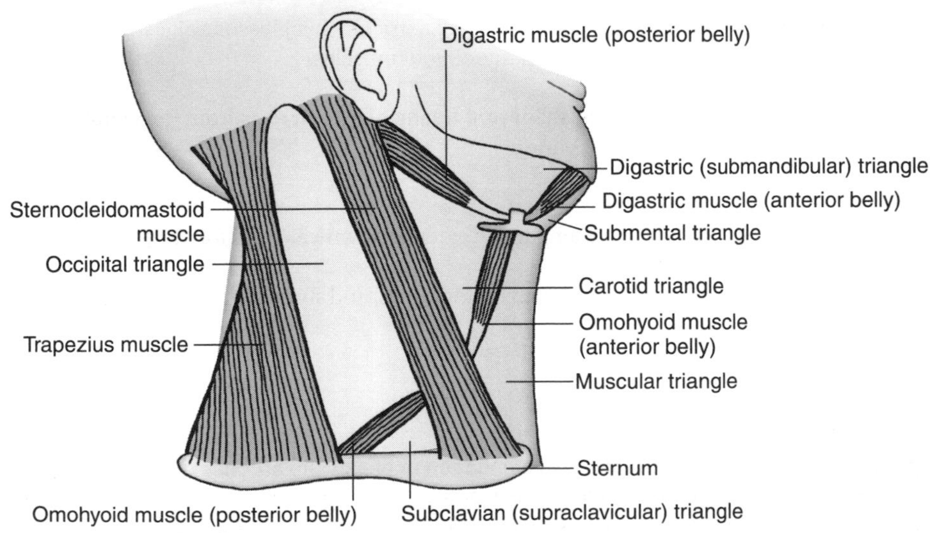

FIGURE 8.1. Subdivisions of the cervical triangle.

- Contains the accessory nerve, cutaneous branches of the cervical plexus, external jugular vein, transverse cervical and suprascapular vessels, subclavian vein (occasionally) and artery, posterior (inferior) belly of the omohyoid, and roots and trunks of the brachial plexus.
- Also contains the nerve to the subclavius and the dorsal scapular, suprascapular, and long thoracic nerves.
- Is further divided into the occipital and subclavian (supraclavicular or omoclavicular) triangles by the omohyoid posterior belly.

B. Anterior Triangle

- Is bounded by the anterior border of the sternocleidomastoid, the anterior midline of the neck, and the inferior border of the mandible.
- Has a roof formed by the **platysma** and the investing layer of the **deep cervical fascia**.
- Is further divided by the omohyoid anterior belly and the **digastric** anterior and posterior bellies into the digastric (submandibular), **submental** (suprahyoid), **carotid**, and **muscular** (inferior carotid) triangles.

CLINICAL CORRELATES

Torticollis (wryneck) is a spasmodic **contraction or shortening of the neck muscles**, producing twisting of the neck with the chin pointing upward and to the opposite side. It is due to injury to the sternocleidomastoid muscle or avulsion of the accessory nerve at the time of birth and unilateral fibrosis in the muscle, which cannot lengthen with the growing neck (congenital torticollis).

C. Hyoid Bone

- Is a U-shaped bone consisting of a median **body**, paired **lesser horns** (cornua) laterally, and paired **greater horns** (cornua) posteriorly.

1. Body

- Provides for attachments for the geniohyoid, mylohyoid, omohyoid, and sternohyoid muscles.

2. Greater Horn

- Provides attachments for the middle constrictor, hyoglossus, digastric (anterior and posterior) bellies, stylohyoid, and thyrohyoid muscles.

3. Lesser Horn

- Provides attachment for the **stylohyoid ligament**, which runs from the **styloid process** to the lesser horn of the hyoid bone.

D. Styloid Process

- Is a slender projection of variable length and extends downward and forward from the temporal bone.
- Gives origin to three muscles (stylohyoid, styloglossus, and stylopharyngeus) and two ligaments (stylohyoid and stylomandibular).

CLINICAL CORRELATES

Eagle's syndrome is an elongation of the styloid process or excessive calcification of the styloid process or stylohyoid ligament that causes neck, throat, or facial pain and dysphagia (difficulty in swallowing). The pain may occur due to compression of the glossopharyngeal nerve, which winds around the styloid process or stylohyoid ligament as it descends to supply the tongue, pharynx, and neck. Also, the pain may be caused by pressure on the internal and external carotid arteries by a deviated and elongated styloid process. Its treatment is styloidectomy.

II. MUSCLES (Figure 8.2; Table 8.1)

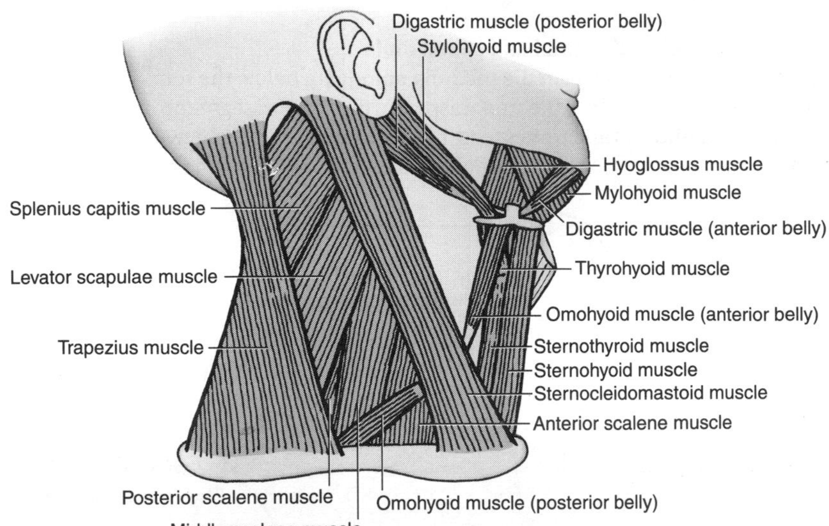

FIGURE 8.2. Muscles of the cervical triangle.

table 8.1 Muscles of the Neck

Muscle	Origin	Insertion	Nerve	Action
Cervical muscles				
Platysma	Superficial fascia over upper part of deltoid and pectoralis major	Mandible; skin and muscles over mandible and angle of mouth	Facial nerve	Depresses lower jaw and lip and angle of mouth; wrinkles skin of neck
Sternocleidomastoid	Manubrium sterni and medial one-third of clavicle	Mastoid process and lateral half of superior nuchal line	Spinal accessory nerve; C2–C8 (sensory)	Singly turns face toward opposite side; together flex head, raise thorax
Suprahyoid muscles				
Digastric	Anterior belly from digastric fossa of mandible; posterior belly from mastoid notch	Intermediate tendon attached to body of hyoid	Posterior belly by facial nerve; anterior belly by mylohyoid nerve of trigeminal nerve	Elevates hyoid and floor of mouth; depresses mandible
Mylohyoid	Mylohyoid line of mandible	Median raphe and body of hyoid bone	Mylohyoid nerve of trigeminal nerve	Elevates hyoid and floor of mouth; depresses mandible
Stylohyoid	Styloid process	Body of hyoid	Facial nerve	Elevates hyoid
Geniohyoid	Genial tubercle of mandible	Body of hyoid	C1 via hypoglossal nerve	Elevates hyoid and floor of mouth
Infrahyoid muscles				
Sternohyoid	Manubrium sterni and medial end of clavicle	Body of hyoid	Ansa cervicalis	Depresses hyoid and larynx
Sternothyroid	Manubrium sterni; first costal cartilage	Oblique line of thyroid cartilage	Ansa cervicalis	Depresses hyoid and larynx
Thyrohyoid	Oblique line of thyroid cartilage	Body and greater horn of hyoid	C1 via hypoglossal nerve	Depresses hyoid and elevates larynx
Omohyoid	Inferior belly from medial lip of suprascapular notch and suprascapular ligament; superior belly from intermediate tendon	Inferior belly to intermediate tendon; superior belly to body of hyoid	Ansa cervicalis	Depresses and retracts hyoid and larynx

III. NERVES (Figures 8.3 to 8.4)

A. Accessory Nerve

- Is formed by the **union of cranial and spinal roots**.
- Has cranial roots that arise from the medulla oblongata below the roots of the vagus.
- Has spinal roots that arise from the lateral aspect of the cervical segment of the spinal cord between C1 and C3 (or C1 and C7) and unites to form a trunk that ascends between the dorsal and ventral roots of the spinal nerves in the vertebral canal and passes through the foramen magnum.

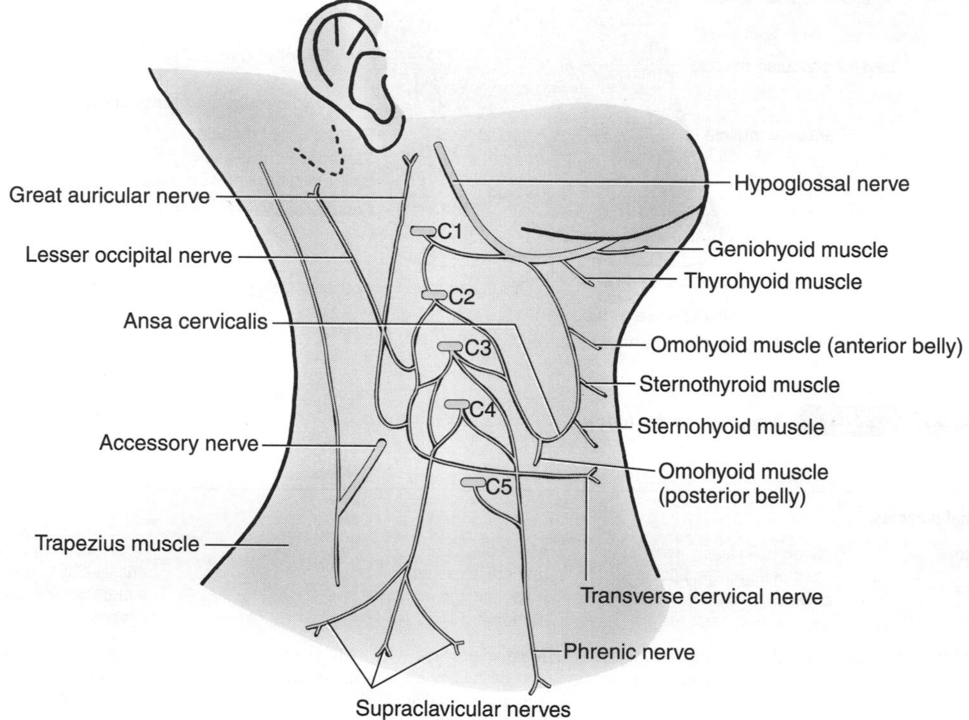

FIGURE 8.3. Cervical plexus.

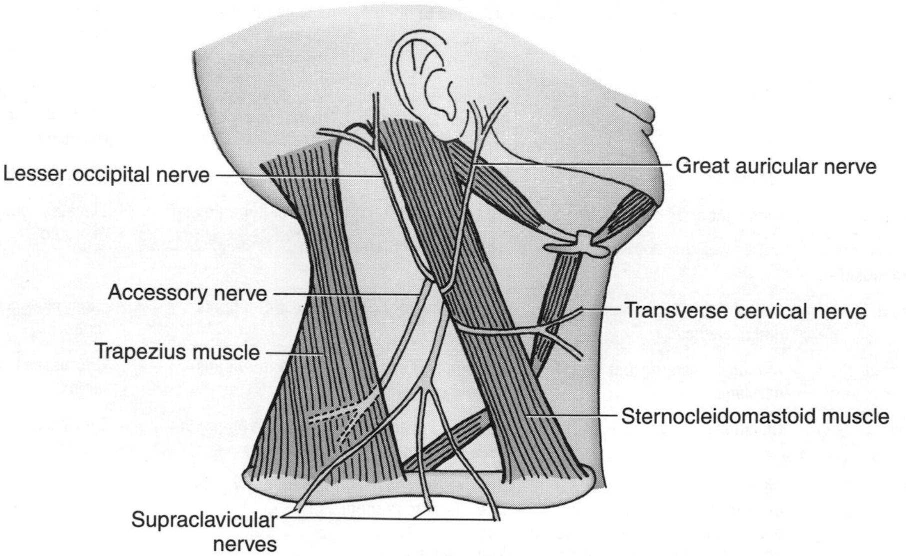

FIGURE 8.4. Cutaneous branches of the cervical plexus.

- Has both spinal and cranial portions, which traverse the jugular foramen, where they interchange fibers. The cranial portion contains motor fibers that join the vagus nerve and innervate the soft palate, pharyngeal constrictors, and larynx. The spinal portion innervates the sternocleidomastoid and trapezius muscles.
- Lies on the levator scapulae in the posterior cervical triangle and then passes deep to the trapezius.

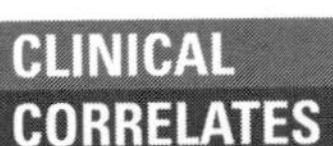

Lesion of the accessory nerve in the neck denervates the trapezius, leading to atrophy of the muscle. It causes a downward displacement or **drooping of the shoulder**.

B. Cervical Plexus (Figures 8.3 to 8.4)

- Is formed by the ventral primary rami of C1 to C4.

1. Cutaneous Branches

(a) Lesser Occipital Nerve (C2)

- Ascends along the posterior border of the sternocleidomastoid to the scalp behind the auricle.

(b) Great Auricular Nerve (C2–C3)

- Ascends on the sternocleidomastoid to innervate the skin behind the auricle and on the parotid gland.

(c) Transverse Cervical Nerve (C2–C3)

- Turns around the posterior border of the sternocleidomastoid and innervates the skin of the anterior cervical triangle.

(d) Supraclavicular Nerve (C3–C4)

- Emerges as a common trunk from under the sternocleidomastoid and then divides into anterior, middle, and lateral branches to the skin over the clavicle and the shoulder.

2. Motor Branches

(a) Ansa Cervicalis

- Is a **nerve loop** formed by the union of the superior root (C1 or C1 and C2; **descendens hypoglossi**) and the inferior root (C2 and C3; **descendens cervicalis**).
- Lies superficial to or within the carotid sheath in the anterior cervical triangle.
- Innervates the infrahyoid (or strap) muscles, such as the omohyoid, sternohyoid, and sternothyroid muscles, with the exception of the thyrohyoid muscle, which is innervated by C1 via the hypoglossal nerve.

(b) Phrenic Nerve (C3–C5)

- Arises from the third, fourth, and fifth cervical nerves but chiefly from the fourth cervical nerve; contains motor, sensory, and sympathetic nerve fibers; and provides the motor supply to the **diaphragm** and sensation to its central part.
- Descends on the anterior surface of the anterior scalene muscle under cover of the sternocleidomastoid muscle.
- Passes between the subclavian artery and vein at the root of the neck and enters the thorax by crossing in front of the origin of the internal thoracic artery, where it joins the pericardiacophrenic branch of this artery.
- Passes anterior to the root of the lung and between the mediastinal pleura and fibrous pericardium to supply sensory fibers to these structures.

(c) Twigs From the Plexus

- Supply the longus capitis and cervicis or colli, sternocleidomastoid, trapezius, levator scapulae, and scalene muscles.

(d) Accessory Phrenic Nerve (C5)

- Occasionally arises as a contribution of C5 to the phrenic nerve or a branch of the nerve to the subclavius (C5), descends lateral to the phrenic nerve, enters the thorax by passing posterior to the subclavian vein, and joins the phrenic nerve below the first rib to supply the diaphragm.

C. Brachial Plexus (See Figure 7.7)

- Is formed by the union of the ventral primary rami of C5 to T1 and passes between the anterior scalene and middle scalene muscles.

1. **Its Roots Give Rise to the:**
   - (a) **Dorsal Scapular Nerve (C5)**
     - Emerges from behind the anterior scalene muscle and runs downward and backward through the middle scalene muscle and then deep to the trapezius.
     - Passes deep to or through the levator scapulae and descends along with the dorsal scapular artery on the deep surface of the rhomboid muscles along the medial border of the scapula, innervating the levator scapulae and rhomboid muscles.
   - (b) **Long Thoracic Nerve (C5–C7)**
     - Pierces the middle scalene muscle, descends behind the brachial plexus, and enters the axilla to innervate the serratus anterior.
2. **Its Upper Trunk Gives Rise to the:**
   - (a) **Suprascapular Nerve (C5–C6)**
     - Passes deep to the trapezius and joins the suprascapular artery in a course toward the shoulder.
     - Passes through the **scapular notch** under the superior transverse scapular ligament.
     - Supplies the supraspinatus and infraspinatus muscles.
   - (b) **Nerve to the Subclavius Muscle (C5)**
     - Descends in front of the plexus and behind the clavicle to innervate the subclavius.
     - Communicates with the phrenic nerve as the **accessory phrenic nerve** in many cases.

CLINICAL CORRELATES

Injury to the upper trunk of the brachial plexus may be caused by a violent separation of the head from the shoulder such as occurs in a fall from a motorcycle. The arm is in medial rotation due to paralysis of the lateral rotators, resulting in **waiter's tip hand**. It may be caused by stretching an infant's neck during a difficult delivery. This is referred to as **birth palsy** or obstetric paralysis.

IV. BLOOD VESSELS (Figure 8.5)

A. Subclavian Artery

- Is a branch of the **brachiocephalic trunk** on the right but arises directly from the **arch of the aorta** on the left.
- Is divided into three parts by the anterior scalene muscle: the first part passes from the origin of the vessel to the medial margin of the anterior scalene; the second part lies behind this muscle; and the third part passes from the lateral margin of the muscle to the outer border of the first rib.
- Its branches include the following:

1. **Vertebral Artery**
   - Arises from the first part of the subclavian artery and ascends between the anterior scalene and longus colli muscles.
   - Ascends through the transverse foramina of vertebrae C1 to C6, winds around the superior articular process of the atlas, and passes through the foramen magnum into the cranial cavity.
2. **Thyrocervical Trunk**
   - Is a short trunk from the first part of the subclavian artery that divides into the following arteries:
   - (a) **Inferior Thyroid Artery**
     - Ascends in front of the anterior scalene muscle, turns medially behind the carotid sheath but in front of the vertebral vessels, and then arches downward to the lower pole of the thyroid gland.
     - Gives rise to an ascending cervical artery, which ascends on the anterior scalene muscle medial to the phrenic nerve.
   - (b) **Transverse Cervical Artery**
     - Runs laterally across the anterior scalene muscle, phrenic nerve, and trunks of the brachial plexus, passing deep to the trapezius.

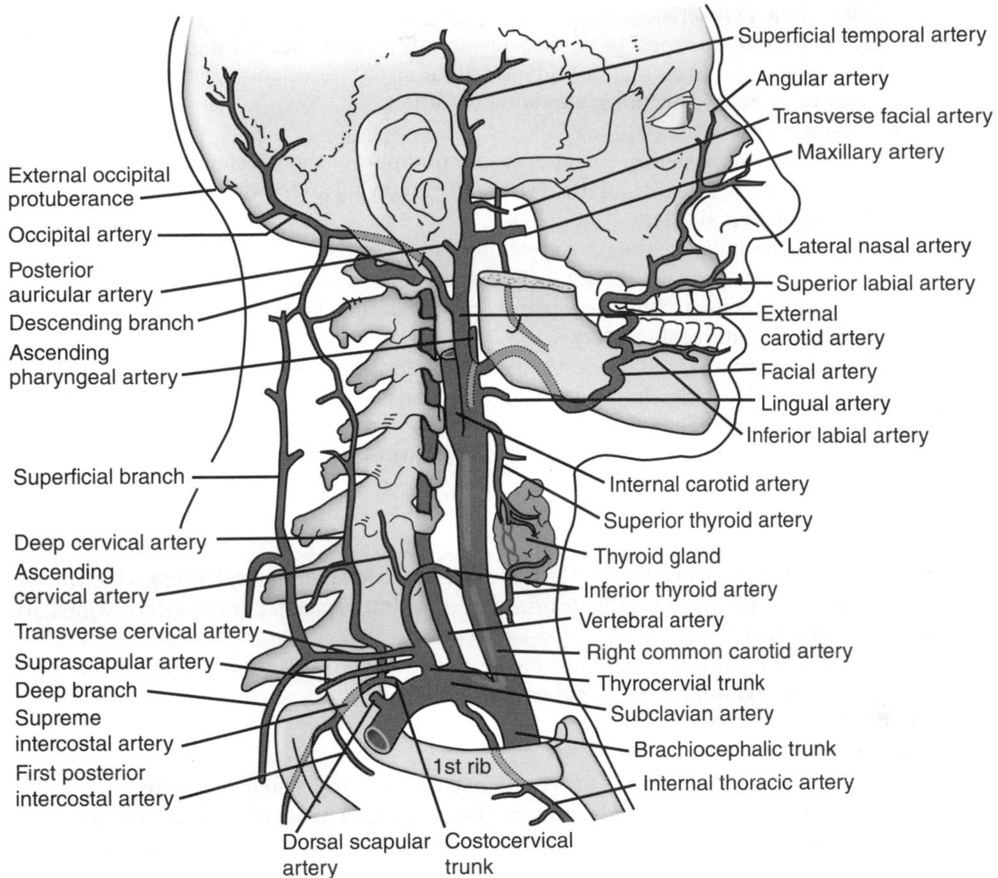

FIGURE 8.5. Subclavian and carotid arteries and their branches.

- Divides into a superficial branch and a deep branch, which takes the place of the **dorsal (descending) scapular artery**. In the absence of the deep branch, the superficial branch is known as the **superficial cervical artery**.

(c) Suprascapular Artery

- Passes in front of the anterior scalene muscle and the brachial plexus parallel to but below the transverse cervical artery.
- Passes superior to the superior transverse scapular ligament, whereas the suprascapular nerve passes inferior to this ligament.

CLINICAL CORRELATES

Thoracic outlet (neurovascular compression) syndrome is a compression of the lower trunk of the brachial plexus and the subclavian vessels in the thoracic outlet (space between the clavicle and the first rib). It is caused by **abnormal insertion** of the anterior and middle scalene muscles, causing ischemic muscle pain in the upper limb, by the **cervical rib** (cartilagenous accessary rib attached to vertebra C7), compressing the subclavian artery, and by the **fractured clavicle**, causing subclavian venous bleeding, which leads to pulmonary embolism.

Subclavian steal syndrome is a cerebral and brain stem ischemia caused by reversal of blood flow from the basilar artery through the vertebral artery into the subclavian artery in the presence of **occlusive disease of the subclavian artery** proximal to the origin of the vertebral artery. When there is very little blood flow through the vertebral artery, it may **steal blood flow from the carotid**, circle of Willis, and basilar circulation and divert it through the vertebral artery into the subclavian artery and into the arm, causing vertebrobasilar insufficiency and thus brain stem ischemia and stroke. Symptoms are dizziness, ataxia, vertigo, visual disturbance, motor deficit, confusion, aphasia, headache, syncope, arm weakness, and arm claudication with exercise. It can be treated by a carotid–subclavian bypass.

3. **Internal Thoracic Artery**
   - Arises from the first part of the subclavian artery, descends through the thorax behind the upper six costal cartilages, and ends at the sixth intercostal space by dividing into the **superior epigastric and musculophrenic arteries.**
4. **Costocervical Trunk**
   - Arises from the posterior aspect of the second part of the subclavian artery behind the anterior scalene muscle and divides into the following arteries:
   - **(a) Deep Cervical Artery**
     - Passes between the transverse process of vertebra C7 and the neck of the first rib, ascends between the semispinalis capitis and semispinalis cervicis muscles, and anastomoses with the deep branch of the descending branch of the occipital artery.
   - **(b) Superior Intercostal Artery**
     - Descends behind the cervical pleura anterior to the necks of the first two ribs and gives rise to the first two posterior intercostal arteries.
5. **Dorsal (Descending) Scapular Artery**
   - Arises from the third part of the subclavian artery or arises as the deep (descending) branch of the transverse cervical artery.

B. Common Carotid Arteries

- Have different origins on the right and left sides: the **right common carotid artery**, which begins at the bifurcation of the brachiocephalic artery, and the **left common carotid artery**, which arises from the aortic arch.
- Ascend within the carotid sheath and divide at the level of the upper border of the thyroid cartilage into the **external and internal carotid arteries.**

1. **Receptors**
   - **(a) Carotid Body**
     - Lies at the bifurcation of the common carotid artery as an ovoid body.
     - Is a **chemoreceptor** that is stimulated by chemical changes (e.g., lack of oxygen, excess of carbon dioxide, and increased hydrogen ion concentration) in the circulating blood that help control respiration.
     - Is innervated by the **nerve to the carotid body**, which arises from the pharyngeal branch of the vagus nerve, and by the **carotid sinus branch** of the glossopharyngeal nerve.
   - **(b) Carotid Sinus**
     - Is a **spindle-shaped dilatation** located at the origin of the internal carotid artery, which functions as a **pressoreceptor (baroreceptor)**, and is stimulated by changes in blood pressure. When stimulated, it causes a slowing of the heart rate, vasodilation, and a decrease in blood pressure.
     - Is innervated primarily by the carotid sinus branch of the glossopharyngeal nerve but is also innervated by the nerve to the carotid body of the vagus nerve.

CLINICAL CORRELATES

Carotid sinus syncope is a temporary loss of consciousness or fainting caused by diminished cerebral blood flow. It results from hypersensitivity of the carotid sinus, and attacks may be produced by pressure on a sensitive carotid sinus such as taking the carotid pulse near the superior border of the thyroid cartilage.

Carotid endarterectomy is the excision of atherosclerotic thickening of intima of the internal carotid artery for the prevention of stroke in patients with symptoms of obstructive disease of the carotid artery.

2. **Internal Carotid Artery**
   - Has no branches in the neck, ascends within the carotid sheath in company with the vagus nerve and the internal jugular vein, and enters the cranium through the **carotid canal** in the petrous part of the temporal bone.
   - In the middle cranial fossa, it gives rise to the **ophthalmic artery** and the **anterior and middle cerebral arteries** and participates in the formation of the circulus arteriosus

(circle of Willis), which is an important polygonal anastomosis between four arteries: the two vertebrals and the two carotids. It is formed by the posterior cerebral, posterior communicating, internal carotid, anterior cerebral, and anterior communicating arteries.

3. External Carotid Artery

- Extends from the level of the upper border of the thyroid cartilage to the neck of the mandible, where it ends in the parotid gland by dividing into the maxillary and superficial temporal arteries.
- Has eight named branches:

(a) Superior Thyroid Artery

- Arises below the level of the greater horn of the hyoid bone.
- Descends obliquely forward in the carotid triangle and passes deep to the infrahyoid muscles to reach the superior pole of the thyroid gland.
- Gives rise to an infrahyoid, sternocleidomastoid, superior laryngeal, cricothyroid, and several glandular branches.

(b) Lingual Artery

- Arises at the level of the tip of the greater horn of the hyoid bone and passes deep to the hyoglossus to reach the tongue.
- Gives rise to suprahyoid, dorsal lingual, sublingual, and deep lingual branches.

(c) Facial Artery

- Arises just above the lingual artery and ascends forward, deep to the posterior belly of the digastric and stylohyoid muscles.
- Hooks around the lower border of the mandible at the anterior margin of the masseter to enter the face.

(d) Ascending Pharyngeal Artery

- Arises from the deep surface of the external carotid artery in the carotid triangle and ascends between the internal carotid artery and the wall of the pharynx.
- Gives rise to pharyngeal, palatine, inferior tympanic, and meningeal branches.

(e) Occipital Artery

- Arises from the posterior surface of the external carotid artery, just above the level of the hyoid bone.
- Passes deep to the digastric posterior belly, occupies the groove on the mastoid process, and appears on the skin above the occipital triangle.
- Gives rise to the following:

1. Sternocleidomastoid Branch

- Descends inferiorly and posteriorly over the hypoglossal nerve and enters the substance of the muscle.
- Anastomoses with the sternocleidomastoid branch of the superior thyroid artery.

2. Descending Branch

- Its superficial branch anastomoses with the superficial branch of the transverse cervical artery.
- Its deep branch anastomoses with the deep cervical artery of the costocervical trunk.

(f) Posterior Auricular Artery

- Arises from the posterior surface of the external carotid artery just above the digastric posterior belly.
- Ascends superficial to the styloid process and deep to the parotid gland and ends between the mastoid process and the external acoustic meatus.
- Gives rise to stylomastoid, auricular, and occipital branches.

(g) Maxillary Artery

- Arises behind the neck of the mandible as the larger terminal branch of the external carotid artery.
- Runs deep to the neck of the mandible and enters the infratemporal fossa.

(h) Superficial Temporal Artery

- Arises behind the neck of the mandible as the smaller terminal branch of the external carotid artery.

- Gives rise to the **transverse facial artery**, which runs between the zygomatic arch above and the parotid duct below.
- Ascends in front of the external acoustic meatus into the scalp, accompanying the auriculotemporal nerve and the superficial temporal vein.

CLINICAL CORRELATES

Temporal (giant cell) arteritis is granulomatous inflammation with multinucleated giant cells, affecting the medium-sized arteries, especially the temporal artery. Symptoms include severe headache, excruciating pain in the temporal area, temporal artery tenderness, visual impairment, transient diplopia, jaw claudication, fever, fatigue, and weight loss. Its cause is unknown, but it is diagnosed by a temporal artery biopsy and can be treated with corticosteroids such as prednisone.

C. Veins (Figure 8.6)

1. Retromandibular Vein

- Is formed by the superficial temporal and maxillary veins.
- Divides into an anterior branch, which joins the facial vein to form the common facial vein, and a posterior branch, which joins the posterior auricular vein to form the external jugular vein.

2. External Jugular Vein

- Is formed by the union of the **posterior auricular vein** and the posterior branch of the **retromandibular vein**.
- Crosses the sternomastoid obliquely under the platysma and ends in the subclavian (or sometimes the internal jugular) vein.
- Receives the suprascapular, transverse cervical, and anterior jugular veins.

3. Internal Jugular Vein (Figure 8.7)

- Begins in the **jugular foramen** as a continuation of the sigmoid sinus, descends in the carotid sheath, and ends in the **brachiocephalic vein**.
- Has the superior bulb at its beginning and the inferior bulb just above its termination.
- Receives the facial, lingual, and superior and middle thyroid veins.

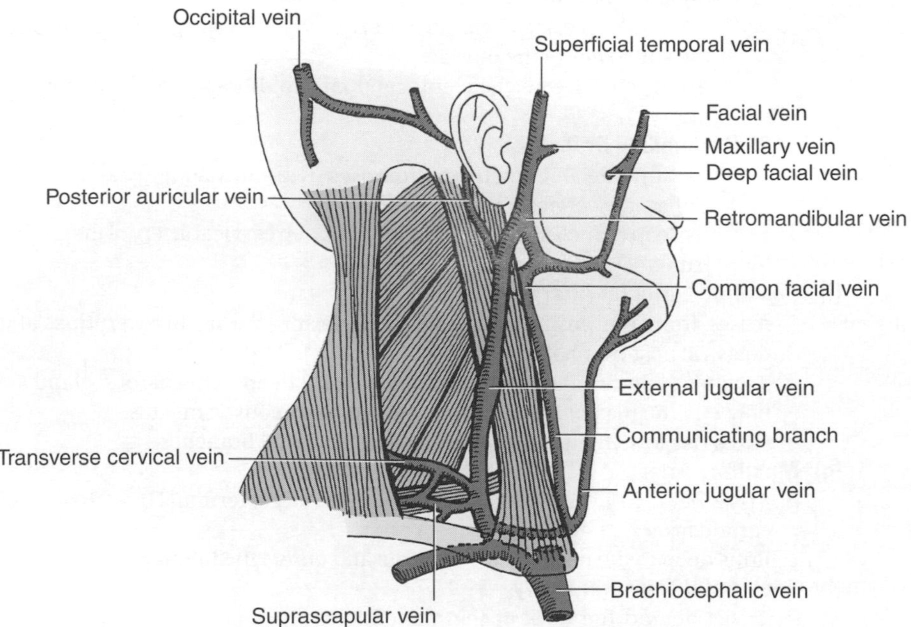

FIGURE 8.6. Veins of the cervical triangle.

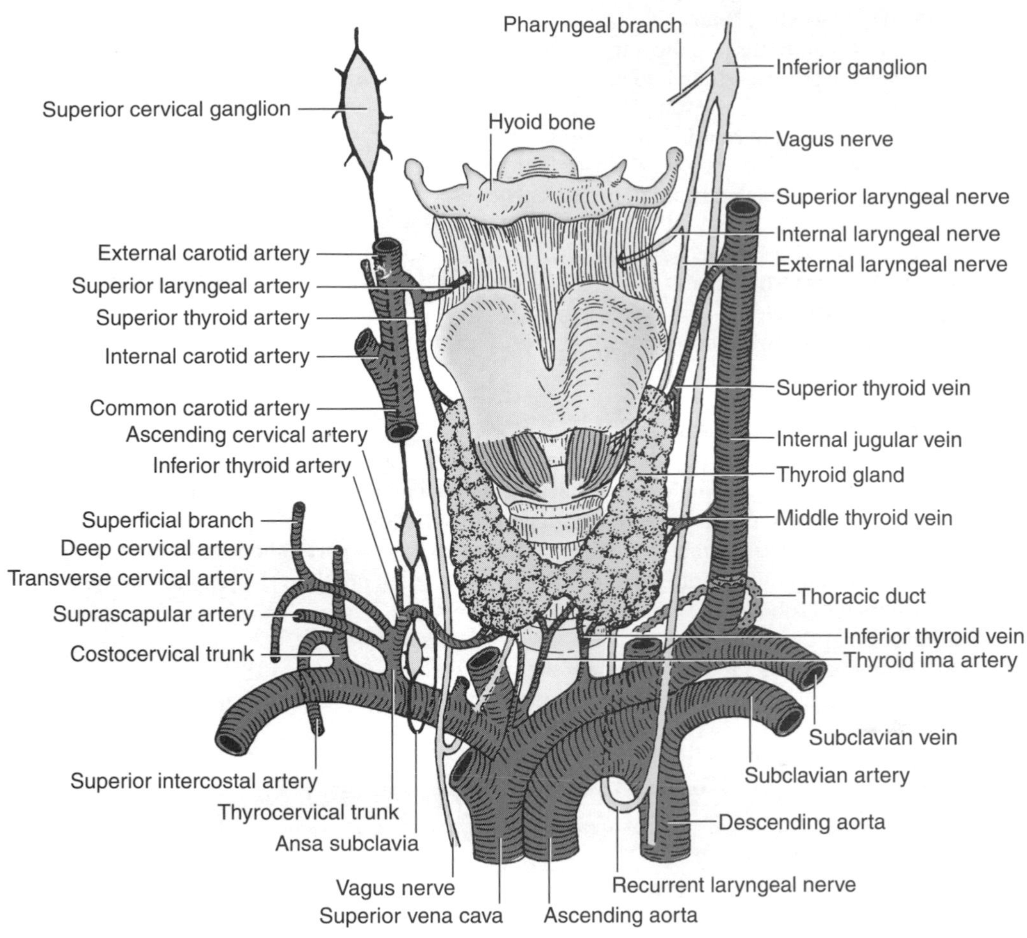

FIGURE 8.7. Deep structures of the neck.

CLINICAL CORRELATES **Central venous line** is an intravenous needle and catheter placed into a large vein such as the internal jugular or subclavian vein to give fluids or medication. A **central line** is inserted in the apex of the triangular interval between the clavicle and the clavicular and sternal heads of the sternocleidomastoid muscle into the **internal jugular vein** through which the catheter is threaded into the superior vena cava (a large central vein in the chest). The needle is then directed inferolaterally. Air embolism or laceration of the internal jugular vein is a possible complication of catheterization. A **central line** may also be inserted into the retroclavicular portion of the **right subclavian vein**, and it should be guided medially along the long axis of the clavicle to reach the posterior surface where the vein runs over the first rib. The lung is vulnerable to injury, and pneumothorax and arterial puncture, causing hemothorax, are potential complications of a subclavian catheterization.

V. LYMPHATICS

A. Superficial Lymph Nodes of the Head

- Lymph vessels from the face, scalp, and ear drain into the occipital, retroauricular, parotid, buccal (facial), submandibular, submental, and superficial cervical nodes, which in turn drain into the **deep cervical nodes** (including the jugulodigastric and juguloomohyoid nodes).

B. Deep Lymph Nodes of the Head

- The middle ear drains into the retropharyngeal and upper deep cervical nodes; the nasal cavity and paranasal sinuses drain into the submandibular, retropharyngeal, and upper deep cervical; the tongue drains into the submental, submandibular, and upper and lower cervical; the larynx drains into the upper and lower deep cervical; the pharynx drains into the retropharyngeal and upper and lower deep cervical; and the thyroid gland drains into the lower deep cervical, prelaryngeal, pretracheal, and paratracheal nodes.

C. Superficial Cervical Lymph Nodes

- Lie along the **external jugular vein** in the posterior triangle and along the **anterior jugular vein** in the anterior triangle.
- Drain into the deep cervical nodes.

D. Deep Cervical Lymph Nodes

1. Superior Deep Cervical Nodes

- Lie along the **internal jugular vein** in the carotid triangle of the neck.
- Receive afferent lymphatics from the back of the head and neck, tongue, palate, nasal cavity, larynx, pharynx, trachea, thyroid gland, and esophagus.
- Have efferent vessels that join those of the inferior deep cervical nodes to form the **jugular trunk**, which empties into the thoracic duct on the left and into the junction of the internal jugular and subclavian veins on the right.

2. Inferior Deep Cervical Nodes

- Lie on the **internal jugular vein** near the subclavian vein.
- Receive afferent lymphatics from the anterior jugular, transverse cervical, and apical axillary nodes.

DEEP NECK AND PREVERTEBRAL REGION

I. DEEP STRUCTURES OF THE NECK (Figure 8.7)

A. Trachea

- Begins at the inferior border of the cricoid cartilage (C6).
- Has **16 to 20 incomplete hyaline cartilaginous rings** that open posteriorly to prevent the trachea from collapsing.

CLINICAL CORRELATES

Tracheotomy (tracheostomy) is the procedure of creating an opening through the trachea by first making an incision between the third and fourth rings of cartilage to allow entry of a tube into the airway, usually as an emergent procedure to reestablish airway or in a patient who has been on life support for a prolonged period of time with an endotracheal tube and to decrease the risk of tracheomalacia.

B. Esophagus

- Is a muscular tube (approximately 10 in. long), begins at the lower border of the pharynx at the level of the cricoid cartilage (C6), descends behind the trachea, and ends in the stomach at T11.
- The cricopharyngeus muscle, the sphincter of the upper esophageal opening, remains closed except during deglutition (swallowing) and emesis (vomiting).
- Is innervated by the recurrent laryngeal nerves and the sympathetic trunks and receives blood from branches of the inferior thyroid arteries.

C. Thyroid Gland (Figure 8.7)

- Is an endocrine gland that produces **thyroxine** and **thyrocalcitonin**, which are essential for metabolism and growth. The thyroid takes iodine from food to produce thyroid hormones and is controlled by thyroid-stimulating hormone produced by the pituitary gland.

- Consists of right and left lobes connected by the **isthmus**, which usually crosses the second and third (or second, third, and fourth) tracheal rings. An inconstant **pyramidal lobe**, a remnant of the thyroglossal duct, extends upward from the isthmus, usually to the left of the midline, and may be anchored to the hyoid bone by a fibrous or muscular band known as the **levator glandulae thyroideae**.
- Is supplied by the superior and inferior thyroid arteries and sometimes the **thyroid ima artery**, an inconsistent branch from the brachiocephalic trunk.
- Drains via the superior and middle thyroid veins to the internal jugular vein and via the inferior thyroid vein to the brachiocephalic vein.

CLINICAL CORRELATES **Goiter** is an **enlargement of the thyroid gland**, which is commonly caused by **iodine deficiency** (because iodine is vital to the formation of thyroid hormone), **hyperthyroidism** (overproduction of thyroid hormones), or **hypothyroidism** (which causes the gland to swell in its attempt to produce more hormones). The enlarged gland compresses the trachea, larynx, esophagus, and recurrent laryngeal nerve, causing symptoms of breathing difficulties (dyspnea), loss of speech, cough or wheezing, swallowing difficulties (dysphagia), neck vein distention, and dizziness. The goiter can be treated with radioactive iodine to shrink the gland or with thyroidectomy.

Graves disease is an autoimmune disease in which the immune system overstimulates the thyroid gland, causing **hyperthyroidism** that causes **goiter** and **exophthalmos** (or **proptosis**). The most common symptoms include insomnia, irritability, weight loss, increased perspiration, muscle weakness, palpitations, nervousness, and hand tremors. **Hashimoto disease** (chronic **thyroiditis**) is an autoimmune disease in which the immune system destroys the thyroid gland, resulting in **hypothyroidism** and goiter.

Papillary carcinoma of the thyroid is a malignancy of the thyroid and is the most common type of thyroid carcinoma, accounting for approximately 70% of all thyroid tumors. The cancer occurs more in females, and its symptoms include a lump on the side of the neck, hoarseness of the voice, and difficulty swallowing. Its treatment is surgical removal of the tumor, and after surgery, most patients are treated with radioactive iodine and should take thyroid hormone for life.

Thyroidectomy is a surgical removal of the thyroid gland, and during surgery, the thyroid ima artery and inferior thyroid veins are vulnerable to injury. Potential complications may include **hemorrhage** from injury of the anterior jugular veins; **nerve paralysis**, particularly of the recurrent laryngeal nerves; **pneumothorax** resulting from damage of the cervical dome of the pleura; and **esophageal injury** due to its immediate posterior location to the trachea.

D. Parathyroid Glands

- Are endocrine glands that play a vital role in the regulation of calcium and phosphorus metabolism and are controlled by the pituitary and hypothalamus.
- Secrete parathyroid hormone (PTH), which is essential to life because low calcium levels lead to lethal neuromuscular disorders.
- Usually consist of **four** (two to six) **small ovoid bodies** that lie against the dorsum of the thyroid under its sheath but with their own capsule.
- Are supplied chiefly by the inferior thyroid artery.

CLINICAL CORRELATES **Inadvertent parathyroidectomy** may occur during thyroidectomy, which would result in decreased production of PTH and lead to low calcium levels, which in turn would lead to muscle spasms (tetany) as well as high levels of phosphorus and low levels of vitamin D.

Cricothyrotomy is an incision through the skin and cricothyroid membrane and insertion of a tracheotomy tube into the trachea for relief of acute respiratory obstruction. When making a skin incision, care must be taken not to injure the anterior jugular veins, which lie near the midline of the neck. It is preferable for nonsurgeons to perform a tracheostomy for emergency respiratory obstructions.

E. Thyroid Cartilage

- Is a hyaline cartilage that forms a laryngeal prominence known as the **Adam's apple**, which is particularly apparent in males.
- Has a superior horn that is joined to the tip of the greater horn of the hyoid bone by the lateral thyroid ligament and an inferior horn that articulates with the cricoid cartilage.

F. Vagus Nerve

- Runs through the jugular foramen and gives rise to the superior laryngeal nerve, which is divided into the external and internal laryngeal nerves.

1. External Laryngeal Nerve

- Runs along with the superior thyroid artery.
- Supplies the cricothyroid and inferior pharyngeal constrictor muscles.

2. Internal Laryngeal Nerve

- Accompanies the superior laryngeal artery.
- Supplies the sensory fibers to the larynx above the vocal cord and taste fibers to the epiglottis.

G. Sympathetic Trunk

- Is covered by the prevertebral fascia (the prevertebral fascia splits to enclose the sympathetic trunk).
- Runs behind the carotid sheath and in front of the longus colli and longus capitis muscles.
- Contains preganglionic and postganglionic sympathetic fibers, cell bodies of the postganglionic sympathetic fibers, and visceral afferent fibers with cell bodies in the upper thoracic dorsal root ganglia.
- Emits gray rami communicantes but receives no white rami communicantes in the cervical region.
- Bears the following cervical ganglia:

1. Superior Cervical Ganglion

- Lies in front of the transverse processes of vertebrae C1 to C2, posterior to the internal carotid artery and anterior to the longus capitis.
- Contains cell bodies of postganglionic sympathetic fibers that pass to the visceral structures of the head and neck.
- Gives rise to the **internal carotid nerve** to form the internal carotid plexus; the **external carotid nerve** to form the external carotid plexus; the pharyngeal branches that join the **pharyngeal branches** of the glossopharyngeal and vagus nerves to form the pharyngeal plexus; and the **superior cervical cardiac nerve** to the heart.

2. Middle Cervical Ganglion

- Lies at the level of the cricoid cartilage (vertebra C6).
- Gives rise to a **middle cervical cardiac nerve**, which is the largest of the three cervical sympathetic cardiac nerves.

3. Inferior Cervical Ganglion

- Fuses with the first thoracic ganglion to become the **cervicothoracic (stellate) ganglion**.
- Lies in front of the neck of the first rib and the transverse process of vertebra C7 and behind the dome of the pleura and the vertebral artery.
- Gives rise to the inferior cervical cardiac nerve.

CLINICAL CORRELATES

Horner syndrome is caused by thyroid carcinoma, which may cause a lesion of the cervical sympathetic trunk; by Pancoast tumor at the apex of the lungs, which injures the stellate ganglion; or by a penetrating injury to the neck, injuring cervical sympathetic nerves. This syndrome is characterized by presence of ptosis, miosis, enophthalmos, anhidrosis, and vasodilation. (These are explained in the sections pertaining to the eye. See the section on the orbit.)

Stellate ganglion block is performed under fluoroscopy by inserting the needle at the level of the C6 vertebra to avoid piercing the pleura, although the ganglion lies at the level of the C7 vertebra. The needle of the anesthetic syringe is inserted between the trachea and the carotid sheath through the skin over the anterior tubercle of the transverse process of the C6 vertebra (Chassaignac or carotid tubercle) and then directed medially and inferiorly. Once needle position close to the ganglion is confirmed, the local anesthetic is injected beneath the prevertebral fascia.

4. Ansa Subclavia

- Is the cord connecting the middle and inferior cervical sympathetic ganglia, forming a loop around the first part of the subclavian artery.

H. Thoracic Duct

- Ascends through the posterior mediastinum between the aorta and azygos vein.
- Arches laterally over the apex of the left pleura, posterior to the left carotid sheath, and anterior to the sympathetic trunk and vertebral and subclavian arteries; runs behind the left internal jugular vein; and then usually empties into the left brachiocephalic vein at the junction of the left internal jugular and subclavian veins.

II. DEEP CERVICAL FASCIAE (Figure 8.8)

A. Superficial (Investing) Layer of Deep Cervical Fascia

- Surrounds the deeper parts of the neck.
- Splits to enclose the sternocleidomastoid and trapezius muscles.
- Is attached superiorly along the mandible, mastoid process, external occipital protuberance, and superior nuchal line of the occipital bone.
- Is attached inferiorly along the acromion and spine of the scapula, clavicle, and manubrium sterni.

B. Prevertebral Layer of Deep Cervical Fascia

- Is cylindrical and encloses the **vertebral column** and its associated muscles.
- Covers the scalene muscles and the deep muscles of the back.

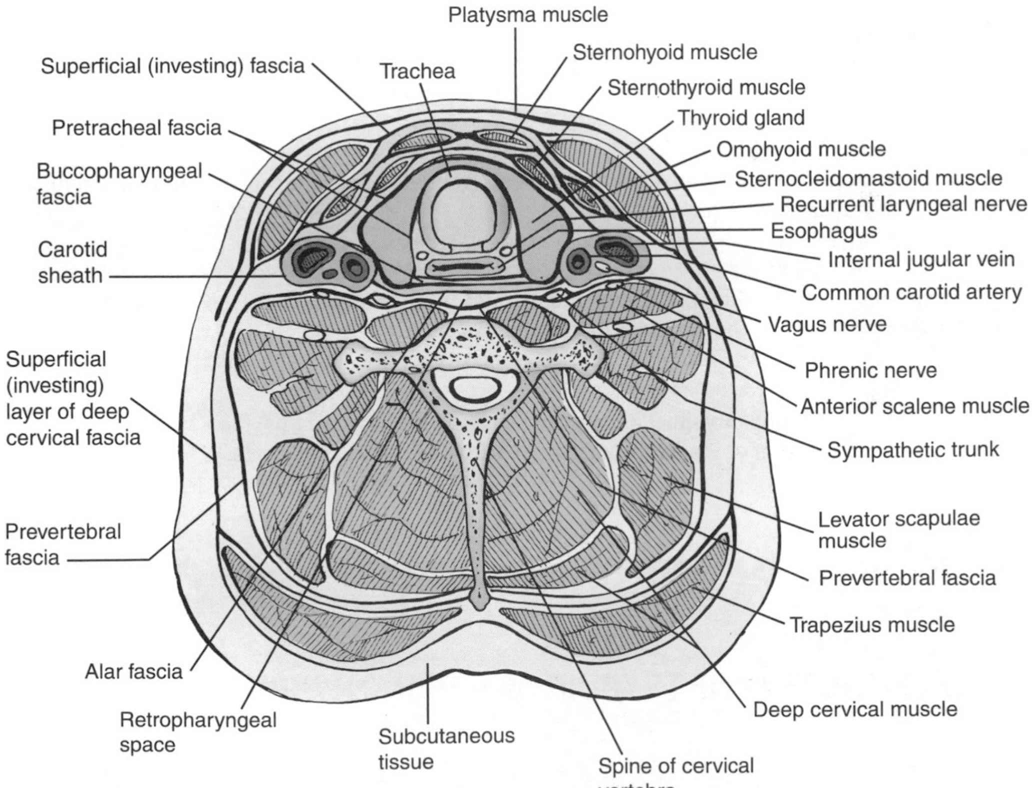

FIGURE 8.8. Cross section of the neck.

- Attaches to the external occipital protuberance and the basilar part of the occipital bone and becomes continuous with the **endothoracic fascia** and the **anterior longitudinal ligament** of the bodies of the vertebrae in the thorax.

CLINICAL CORRELATES **Danger space** is the space between the anterior (alar part) and posterior layers of prevertebral fascia because of its extension from the base of the skull to the diaphragm, providing a route for the spread of infection.

C. Carotid Sheath

- Contains the **common** and **internal carotid arteries, internal jugular vein**, and **vagus nerve**.
- Does not contain the sympathetic trunk, which lies posterior to the carotid sheath and is enclosed in the prevertebral fascia.
- Blends with the prevertebral, pretracheal, and investing layers and also attaches to the base of the skull.

D. Pretracheal Layer of Deep Cervical Fascia

- Invests the **larynx** and **trachea**, encloses the **thyroid gland**, is continuous with the buccopharyngeal facia, and contributes to the formation of the carotid sheath.
- Attaches superiorly to the thyroid and cricoid cartilages and inferiorly to the pericardium.

E. Alar Fascia

- Is an ancillary layer of the deep cervical fascia between the pretracheal (or buccopharyngeal) and prevertebral fasciae and forms a subdivision of the retropharyngeal space.
- Blends with the carotid sheath laterally and extends from the base of the skull to the level of the seventh cervical vertebra, where it merges with the pretracheal fascia.

F. Buccopharyngeal Fascia

- Covers the buccinator muscles and the pharynx and blends with the pretracheal fascia.
- Is attached to the pharyngeal tubercle and the pterygomandibular raphe.

G. Pharyngobasilar Fascia

- Is the **fibrous coat in the wall of the pharynx** and is situated between the mucous membrane and the pharyngeal constrictor muscles.

H. Retropharyngeal Space

- Is the space between the prevertebral fascia and buccopharyngeal fascia, extending from the base of the skull into the posterior mediastinum.

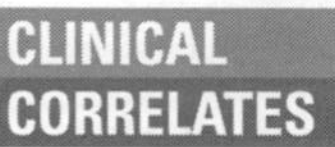

Retropharyngeal abscess or infection may spread from the neck into the posterior mediastinum through the retropharyngeal space.

III. PREVERTEBRAL OR DEEP NECK MUSCLES (Table 8.2)

IV. DEVELOPMENT OF THYROID AND PARATHYROID GLAND

A. Thyroid Gland

- Develops from the thyroid diverticulum, which forms from the **endoderm** in the floor of the foregut (pharynx) and divides into right and left lobes that are connected by the isthmus of the gland.

table 8.2 Prevertebral or Deep Neck Muscles

Muscle	Origin	Insertion	Nerve	Action
Lateral vertebral				
Anterior scalene	Transverse processes of CV3–CV6	Scalene tubercle on first rib	Lower cervical (C5–C8)	Elevates first rib; bends neck
Middle scalene	Transverse processes of CV2–CV7	Upper surface of first rib	Lower cervical (C5–C8)	Elevates first rib; bends neck
Posterior scalene	Transverse processes of CV4–CV6	Outer surface of second rib	Lower cervical (C6–C8)	Elevates second rib; bends neck
Anterior vertebral				
Longus capitis	Transverse process of CV3–CV6	Basilar part of occipital bone	C1–C4	Flexes and rotates head
Longus colli (L. cervicis)	Transverse processes and bodies of CV3–TV3	Anterior tubercle of atlas; bodies of CV2–CV4; transverse process of CV5–CV6	C2–C6	Flexes and rotates neck
Rectus capitis anterior	Lateral mass of atlas	Basilar part of occipital bone	C1–C2	Flexes and rotates head
Rectus capitis lateralis	Transverse process of atlas	Jugular process of occipital bone	C1–C2	Flexes head laterally

- Descends caudally into the neck, passing ventral to the hyoid bone and laryngeal cartilages. During migration, the developing gland remains connected to the tongue by the **thyroglossal duct**, which is an endodermal tube and extends between the thyroid primordium and posterior part of the tongue. This duct is later obliterated, and the site of the duct is marked by the **foramen cecum**.
- Parafollicular cells are derived from the neural crest via the ultimobranchial (end gill) body in the fourth pharyngeal pouch and then migrate into the thyroid gland.

CLINICAL CORRELATES **Thyroglossal duct cyst** is a cyst in the midline of the neck, resulting from lack of closure of a segment of the thyroglossal duct. It occurs most commonly in the region below the hyoid bone. As the cyst enlarges, it is prone to infection. Occasionally, a **thyroglossal cyst** ruptures spontaneously, producing a sinus as a result of an infection of the cyst.

B. Parathyroid Gland

- Inferior parathyroid glands develop as the result of proliferation of endodermal cells in the third pharyngeal pouch.
- Superior parathyroid glands develop as the result of proliferation of endodermal cells in the fourth pharyngeal pouch.

FACE AND SCALP

I. MUSCLES OF FACIAL EXPRESSION (Figure 8.9; Table 8.3)

II. NERVE SUPPLY TO THE FACE AND SCALP (Figures 8.10 to 8.11)

A. Facial Nerve (Figure 8.12)

- Comes through the **stylomastoid foramen** and appears posterior to the parotid gland.

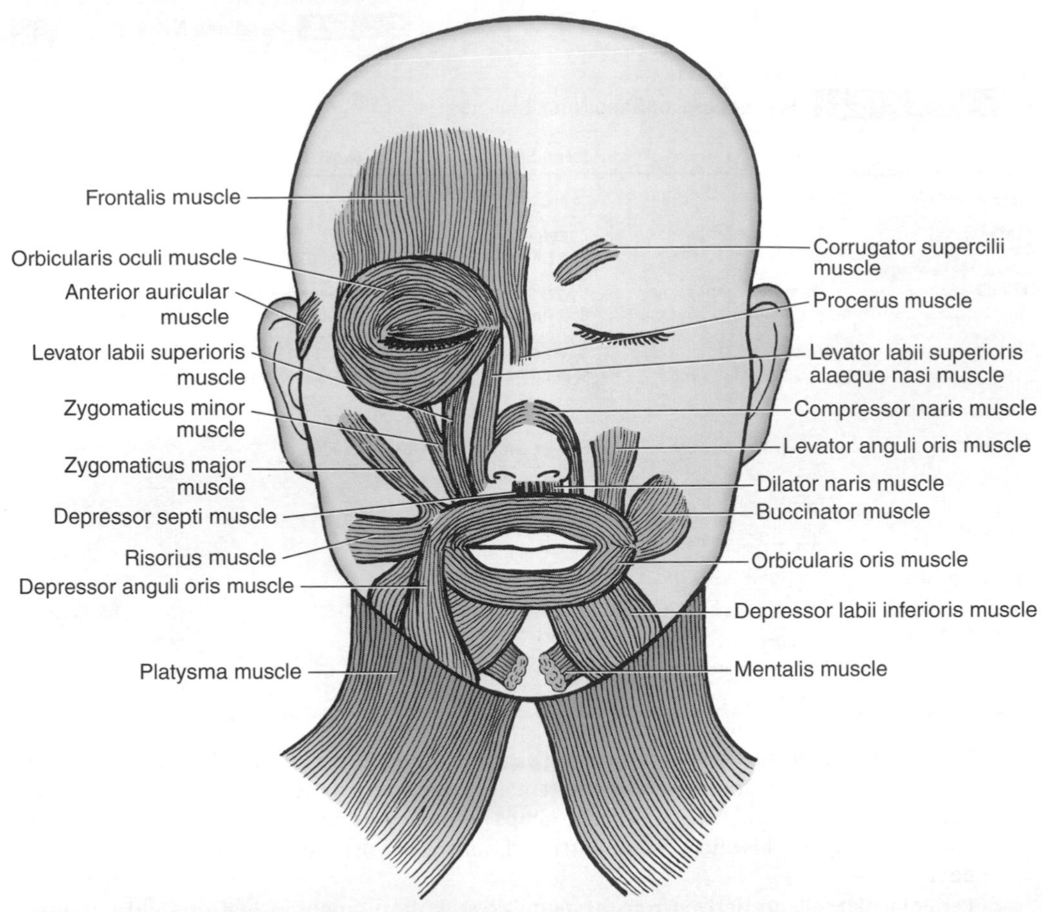

FIGURE 8.9. Muscles of facial expression.

table 8.3 Muscles of Facial Expression

Muscle	Origin	Insertion	Nerve	Action
Occipitofrontalis	Superior nuchal line; upper orbital margin	Epicranial aponeurosis	Facial	Elevates eyebrows; wrinkles forehead (surprise)
Corrugator supercilii	Medial supraorbital margin	Skin of medial eyebrow	Facial	Draws eyebrows downward medially (anger, frowning)
Orbicularis oculi	Medial orbital margin; medial palpebral ligament; lacrimal bone	Skin and rim of orbit; tarsal plate; lateral palpebral raphe	Facial	Closes eyelids: orbital part tightly (wink); palpebral part gently
Procerus	Nasal bone and cartilage	Skin between eyebrows	Facial	Wrinkles skin over bones (sadness)
Nasalis	Maxilla lateral to incisive fossa	Bridge on nose (transverse part); Ala (alar part)	Facial	Compresses nostrils (transverse part); dilates nostrils (alar part)
Depressor septi	Incisive fossa of maxilla	Ala and nasal septum	Facial	Constricts nares
Orbicularis oris	Maxilla above incisor teeth	Skin of lip	Facial	Closes lips or purse
Levator anguli oris	Canine fossa of maxilla	Angle of mouth	Facial	Elevates angle of mouth medially (disgust)
Levator labii superioris	Maxilla above infraorbital foramen	Skin of upper lip	Facial	Elevates upper lip; dilates nares (disgust)
Levator labii superioris alaeque nasi	Frontal process of maxilla	Skin of upper lip	Facial	Elevates ala of nose and upper lip

table 8.3 Muscles of Facial Expression *(continued)*

Muscle	Origin	Insertion	Nerve	Action
Zygomaticus major	Zygomatic arch	Angle of mouth	Facial	Draws angle of mouth backward and upward (smile)
Zygomaticus minor	Zygomatic arch	Angle of mouth	Facial	Elevates upper lip
Depressor labii inferioris	Mandible below mental foramen	Orbicularis oris and skin of lower lip	Facial	Depresses lower lip
Depressor anguli oris	Oblique line of mandible	Angle of mouth	Facial	Depresses angle of mouth (frowning)
Risorius	Fascia over masseter	Angle of mouth	Facial	Retracts angle of mouth (grimace)
Buccinator	Mandible; pterygomandibular raphe; alveolar processes	Angle of mouth	Facial	Compresses cheek to keep it taut
Mentalis	Incisive fossa of mandible	Skin of chin	Facial	Elevates and protrudes lower lip (doubt)
Auricularis anterior, superior, and posterior	Temporal fascia; epicranial aponeurosis; mastoid process	Anterior, superior, and posterior sides of auricle	Facial	Retract and elevate ear

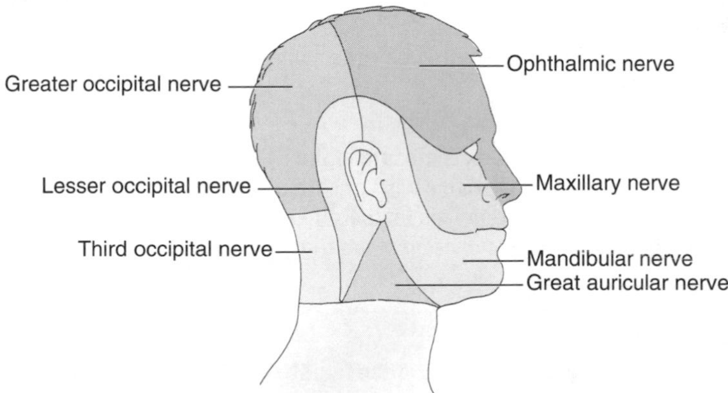

FIGURE 8.10. Sensory innervation of the face.

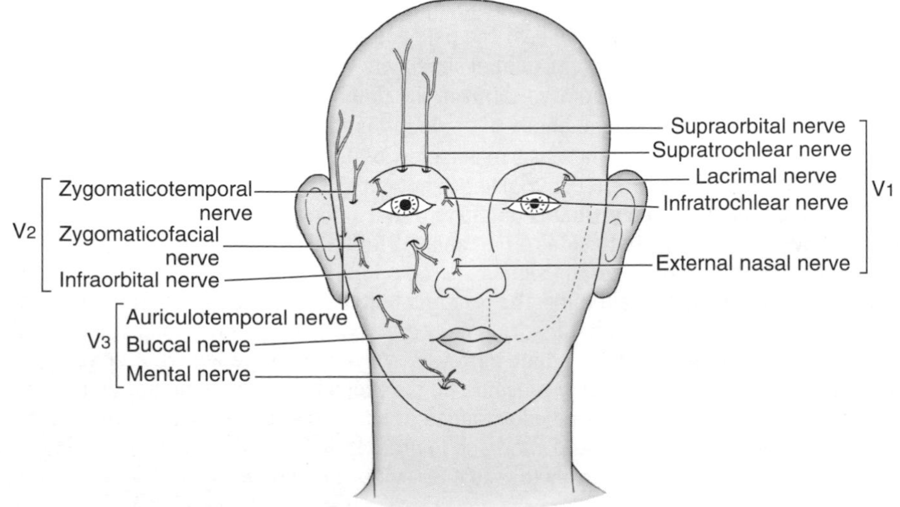

FIGURE 8.11. Cutaneous innervation of the face and scalp.

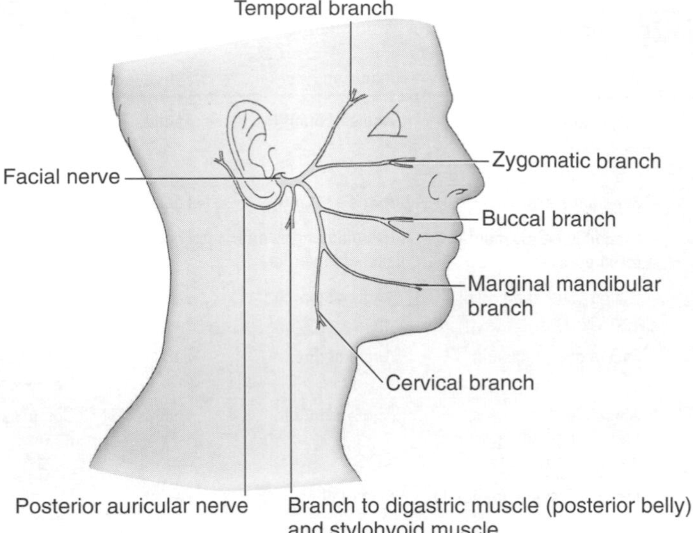

FIGURE 8.12. Distribution of the facial nerve.

- Enters the parotid gland to give rise to five terminal branches—the **temporal, zygomatic, buccal, mandibular, and cervical branches**—that radiate forward in the face.
- Innervates the muscles of facial expression and sends the posterior auricular branch to the muscles of the auricle and the occipitalis muscle.
- Also innervates the digastric posterior belly and stylohyoid muscles.

CLINICAL CORRELATES

Corneal blink reflex is **closure of the eyelids** in response to blowing on the cornea or touching it with a wisp of cotton. It is caused by bilateral contraction of the orbicularis oculi muscles. Its efferent limb (of the reflex arc) is the facial nerve; its afferent limb is the nasociliary nerve of the ophthalmic division of the trigeminal nerve.

CLINICAL CORRELATES

Bell palsy is a **paralysis of the facial muscles** on the affected side because of a lesion of the facial nerve. Symptoms usually begin suddenly and peak within 48 hours, but pain in or behind the ear can precede the palsy by a day or two. The palsy manifests as an inability to wrinkle the forehead, drooping of the eyebrow, sagging of the lower eyelid, and inability to close or blink the eye, sagging corners of the mouth, inability to smile, whistle, or blow, and tingling around the lips. The palsy causes decreased lacrimation (as a result of a lesion of the greater petrosal nerve), painful sensitivity to sounds (damage of nerve to the stapedius), loss of taste in the anterior two-thirds of the tongue (lesion of chorda tympani), and deviation of the lower jaw and tongue (injury of nerve to the digastric posterior belly). A central lesion of the facial nerve results in paralysis of muscles in the lower face on the contralateral (opposite) side; consequently, forehead wrinkling is not impaired. Therefore, the patient with peripheral **facial palsy** shows **no wrinkles** on the affected side, but the patient with a **stroke** or a **brain tumor** shows wrinkles on both sides. The cause of Bell palsy is unknown (idiopathic), but in some cases may be attributed to herpes simplex (viral) infection and less commonly, a lesion of the facial nerve, a stroke, or a brain tumor. Its treatment includes a course of steroid treatment–60 to 80 mg of prednisone (anti-inflammatory drug) daily during the first 5 days, followed by tapering doses over the next 5 days–may help reduce paralysis and expedite recovery by reducing inflammation and swelling and relieving pressure on the facial nerve for some patients. Treatment also includes antiviral drugs, such as acyclovir alone or in combination with steroids. The patient is advised to avoid exposure to cold and wind and to protect the eyes from drying out with artificial tears and eye patches. Recovery is likely to take a few weeks to months.

B. Trigeminal Nerve

- Provides sensory innervation to the **skin of the face**.

1. Ophthalmic Division

- Innervates the area above the upper eyelid and dorsum of the nose.
- Supplies the face as the **supraorbital**, **supratrochlear**, **infratrochlear**, **external nasal**, and **lacrimal nerves**.

2. Maxillary Division

- Innervates the face below the level of the eyes and above the upper lip.
- Supplies the face as the zygomaticofacial, zygomaticotemporal, and infraorbital nerves.

3. Mandibular Division

- Innervates the face below the level of the lower lip.
- Supplies the face as the auriculotemporal, buccal, and mental nerves.

CLINICAL CORRELATES

Trigeminal neuralgia (tic douloureux) is marked by **paroxysmal pain** along the course of the trigeminal nerve, especially radiating to the maxillary or mandibular area. The common causes of this disorder are aberrant blood vessels, aneurysms, chronic meningeal inflammation, brain tumors compressing on the trigeminal nerve at the base of the brain, and other lesions such as multiple sclerosis. Carbamazepine is regarded as the treatment of choice, but the synergistic combination of carbamazepine and baclofen may provide relief from episodic pain. If medical treatments are not effective, the neuralgia may be alleviated by sectioning the sensory root of the trigeminal nerve in the trigeminal (Meckel) cave in the middle cranial fossa.

III. BLOOD VESSELS OF THE FACE AND SCALP (Figures 8.13 to 8.14)

A. Facial Artery

- Arises from the **external carotid artery** just above the upper border of the hyoid bone.
- Passes deep to the mandible, winds around the lower border of the mandible, and runs upward and forward on the face.
- Gives rise to the ascending palatine, tonsillar, glandular, and submental branches in the neck and the inferior labial, superior labial, and lateral nasal branches in the face.

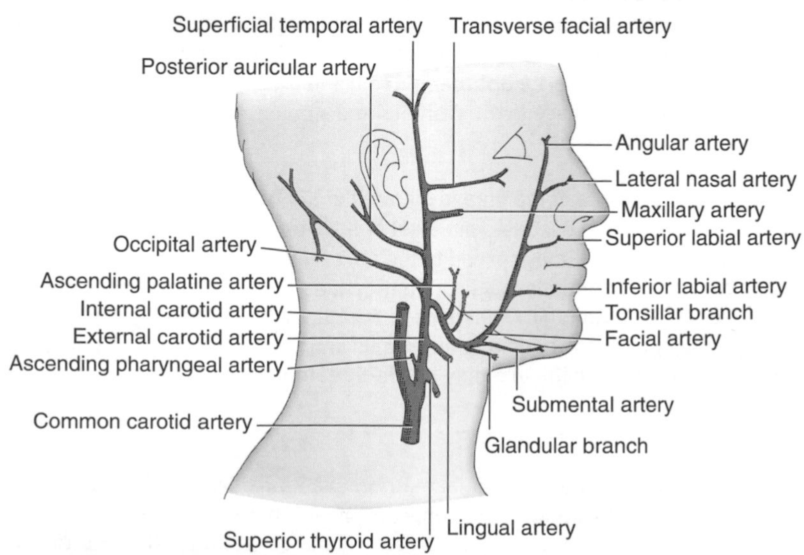

FIGURE 8.13. Blood supply to the face and scalp.

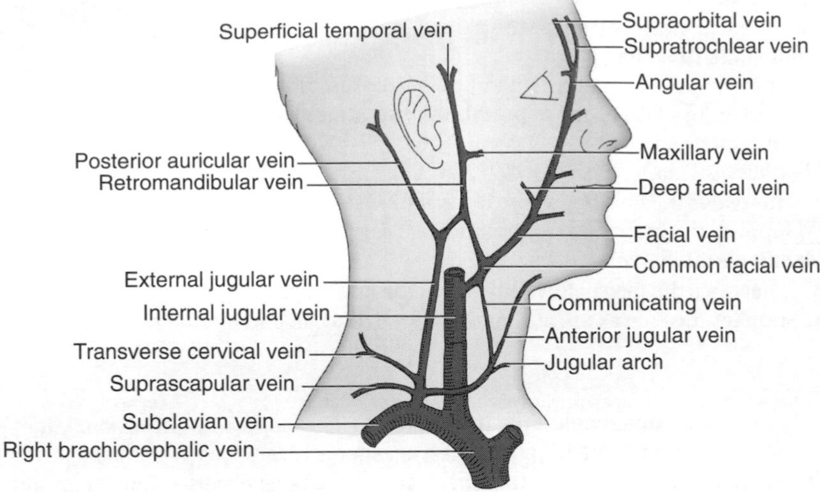

FIGURE 8.14. Veins of the head and neck.

- Terminates as an angular artery that anastomoses with the palpebral and dorsal nasal branches of the ophthalmic artery to establish communication between the external and internal carotid arteries.

B. Superficial Temporal Artery

- Arises behind the neck of the mandible as the smaller terminal branch of the external carotid artery and ascends anterior to the external acoustic meatus into the scalp.
- Accompanies the auriculotemporal nerve along its anterior surface.
- Gives rise to the **transverse facial artery**, which passes forward across the masseter between the zygomatic arch above and the parotid duct below.
- Also gives rise to zygomaticoorbital, middle temporal, anterior auricular, frontal, and parietal branches.

C. Facial Vein

- Begins as an angular vein by the confluence of the supraorbital and supratrochlear veins. The angular vein is continued at the lower margin of the orbital margin into the facial vein.
- Receives tributaries corresponding to the branches of the facial artery and also receives the **infraorbital and deep facial veins**.
- Drains either directly into the internal jugular vein or by joining the anterior branch of the retromandibular vein to form the **common facial vein**, which then enters the internal jugular vein.
- Communicates with the superior ophthalmic vein and thus with the **cavernous sinus**, allowing a route of infection from the face to the cranial dural sinus.

CLINICAL CORRELATES

Danger area of the face is the **area of the face near the nose** drained by the facial veins. Pustules (pimples) or boils or other skin infections, particularly on the side of the nose and upper lip, may spread to the cavernous venous sinus via the facial vein, pterygoid venous plexus, and ophthalmic veins. **Septicemia** (blood infection) is a systemic disease caused by the presence of pathogenic organisms or their **toxins** in the bloodstream and is often associated with severe infections, leading to meningitis and cavernous sinus thrombosis, both of which may cause neurologic damage and may be life-threatening.

D. Retromandibular Vein

- Is formed by the union of the superficial temporal and maxillary veins behind the mandible.
- Divides into an **anterior branch**, which joins the facial vein to form the common facial vein, and a **posterior branch**, which joins the posterior auricular vein to form the external jugular vein.

IV. SCALP

A. Layers (Figure 8.15)

1. Skin

- Provided with abundant hairs and contains numerous sebaceous glands.

2. Connective Tissue (Dense Subcutaneous Tissue)

- Is composed of dense connective tissue, which contains numerous blood vessels and nerves, sweat glands, and hair follicles. The arteries nourish the hair follicles and anastomose freely and are held by the dense connective tissue around them, and thus, they tend to remain open when cut, causing profuse bleeding.

3. Aponeurosis Epicranialis (Galea Aponeurotica)

- Is a **tendinous sheet** that covers the vault of the skull and unites the occipital and frontal bellies of the occipitofrontal muscles.

4. Loose Connective Tissue

- Forms the loose and scanty **subaponeurotic space** and contains the emissary veins.
- Is termed a **dangerous area** because infection (blood and pus) can spread easily in it or from the scalp to the intracranial sinuses by way of the emissary veins.

5. Pericranium

- Is the **periosteum** over the surface of the skull.

CLINICAL CORRELATES

Scalp hemorrhage results from laceration of arteries in the dense connective tissue layer that is unable to contract or retract and thus remain open, leading to profuse bleeding. **Deep scalp wounds** gape widely when the epicranial aponeurosis is lacerated in the coronal plane because of the pull of the frontal and occipital bellies of the epicranius muscle in opposite directions. **Scalp infection** localized in the loose connective tissue layer spreads across the calvaria to the intracranial dural venous sinuses through emissary veins, causing **meningitis** or **septicemia**.

B. Innervation and Blood Supply (Figure 8.16)

- Is innervated by the supratrochlear, supraorbital, zygomaticotemporal, auriculotemporal, lesser occipital, greater occipital, and third occipital nerves.
- Is supplied by the supratrochlear and supraorbital branches of the internal carotid and by the superficial temporal, posterior auricular, and occipital branches of the external carotid arteries.

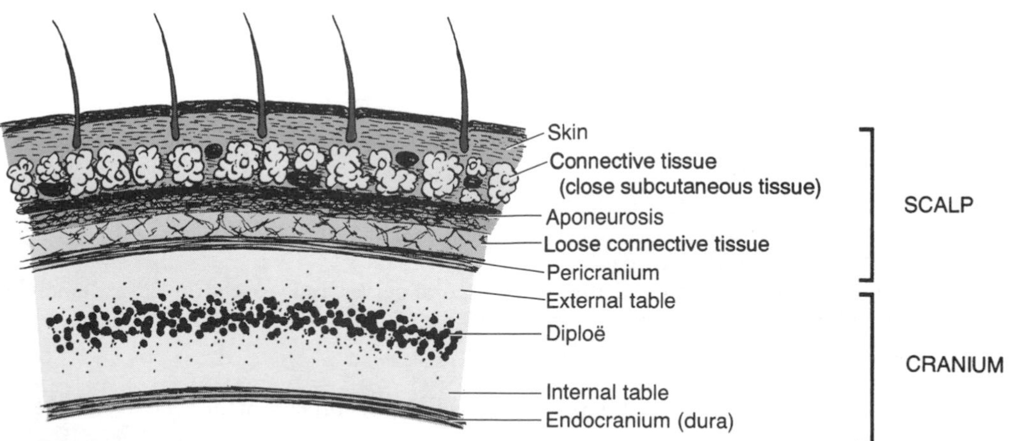

FIGURE 8.15. Layers of the scalp and cranium.

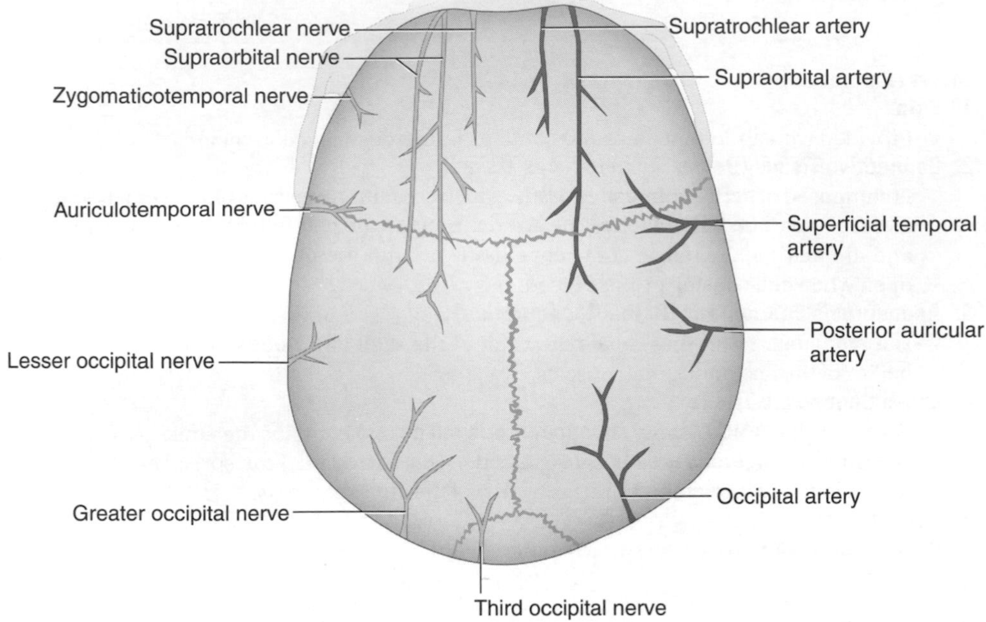

FIGURE 8.16. Nerves and arteries of the scalp.

TEMPORAL AND INFRATEMPORAL FOSSAE

I. INTRODUCTION

A. Infratemporal Fossa (Figures 8.17 to 8.18)

- Contains the lower portion of the temporalis muscle, the lateral and medial pterygoid muscles, the pterygoid plexus of veins, the mandibular nerve and its branches, the maxillary artery and its branches, the chorda tympani, and the otic ganglion.
- Has the following boundaries:
  1. **Anterior**
     - Posterior surface of the maxilla.
  2. **Posterior**
     - Styloid and mastoid processes.
  3. **Medial**
     - Lateral pterygoid plate of the sphenoid bone.
  4. **Lateral**
     - Ramus and coronoid process of the mandible.
  5. **Roof**
     - Greater wing of the sphenoid and infratemporal crest.

B. Temporal Fossa (See Figures 8.17 to 8.18)

- Contains the temporalis muscle, the deep temporal nerves and vessels, the auriculotemporal nerve, and the superficial temporal vessels.
- Has the following boundaries:
  1. **Anterior**
     - Zygomatic process of the frontal bone and the frontal process of the zygomatic bone.
  2. **Posterior**
     - Temporal line.

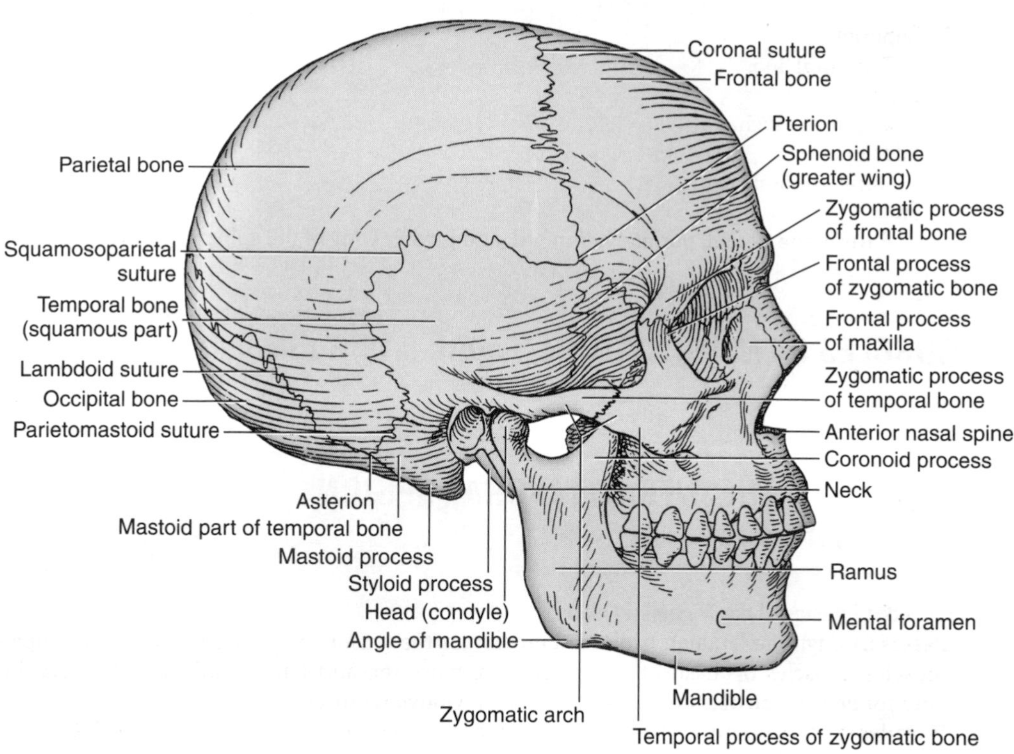

FIGURE 8.17. Lateral view of the skull.

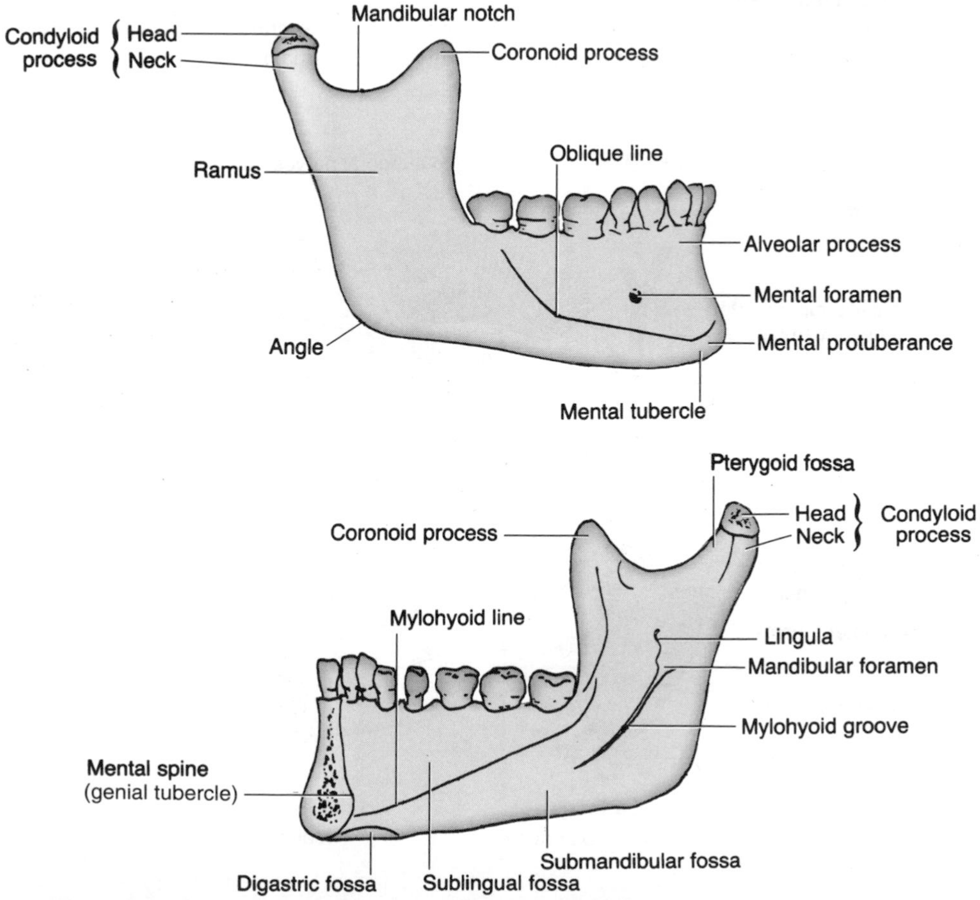

FIGURE 8.18. External (buccal) and internal (lingual) surfaces of the mandible.

3. **Superior**
   - Temporal line.
4. **Lateral**
   - Zygomatic arch.
5. **Inferior**
   - Infratemporal crest.
6. **Floor**
   - Parts of the frontal, parietal, temporal, and greater wing of the sphenoid bone.

II. MUSCLES OF MASTICATION (Figure 8.19; Table 8.4)

III. NERVES OF THE INFRATEMPORAL REGION (See Figure 8.19)

A. Mandibular Division of the Trigeminal Nerve

- Passes through the **foramen ovale** and innervates the tensor veli palatini and tensor tympani muscles, muscles of mastication (temporalis, masseter, and lateral and medial pterygoid), anterior belly of the digastric muscle, and the mylohyoid muscle.
- Provides sensory innervation to the lower **teeth** and **gum** and to the lower part of the **face** below the lower lip and the mouth.
- Gives rise to the following branches:
  1. **Meningeal Branch**
     - Accompanies the middle meningeal artery, enters the cranium through the **foramen spinosum**, and supplies the meninges of the middle cranial fossa.

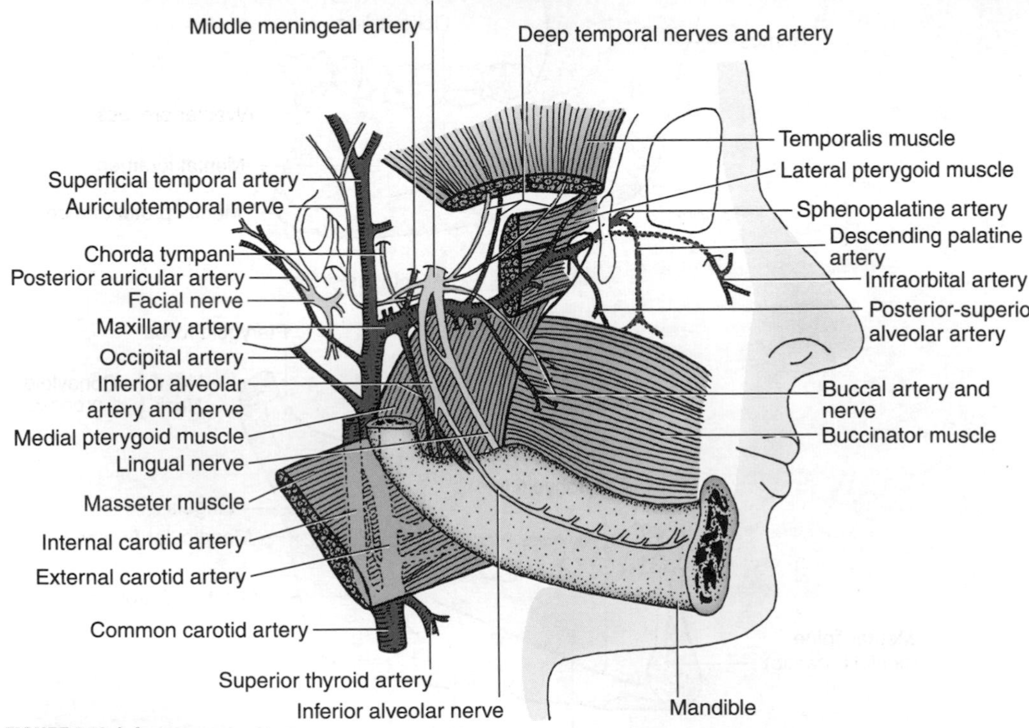

FIGURE 8.19. Infratemporal region.

table 8.4 Muscles of Mastication*

Muscle	Origin	Insertion	Nerve	Action on Mandible
Temporalis	Temporal fossa	Coronoid process and ramus of mandible	Trigeminal	Elevates; retracts
Masseter	Lower border and medial surface of zygomatic arch	Lateral surface of coronoid process, ramus and angle of mandible	Trigeminal	Elevates (superficial part); retracts (deep part)
Lateral pterygoid	Superior head from infratemporal surface of sphenoid; inferior head from lateral surface of lateral pterygoid plate of sphenoid	Neck of mandible; articular disk and capsule of temporomandibular joint	Trigeminal	Depresses (superior head); protracts (inferior head)
Medial pterygoid	Tuber of maxilla (superficial head); medial surface of lateral pterygoid plate; pyramidal process of palatine bone (deep head)	Medial surface of angle and ramus of mandible	Trigeminal	Elevates; protracts

*The jaws are opened by the lateral pterygoid muscle and are closed by the temporalis, masseter, and medial pterygoid muscles.

2. **Muscular Branches**
   - Include masseteric, deep temporal, medial, and lateral pterygoid nerves.
3. **Buccal Nerve**
   - Descends between the two heads of the lateral pterygoid muscle.
   - Innervates skin and fascia on the buccinator muscle and penetrates this muscle to supply the mucous membrane of the cheek and gums.
4. **Auriculotemporal Nerve**
   - Arises from two roots that encircle the middle meningeal artery.
   - Carries **postganglionic parasympathetic** and **sympathetic** general visceral efferent (GVE) fibers to the parotid gland and sensory general somatic afferent (GSA) fibers to the temporomandibular joint and the skin of the auricle and the scalp.

CLINICAL CORRELATES

Frey syndrome produces **flushing and sweating instead of salivation** in response to taste of food after injury of the **auriculotemporal nerve**, which carries parasympathetic secretomotor fibers to the parotid gland and sympathetic fibers to the sweat glands. When the nerve is severed, the fibers can regenerate along each other's pathways and innervate the wrong gland. It can occur after parotid surgery and may be treated by cutting the tympanic plexus in the middle ear.

5. **Lingual Nerve**
   - Descends deep to the lateral pterygoid muscle, where it joins the **chorda tympani**, which conveys the **parasympathetic preganglionic** (secretomotor) fibers to the submandibular ganglion and **taste** fibers from the anterior two-thirds of the tongue.
   - Supplies **general sensation** for the anterior two-thirds of the tongue.
   - Lies anterior to the inferior alveolar nerve on the medial pterygoid muscle, deep to the ramus of the mandible.
   - Crosses lateral to the styloglossus and hyoglossus muscles, passes deep to the mylohyoid muscle, and descends lateral to and loops under the submandibular duct.
6. **Inferior Alveolar Nerve**
   - Passes deep to the lateral pterygoid muscle and then between the sphenomandibular ligament and the ramus of the mandible.
   - Enters the mandibular canal through the mandibular foramen and supplies the tissues of the chin and lower teeth and gum.
   - Gives rise to the following branches:
     1. **Mylohyoid nerve**, which innervates the mylohyoid and the anterior belly of the digastric muscle.
     2. **Inferior dental branch**, which innervates lower teeth.

3. **Mental nerve**, which innervates the skin over the chin.
4. **Incisive branch**, which innervates the canine and incisor teeth.

B. Otic Ganglion

- Lies in the infratemporal fossa, just below the foramen ovale between the mandibular nerve and the tensor veli palatini.
- Receives preganglionic parasympathetic fibers that run in the glossopharyngeal nerve, tympanic nerve and plexus, and lesser petrosal nerve and synapse in this ganglion.
- Contains cell bodies of postganglionic parasympathetic fibers that run in the **auriculotemporal nerve** to innervate the parotid gland.

IV. BLOOD VESSELS OF THE INFRATEMPORAL REGION (FIGURE 8.19)

A. Maxillary Artery

- Arises from the external carotid artery at the posterior border of the ramus of the mandible.
- Divides into three parts:

1. Mandibular Part

- Runs anteriorly between the neck of the mandible and the sphenomandibular ligament and gives rise to the following branches:

(a) Deep Auricular Artery

- Supplies the external acoustic meatus.

(b) Anterior Tympanic Artery

- Supplies the tympanic cavity and tympanic membrane.

(c) Middle Meningeal Artery

- Is embraced by two roots of the auriculotemporal nerve, enters the middle cranial fossa through the **foramen spinosum**, and runs between the dura mater and the periosteum.

CLINICAL CORRELATES **Rupture of the middle meningeal artery** may be caused by fracture of the squamous part of the temporal bone as it runs through the foramen spinosum and just deep to the inner surface of the temporal bone. It causes **epidural hematoma** with increased intracranial pressure.

(d) Accessory Meningeal Artery

- Passes through the foramen ovale.

(e) Inferior Alveolar Artery

- Follows the inferior alveolar nerve, gives off the mylohyoid branch, and enters the mandibular canal through the mandibular foramen and supplies the tissues of the chin and lower teeth.

2. Pterygoid Part

- Runs anteriorly deep to the temporalis and superficial or deep to the lateral pterygoid muscle.
- Branches the anterior and posterior deep temporal, pterygoid, masseteric, and buccal arteries, which supply chiefly the muscles of mastication.

3. Pterygopalatine Part

- Runs between the two heads of the lateral pterygoid muscle and then through the pterygomaxillary fissure into the pterygopalatine fossa, and has the following arteries:

(a) Posterior–Superior Alveolar Arteries

- Run downward on the posterior surface of the maxilla and supply the molar and premolar teeth and the maxillary sinus.

(b) Infraorbital Artery

- Enters the orbit through the inferior orbital fissure, traverses the infraorbital groove and canal, and emerges on the face through the infraorbital foramen.
- Divides into branches to supply the lower eyelid, lacrimal sac, upper lip, and cheek.
- Gives rise to **anterior and middle superior alveolar branches** to the upper canine and incisor teeth and the maxillary sinus.

(c) Descending Palatine Artery

- Descends in the palatine canal and supplies the soft and hard palates.
- Gives rise to the **greater** and **lesser palatine arteries**, which pass through the greater and lesser palatine foramina, respectively. The lesser palatine artery supplies the soft palate. The greater palatine artery supplies the hard palate and sends a branch to anastomose with the terminal (nasopalatine) branch of the sphenopalatine artery in the incisive canal or on the nasal septum.

(d) Artery of the Pterygoid Canal

- Passes through the pterygoid canal and supplies the upper part of the pharynx, auditory tube, and tympanic cavity.

(e) Pharyngeal Artery

- Supplies the roof of the nose and pharynx, sphenoid sinus, and auditory tube.

(f) Sphenopalatine Artery

- Enters the nasal cavity through the sphenopalatine foramen in company with the nasopalatine branch of the maxillary nerve.
- Is the principal artery to the nasal cavity, supplying the conchae, meatus, and paranasal sinuses and may cause **epistaxis** (nosebleed) when damaged.

B. Pterygoid Venous Plexus (Figure 8.20)

- Lies on the lateral surface of the medial pterygoid muscle, receives veins corresponding to the branches of the maxillary artery, and drains into the maxillary vein.
- Communicates with the **cavernous sinus** by emissary veins (which pass through the foramen ovale), the **inferior ophthalmic vein** by a vein (which runs through the infraorbital fissure), and the **facial vein** by the deep facial vein.

C. Retromandibular Vein

- Is formed by the superficial temporal vein and the maxillary vein. It divides into an anterior branch, which joins the facial vein to form the common facial vein, and a posterior branch, which joins the posterior auricular vein to form the external jugular vein.

V. PAROTID GLAND

- Is the largest of the three glands and occupies the **retromandibular space** between the ramus of the mandible in front and the mastoid process and the sternocleidomastoid muscle behind.
- Is invested with a dense fibrous capsule, the parotid sheath, derived from the investing layer of the deep cervical fascia.
- Is separated from the submandibular gland by a facial extension and the **stylomandibular ligament**, which extends from the styloid process to the angle of the mandible. (Therefore, pus does not readily exchange between these two glands.)
- Has the parotid (Stensen) duct, which crosses the masseter, pierces the buccinator muscle, and opens into the vestibule of the oral cavity opposite the second upper molar tooth.
- Is innervated by parasympathetic (secretomotor) fibers of the glossopharyngeal nerve by way of the **lesser petrosal nerve**, **otic ganglion**, and **auriculotemporal nerve**.
- Secretes a copious watery saliva by parasympathetic stimulation and produces a small amount of viscous saliva by sympathetic stimulation.
- Complete surgical removal of the parotid may damage the facial nerve.

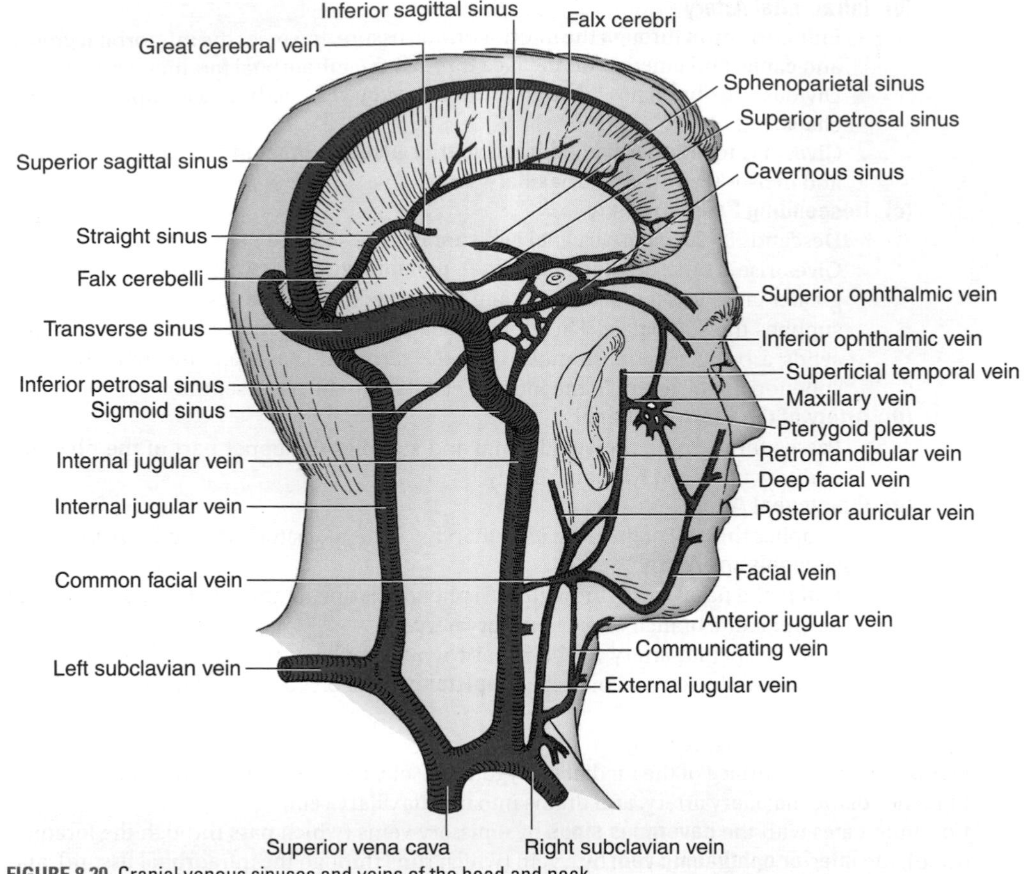

FIGURE 8.20. Cranial venous sinuses and veins of the head and neck.

CLINICAL CORRELATES

Mumps (epidemic parotitis) is a highly contagious disease caused by a **viral infection**. It can be spread to other people by breathing, coughing, kissing, sneezing, and talking. It irritates the auriculotemporal nerve, causing severe pain because of **inflammation** and **swelling of the parotid gland** and **stretching of its capsule**, and pain is exacerbated by compression from swallowing or chewing. Other symptoms include chills, headache, fever, and sore throat. It may be accompanied by meningitis, encephalitis, and inflammation and swelling of the testes (orchitis) or ovaries, causing **sterility** if it occurs after puberty.

VI. JOINTS AND LIGAMENTS OF THE INFRATEMPORAL REGION

A. Temporomandibular Joint

- Is a combined **gliding** and **hinge** type of the **synovial joint** (ginglymoid-diarthrodial compound synovial joint) and has **two** (superior and inferior) **synovial cavities** divided by an **articular disk**, which is a **dense fibrous tissue**. Its articular surfaces of the bones are covered by **fibrocartilage**.
- Consists of an upper **gliding joint** between the articular tubercle and mandibular fossa above and the articular disk below where forward gliding or **protrusion** and backward gliding or **retraction** (translation by dentists) take place, and a lower **hinge joint** between the disk and the mandibular head (condyle) where elevation or **closing** and depression or **opening** of the jaw take place. During yawning, the disk and the head of the mandible glide across the articular tubercle.

- Has an **articular capsule** that extends from the articular tubercle and the margins of the mandibular fossa to the neck of the mandible.
- Is reinforced by the **lateral** (temporomandibular) **ligament**, which extends from the tubercle on the zygoma to the neck of the mandible, and the **sphenomandibular ligament**, which extends from the spine of the sphenoid bone to the lingula of the mandible.
- Is innervated by the **auriculotemporal** and **masseteric** branches of the mandibular nerve.
- Is supplied by the superficial temporal, maxillary (middle meningeal and anterior tympanic branches), and ascending pharyngeal arteries.

CLINICAL CORRELATES **Dislocation of the temporomandibular joint** occurs anteriorly as the mandible head glides across the articular tubercle during yawning and laughing. A blow to the chin with the mouth closed may drive the head of the mandible posteriorly and superiorly, causing fracture of the bony auditory canal and the floor of the middle cranial fossa.

B. Pterygomandibular Raphe

- Is a **ligamentous band** (or a tendinous inscription) between the buccinator muscle and the superior pharyngeal constrictor.
- Extends between the pterygoid hamulus superiorly and the posterior end of the mylohyoid line of the mandible inferiorly.

C. Stylomandibular Ligament

- Extends from the styloid process to the posterior border of the ramus of the mandible, near the angle of the mandible, separating the parotid from the submandibular gland.

SKULL AND CRANIAL CAVITY

I. SKULL (Figures 8.17, 8.21, and 8.22)

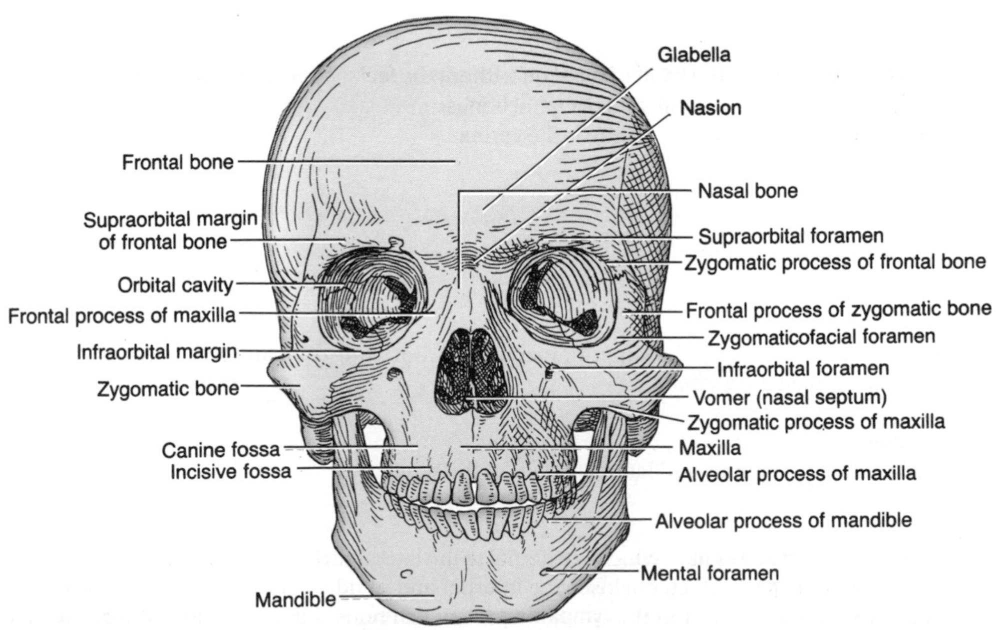

FIGURE 8.21. Anterior view of the skull.

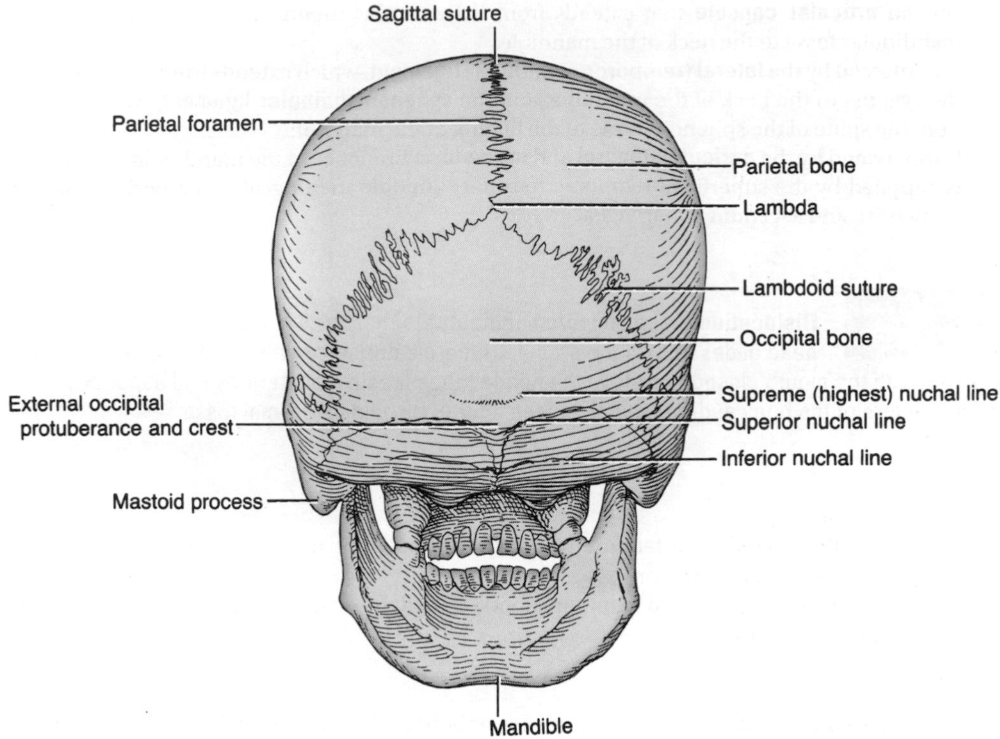

FIGURE 8.22. Posterior view of the skull.

- Is the skeleton of the head and may be divided into two types of bones: 8 **cranial bones** for enclosing the brain (unpaired frontal, occipital, ethmoid, and sphenoid bones and paired parietal and temporal bones), which **can be seen in the cranial cavity**, and 14 **facial bones** (paired lacrimal, nasal, palatine, inferior turbinate, maxillary, and zygomatic bones and unpaired vomer and mandible).

A. Cranium

- Is sometimes restricted to the skull without the mandible.

B. Calvaria

- Is the **skullcap**, which is the vault of the skull without the facial bones. It consists of the superior portions of the frontal, parietal, and occipital bones.
- Its highest point on the sagittal suture is the **vertex**.

II. BONES OF THE CRANIUM

A. Frontal Bone

- Underlies the forehead and the superior margin and roof of the orbit and has a smooth median prominence called the **glabella**.

B. Parietal Bone

- Forms part of the superior and lateral surface of the skull.

C. Temporal Bone

- Consists of the **squamous part**, which is external to the lateral surface of the temporal lobe of the brain; the **petrous part**, which encloses the internal and middle ears; the **mastoid part**, which contains mastoid air cells; and the **tympanic part**, which houses the external auditory meatus and the tympanic cavity.

D. Occipital Bone

- Consists of **squamous, basilar**, and **two lateral condylar parts.**
- Encloses the foramen magnum and forms the cerebral and cerebellar fossae.

E. Sphenoid Bone

- Consists of the body (which houses the sphenoid sinus), the greater and lesser wings, and the **pterygoid process**.

F. Ethmoid Bone

- Is located between the orbits and consists of the **cribriform plate, perpendicular plate**, and two lateral masses enclosing ethmoid air cells.

III. SUTURES OF THE SKULL

- Are the immovable fibrous joints between the bones of the skull.

A. Coronal Suture

- Lies between the frontal bone and the two parietal bones.

B. Sagittal Suture

- Lies between the two parietal bones.

C. Squamous (Squamoparietal) Suture

- Lies between the parietal bone and the squamous part of the temporal bone.

D. Lambdoid Suture

- Lies between the two parietal bones and the occipital bone.

E. Junctions of the Cranial Sutures

1. **Lambda**
   - Intersection of the lambdoid and sagittal sutures.
2. **Bregma**
   - Intersection of the sagittal and coronal sutures.
3. **Pterion**
   - A craniometric point at the junction of the frontal, parietal, and temporal bones and the great wing of the sphenoid bone.
4. **Asterion**
   - A craniometric point at the junction of the parietal, occipital, and temporal (mastoid part) bones.
5. **Nasion**
   - A point on the middle of the nasofrontal suture (intersection of the frontal and two nasal bones).
6. **Inion**
   - Most prominent point of the external occipital protuberance, which is used as a fixed point in craniometry.

CLINICAL CORRELATES

Skull fracture: Fracture at the **pterion** may rupture the middle meningeal artery, and a depressed fracture may compress the underlying brain. A fracture of the petrous portion of the **temporal bone** may cause blood or cerebrospinal fluid (CSF) to escape from the ear, hearing loss, and facial nerve damage. Fracture of the **anterior cranial fossa** causes anosmia, periorbital bruising (raccoon eyes), and CSF leakage from the nose (rhinorrhea). A blow to the top of the head may fracture the skull base with related cranial nerve (CN) injury, CSF leakage from a dura–arachnoid tear, and dural sinus thrombosis. **Tripod fracture** is a facial fracture involving the three supports of the malar (cheek or zygomatic) bone, including the zygomatic processes of the temporal, frontal, and maxillary bones.

IV. FORAMINA IN THE SKULL (Figures 8.23 to 8.24)

- Include the following, which are presented here with the structures that pass through them:

A. Anterior Cranial Fossa

1. Cribriform plate

- Olfactory nerves.

2. Foramen cecum

- Occasional small emissary vein from nasal mucosa to superior sagittal sinus.

3. Anterior and posterior ethmoidal foramina

- Anterior and posterior ethmoidal nerves, arteries, and veins.

B. Middle Cranial Fossa

1. Optic canal

- Optic nerve, ophthalmic artery, and central artery and vein of the retina.

2. Superior orbital fissure

- Oculomotor, trochlear, and abducens nerves; ophthalmic division of trigeminal nerve; and ophthalmic veins.

3. Foramen rotundum

- Maxillary division of trigeminal nerve.

4. Foramen ovale

- Mandibular division of trigeminal nerve, accessory meningeal artery, and occasionally lesser petrosal nerve.

5. Foramen spinosum

- Middle meningeal artery.

6. Foramen lacerum

- Nothing passes through this foramen, but the upper part is traversed by the internal carotid artery and greater and deep petrosal nerves en route to the pterygoid canal.

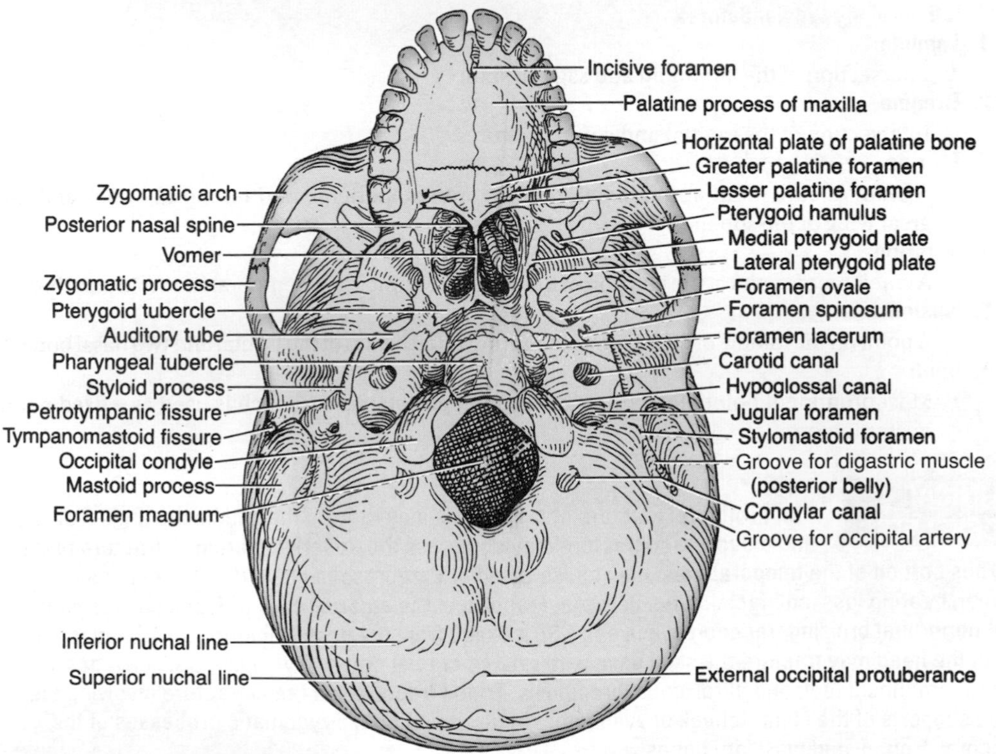

FIGURE 8.23. Base of the skull.

7. **Carotid canal**
   - Internal carotid artery and sympathetic nerves (carotid plexus).
8. **Hiatus of facial canal**
   - Greater petrosal nerve.

C. Posterior Cranial Fossa

1. **Internal auditory meatus**
   - Facial and vestibulocochlear nerves and labyrinthine artery.
2. **Jugular foramen**
   - Glossopharyngeal, vagus, and spinal accessory nerves and beginning of internal jugular vein.
3. **Hypoglossal canal**
   - Hypoglossal nerve and meningeal artery.
4. **Foramen magnum**
   - Spinal cord, spinal accessory nerve, vertebral arteries, venous plexus of vertebral canal, and anterior and posterior spinal arteries.
5. **Condyloid foramen**
   - Condyloid emissary vein.
6. **Mastoid foramen**
   - Branch of occipital artery to dura mater and mastoid emissary vein.

D. Foramina in the Front of the Skull (Figure 8.21)

1. **Zygomaticofacial foramen**
   - Zygomaticofacial nerve.
2. **Supraorbital notch or foramen**
   - Supraorbital nerve and vessels.
3. **Infraorbital foramen**
   - Infraorbital nerve and vessels.
4. **Mental foramen**
   - Mental nerve and vessels.

E. Foramina in the Base of the Skull (Figure 8.23)

1. **Petrotympanic fissure**
   - Chorda tympani and often anterior tympanic artery.
2. **Stylomastoid foramen**
   - Facial nerve.

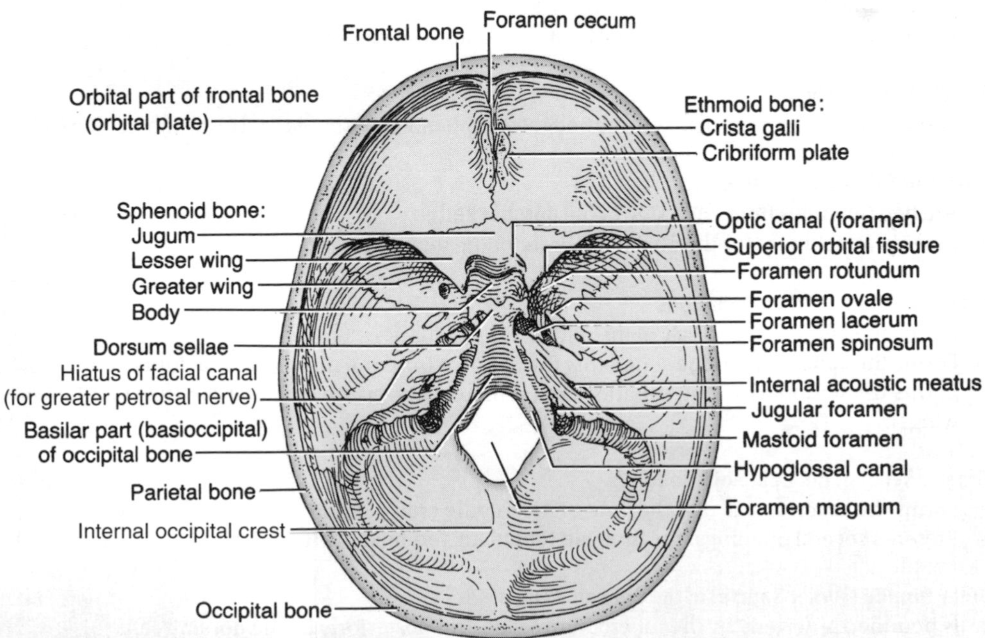

FIGURE 8.24. Interior of the base of the skull.

3. **Incisive canal**
   - Nasopalatine nerve and terminal part of the sphenopalatine or greater palatine vessels.
4. **Greater palatine foramen**
   - Greater palatine nerve and vessels.
5. **Lesser palatine foramen**
   - Lesser palatine nerve and vessels.
6. **Palatine canal**
   - Descending palatine vessels and the greater and lesser palatine nerves.
7. **Pterygoid canal**
   - Runs from the anterior wall of the foramen lacerum to the pterygopalatine fossa and transmits the nerve of the pterygoid canal (vidian nerve).
8. **Sphenopalatine foramen**
   - Sphenopalatine vessels and nasopalatine nerve.

V. STRUCTURES IN THE CRANIAL FOSSAE (Figure 8.24)

A. Foramen Cecum

- Is a small pit in front of the crista galli between the ethmoid and frontal bones.
- May transmit an emissary vein from the nasal mucosa and the frontal sinus to the superior sagittal sinus.

B. Crista Galli

- Is the triangular midline process of the ethmoid bone extending upward from the cribriform plate.
- Provides attachment for the **falx cerebri**.

C. Cribriform Plate of the Ethmoid Bone

- Is perforated by 15 to 20 foramina, supports the olfactory bulb, and transmits olfactory nerves from the olfactory mucosa to the olfactory bulb.

D. Anterior Clinoid Processes

- Are two anterior processes of the lesser wing of the sphenoid bone, which are located in the middle cranial fossa.
- Provide attachment for the free border of the tentorium cerebelli.

E. Middle Clinoid Process

- Is a small inconstant eminence on the body of the sphenoid, posterolateral to the tuberculum sellae.

F. Posterior Clinoid Processes

- Are two tubercles from each side of the **dorsum sellae**.
- Provide attachment for the attached border of the tentorium cerebelli.

G. Lesser Wing of the Sphenoid Bone

- Forms the anterior boundary of the middle cranial fossa.
- Forms the **sphenoidal ridge** separating the anterior from the middle cranial fossa.
- Forms the boundary of the superior orbital fissure (the space between the lesser and greater wings).

H. Greater Wing of the Sphenoid Bone

- Forms the anterior wall and the floor of the middle cranial fossa.
- Presents several openings: the **foramen rotundum**, **foramen ovale**, and **foramen spinosum**.

I. Sella Turcica (Turk's Saddle) of the Sphenoid Bone

- Is bounded anteriorly by the tuberculum sellae and posteriorly by the dorsum sellae.

- Has a deep central depression known as the **hypophyseal fossa**, which accommodates the pituitary gland or the hypophysis.
- Lies directly above the sphenoid sinus located within the body of the sphenoid bone; its dural roof is formed by the **diaphragma sellae**.

J. Jugum Sphenoidale

- Is a portion of the body of the sphenoid bone connecting the two lesser wings and forms the roof for the **sphenoidal air sinus**.

K. Clivus

- Is the downward sloping surface from the dorsum sellae to the foramen magnum.
- Is formed by a part of the body of the **sphenoid** and a portion of the basilar part of the occipital bone.

VI. MENINGES OF THE BRAIN (Figure 8.25)

A. Pia Mater

- Is a delicate investment that is closely applied to the brain and dips into fissures and sulci.
- Enmeshes blood vessels on the surfaces of the brain.

CLINICAL CORRELATES **Pial hemorrhage** is due to damage to the small vessels of the pia and brain tissue. **Cerebral hemorrhage** is caused by rupture of the thin-walled lenticulostriate artery, a branch of the middle cerebral artery, producing hemiplegia (paralysis of one side of the body).

B. Arachnoid Layer

- Is a filmy, transparent, spidery layer that is connected to the pia mater by weblike trabeculations.
- Is separated from the pia mater by the **subarachnoid space**, which is filled with CSF.
- May contain blood after hemorrhage of a cerebral artery.
- Projects into the venous sinuses to form **arachnoid villi**, which serve as sites where CSF diffuses into the venous blood.

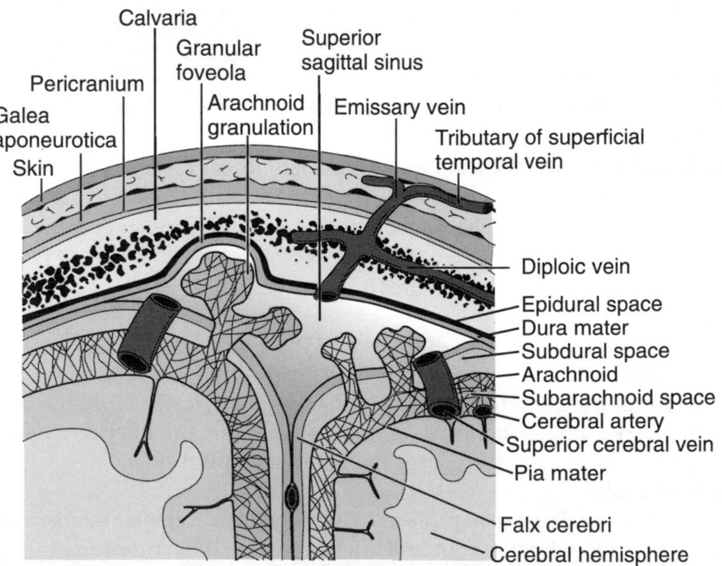

FIGURE 8.25. Scalp, calvaria, meninges, and dural venous sinuses.

1. **Cerebrospinal Fluid**
   - Is formed by **vascular choroid plexuses** in the ventricles of the brain and is contained in the subarachnoid space.
   - Circulates through the ventricles, enters the subarachnoid space, and eventually filters into the venous system.
2. **Arachnoid Granulations**
   - Are tuftlike collections of highly folded arachnoid (aggregations of arachnoid villi) that project into the superior sagittal sinus and the lateral lacunae, which are lateral extensions of the superior sagittal sinus.
   - Absorb CSF into the dural sinuses and often produce erosion or pitting of the inner surface of the calvaria, forming the **granular pit**.

CLINICAL CORRELATES

Subarachnoid hemorrhage is due to rupture of cerebral arteries and veins that cross the subarachnoid space. It may be caused by rupture of an aneurysm on the circle of Willis or, less commonly, by a hemangioma (proliferation of blood vessels leads to a mass that resembles a neoplasm).

C. Dura Mater
- Is the tough, fibrous, outermost layer of the meninges external to the **subdural space**, the space between the arachnoid and the dura.
- Lies internal to the **epidural space**, a potential space that contains the middle meningeal arteries in the cranial cavity.
- Forms the **dural venous sinuses**, spaces between the periosteal and meningeal layers or between duplications of the meningeal layers.
- **Subdural hematoma** is due to rupture of bridging cerebral veins as they pass from the brain surface into the venous sinuses that result from a blow on the front or the back of the head, causing displacement of the brain.

CLINICAL CORRELATES

Epidural hematoma is due to rupture of the middle meningeal arteries or veins caused by trauma near the pterion, fracture of the greater wing of the sphenoid, or a torn dural venous sinus. An epidural hematoma may put pressure on the brain and form a biconvex pattern on computed tomography (CT) scan or magnetic resonance imaging (MRI).

3. **Innervation of the Dura Mater**
   - **Anterior and posterior ethmoidal branches** of the ophthalmic division of the trigeminal nerve in the anterior cranial fossa.
   - **Meningeal branches of the maxillary** and mandibular divisions of the trigeminal nerve in the middle cranial fossa.
   - **Meningeal branches of the vagus** and hypoglossal (originate from C1) nerves in the posterior cranial fossa.
4. **Projections of the Dura Mater** (Figures 8.20 and 8.25)
   - **(a) Falx Cerebri**
     - Is the sickle-shaped double layer of the dura mater, lying between the cerebral hemispheres.
     - Is attached anteriorly to the crista galli and posteriorly to the tentorium cerebelli.
     - Has a free inferior concave border that contains the **inferior sagittal sinus**, and its upper convex margin encloses the **superior sagittal sinus**.
   - **(b) Falx Cerebelli**
     - Is a small sickle-shaped projection between the cerebellar hemispheres.
     - Is attached to the posterior and inferior parts of the tentorium.
     - Contains the **occipital sinus** in its posterior border.

(c) Tentorium Cerebelli

- Is a crescentic fold of dura mater that supports the occipital lobes of the cerebral hemispheres and covers the cerebellum.
- Has a free internal concave border, which bounds the **tentorial notch**, whereas its external convex border encloses the **transverse sinus** posteriorly and the **superior petrosal sinus** anteriorly. The free border is anchored to the anterior clinoid process, whereas the attached border is attached to the posterior clinoid process.

(d) Diaphragma Sellae

- Is a circular, horizontal fold of dura that forms the roof of the sella turcica, covering the pituitary gland or the hypophysis.
- Has a central aperture for the hypophyseal stalk or infundibulum.

VII. CRANIAL VENOUS CHANNELS (Figures 8.20 and 8.26)

A. Superior Sagittal Sinus

- Lies in the midline along the convex border of the falx cerebri.
- Begins at the crista galli and receives the cerebral, diploic meningeal, and parietal emissary veins.

B. Inferior Sagittal Sinus

- Lies in the free edge of the falx cerebri and is joined by the **great cerebral vein of Galen** to form the straight sinus.

C. Straight Sinus

- Runs along the line of attachment of the falx cerebri to the tentorium cerebelli.
- Is formed by union of the inferior sagittal sinus and the great vein of Galen.

D. Transverse Sinus

- Runs laterally from the confluence of sinuses along the edge of the tentorium cerebelli.

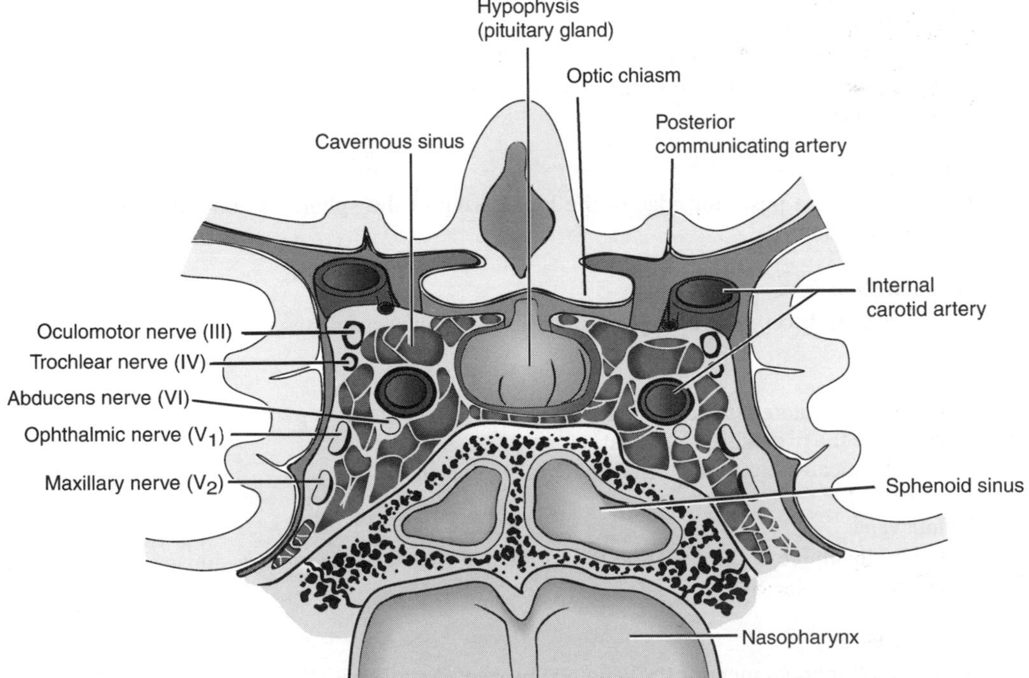

FIGURE 8.26. Frontal section through the cavernous sinus.

E. Sigmoid Sinus

- Is a continuation of the transverse sinus; arches downward and medially in an **S-shaped** groove on the mastoid part of the temporal bone.
- Enters the superior bulb of the internal jugular vein.

F. Cavernous Sinuses

- Are located on each side of the sella turcica and the body of the sphenoid bone and lie between the meningeal and periosteal layers of the dura mater.
- The internal carotid artery and the abducens nerve pass through these sinuses. In addition, the oculomotor, trochlear, ophthalmic, and maxillary nerves pass forward in the lateral wall of these sinuses.
- Communicate with the pterygoid venous plexus by emissary veins and receive the superior ophthalmic vein.

CLINICAL CORRELATES

Cavernous sinus thrombosis is the formation of blood clot within the cavernous sinus and is caused by bacterial infections induced commonly by *Staphylococcus*. The common cause is usually from a spreading infection in the nose, sinuses, ears, or teeth. Cavernous sinus thrombosis may produce headache, **papilledema** (edema of the optic disk or nerve due to increased intracranial pressure), **exophthalmos** or proptosis (protrusion of the eyeball), **diplopia** (double vision), **vision loss** (due to damage of the optic nerve or central artery and vein of the retina), **ophthalmoplegia** (paralysis of the eye movement muscles), chemosis (swelling of the conjunctivae), **sluggish pupillary responses** (due to damage of sympathetic and parasympathetic nerves), **meningitis,**and paralysis of the CNs that course through the cavernous sinus. It can be treated with high-dose antibiotics, and sometimes surgery is needed to drain the infected sinuses. Corticosteroids used as adjunctive therapy may reduce edema and inflammation.

G. Superior Petrosal Sinus

- Lies in the margin of the tentorium cerebelli, running from the posterior end of the cavernous sinus to the transverse sinus.

H. Inferior Petrosal Sinus

- Drains the cavernous sinus into the bulb of the internal jugular vein.
- Runs in a groove between the petrous part of the temporal bone and the basilar part of the occipital bone.

I. Sphenoparietal Sinus

- Lies along the posterior edge of the lesser wing of the sphenoid bone and drains into the cavernous sinus.

J. Occipital Sinus

- Lies in the falx cerebelli and drains into the confluence of sinuses.

K. Basilar Plexus

- Consists of interconnecting venous channels on the basilar part of the occipital bone and connects the two inferior petrosal sinuses.
- Communicates with the internal vertebral venous plexus.

L. Diploic Veins

- Lie in the **diploë** of the skull and are connected with the cranial dura sinuses by the emissary veins.

M. Emissary Veins

- Are small veins connecting the venous sinuses of the dura with the diploic veins and the veins of the scalp.

VIII. BLOOD SUPPLY OF THE BRAIN (Figure 8.27)

A. Internal Carotid Artery

- Enters the carotid canal in the petrous portion of the temporal bone.
- Is separated from the tympanic cavity by a thin bony structure.
- Lies within the cavernous sinus and gives rise to small twigs to the wall of the cavernous sinus, to the hypophysis, and to the semilunar ganglion of the trigeminal nerve.
- Pierces the dural roof of the cavernous sinus between the anterior clinoid process and the middle clinoid process, which is a small projection posterolateral to the tuberculum sellae.
- Forms a carotid **siphon** (a bent tube with two arms of unequal length), which is the petrosal part just before it enters the cranial cavity.

1. Ophthalmic Artery

- Enters the orbit via the optic canal with the optic nerve.

2. Posterior Communicating Artery

- Arises from the carotid siphon and joins the posterior cerebral artery.
- Runs backward below the optic tract and supplies the optic chiasma and tract and hypothalamus.

3. Anterior Choroidal Artery

- Supplies the choroid plexus of the lateral ventricles, optic tract and radiations, and lateral geniculate body.

4. Anterior Cerebral Artery

- Enters the longitudinal fissure of the cerebrum, supplies the optic chiasma and medial surface of the frontal and parietal lobes of the brain, and unites each by the short anterior communicating artery.

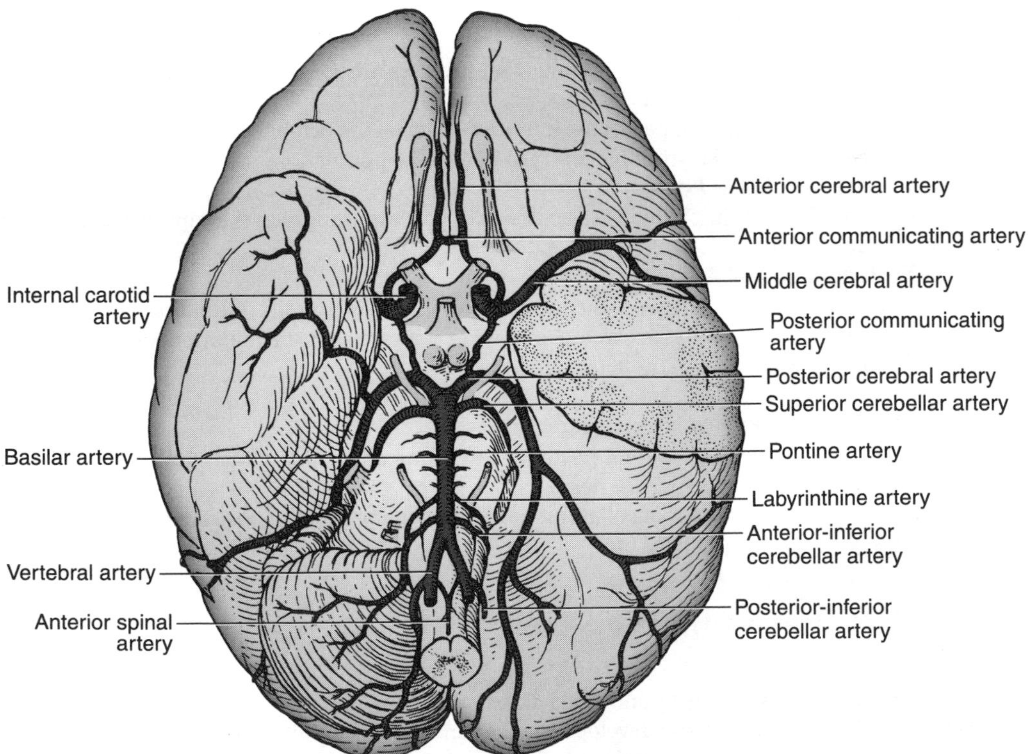

FIGURE 8.27. Arterial circle on the inferior surface of the brain.

5. **Middle Cerebral Artery**
   - Passes laterally in the lateral cerebral fissure and supplies the lateral convexity of the cerebral hemisphere.

B. Vertebral Arteries

- Arise from the first part of the subclavian artery and ascend through the transverse foramina of the vertebrae C1 to C6.
- Curve posteriorly behind the lateral mass of the atlas, pierce the dura mater into the vertebral canal, and then enter the cranial cavity through the foramen magnum.
- Join to form the **basilar artery**.
- Give rise to the following:

1. **Anterior Spinal Artery**
   - Arises as two roots from the vertebral arteries shortly before the junction of the vertebral arteries.
   - Descends in front of the medulla, and the two roots unite to form a single median trunk at the level of the foramen magnum.
2. **Posterior Spinal Artery**
   - Arises from the vertebral artery or the posterior–inferior cerebellar artery.
   - Descends on the side of the medulla, and the right and left roots unite at the lower cervical region.
3. **Posterior–Inferior Cerebellar Artery**
   - Is the largest branch of the vertebral artery, distributes to the posterior–inferior surface of the cerebellum, and gives rise to the posterior spinal artery.

C. Basilar Artery

- Is formed by the union of the two vertebral arteries at the lower border of the pons.
- Ends near the upper border of the pons by dividing into the right and left posterior cerebral arteries.

1. **Pontine Arteries**
   - Are several in number and supply the pons.
2. **Labyrinthine Artery**
   - Enters the internal auditory meatus and supplies the cochlea and vestibular apparatus.
3. **Anterior–Inferior Cerebellar Artery**
   - Supplies the anterior part of the inferior surface of the cerebellum.
   - Gives rise to the labyrinthine artery in 85% of the population.
4. **Superior Cerebellar Artery**
   - Passes laterally just behind the oculomotor nerve and supplies the superior surface of the cerebellum.
5. **Posterior Cerebral Artery**
   - Is formed by bifurcation of the basilar artery, passes laterally in front of the oculomotor nerve, winds around the cerebral peduncle, and supplies the midbrain and the temporal and occipital lobes of the cerebrum.

D. Circle of Willis (Circulus Arteriosus) (Figure 8.28)

- Is formed by the posterior cerebral, posterior communicating, internal carotid, anterior cerebral, and anterior communicating arteries.
- Forms an important means of **collateral circulation** in the event of obstruction.

IX. DEVELOPMENT OF THE SKULL

- **Cranial base** develops mainly by endochondral ossification.
- **Cranial vault** and facial skeleton develop by intramembranous ossification.
- **Sutures** are important sites of growth and allow bones to overlap (molding) during birth.

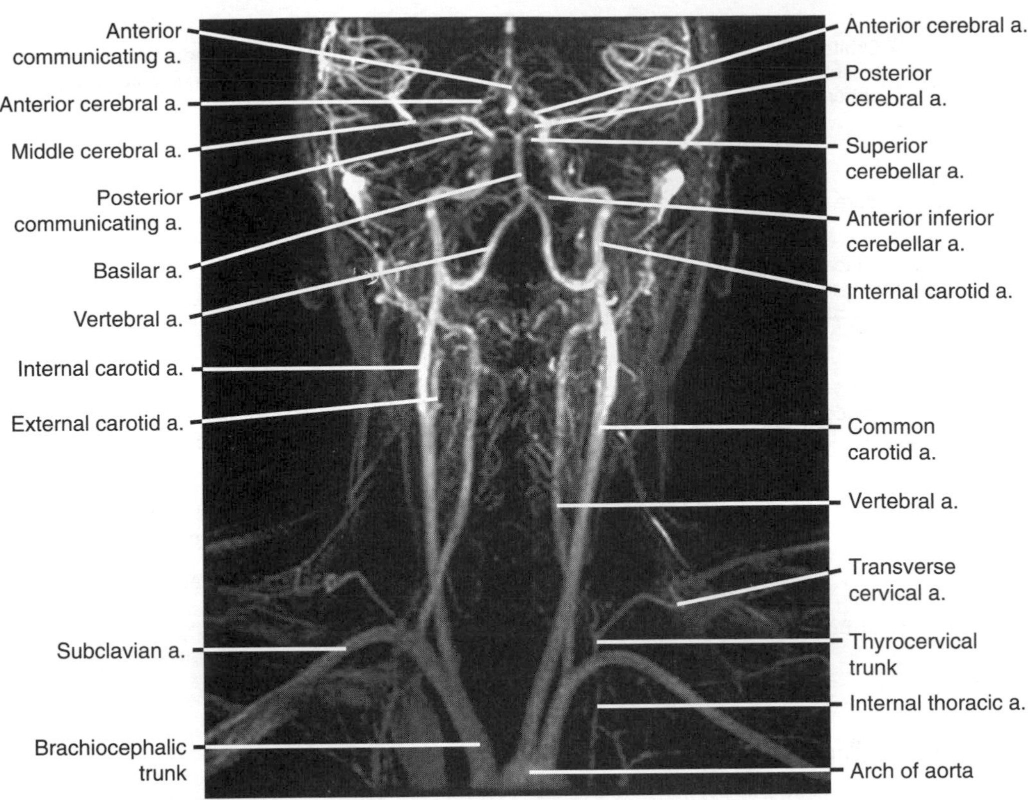

FIGURE 8.28. Formation of the circle of Willis.

NERVES OF THE HEAD AND NECK

I. CRANIAL AND AUTONOMIC NERVES (See Chapter 9)

II. AUTONOMIC NERVES (See Chapter 9)

ORBIT

I. BONY ORBIT (Figure 8.29)

A. Orbital Margin

- Is formed by the frontal, maxillary, and zygomatic bones.

B. Walls of the Orbit

1. Superior Wall or Roof

- Orbital part of frontal bone and lesser wing of sphenoid bone.

2. Lateral Wall

- Zygomatic bone (frontal process) and greater wing of sphenoid bone.

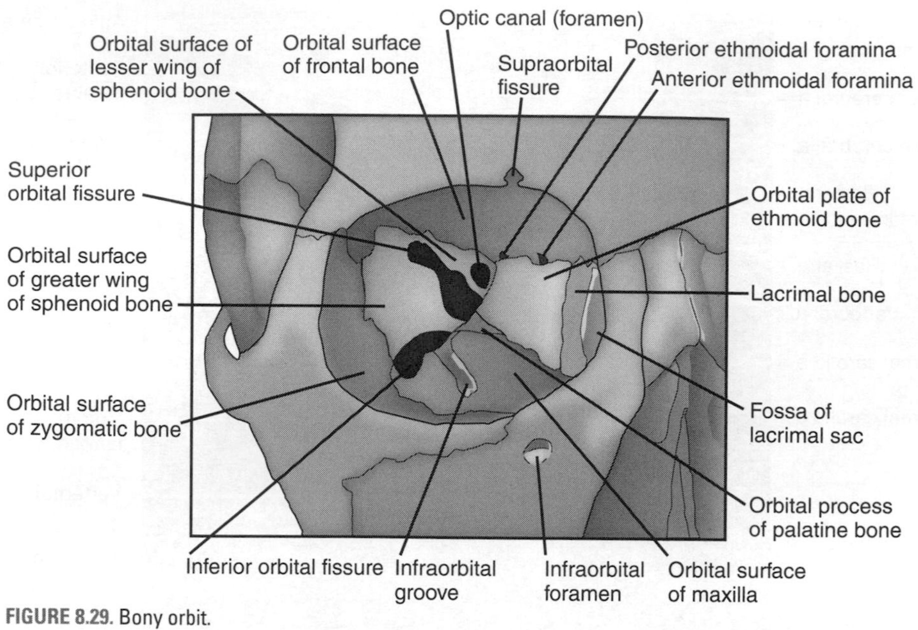

FIGURE 8.29. Bony orbit.

3. **Inferior Wall or Floor**
   - Maxilla (orbital surface), zygomatic, and palatine bones.
4. **Medial Wall**
   - Ethmoid (orbital plate), frontal, lacrimal, and sphenoid (body) bones.

C. Fissures, Canals, and Foramina

1. **Superior Orbital Fissure**
   - Communicates with the middle cranial fossa and is bounded by the greater and lesser wings of the sphenoid.
   - Transmits the oculomotor, trochlear, abducens, and ophthalmic nerves (three branches) and the ophthalmic veins.
2. **Inferior Orbital Fissure**
   - Communicates with the infratemporal and pterygopalatine fossae.
   - Is bounded by the greater wing of the sphenoid (above) and the maxillary and palatine bones (below). It is bridged by the orbitalis (smooth) muscle.
   - Transmits the maxillary (or infraorbital) nerve and its zygomatic branch and the infraorbital vessels.
3. **Optic Canal**
   - Connects the orbit with the middle cranial fossa.
   - Is formed by the two roots of the lesser wing of the sphenoid, lies in the posterior part of the roof of the orbit, and transmits the optic nerve and ophthalmic artery.
4. **Infraorbital Groove and Infraorbital Foramen**
   - Transmit the infraorbital nerve and vessels.
5. **Supraorbital Notch or Foramen**
   - Transmits the supraorbital nerve and vessels.
6. **Anterior and Posterior Ethmoidal Foramina**
   - Transmit the anterior and posterior ethmoidal nerves and vessels, respectively.
7. **Nasolacrimal Canal**
   - Is formed by the maxilla, lacrimal bone, and inferior nasal concha.
   - Transmits the nasolacrimal duct from the lacrimal sac to the inferior nasal meatus.

CLINICAL CORRELATES **Fracture of the orbital floor** involving the maxillary sinus commonly occurs as a result of a blunt force to the face. This fracture causes displacement of the eyeball, causing symptoms of **double vision** (diplopia), and also causes an injury to the infraorbital nerve, producing loss of sensation of the skin of the cheek and the gum. This fracture may cause entrapment of the inferior rectus muscle, which may limit upward gaze.

II. NERVES (Figures 8.30 to 8.32)

A. Ophthalmic Nerve

- Enters the orbit through the superior orbital fissure and divides into three branches:

1. Lacrimal Nerve

- Enters the orbit through the superior orbital fissure.
- Enters the lacrimal gland, giving rise to branches to the lacrimal gland, the conjunctiva, and the skin of the upper eyelid.
- Its terminal part is joined by the zygomaticotemporal nerve that carries postganglionic parasympathetic and sympathetic GVE fibers.

2. Frontal Nerve

- Enters the orbit through the superior orbital fissure.
- Runs superior to the levator palpebrae superioris.
- Divides into the **supraorbital nerve**, which passes through the supraorbital **notch or foramen** and supplies the scalp, forehead, frontal sinus, and upper eyelid, and the **supratrochlear nerve**, which passes through the trochlea and supplies the scalp, forehead, and upper eyelid.

3. Nasociliary Nerve

- Is the sensory nerve for the eye and mediates the afferent limb of the corneal reflex.
- Enters the orbit through the superior orbital fissure, within the common tendinous ring.
- Gives rise to the following:
  1. **A communicating branch** to the ciliary ganglion.
  2. **Short ciliary nerves**, which carry postganglionic parasympathetic fibers to the ciliary muscle and sphincter pupillae and postganglionic sympathetic fibers to the dilator pupillae, and afferent fibers from the iris and cornea.

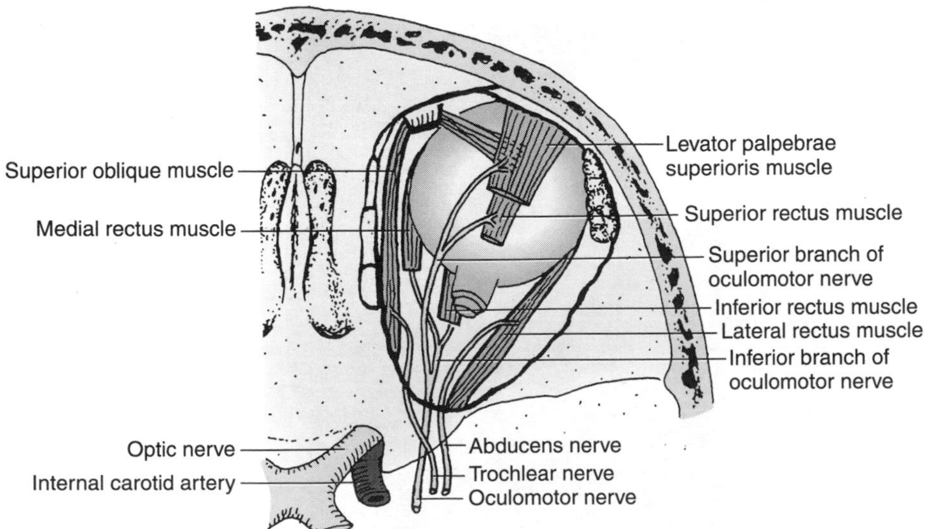

FIGURE 8.30. Motor nerves of the orbit.

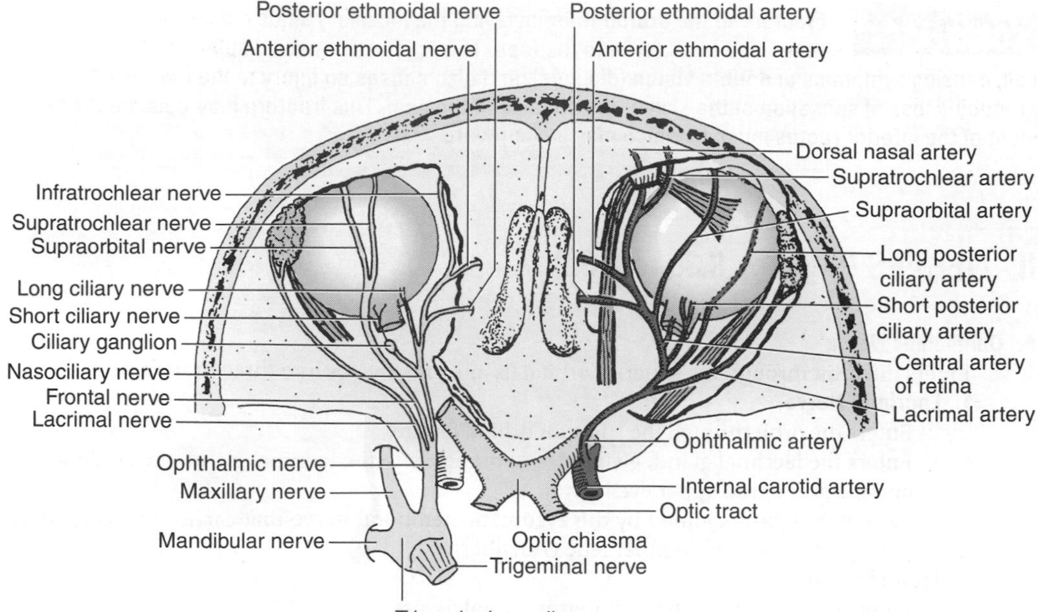

FIGURE 8.31. Branches of the ophthalmic nerve and ophthalmic artery.

3. **Long ciliary nerves**, which transmit postganglionic sympathetic fibers to the dilator pupillae and afferent fibers from the iris and cornea.
4. **The posterior ethmoidal nerve**, which passes through the posterior ethmoidal foramen to the sphenoidal and posterior ethmoidal sinuses.
5. **The anterior ethmoidal nerve**, which passes through the anterior ethmoidal foramen to supply the anterior ethmoidal air cells. It divides into **internal nasal branches**, which supply the septum and lateral walls of the nasal cavity, and **external nasal branches**, which supply the skin of the tip of the nose.
6. **The infratrochlear nerve**, which innervates the eyelids, conjunctiva, skin of the nose, and lacrimal sac.

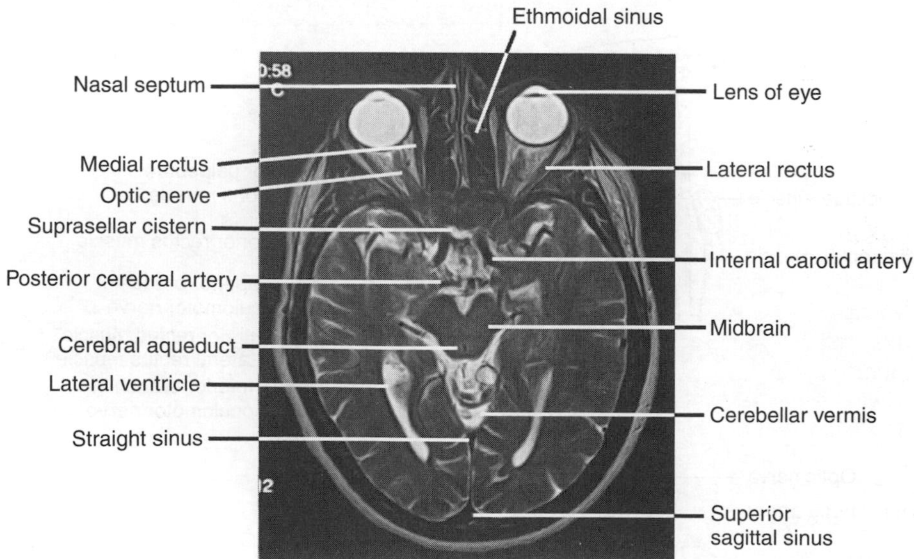

FIGURE 8.32. Axial MRI scan of the head.

B. Optic Nerve

- Consists of the axons of the ganglion cells of the retina and leaves the orbit by passing through the **optic canal**.
- Carries special somatic afferent fibers for vision from the retina to the brain and mediates the **afferent limb** of the **pupillary light reflex**.
- Joins the optic nerve from the corresponding eye to form the optic chiasma.

CLINICAL CORRELATES

Hemianopia (hemianopsia) is a condition characterized by loss of vision (blindness) in one-half of the visual field of each eye. Blindness may occur as the result of a lesion of the **optic nerve**. Types of hemianopia are (a) **bitemporal (heteronymous) hemianopia**, loss of vision in the temporal visual field of both eyes resulting from a lesion of the optic chiasma caused by a pituitary tumor; (b) **right nasal hemianopia**, blindness in the nasal field of vision of the right eye as the result of a **right perichiasmal lesion** such as an aneurysm of the internal carotid artery; and (c) **left homonymous hemianopia**, loss of sight in the left half of the visual field of both eyes resulting from a lesion of the **right optic tract** or **optic radiation**.

CLINICAL CORRELATES

Papilledema (choked disk) is an edema of the optic disk or optic nerve, often resulting from increased intracranial pressure and increased CSF pressure or thrombosis of the central vein of the retina, slowing venous return from the retina.

C. Oculomotor Nerve

- Enters the orbit through the superior orbital fissure and divides into a **superior division**, which innervates the superior rectus and levator palpebrae superioris muscles, and an **inferior division**, which innervates the medial rectus, inferior rectus, and inferior oblique muscles.
- Its inferior division also carries preganglionic parasympathetic fibers (with cell bodies located in the Edinger–Westphal nucleus) to the **ciliary ganglion**.

D. Trochlear Nerve

- Passes through the lateral wall of the cavernous sinus, and enters the orbit through the superior orbital fissure, and innervates the superior oblique muscle.

E. Abducens Nerve

- Enters the orbit through the superior orbital fissure and supplies the lateral rectus muscle.

F. Ciliary Ganglion

- Is a parasympathetic ganglion situated behind the eyeball, between the optic nerve and the lateral rectus muscle (see Nerves of the Head and Neck: II. A, Chapter 9).

III. BLOOD VESSELS (Figure 8.31)

A. Ophthalmic Artery

- Is a branch of the internal carotid artery and enters the orbit through the **optic canal** beneath the optic nerve.
- Gives rise to the **ocular and orbital vessels**, which include the following:

1. Central Artery of the Retina

- Is the **most important branch** of the ophthalmic artery.
- Travels in the optic nerve; it divides into superior and inferior branches to the optic disk, and each of those further divides into temporal and nasal branches.
- Is an end artery that does not anastomose with other arteries, and thus, its **occlusion results in blindness**.

2. **Long Posterior Ciliary Arteries**
   - Pierce the sclera and supply the ciliary body and the iris.
3. **Short Posterior Ciliary Arteries**
   - Pierce the sclera and supply the choroid.
4. **Lacrimal Artery**
   - Passes along the superior border of the lateral rectus and supplies the lacrimal gland, conjunctiva, and eyelids.
   - Gives rise to two **lateral palpebral arteries**, which contribute to arcades in the upper and lower eyelids.
5. **Medial Palpebral Arteries**
   - Contribute to arcades in the upper and lower eyelids.
6. **Muscular Branches**
   - Supply orbital muscles and give off the anterior ciliary arteries, which supply the iris.
7. **Supraorbital Artery**
   - Passes through the supraorbital notch (or foramen) and supplies the forehead and the scalp.
8. **Posterior Ethmoidal Artery**
   - Passes through the posterior ethmoidal foramen to the posterior ethmoidal air cells.
9. **Anterior Ethmoidal Artery**
   - Passes through the anterior ethmoidal foramen to the anterior and middle ethmoidal air cells, frontal sinus, nasal cavity, and external nose.
10. **Supratrochlear Artery**
   - Passes to the supraorbital margin and supplies the forehead and the scalp.
11. **Dorsal Nasal Artery**
   - Supplies the side of the nose and the lacrimal sac.

B. Ophthalmic Veins (Figure 8.33)

1. **Superior Ophthalmic Vein**
   - Is formed by the union of the supraorbital, supratrochlear, and angular veins.
   - Receives branches corresponding to most of those of the ophthalmic artery and, in addition, receives the inferior ophthalmic vein before draining into the cavernous sinus.
2. **Inferior Ophthalmic Vein**
   - Begins by the union of small veins in the floor of the orbit.
   - Communicates with the pterygoid venous plexus and often with the infraorbital vein and terminates directly or indirectly in the cavernous sinus.

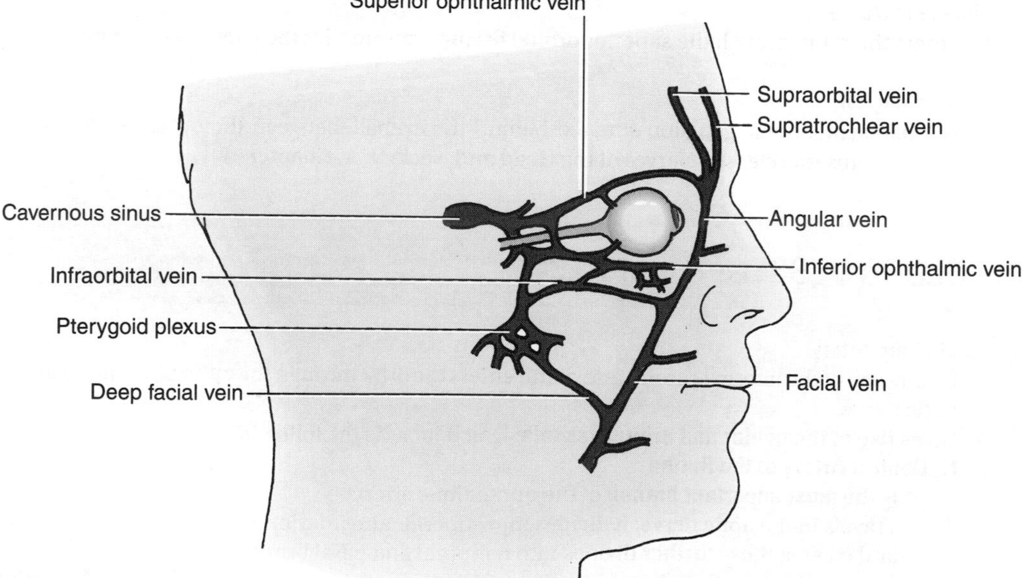

FIGURE 8.33. Ophthalmic veins.

IV. MUSCLES OF EYE MOVEMENT (Figures 8.30, 8.34, 8.35; Table 8.5)

CLINICAL CORRELATES **Diplopia (double vision)** is caused by **paralysis of one or more extraocular muscles,** resulting from injury of the nerves supplying them.

Strabismus (squint eye or crossed eye) is a condition in which the eyes are not aligned properly and point (look) in different directions. It occurs when the eye deviates medially (**internal strabismus** or esotropia) or deviate laterally (**external strabismus** or exotropia) as a result of weakness or paralysis of extrinsic eye muscle due to damage to the oculomotor or abducens nerve. Its symptoms include misaligned eyes, double vision, and a loss of depth perception. Treatments include eyeglasses, prisms, vision therapy, or eye muscle surgery.

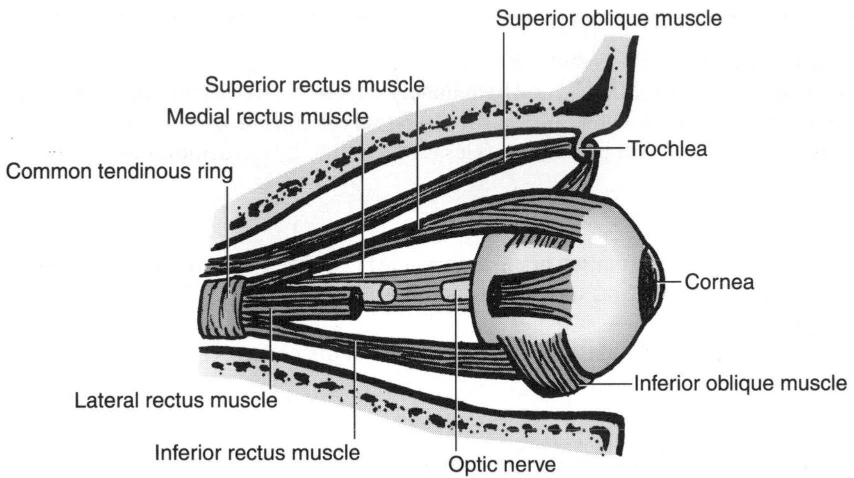

FIGURE 8.34. Muscles of the orbit.

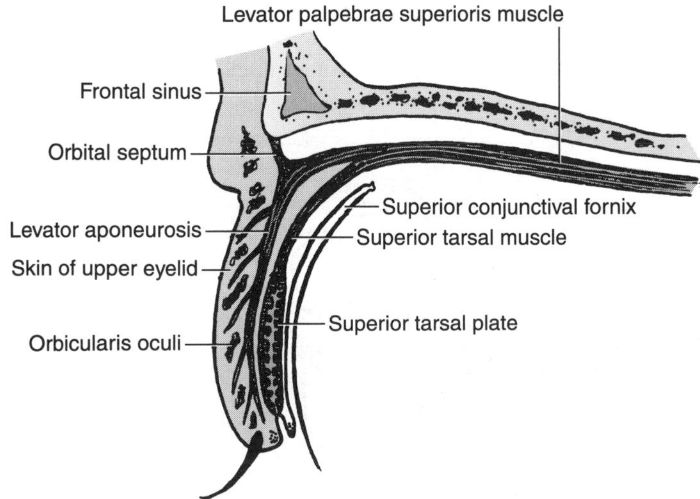

FIGURE 8.35. Structure of the upper eyelid.

table 8.5 Muscles of Eye Movement

Muscle	Origin	Insertion	Nerve	Actions on Eyeball
Superior rectus	Common tendinous ring	Sclera just behind cornea	Oculomotor	Elevates; intorts
Inferior rectus	Common tendinous ring	Sclera just behind cornea	Oculomotor	Depresses; extorts
Medial rectus	Common tendinous ring	Sclera just behind cornea	Oculomotor	Adducts
Lateral rectus	Common tendinous ring	Sclera just behind cornea	Abducens	Abducts
Levator palpebrae superioris	Lesser wing of sphenoid above and anterior to optic canal	Tarsal plate and skin of upper eyelid	Oculomotor, sympathetic	Elevates upper eyelid
Superior oblique	Body of sphenoid bone above optic canal	Sclera beneath superior rectus	Trochlear	Rotates upper pole of eyeball medially (intorts) so that cornea looks downward and laterally
Inferior oblique	Floor of orbit lateral to lacrimal groove	Sclera beneath lateral rectus	Oculomotor	Rotates upper pole of eyeball laterally (extorts) so that cornea looks upward and laterally

A. Innervation of Muscles of the Eyeball (Figure 8.30)

- Can be summarized as **SO_4**, **LR_6**, and **$Remainder_3$**, which means that the superior oblique muscle is innervated by the trochlear nerve, the lateral rectus muscle is innervated by the abducens nerve, and the **remainder** of these muscles is innervated by the oculomotor nerve.

B. Movements of the Eye

1. Intorsion

- Is a **medial (inward) rotation** of the upper pole (12 o'clock position) of the cornea, caused by the superior oblique and superior rectus muscles.

2. Extorsion

- Is a **lateral (outward) rotation** of the upper pole of the cornea, caused by the inferior oblique and inferior rectus muscles.

C. Common Tendinous Ring (Figure 8.36)

- Is a **fibrous ring** that surrounds the optic canal and the medial part of the superior orbital fissure.
- Is the site of origin of the four rectus muscles of the eye and transmits the following structures:

1. **Oculomotor, nasociliary, and abducens nerves**, which enter the orbit through the superior orbital fissure and the common tendinous ring.

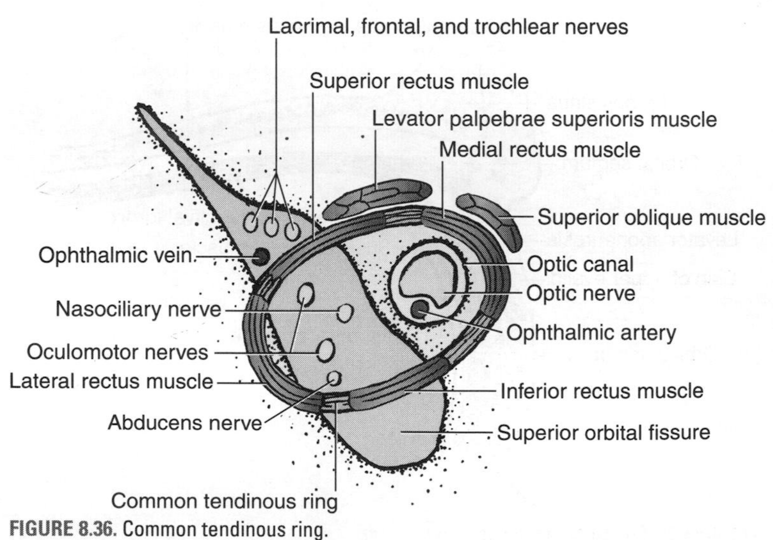

FIGURE 8.36. Common tendinous ring.

2. **Optic nerve, ophthalmic artery, and central artery and vein of the retina**, which enter the orbit through the optic canal and the tendinous ring.
3. **Superior ophthalmic vein plus the trochlear, frontal, and lacrimal nerves**, which enter the orbit through the superior orbital fissure but outside the tendinous ring.

V. LACRIMAL APPARATUS (Figure 8.37)

A. Lacrimal Gland

- Lies in the upper lateral region of the orbit on the lateral rectus and the levator palpebrae superioris muscles.
- Is drained by 12 **lacrimal ducts**, which open into the superior conjunctival fornix.

B. Lacrimal Canaliculi

- Are two curved canals that begin as a lacrimal punctum (or pore) in the margin of the eyelid and open into the lacrimal sac.

C. Lacrimal Sac

- Is the upper dilated end of the **nasolacrimal duct**, which opens into the inferior meatus of the nasal cavity.

D. Tears

- Are produced by the **lacrimal gland.**
- Pass through excretory ductules into the superior conjunctival fornix.
- Are spread evenly over the eyeball by blinking movements and accumulate in the area of the **lacrimal lake.**
- Enter the lacrimal canaliculi through their lacrimal puncta (which is on the summit of the lacrimal papilla) before draining into the lacrimal sac, nasolacrimal duct, and finally, the inferior nasal meatus.

CLINICAL CORRELATES

Crocodile tears syndrome (Bogorad syndrome) is **spontaneous lacrimation during eating** caused by a lesion of the facial nerve proximal to the geniculate ganglion. It follows facial paralysis and is due to misdirection of regenerating parasympathetic fibers, which formerly innervated the salivary (submandibular and sublingual) glands, to the lacrimal glands.

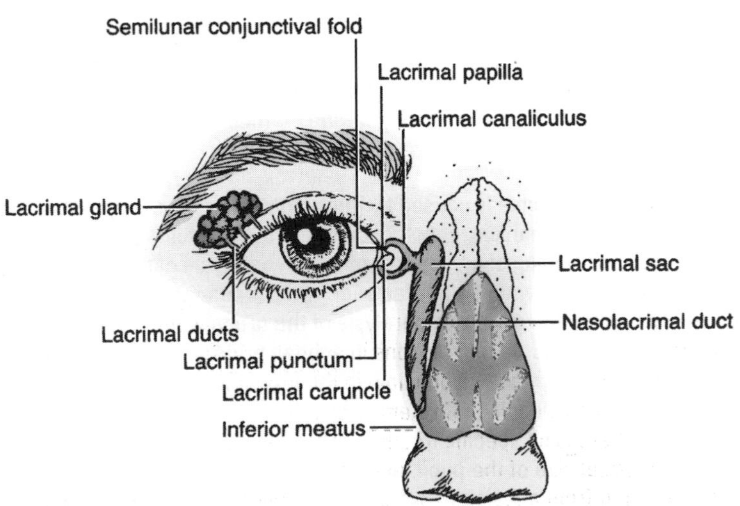

FIGURE 8.37. Lacrimal apparatus.

VI. EYEBALL (Figures 8.30 to 8.32)

A. External White Fibrous Coat

- Consists of the sclera and the cornea.

1. Sclera

- Is a tough white fibrous tunic enveloping the posterior five-sixths of the eye.

2. Cornea

- Is a transparent structure forming the anterior one-sixth of the external coat.
- Is responsible for the refraction of light entering the eye.

B. Middle Vascular Pigmented Coat

- Consists of the choroid, ciliary body, and iris.

1. Choroid

- Consists of an outer pigmented (dark brown) layer and an inner highly vascular layer, which invests the posterior five-sixths of the eyeball.
- **Nourishes the retina** and darkens the eye.

2. Ciliary Body

- Is a **thickened portion of the vascular coat** between the choroid and the iris and consists of the ciliary ring, ciliary processes, and ciliary muscle.
  1. The **ciliary processes** are radiating pigmented ridges that encircle the margin of the lens.
  2. The **ciliary muscle** consists of meridional and circular fibers of smooth muscle innervated by parasympathetic fibers. It contracts to pull the **ciliary ring** and ciliary processes, relaxing the suspensory ligament of the lens and allowing it to increase its convexity.

CLINICAL CORRELATES

Accommodation is the adjustment or adaptation of the eye to focus on a near object. It occurs with contraction of the ciliary muscle, causing a relaxation of the suspensory ligament (ciliary zonular fibers) and an increase in thickness, convexity, and refractive power of the lens. It is mediated by parasympathetic fibers running within the oculomotor nerve.

Argyll–Robertson pupil is a miotic pupil that responds to accommodation (constricts on near focus) but fails to respond to light. It is caused by a lesion in the midbrain and seen in neurosyphilis (or syphilis) and in diabetes.

Pupillary light reflex is constriction of the pupil in response to light stimulation (direct reflex), and the contralateral pupil also constricts (consensual reflex). It is mediated by parasympathetic nerve fibers in the oculomotor nerve (efferent limb), and its afferent limb is the optic nerve.

3. Iris

- Is a thin, contractile, circular, pigmented diaphragm with a central aperture, the **pupil**.
- Contains circular muscle fibers (**sphincter pupillae**), which are innervated by **parasympathetic** fibers, and radial fibers (**dilator pupillae**), which are innervated by **sympathetic** fibers.

CLINICAL CORRELATES

Horner syndrome is caused by **injury to cervical sympathetic nerves** and characterized by (a) **miosis**, constriction of the pupil resulting from paralysis of the dilator muscle of the iris; (b) **ptosis**, drooping of an upper eyelid from paralysis of the smooth muscle component (superior tarsal plate) of the levator palpebrae superioris; (c) **enophthalmos**, retraction (backward displacement) of an eyeball into the orbit from paralysis of the orbitalis muscle, which is smooth muscle and bridges the inferior orbital fissure and functions in eyeball protrusion; (d) **anhidrosis**, absence of sweating; and (e) **vasodilation**, increased blood flow in the face and neck (flushing). Common causes of lesions to cervical sympathetics include brain stem stroke, tuberculosis, Pancoast tumor, trauma, and injury to carotid arteries. There is no specific treatment that improves or reverses the condition.

Anisocoria is an unequal size of the pupil; **miosis** is a constricted pupil caused by paralysis of the dilator pupillae resulting from a lesion of sympathetic nerve; **mydriasis** is a dilated pupil caused by paralysis of the sphincter pupillae resulting from a lesion of the parasympathetic nerve.

C. Internal Nervous Coat

- Consists of the **retina**, which has an outer pigmented layer and an inner nervous layer.
- Has a posterior part that is photosensitive; its anterior part, which is not photosensitive, constitutes the inner lining of the ciliary body and the posterior part of the iris.

1. Optic Disk (Blind Spot)

- Consists of **optic nerve fibers** formed by axons of the ganglion cells. These cells are connected to the rods and cones by bipolar neurons.
- Is located nasal (or medial) to the fovea centralis and the posterior pole of the eye, has no receptors, and is insensitive to light.
- Has a depression in its center termed the **physiologic cup**.

2. Macula (Yellow Spot or Macula Lutea)

- Is a yellowish area near the center of the retina on the temporal side of the optic disk for the most distinct vision.
- Contains the fovea centralis.

3. Fovea Centralis

- Is a central depression (foveola) in the macula.
- Is avascular and is nourished by the choriocapillary lamina of the choroid.
- Has cones only (no rods), each of which is connected with only one ganglion cell, and functions in detailed vision.

4. Rods

- Are approximately 120 million in number and are most numerous approximately 0.5 cm from the fovea centralis.
- Contain **rhodopsin**, a visual purple pigment.
- Are specialized for vision in dim light.

5. Cones

- Are 7 million in number and are most numerous in the foveal region.
- Are associated with **visual acuity** and **color vision**.

CLINICAL CORRELATES

Myopia (nearsightedness) is a condition in which the focus of objects lies in front of the retina, resulting from elongation of the eyeball. **Hyperopia** (farsightedness) is a condition in which the focus of objects lies behind the retina.

Retinal detachment is a separation of the sensory layer from the pigment layer of the retina. It may occur in trauma such as a blow to the head and can be reattached surgically by photocoagulation by laser beam.

Retinitis pigmentosa is an inherited disorder that causes a **degeneration of photoreceptor cells** in the retina or a progressive retinal atrophy, characterized by **constricted visual fields (tunnel vision** or **loss of peripheral vision)**, nyctalopia (night blindness), attenuation (thinning) of the retinal vessels, and pigment infiltration of the inner retinal layers.

Macular degeneration (often called age-related macular degeneration) is a degenerative change in the macula in the center of the retina. A patient with this condition sees the edges of images but has **no central vision** (a **ring of peripheral vision**). It occurs in dry and wet forms. The dry type (nonneovascular) is the most common form; in this type, the **light-sensitive layer** of cells in the macula become **thinned** and causes more gradual loss of vision. The wet type (neovascular) is caused by the **growth of abnormal blood vessels** from the choroid underneath the macula. These abnormal blood vessels tend to hemorrhage or **leak**, resulting in the formation of scar tissue if left untreated. There is no treatment for dry macular degeneration. Laser treatments are effective at preventing or slowing the progress of wet type degeneration by sealing the leaking blood vessels, but no treatment restores vision loss.

Diabetic retinopathy is a degenerative disease of the retina and a leading cause of blindness associated with diabetes mellitus. The background type (the earliest phase) is marked by microaneurysms, intraretinal dotlike hemorrhages, exudates (as a result of **leaky vessels**), cotton-wool spots, and **macular edema**. The proliferative type is characterized by neovascularization (proliferation of new, abnormal vessel growth) of the retina and optic disk, which may project into the vitreous, proliferation of fibrous tissue, vitreous hemorrhage, and retinal detachment. It can be treated with laser photocoagulation to seal off leaking blood vessels and destroy new growth.

D. Refractive Media

- Consist of the cornea, aqueous humor, lens, and vitreous body.

1. **Cornea (See Orbit: VI. A.2.)**
2. **Aqueous Humor**
   - Is formed by the ciliary processes and provides nutrients for the avascular cornea and lens.
   - Passes through the pupil from the **posterior chamber** (between the iris and the lens) into the **anterior chamber** (between the cornea and the iris) and is drained into the scleral venous plexus through the canal of Schlemm at the iridocorneal angle.
   - Its impaired drainage causes an increased intraocular pressure, leading to atrophy of the retina and blindness.

CLINICAL CORRELATES **Glaucoma** is characterized by **increased intraocular pressure** resulting from **impaired drainage of aqueous humor** (which is produced by the ciliary processes) into the venous system through the scleral venous sinus (**Schlemm canal**), which is a circular vascular channel at the corneoscleral junction or limbus. The increased pressure causes **impaired retinal blood flow**, producing retinal ischemia or atrophy of the retina; degeneration of the nerve fibers in the retina, particularly at the optic disk; defects in the visual field; and blindness. Glaucoma can be treated by surgical iridectomy or laser iridotomy for drainage of aqueous humor or by use of drugs to inhibit the secretion of aqueous humor.

3. **Lens**
   - Is a transparent **avascular biconvex structure** enclosed in an elastic capsule.
   - Is held in position by radially arranged **zonular fibers** (suspensory ligament of the lens), which are attached medially to the lens capsule and laterally to the ciliary processes.
   - Flattens to focus on distant objects by pulling the zonular fibers and becomes a globular shape to accommodate the eye for near objects by contracting the ciliary muscle and thus relaxing zonular fibers.

CLINICAL CORRELATES **Cataract** is a clouding **(opacity or milky white) of the crystalline eye lens or of its capsule**, which must be removed. It results in little light being transmitted to the retina, causing blurred images and poor vision.
Presbyopia is a condition involving a **reduced ability to focus on near objects**. It is caused by the loss of elasticity of the crystalline lens, occurs in advanced age and is corrected with bifocal lenses.

4. **Vitreous Body**
   - Is a transparent gel called **vitreous humor**, which fills the eyeball posterior to the lens (vitreous chamber between the lens and the retina).
   - Holds the retina in place and provides support for the lens.

VII. DEVELOPMENT OF THE EYE

- The eye forms from a neuroectodermal evagination (optic cup and optic stalk) of the wall of the brain (diencephalon) and from the surface ectoderm (lens placode), mesoderm, and neural crest cells.

A. Neuroectoderm of the Diencephalon

- Evaginates to form the **optic vesicle**, which in turn invaginates to form the optic cup and optic stalk. This induces the ectoderm to thicken and form the lens placode.

1. **Optic cup** forms the retina, iris, and ciliary body.
2. **Optic stalk** forms the optic nerve.

B. Surface Ectoderm

- Invaginates to form the **lens placode**, which forms the lens and anterior epithelium of cornea.

C. Mesoderm

- Forms the sclera, portions of the cornea, vitreous body, and extraocular muscles.

D. Neural Crest Cells

- Form the choroids, sphincter pupillae muscle, dilator pupillae muscle, and ciliary muscle.

E. Hyaloid Artery and Vein

- Form the central artery and vein of the retina.

ORAL CAVITY AND PALATE

I. ORAL CAVITY (Figure 8.38)

- Consists of the vestibule and the oral cavity proper.

A. Oral Vestibule

- Is bounded by lips and cheeks externally and teeth and gums internally and receives opening of parotid duct at the parotid papilla opposite second maxillary molar.

B. Oral Cavity Proper

- Is bounded anteriorly and laterally by teeth and gums; its **roof** is formed by the palate, and its **floor** is formed by the tongue and the mucosa, supported by the geniohyoid and mylohyoid muscles.
- Communicates posteriorly with the oropharynx.

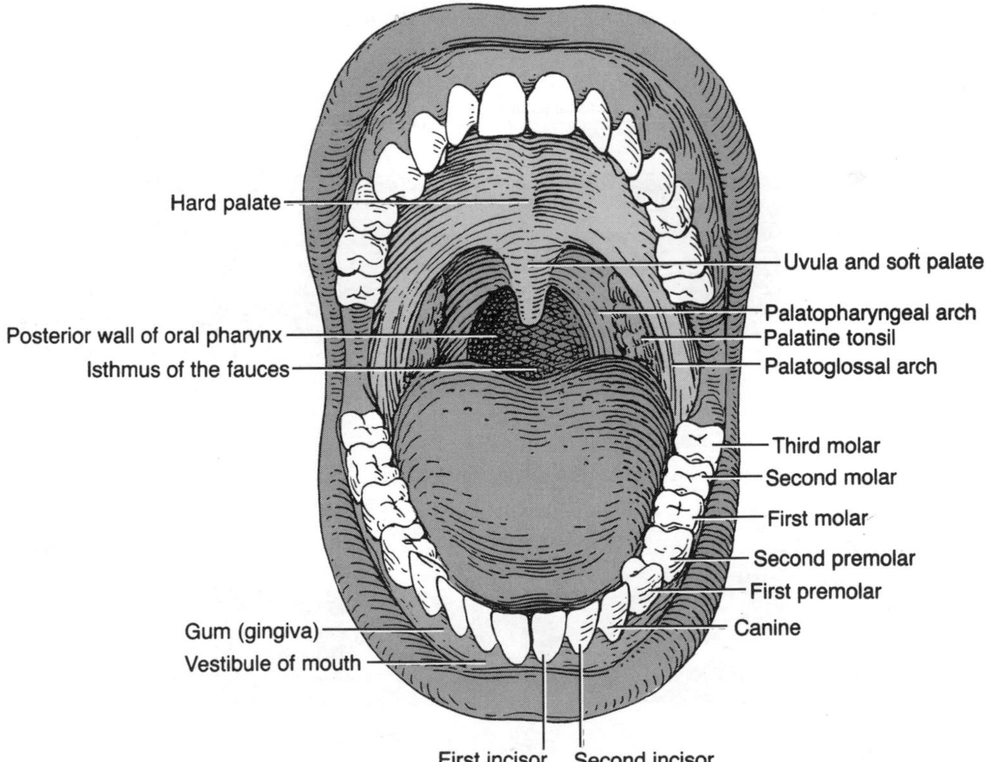

FIGURE 8.38. Oral cavity.

II. PALATE (Figures 8.38 to 8.39)

- Forms the roof of the mouth and the floor of the nasal cavity.

A. Hard Palate

- Is the anterior four-fifths of the palate and forms a **bony framework covered with a mucous membrane** between the nasal and oral cavities.
- Consists of the **palatine processes** of the maxillae and horizontal plates of the palatine bones.
- Contains the incisive foramen in its median plane anteriorly and the greater and lesser palatine foramina posteriorly.
- Receives sensory innervation through the greater palatine and nasopalatine nerves and blood from the greater palatine artery.

B. Soft Palate

- Is a **fibromuscular fold** extending from the posterior border of the hard palate and makes up one-fifth of the palate.
- Moves posteriorly against the pharyngeal wall to close the oropharyngeal (faucial) isthmus when swallowing or speaking.
- Is continuous with the **palatoglossal** and **palatopharyngeal folds**.
- Receives blood from the greater and lesser palatine arteries of the descending palatine artery of the maxillary artery, the ascending palatine artery of the facial artery, and the palatine branch of the ascending pharyngeal artery.
- Receives sensory innervation through the lesser palatine nerves and receives skeletal motor innervation from the vagus nerve. A lesion of the vagus nerve deviates the uvula to the opposite side.

CLINICAL CORRELATES

Lesion of the vagus nerve causes deviation of the uvula toward the opposite side of the lesion on phonation because of paralysis of the musculus uvulae. This muscle is innervated by the vagus nerve and elevates the uvula.

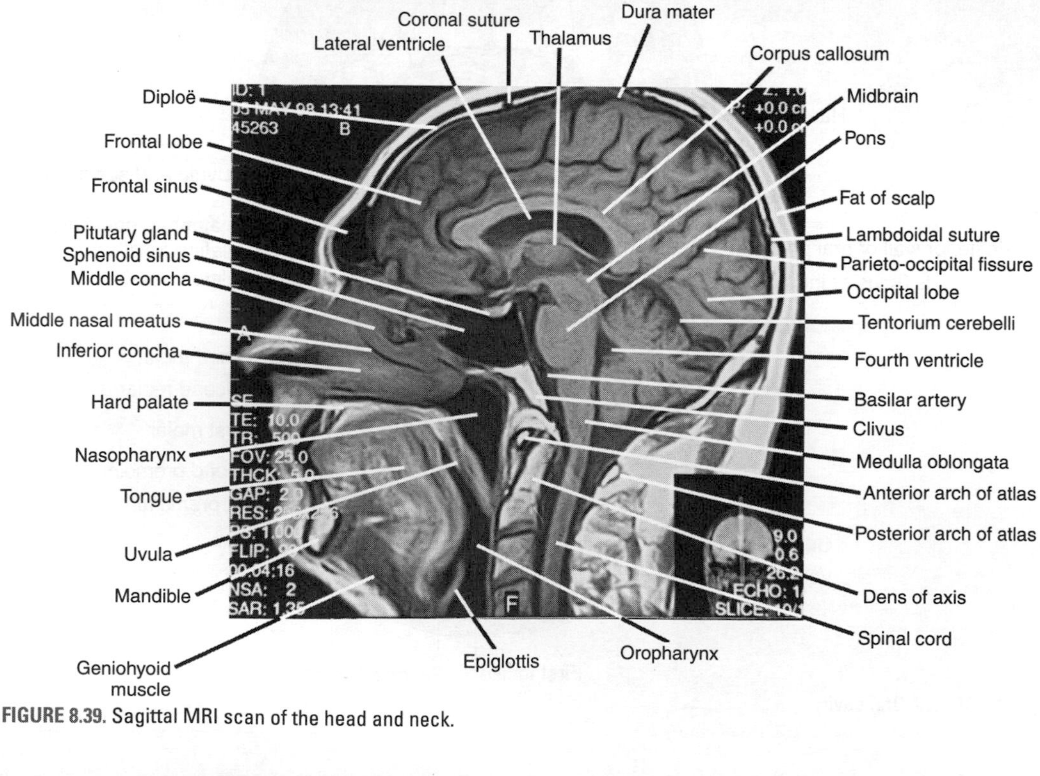

FIGURE 8.39. Sagittal MRI scan of the head and neck.

table 8.6 Muscles of the Palate

Muscle	Origin	Insertion	Nerve	Action
Tensor veli palatini	Scaphoid fossa; spine of sphenoid; cartilage of auditory tube	Tendon hooks around hamulus of medial pterygoid plate to insert into aponeurosis of soft palate	Mandibular branch of trigeminal nerve	Tenses soft palate
Levator veli palatini	Petrous part of temporal bone; cartilage of auditory tube	Aponeurosis of soft palate	Vagus nerve via pharyngeal plexus	Elevates soft palate
Palatoglossus	Aponeurosis of soft palate	Dorsolateral side of tongue	Vagus nerve via pharyngeal plexus	Elevates tongue
Palatopharyngeus	Aponeurosis of soft palate	Thyroid cartilage and side of pharynx	Vagus nerve via pharyngeal plexus	Elevates pharynx; closes nasopharynx
Musculus uvulae	Posterior nasal spine of palatine bone; palatine aponeurosis	Mucous membrane of uvula	Vagus nerve via pharyngeal plexus	Elevates uvula

C. Muscles of the Palate (Table 8.6)

III. TONGUE (Figures 8.38 and 8.40)

- Is attached by muscles to the hyoid bone, mandible, styloid process, palate, and pharynx.
- Is divided by a V-shaped **sulcus terminalis** into two parts—an anterior two-thirds and a posterior one-third—which differ developmentally, structurally, and in innervation.
- The **foramen cecum** is located at the apex of the "V" and indicates the site of origin of the embryonic **thyroglossal duct**.

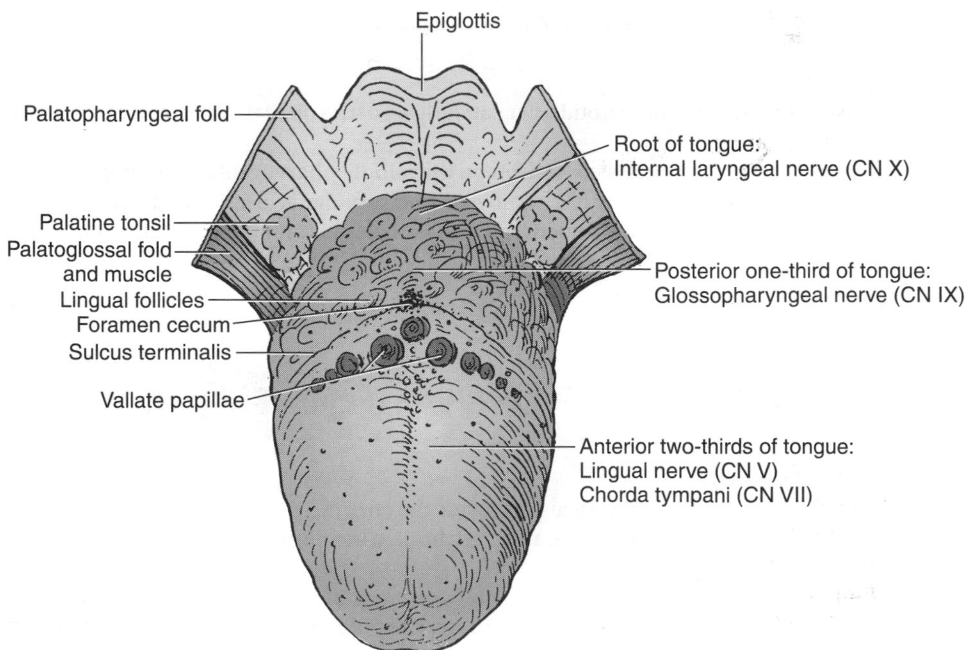

FIGURE 8.40. Tongue.

CLINICAL CORRELATES **Tongue-tie (ankyloglossia)** is an **abnormal shortness of frenulum linguae**, resulting in limitation of its movement and thus a severe speech impediment. It can be corrected surgically by cutting the frenulum.

A. Lingual Papillae

- Are small, nipple-shaped projections on the anterior two-thirds of the dorsum of the tongue.
- Are divided into the vallate, fungiform, filiform, and foliate papillae.

1. Vallate Papillae

- Are arranged in the form of a **"V"** in front of the sulcus terminalis.
- Are studded with numerous taste buds and are innervated by the glossopharyngeal nerve.

2. Fungiform Papillae

- Are mushroom-shaped projections with red heads and are scattered on the sides and the apex of the tongue.

3. Filiform Papillae

- Are numerous, slender, conical projections that are arranged in rows parallel to the sulcus terminalis.

4. Foliate Papillae

- Are found in certain animals but are rudimentary in humans.

B. Lingual Tonsil

- Is the collection of **nodular masses of lymphoid follicles** on the posterior one-third of the dorsum of the tongue.

C. Lingual Innervation

- The extrinsic and intrinsic muscles of the tongue are innervated by the **hypoglossal nerve** except for the palatoglossus, which is innervated by the vagus nerve. A lesion of the hypoglossal nerve deviates the tongue toward the injured side.
- The anterior two-thirds of the tongue receives general sensory innervation from the **lingual nerve** and taste sensation from the **chorda tympani**.
- The posterior one-third of the tongue and the vallate papillae receive both general and taste innervation from the **glossopharyngeal nerve**.
- The epiglottic region of the tongue and the epiglottis receive both general and taste innervation from the **internal laryngeal branch** of the vagus nerve.

D. Lingual Artery

- Arises from the external carotid artery at the level of the tip of the greater horn of the hyoid bone in the carotid triangle.
- Passes deep to the hyoglossus and lies on the middle pharyngeal constrictor muscle.
- Gives rise to the suprahyoid, dorsal lingual, and sublingual arteries and terminates as the **deep lingual artery**, which ascends between the genioglossus and inferior longitudinal muscles.

E. Muscles of the Tongue (Table 8.7)

IV. TEETH AND GUMS OR GINGIVAE (Figure 8.38)

A. Structure of the Teeth

- **Enamel** is the hardest substance that covers the crown.
- **Dentin** is a hard substance that is nurtured through the fine dental tubules of odontoblasts lining the central pulp space.
- **Pulp** fills the central cavity, which is continuous with the root canal. It contains numerous blood vessels, nerves, and lymphatics, which enter the pulp through an apical foramen at the apex of the root.

table 8.7 Muscles of the Tongue

Muscle	Origin	Insertion	Nerve	Action
Styloglossus	Styloid process	Side and inferior aspect of tongue	Hypoglossal nerve	Retracts and elevates tongue
Hyoglossus	Body and greater horn of hyoid bone	Side and inferior aspect of tongue	Hypoglossal nerve	Depresses and retracts tongue
Genioglossus	Genial tubercle of mandible	Inferior aspect of tongue; body of hyoid bone	Hypoglossal nerve	Protrudes and depresses tongue
Palatoglossus	Aponeurosis of soft palate	Dorsolateral side of tongue	Vagus nerve via pharyngeal plexus	Elevates tongue

B. Parts of the Teeth

- **Crown** projects above the gingival surface and is covered by enamel.
- **Neck** is the constricted area at the junction of the crown and root.
- **Root**, embedded in the alveolar part of the maxilla or mandible, is covered with cement, which is connected to the bone of the alveolus by a layer of modified periosteum, the periodontal ligament. Each maxillary molar generally has three roots, and each mandibular molar has two roots.

C. Basic Types of Teeth

- **Incisors**, which are chisel-shaped teeth that have a single root, are used for cutting or biting.
- **Canines**, which have a single prominent cone and a single root, are used for tearing.
- **Premolars**, which usually have two cusps, are used for grinding. The upper first premolar tooth may be bifid, and all others each have a single root.
- **Molars**, which usually have three (sometimes three to five) cusps, are used for grinding. The upper molar teeth have three roots, and the lower one has two roots.

D. Two Sets of Teeth

- **Deciduous (primary) teeth**: two incisors, one canine, and two molars in each quadrant, for a total of 20.
- **Permanent teeth:** two incisors, one canine, two premolars, and three molars in each quadrant, for a total of 32.

E. Innervation of the Teeth and Gums (Figure 8.41)

1. Maxillary Teeth

- Innervated by the anterior, middle, and posterior–superior alveolar branches of the maxillary nerve.

2. Mandibular Teeth

- Innervated by the inferior alveolar branch of the mandibular nerve.

CLINICAL CORRELATES

Abscess or infection of the maxillary teeth irritates the **maxillary nerve**, causing upper **toothache**. It may result in symptoms of **sinusitis**, with pain referred to the distribution of the maxillary nerve.

Abscess or infection of the mandibular teeth might spread through the lower jaw to emerge on the face or in the floor of the mouth. It irritates the **mandibular nerve**, causing **pain** that may be **referred to the ear** because this nerve also innervates a part of the ear.

3. Maxillary Gingiva

- **Outer (buccal) surface** is innervated by posterior, middle, and anterior–superior alveolar and infraorbital nerves.
- **Inner (lingual) surface** is innervated by greater palatine and nasopalatine nerves.

4. Mandibular Gingiva

- **Outer (buccal) surface** is innervated by buccal and mental nerves.
- **Inner (lingual) surface** is innervated by lingual nerves.

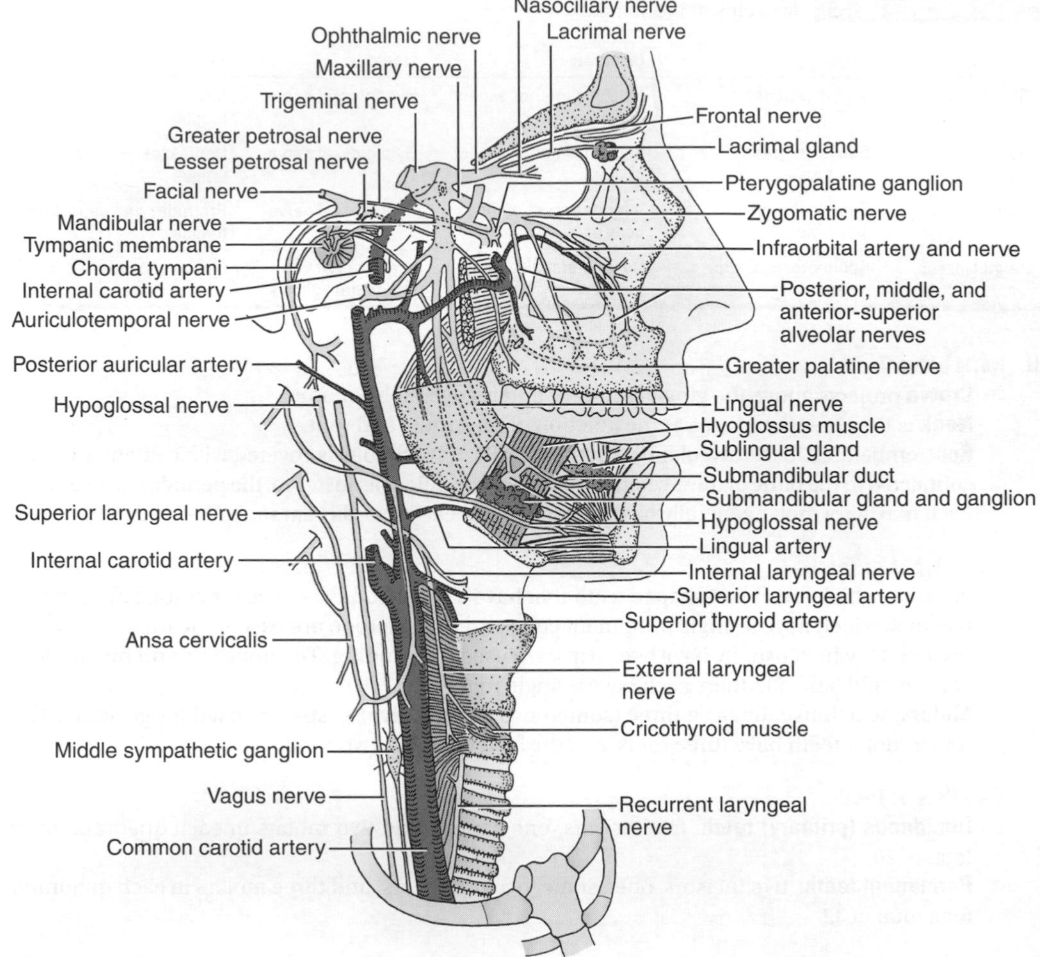

FIGURE 8.41. Branches of the trigeminal nerve and their relationship with other structures.

V. SALIVARY GLANDS (Figure 8.41)

A. Submandibular Gland

- Is ensheathed by the investing layer of the deep cervical fascia and lies in the **submandibular triangle.**
- Its superficial portion is situated superficial to the mylohyoid muscle.
- Its deep portion is located between the hyoglossus and styloglossus muscles medially and the mylohyoid muscle laterally and between the lingual nerve above and the hypoglossal nerve below.
- **Wharton duct** arises from the deep portion and runs forward between the mylohyoid and the hyoglossus, where it runs medial to and then superior to the lingual nerve. It then runs between the sublingual gland and the genioglossus and empties at the summit of the sublingual papilla (caruncle) at the side of the frenulum of the tongue.
- Is innervated by parasympathetic secretomotor fibers from the facial nerve, which run in the chorda tympani and in the lingual nerve and synapse in the submandibular ganglion.

B. Sublingual Gland

- Is located in the floor of the mouth between the mucous membrane above and the mylohyoid muscle below.

- Surrounds the terminal portion of the submandibular duct.
- Empties mostly into the floor of the mouth along the sublingual fold by 12 short ducts, some of which enter the submandibular duct.
- Is supplied by postganglionic parasympathetic (secretomotor) fibers from the submandibular ganglion either directly or through the lingual nerve.

CLINICAL CORRELATES **Ludwig angina** is an **infection of the floor of the mouth** (submandibular space) with secondary involvement of the sublingual and submental spaces, usually resulting from a dental infection. Symptoms include painful swelling of the floor of the mouth, elevation of the tongue, dysphagia (difficulty in swallowing), dysphonia (impairment of voice production), edema of the glottis, fever, and rapid breathing.

VI. DEVELOPMENT OF THE PALATE

A. Primary Palate

- Is formed by the medial nasal prominences at the midline. Posterior to the primary palate, the maxillary process on each side sends a horizontal plate (palatal process); these plates fuse to form the secondary palate and also unite with the primary palate and the developing nasal septum.

B. Secondary Palate

- Is formed by fusion of the lateral palatine processes (palatal shelves) that develop from the maxillary prominences.

C. Definitive Palate

- Is formed by fusion of the primary and secondary palates at the incisive foramen.

CLINICAL CORRELATES **Cleft palate** occurs when the palatine shelves fail to fuse with each other or the primary palate. **Cleft lip** occurs when the maxillary prominence and the medial nasal prominence fail to fuse.

VII. DEVELOPMENT OF THE TONGUE

A. The Anterior Two-Thirds of the Tongue

- Develop from one median lingual swelling (tongue bud) and two lateral lingual swellings (tongue buds) in the pharyngeal arch 1. Overgrowth of the lateral swellings forms the anterior two-thirds of the tongue.
- Receives general sensation (GSA) carried by the lingual branch of CN V and taste sensation (special visceral afferent [SVA]) carried by the chorda tympani branch of CN VII.

B. The Posterior One-Third of the Tongue

- Develops from the copula or hypobranchial eminence that is formed by mesoderm of the pharyngeal arches 3 and 4.
- Receives general sensation and taste sensation carried by CN IX.

C. Muscles of the Tongue

- Intrinsic and extrinsic muscles (styloglossus, hyoglossus, genioglossus, and palatoglossus) are derived from myoblasts that migrate to the tongue region from occipital somites. Motor innervation is supplied by CN XII, except for the palatoglossus muscle, which is innervated by CN X.

VIII. DEVELOPMENT OF TEETH

- Teeth are formed by **ectoderm** and **neural crest-derived mesenchyme.**
- The **dental lamina** develops from the oral epithelium (ectoderm) as a downgrowth into the underlying mesenchyme (is of neural crest origin), and gives rise to the tooth buds, which develop into a cup-shaped enamel organ.
- The **enamel organs** are derived from **ectoderm** and develop first for the deciduous teeth, then the permanent teeth, and gives rise to the amenoblasts, which form enamel.
- The **dental papillae** are formed by a condensation of neural crest mesenchyme that underlie the enamel organs, and give rise to the odontoblasts (which form dentin) and dental pulp.
- The **dental sacs** are formed by a condensation of neural crest mesenchyme surrounding the dental papillae, and give rise to cementoblasts (which form cementum) and the periodontal ligaments.

IX. DEVELOPMENT OF SALIVARY GLANDS

- Salivary glands originate as thickening of the oral epithelium.
- The parotid glands are probably derived from **ectoderm**, whereas the submandibular and sublingual glands are thought to be derived from **endoderm**.

PHARYNX AND TONSILS

I. PHARYNX (Figures 8.39 and 8.42)

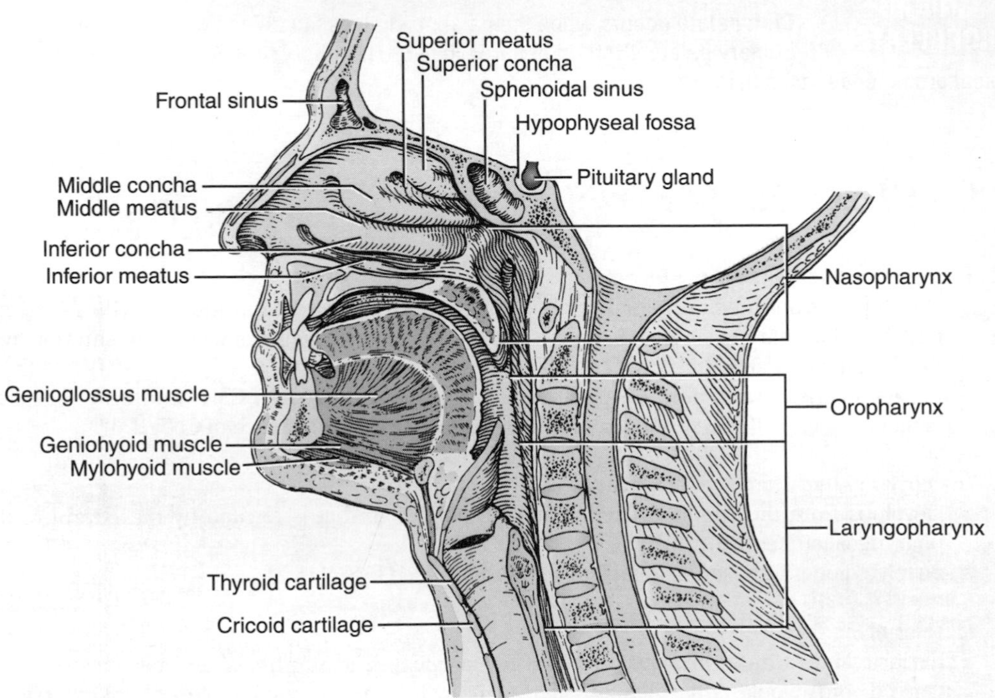

FIGURE 8.42. Pharynx.

- Is a **funnel-shaped fibromuscular** tube that extends from the base of the skull to the inferior border of the cricoid cartilage.
- Conducts food to the esophagus and air to the larynx and lungs.

II. SUBDIVISIONS OF THE PHARYNX

A. Nasopharynx

- Is situated behind the nasal cavity above the soft palate and communicates with the nasal cavities through the **nasal choanae**.
- Contains the **pharyngeal tonsils** in its posterior wall.
- Is connected with the tympanic cavity through the **auditory (eustachian) tube**, which equalizes air pressure on both sides of the tympanic membrane.

B. Oropharynx

- Extends between the soft palate above and the superior border of the epiglottis below and communicates with the mouth through the oropharyngeal isthmus.
- Contains the **palatine tonsils**, which are lodged in the **tonsillar fossae** and are bounded by the palatoglossal and palatopharyngeal folds.

CLINICAL CORRELATES **Pharyngeal tumors** may irritate the glossopharyngeal and vagus nerves. Pain that occurs while swallowing is referred to the ear because these nerves contribute sensory innervation to the external ear.

CLINICAL CORRELATES **Heimlich maneuver** is designed to expel an obstructing bolus of food from the throat of a choking victim by wrapping your arms around the victim's waist from behind and placing a fist with one hand and grasping it with the other on the abdomen between the navel and the costal margin and forcefully pressing into the abdomen with a quick inward and upward thrust to dislodge the obstruction.

C. Laryngopharynx (Hypopharynx)

- Extends from the upper border of the epiglottis to the lower border of the cricoid cartilage.
- Contains the **piriform recesses**, one on each side of the opening of the larynx, in which swallowed foreign bodies may be lodged.

III. INNERVATION AND BLOOD SUPPLY OF THE PHARYNX (Figure 8.43)

A. Pharyngeal Plexus

- Lies on the **middle pharyngeal constrictor**.
- Is formed by the **pharyngeal branches** of the glossopharyngeal and vagus nerves and the sympathetic branches from the superior cervical ganglion.
- Its **vagal branch** innervates all of the muscles of the pharynx with the exception of the stylopharyngeus, which is supplied by the glossopharyngeal nerve.
- Its glossopharyngeal component supplies sensory fibers to the pharyngeal mucosa.

B. Arteries of the Pharynx

- Are the ascending pharyngeal artery, ascending palatine branch of the facial artery, descending palatine arteries, pharyngeal branches of the maxillary artery, and branches of the superior and inferior thyroid arteries.

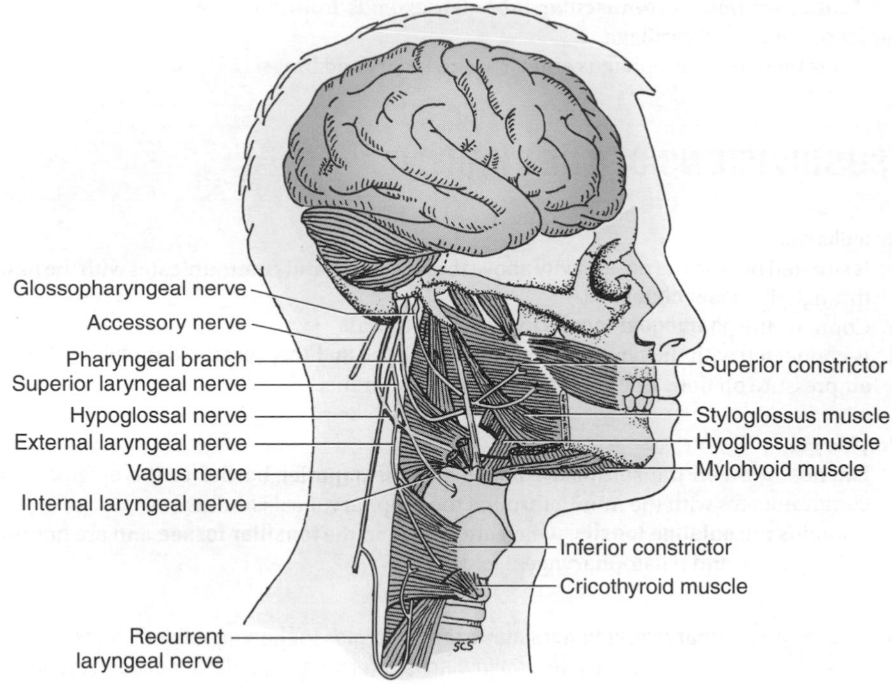

FIGURE 8.43. Nerve supply to the pharynx.

IV. MUSCLES OF THE PHARYNX (Figures 8.44 to 8.45; Table 8.8)

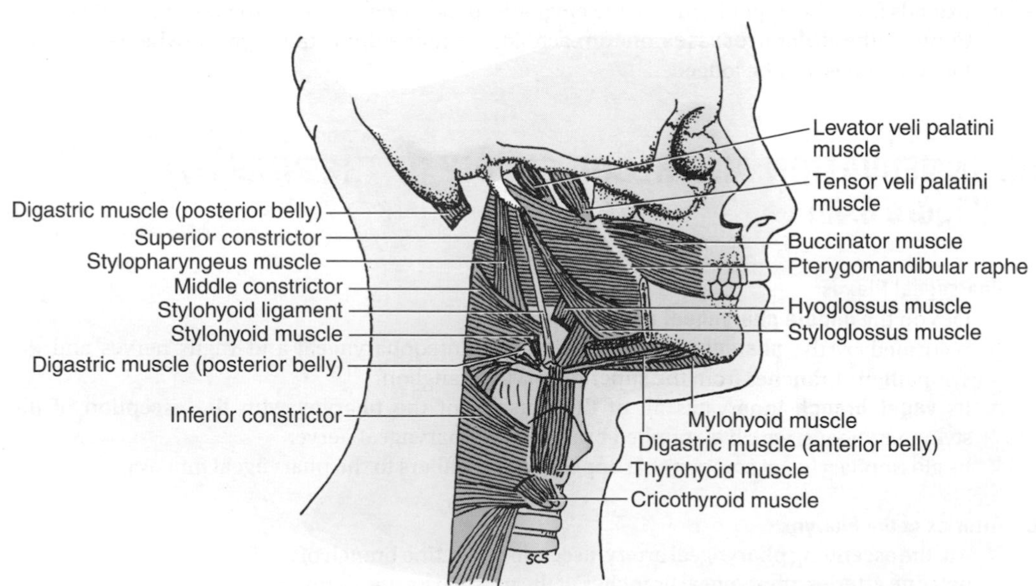

FIGURE 8.44. Muscles of the pharynx

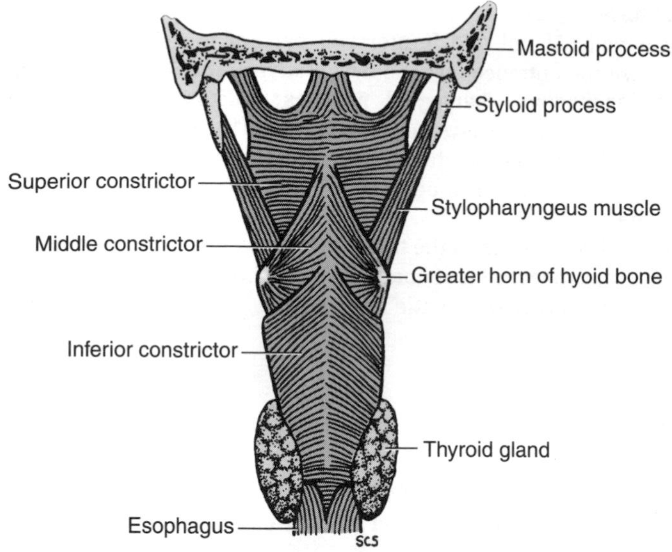

FIGURE 8.45. Pharyngeal constrictors.

V. SWALLOWING (DEGLUTITION)

- Is an act of transferring a food bolus from the mouth through the pharynx and esophagus into the stomach, and may be divided into three phases.

A. Oral Phase

- The **bolus** of food is pushed backward by elevating the tongue by the **styloglossus** and **palatoglossus** through the fauces into the oropharynx.

table 8.8 Muscles of the Pharynx

Muscle	Origin	Insertion	Nerve	Action
Circular muscles				
Superior constrictor	Medial pterygoid plate; pterygoid hamulus; pterygomandibular raphe; mylohyoid line of mandible; side of tongue	Median raphe and pharyngeal tubercle of skull	Vagus nerve via pharyngeal plexus	Constricts upper pharynx
Middle constrictor	Greater and lesser horns of hyoid; stylohyoid ligament	Median raphe	Vagus nerve via pharyngeal plexus	Constricts lower pharynx
Inferior constrictor	Arch of cricoid and oblique line of thyroid cartilages	Median raphe of pharynx	Vagus nerve via pharyngeal plexus, recurrent and external laryngeal nerve	Constricts lower pharynx
Longitudinal muscles				
Stylopharyngeus	Styloid process	Thyroid cartilage and muscles of pharynx	Glossopharyngeal nerve	Elevates pharynx and larynx
Palatopharyngeus	Hard palate; aponeurosis of soft palate	Thyroid cartilage and muscles of pharynx	Vagus nerve via pharyngeal plexus	Elevates pharynx and larynx; closes nasopharynx
Salpingopharyngeus	Cartilage of auditory tube	Muscles of pharynx	Vagus nerve via pharyngeal plexus	Elevates pharynx; opens auditory tube

B. Pharyngeal Phase

- The tensor veli palatini and levator veli palatini muscles elevate the soft palate and uvula to close the entrance into the nasopharynx. The walls of the **pharynx** are raised by the **three longitudinal pharyngeal muscles** (palatopharyngeus, stylopharyngeus, and salpingopharyngeus) to receive the bolus of food. The suprahyoid muscles elevate the hyoid bone and the larynx to close the opening into the larynx, thus passing the bolus over the epiglottis and preventing the food from entering the respiratory passageways.

C. Esophageal Phase

- The sequential contraction of the **three pharyngeal constrictor muscles** (superior, middle, and inferior pharyngeal constrictors) moves the bolus inferiorly into the esophagus, where it is propelled by peristalsis into the stomach.

VI. TONSILS

- Are masses of lymphoid tissue located in the posterior wall of the pharynx (throat), trap bacteria and viruses entering through the throat, and produce antibodies to help protect from infection.

A. Pharyngeal Tonsil

- Is found in the posterior wall and roof of the nasopharynx and is called an adenoid when enlarged.

CLINICAL CORRELATES

Adenoid is hypertrophy or **enlargement of the pharyngeal tonsils** that obstructs passage of air from the nasal cavities through the choanae into the nasopharynx and thus causes **difficulty in nasal breathing** and phonation. It may block the pharyngeal orifices of the auditory tube, and an infection may spread from the nasopharynx through the auditory tube to the middle ear cavity, causing otitis media, which may result in deafness.

B. Palatine Tonsil

- Lies on each side of the oropharynx in an interval between the palatoglossal and palatopharyngeal folds.
- Is highly vascular, receiving blood from the ascending palatine and tonsillar branches of the facial artery, the descending palatine branch of the maxillary artery, a palatine branch of the ascending pharyngeal artery, and the dorsal lingual branches of the lingual artery.
- Is innervated by branches of the glossopharyngeal nerve and the lesser palatine branch of the maxillary nerve.

CLINICAL CORRELATES

Palatine tonsillectomy is surgical removal of a palatine tonsil. During tonsillectomy, the glossopharyngeal nerve may be injured, causing loss of general sensation and taste sensation of the posterior one-third of the tongue. It may cause severe hemorrhage, which may occur from the branches of the facial, ascending pharyngeal, maxillary, and lingual arteries or paratonsillar veins.

Quinsy (peritonsillar abscess) is a painful **pus-filled inflammation** or abscess of the tonsils and surrounding tissues. It develops as a complication of tonsillitis, primarily in adolescents and young adults. The soft palate and uvula are edematous and displaced toward the unaffected side. Symptoms include sore throat, fever, dysphasia (impairment of speech), and trismus (motor disturbance of the trigeminal nerve, especially spasm of the masseter muscle with difficulty in opening the mouth). It can be treated with antibiotics, surgical aspiration, or tonsillectomy.

C. Tubal (Eustachian) Tonsil

- Is a collection of lymphoid nodules near the pharyngeal opening of the auditory tube.

D. Lingual Tonsil

- Is a collection of lymphoid follicles on the posterior portion of the dorsum of the tongue.

E. Waldeyer Tonsillar Ring

- Is a tonsillar ring of lymphoid tissue at the oropharyngeal isthmus, formed by the lingual, palatine (faucial), tubal (eustachian), and pharyngeal tonsil, encircling the back of the throat.

VII. FASCIA AND SPACE OF THE PHARYNX (Figure 8.8)

A. Retropharyngeal Space

- Is a **potential space** between the buccopharyngeal fascia and the prevertebral fascia, extending from the base of the skull to the superior mediastinum.
- Permits movement of the pharynx, larynx, trachea, and esophagus during swallowing.

B. Pharyngobasilar Fascia

- Forms the **submucosa of the pharynx** and blends with the periosteum of the base of the skull.
- Lies internal to the muscular coat of the pharynx; these muscles are covered externally by the buccopharyngeal fascia.

VIII. PHARYNGEAL (BRANCHIAL) APPARATUS

- Consists of the pharyngeal arches, pouches, grooves, and membranes.

A. Pharyngeal (Branchial) Arches (1, 2, 3, 4, 6)

- Are composed of **mesoderm** and **neural crest cells**. (They are formed by migration of neural crest cells around cores of mesoderm covered externally by ectoderm and internally by endoderm.) Each arch has its own cartilaginous, muscular, vascular, and nervous components.

1. **First (Mandibular) Pharyngeal Arch**
   - Forms the Meckel cartilage, which develops the malleus and incus and maxilla, zygomatic and temporal squama, and mandible.
   - Forms muscles of mastication and mylohyoid, digastric anterior belly, tensor veli palatini, and tensor tympani muscles, which are innervated by the CN V (V3).
2. **Second (Hyoid) Pharyngeal Arch**
   - Forms the Reichert cartilage, which develops the stapes, styloid process, lesser cornu, and upper half of the hyoid bone.
   - Forms muscles of facial expression and the digastric posterior belly, stylohyoid, and stapedius muscles, which are innervated by the CN VII.
3. **Third Pharyngeal Arch**
   - Forms the third arch cartilage, which forms the greater cornu and lower half of the hyoid bone.
   - Forms the stylopharyngeus muscle, which is innervated by the CN IX.
4. **Fourth Pharyngeal Arch**
   - Forms the fourth arch cartilage, which forms the laryngeal cartilages.
   - Forms the muscles of the soft palate except the tensor veli palatini, muscles of the pharynx except stylopharyngeus, and the cricopharyngeus muscle, which are innervated by the CN X (superior laryngeal branch).
5. **Sixth Pharyngeal Arch**
   - Forms the sixth arch cartilage, which forms laryngeal cartilages.
   - Forms the intrinsic muscles of the larynx, except cricothyroid, and the upper muscles of the esophagus, which are innervated by the CN X (recurrent laryngeal branch).

B. Pharyngeal Pouches (1, 2, 3, and 4)

- Are evaginations of the foregut **endoderm**.
  1. **Pharyngeal pouch 1** forms the epithelium of the auditory tube and the middle ear cavity.
  2. **Pharyngeal pouch 2** forms the epithelium and crypts of the palatine tonsil.
  3. **Pharyngeal pouch 3** forms the inferior parathyroid gland and thymus.
  4. **Pharyngeal pouch 4** forms the superior parathyroid gland and ultimobranchial body.

C. The Pharyngeal Grooves (1, 2, 3, and 4)

- Are four invaginations of the surface **ectoderm** between adjacent arches.
  1. **Pharyngeal groove 1** gives rise to the epithelium of the external auditory meatus and skin over the tympanic membrane.
  2. Pharyngeal grooves 2, 3, and 4 are obliterated.

D. The Pharyngeal Membranes (1, 2, 3, and 4)

- Are located at the junction of each pharyngeal groove and pouch.
  1. **Pharyngeal membrane 1** gives rise to the tympanic membrane.
  2. **Pharyngeal membranes 2, 3, and 4** are obliterated.

NASAL CAVITY AND PARANASAL SINUSES

I. NASAL CAVITY (Figures 8.39, 8.46, and 8.47)

- Opens on the face through the anterior nasal apertures (**nares, or nostrils**) and communicates with the nasopharynx through a posterior opening, the **choanae**.
- Has a slight dilatation inside the aperture of each nostril, the **vestibule**, which is lined largely with skin containing hair, sebaceous glands, and sweat glands.
- Its function is to warm, clean, humidify, filter the inhaled air for respiration, and help smell and taste.

A. Roof

- Is formed by the nasal, frontal, ethmoid (**cribriform plate**), and sphenoid (body) bones. The cribriform plate transmits the olfactory nerves.

B. Floor

- Is formed by the palatine process of the maxilla and the horizontal plate of the palatine bone.
- Contains the **incisive foramen**, which transmits the nasopalatine nerve and terminal branches of the sphenopalatine artery.

C. Medial Wall (Nasal Septum)

- Is formed primarily by the perpendicular plate of the ethmoid bone, vomer, and septal cartilage.
- Is also formed by processes of the palatine, maxillary, frontal, sphenoid, and nasal bones.

D. Lateral Wall

- Is formed by the superior and middle conchae of the ethmoid bone and the inferior concha.
- Is also formed by the nasal bone, frontal process and nasal surface of the maxilla, lacrimal bone, perpendicular plate of the palatine bone, and medial pterygoid plate of the sphenoid bone.
- Contains the following structures and their openings:
  1. **Sphenoethmoidal Recess**
     - Opening of the sphenoid sinus.
  2. **Superior Meatus**
     - Opening of the posterior ethmoidal air cells.
  3. **Middle Meatus**
     - Opening of the frontal sinus into the infundibulum, openings of the middle ethmoidal air cells on the **ethmoidal bulla**, and openings of the anterior ethmoidal air cells and maxillary sinus in the hiatus semilunaris.

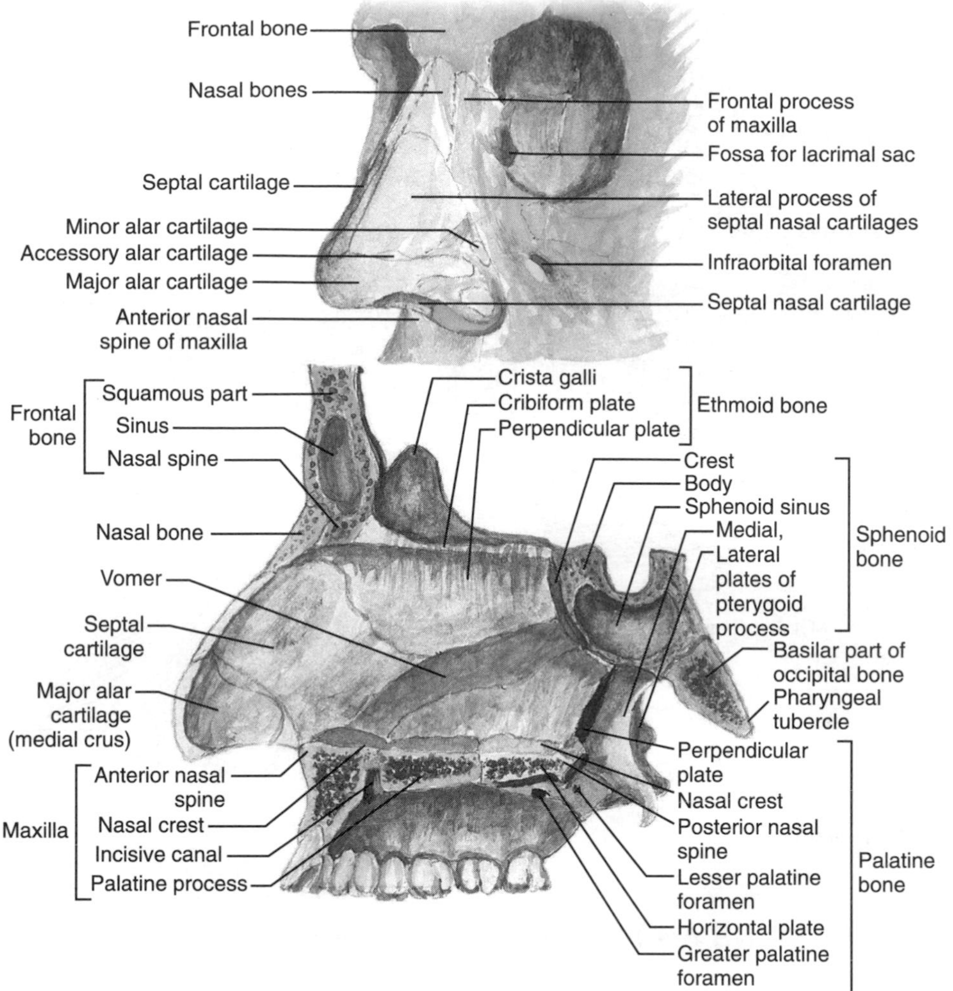

FIGURE 8.46. External nose and nasal septum.

4. **Inferior Meatus**
   - Opening of the **nasolacrimal duct**.
5. **Sphenopalatine Foramen**
   - Opening into the pterygopalatine fossa; transmits the sphenopalatine artery and nasopalatine nerve.

CLINICAL CORRELATES

Nasal polyp is an **inflammatory polyp** that develops from the mucosa of the paranasal sinus, which projects into the nasal cavity and may fill the nasopharynx. The most common cause of nasal polyps is allergic rhinitis. Cortisone or nasal steroid sprays slow polyp growth or will shrink them down temporarily. If medical treatment fails, endoscopic sinus surgery is performed to remove the polyps (polypectomy).

Rhinitis is an inflammation of the nasal mucous membrane, caused by allergies, and has symptoms of runny nose, nasal itching, nasal congestion, and sneezing.

Rhinorrhea (runny nose) is caused by tears draining into the inferior nasal meatus through the nasolacrimal duct. It is also associated with the common cold, hay fever, flu, and allergy, which may cause drainage from the paranasal sinus directly into the nasal cavity.

Rhinoplasty is a type of plastic surgery that changes the shape or size of the nose. **Deviation of the nasal septum** may obstruct the nasal airway and block the openings of the paranasal sinuses.

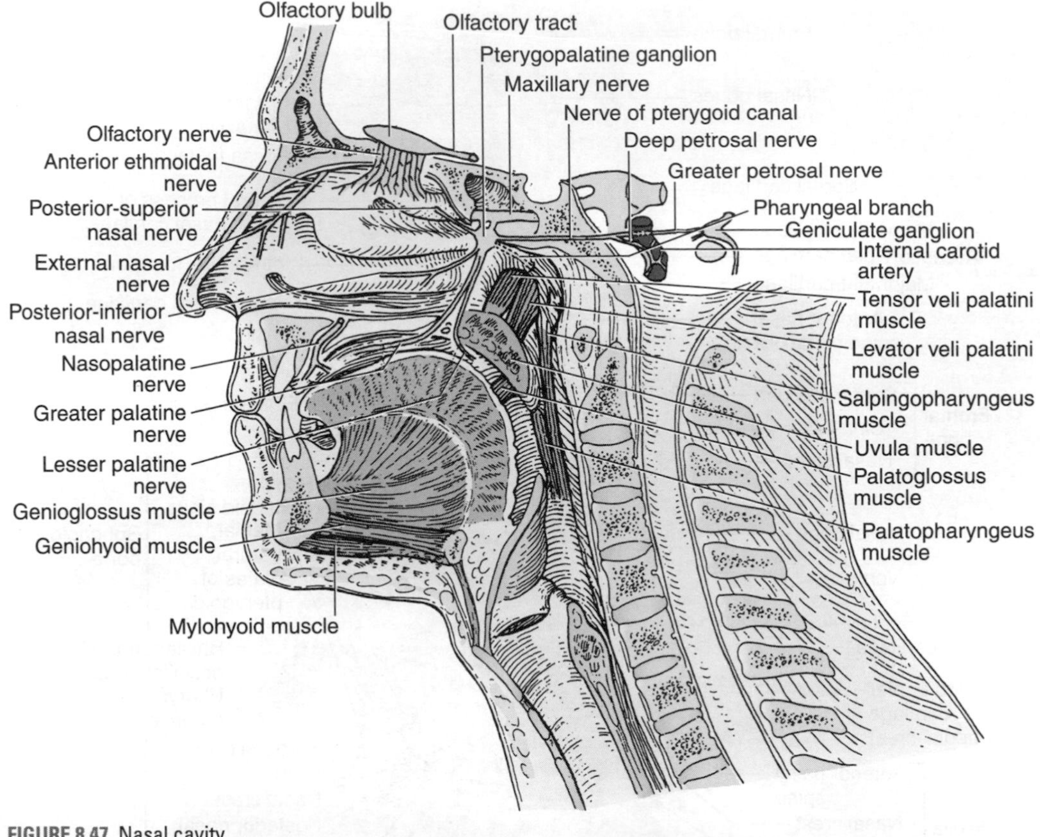

FIGURE 8.47. Nasal cavity.

II. SUBDIVISIONS AND MUCOUS MEMBRANES

A. Vestibule

- Is the dilated part inside the nostril that is bound by the alar cartilages and lined by skin with hairs.

B. Respiratory Region

- Consists of the lower two-thirds of the nasal cavity.
- Warms, moistens, and cleans incoming air with its mucous membrane.

C. Olfactory Region

- Consists of the superior nasal concha and the upper one-third of the nasal septum.
- Is innervated by olfactory nerves, which convey the sense of smell from the olfactory cells and enter the cranial cavity through the cribriform plate of the ethmoid bone to end in the olfactory bulb.

III. BLOOD SUPPLY TO THE NASAL CAVITY

- Occurs via the following routes:
  1. The **lateral nasal branches** of the anterior and posterior ethmoidal arteries of the ophthalmic artery.
  2. The **posterior lateral** nasal and posterior septal branches of the sphenopalatine artery of the maxillary artery.
  3. The **greater palatine branch** (its terminal branch reaches the lower part of the nasal septum through the incisive canal) of the descending palatine artery of the maxillary artery.
  4. The **septal branch** of the superior labial artery of the facial artery and the lateral nasal branch of the facial artery.

CLINICAL CORRELATES

Epistaxis is a **nosebleed** resulting from rupture of the sphenopalatine artery. Nosebleed occurs from nose picking, which tears the veins in the vestibule of the nose. It also occurs from the anterior nasal septum (**Kiesselbach area or plexus**), where branches of the sphenopalatine (from maxillary), greater palatine (from maxillary), anterior ethmoidal (from ophthalmic), and superior labial (from facial) arteries converge. Its treatment includes compression of the nostrils (application of direct pressure to the septal area) and surgical packing.

IV. NERVE SUPPLY TO THE NASAL CAVITY (Figure 8.47)

- **SVA (smell) sensation** is supplied by the olfactory nerves for the olfactory area.
- **GSA sensation** is supplied by the anterior ethmoidal branch of the ophthalmic nerve; the nasopalatine, posterior–superior, and posterior–inferior lateral nasal branches of the maxillary nerve via the pterygopalatine ganglion; and the anterior–superior alveolar branch of the infraorbital nerve.

CLINICAL CORRELATES

Sneeze is an **involuntary, sudden, violent**, and **audible expulsion of air** through the mouth and nose. The afferent limb of the reflex is carried by branches of the maxillary nerve, which convey general sensation from the nasal cavity and palate, and the efferent limb is medicated by the vagus nerve.

V. PARANASAL SINUSES (Figures 8.39 and 8.48)

- Consist of the ethmoidal, frontal, maxillary, and sphenoidal sinuses.
- Are involved in a reduction of weight and resonance for voice.

A. Ethmoidal Sinus

- Consists of numerous **ethmoidal air cells**, which are numerous small cavities within the **ethmoidal labyrinth** between the orbit and the nasal cavity.
- Its infection may erode through the thin orbital plate of the ethmoid bone (lamina papyracea) into the orbit.
- Can be subdivided into the following groups:
  1. **Posterior ethmoidal air cells**, which drain into the superior nasal meatus.
  2. **Middle ethmoidal air cells**, which drain into the summit of the ethmoidal bulla of the middle nasal meatus.
  3. **Anterior ethmoidal air cells**, which drain into the anterior aspect of the hiatus semilunaris in the middle nasal meatus.

CLINICAL CORRELATES

Ethmoidal sinusitis is an inflammation in the ethmoidal sinuses that may erode the medial wall of the orbit, causing an orbital cellulitis that may spread to the cranial cavity.

B. Frontal Sinus

- Lies in the **frontal bone** and opens into the hiatus semilunaris of the middle nasal meatus by way of the frontonasal duct (or infundibulum).
- Is innervated by the supraorbital branch of the ophthalmic nerve.

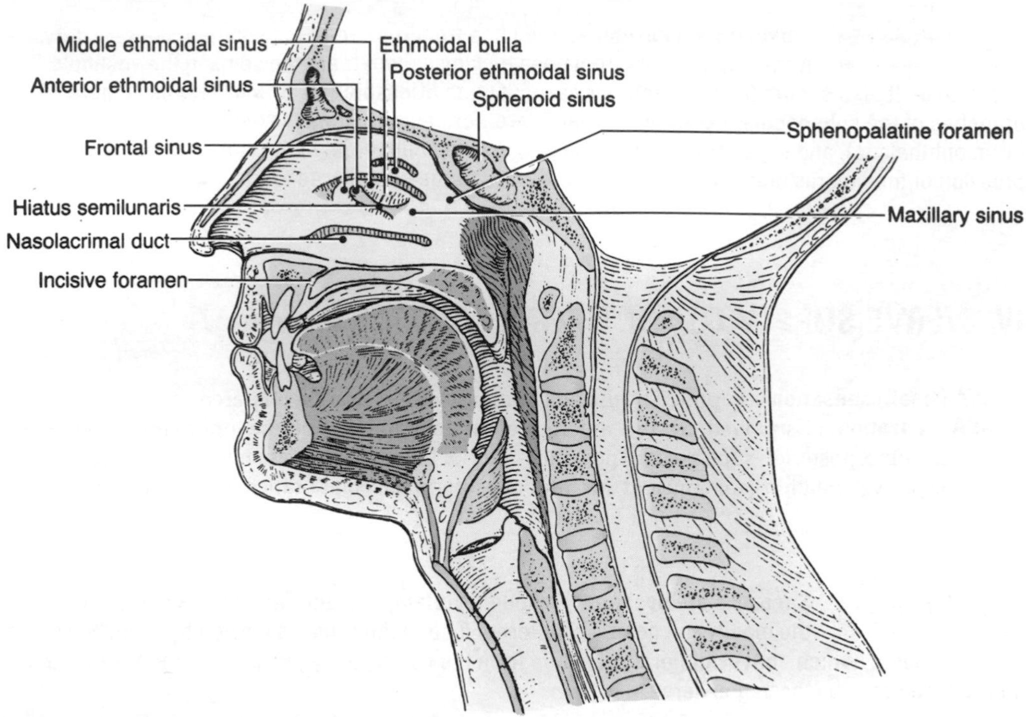

FIGURE 8.48. Openings of the paranasal sinuses.

CLINICAL CORRELATES

Frontal sinusitis is an inflammation in the frontal sinus that may erode the thin bone of the anterior cranial fossa, producing meningitis or brain abscess.

C. Maxillary Sinus

- Is the largest of the paranasal air sinuses and is the only paranasal sinus that may be present at birth.
- Lies in the **maxilla** on each side, lateral to the lateral wall of the nasal cavity and inferior to the floor of the orbit, and drains into the posterior aspect of the hiatus semilunaris in the middle nasal meatus.

CLINICAL CORRELATES

Maxillary sinusitis mimics the clinical signs of maxillary tooth abscess; in most cases, it is related to an infected tooth. Infection may spread from the maxillary sinus to the upper teeth and irritate the nerves to these teeth, causing toothache. It may be confused with toothache because only a thin layer of bone separates the roots of the maxillary teeth from the sinus cavity.

D. Sphenoidal Sinus

- Is contained within the body of the **sphenoid bone**.
- Opens into the **sphenoethmoidal recess** of the nasal cavity.
- Is innervated by branches from the maxillary nerve and by the posterior ethmoidal branch of the nasociliary nerve.
- The pituitary gland lies above this sinus and can be reached by the **transsphenoidal approach**, which follows the nasal septum through the body of the sphenoid. Care must be taken not to damage the cavernous sinus and the internal carotid artery.

CLINICAL CORRELATES

Sphenoidal sinusitis is an infection in the sphenoidal sinus that may spread, may come from the nasal cavity or from the nasopharynx, and may erode the sinus walls to reach the cavernous sinuses, pituitary gland, optic nerve, or brain stem. Close relationships of the sphenoidal sinus with other surrounding structures are clinically important because of potential injury during pituitary surgery and the possible spread of infection to other structures.

VI. DEVELOPMENT OF THE NASAL CAVITY

- **Nasal pits** are ectoderm-lined depressions that result from proliferation of mesenchyme in lateral and medial nasal swellings. The nasal pits deepen, form blind sacs, and rupture to form the nostrils.
- **Oronasal membrane** initially separates nasal cavities from the oral cavity, but its rupture allows communication between nasal and oral cavities through the primitive choanae.
- **Nasal septum** forms as a downgrowth from the medial nasal process.
- **Lateral wall** is formed as the superior, middle, and inferior conchae.
- **Floor of the nasal cavity** is formed by fusion of the medial nasal process (nasal septum) with the palatine processes of the maxilla.
- **Roof of the nose** is formed from the lateral nasal processes.
- **Paranasal sinuses** develop as diverticula of the lateral nasal wall and extend into the maxilla, ethmoid, frontal, and sphenoid bones.

PTERYGOPALATINE FOSSA

I. BOUNDARIES AND OPENINGS

A. Anterior Wall

- Posterior surface of the maxilla or the posterior wall of the maxillary sinus (no openings).

B. Posterior Wall

- Pterygoid process and greater wing of the sphenoid. Openings and their contents include the following:
  1. **Foramen rotundum to middle cranial cavity**: maxillary nerve.
  2. **Pterygoid canal to foramen lacerum**: nerve of the pterygoid canal.
  3. **Palatovaginal (pharyngeal or pterygopalatine) canal to choana**: pharyngeal branch of the maxillary artery and pharyngeal nerve from the pterygopalatine ganglion.

C. Medial Wall

- Perpendicular plate of the palatine. The opening is the **sphenopalatine foramen to the nasal cavity**, which transmits the sphenopalatine artery and nasopalatine nerve.

D. Lateral Wall

- Open (the pterygomaxillary fissure to the infratemporal fossa).

E. Roof

- Greater wing and body of the sphenoid. The opening is the **inferior orbital fissure** to the orbit, which transmits the maxillary nerve.

F. Floor

- Fusion of the maxilla and the pterygoid process of the sphenoid. The opening is the **greater palatine foramen** to the palate, which transmits the greater palatine nerve and vessels.

II. CONTENTS

A. Maxillary Nerve (Figure 8.41)

- Passes through the lateral wall of the cavernous sinus and enters the pterygopalatine fossa through the **foramen rotundum.**
- Is sensory to the skin of the face below the eye but above the upper lip.
- Gives rise to the following branches:

1. Meningeal Branch

- Innervates the dura mater of the middle cranial fossa.

2. Pterygopalatine Nerves (Communicating Branches)

- Are connected to the pterygopalatine ganglion.
- Contain sensory fibers from the trigeminal ganglion.

3. Posterior–Superior Alveolar Nerves

- Descend through the pterygopalatine fissure and enter the posterior–superior alveolar canals.
- Innervate the cheeks, gums, molar teeth, and maxillary sinus.

4. Zygomatic Nerve

- Enters the orbit through the **inferior orbital fissure** and divides into the zygomaticotemporal and zygomaticofacial branches, which supply the skin over the temporal region and over the zygomatic bone, respectively.
- Transmits postganglionic parasympathetic and sympathetic GVE fibers to the lacrimal gland through the zygomaticotemporal branch, which joins the terminal part of the lacrimal nerve.

5. Infraorbital Nerve

- Enters the orbit through the inferior orbital fissure and runs through the infraorbital groove and canal.
- Emerges through the infraorbital foramen and divides in the face into the inferior palpebral, nasal, and superior labial branches.
- Gives rise to the middle and anterior–superior alveolar nerves, which supply the maxillary sinus, teeth, and gums.

6. Branches (Sensory) via the Pterygopalatine Ganglion

- Contain GSA fibers as branches of the maxillary nerve but also carry general visceral afferent (GVA) and GVE fibers from the facial nerve to the nasal mucosa and the palate.

(a) Orbital Branches

- Supply the periosteum of the orbit and the mucous membrane of the posterior ethmoidal and sphenoidal sinuses.

(b) Pharyngeal Branch

- Runs in the pharyngeal (palatovaginal) canal and supplies the roof of the pharynx and the sphenoidal sinuses.

(c) Posterior–Superior Lateral Nasal Branches

- Enter the nasal cavity through the sphenopalatine foramen and innervate the posterior part of the septum, the posterior ethmoidal air cells, and the superior and middle conchae.

(d) Greater Palatine Nerve

- Descends through the palatine canal and emerges through the greater palatine foramen to innervate the hard palate and the inner surface of the maxillary gingiva.
- Gives rise to the posterior–inferior lateral nasal branches.

(e) Lesser Palatine Nerve

- Descends through the palatine canal and emerges through the lesser palatine foramen to innervate the soft palate and the palatine tonsil.
- Contains sensory (GVA and taste) fibers (for the soft palate) that belong to the facial nerve and have their cell bodies in the geniculate ganglion.
- Also contains postganglionic parasympathetic and sympathetic GVE fibers that come from the facial nerve via the greater petrosal and vidian nerves and supply mucous glands in the nasal cavity and the palate.

(f) Nasopalatine Nerve

- Runs obliquely downward and forward on the septum, supplying the septum, and passes through the incisive canal to supply the hard palate and the gum.

B. Pterygopalatine Ganglion (Figures 8.47 and 9.6)

- Is formed by neuron cell bodies of parasympathetic postganglionic GVE fibers and lies in the pterygopalatine fossa just below the maxillary nerve, lateral to the sphenopalatine foramen and anterior to the pterygoid canal.
- Receives preganglionic parasympathetic fibers from the facial nerve by way of the greater petrosal nerve and the nerve of the pterygoid canal.
- Sends postganglionic parasympathetic fibers to the nasal and palatine glands and to the lacrimal gland by way of the maxillary, zygomatic, and lacrimal nerves.
- Also receives postganglionic sympathetic fibers (by way of the deep petrosal nerve and the nerve of the pterygoid canal), which are distributed with the postganglionic parasympathetic fibers.

CLINICAL CORRELATES **Lesion of the nerve of the pterygoid canal** results in vasodilation; a lack of secretion of the lacrimal, nasal, and palatine glands; and a loss of general and taste sensation of the palate.

C. Pterygopalatine Part of the Maxillary Artery

- Supplies blood to the maxilla and maxillary teeth, nasal cavities, and palate.
- Gives rise to the posterior–superior alveolar artery, infraorbital artery (which gives rise to anterior–superior alveolar branches), descending palatine artery (which gives rise to the lesser palatine and greater palatine branches), artery of the pterygoid canal, pharyngeal artery, and sphenopalatine artery.

LARYNX

I. INTRODUCTION

- Is the organ of voice production and the part of the respiratory tract between the lower part of the pharynx and the trachea.
- Acts as a **compound sphincter** to prevent the passage of food or drink into the airway in swallowing and to close the **rima glottidis** during the Valsalva maneuver (buildup of air pressure during coughing, sneezing, micturition, defecation, or parturition).
- Regulates the flow of air to and from the lungs for vocalization (phonation).
- Forms a framework of cartilage for the attachment of ligaments and muscles.

CLINICAL CORRELATES **Laryngitis** is an **inflammation of the mucous membrane of the larynx**. It is characterized by dryness and soreness of the throat, hoarseness, cough, and dysphagia.

II. CARTILAGES (Figure 8.49)

A. Thyroid Cartilage (See Deep Neck and Prevertebral Region: I. E.)

- Is a **single hyaline cartilage** that forms a median elevation called the **laryngeal prominence (Adam's apple)**, which is particularly apparent in males.

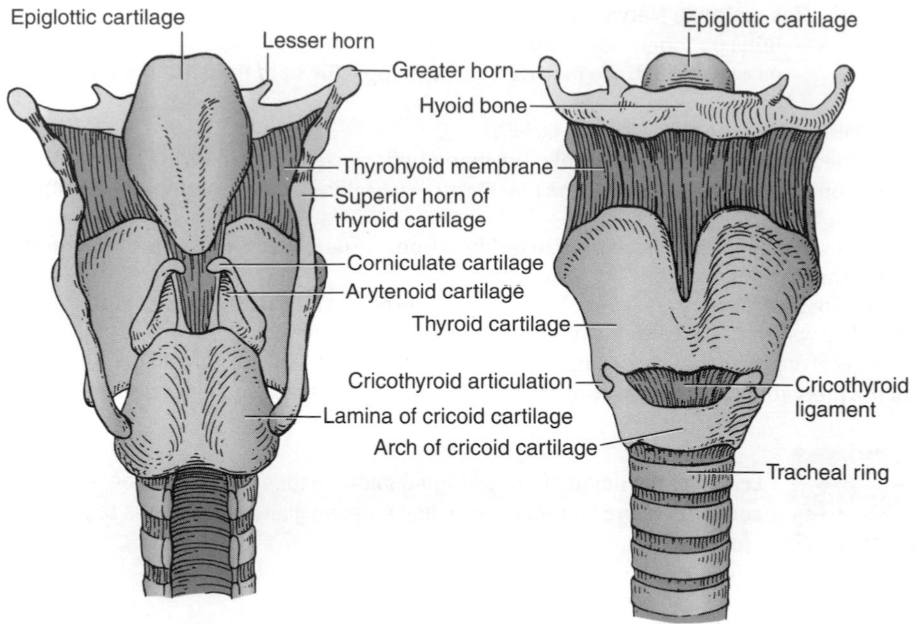

FIGURE 8.49. Cartilages of the larynx.

- Has an **oblique line** on the lateral surface of its lamina that gives attachment for the inferior pharyngeal constrictor, sternothyroid, and thyrohyoid muscles.

B. Cricoid Cartilage

- Is a **single hyaline cartilage** that is shaped like a signet ring.
- Is at the level of CV6 and articulates with the thyroid cartilage. Its lower border marks the end of the pharynx and larynx.

C. Epiglottis

- Is a **single elastic cartilage**.
- Is a spoon-shaped plate that lies behind the root of the tongue and forms the superior part of the anterior wall of the larynx.
- Its lower end is attached to the back of the thyroid cartilage.

CLINICAL CORRELATES **Epiglottitis** is an inflammation or acute mucosal swelling of the epiglottis, which may cause a life-threatening airway obstruction, especially in children.

D. Arytenoid Cartilages

- Are **paired elastic and hyaline cartilages**.
- Are shaped liked pyramids, with bases that articulate with and rotate on the cricoid cartilage.
- Have **vocal processes**, which give attachment to the vocal ligament and vocalis muscle, and **muscular processes**, which give attachment to the thyroarytenoid muscle and the lateral and posterior cricoarytenoid muscles.
- Sits on the **top of the cricoid cartilage** and **rotates** to change the opening of the vocal folds (the rima glottidis).

E. Corniculate Cartilages

- Are **paired elastic cartilages** that lie on the apices of the arytenoid cartilages.
- Are enclosed within the **aryepiglottic folds** of mucous membrane.

F. Cuneiform Cartilages

- Are **paired elastic cartilages** that lie in the aryepiglottic folds anterior to the corniculate cartilages.

III. LIGAMENTS OF THE LARYNX

A. Thyrohyoid Membrane

- Extends from the thyroid cartilage to the medial surface of the hyoid bone.
- Its middle (thicker) part is called the **middle thyrohyoid ligament**, and its lateral portion is pierced by the internal laryngeal nerve and the superior laryngeal vessels.

CLINICAL CORRELATES **Laryngotomy** is an **operative opening into the larynx** through the cricothyroid membrane (cricothyrotomy), through the thyroid cartilage (thyrotomy), or through the thyrohyoid membrane (superior laryngotomy). It is performed when severe edema or an impacted foreign body calls for rapid admission of air into the larynx and trachea.

B. Cricothyroid Ligament

- Extends from the arch of the cricoid cartilage to the thyroid cartilage and the vocal processes of the arytenoid cartilages.

C. Vocal Ligament

- Extends from the posterior surface of the thyroid cartilage to the vocal process of the arytenoid cartilage, and is considered the upper border of the **conus elasticus**.

D. Vestibular (Ventricular) Ligament

- Extends from the thyroid cartilage to the anterior lateral surface of the arytenoid cartilage.

E. Conus Elasticus (Cricovocal Ligament)

- Is the paired lateral portion of the fibroelastic membrane that extends between the superior border of the entire arch of the cricoid cartilage and the vocal ligaments.
- Is formed by the cricothyroid, median cricothyroid, and vocal ligaments.

IV. CAVITIES AND FOLDS (Figure 8.50)

- The laryngeal cavity is divided into three portions by the vestibular and vocal folds: the vestibule, ventricle, and infraglottic cavity.

A. Vestibule

- Extends from the laryngeal inlet to the vestibular (ventricular) folds.

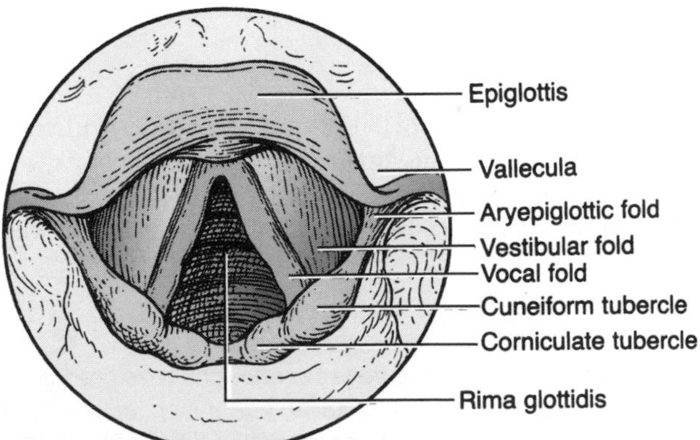

FIGURE 8.50. Interior view of the larynx.

B. Ventricles

- Extend between the vestibular fold and the vocal fold.

C. Infraglottic Cavity

- Extends from the rima glottidis to the lower border of the cricoid cartilage.

D. Rima Glottidis

- Is the space between the vocal folds and arytenoid cartilages.
- Is the narrowest part of the laryngeal cavity.

CLINICAL CORRELATES

Laryngeal obstruction (choking) is caused by aspirated foods, which are usually lodged at the rima glottidis. It can be released by compression of the abdomen to expel air from the lungs and thus dislodge the foods (e.g., the Valsalva maneuver).

Valsalva maneuver is forcible exhalation effort against a closed airway (a closed glottis, nose, or mouth); the resultant increase in intrathoracic pressure impedes venous return to the heart. This maneuver causes a trapping of blood in the great veins, preventing it from entering the right atrium. When the breath is released, there is a drop in intrathoracic pressure, the trapped blood is quickly propelled through the heart producing a reflexic increase in heart rate and blood pressure followed by a drop to normal heart rate shortly thereafter. There is a resultant tachycardia (increase in heart rate) to compensate for decreased cardiac output.

E. Vestibular Folds (False Vocal Cords)

- Extend from the thyroid cartilage above the vocal ligament to the arytenoid cartilage.

F. Vocal Folds (True Vocal Cords)

- Extend from the angle of the thyroid cartilage to the vocal processes of the arytenoid cartilages.
- Contain the **vocal ligament** near their free margin and the **vocalis muscle**, which forms the bulk of the vocal fold.
- Are important in **voice production** because they control the stream of air passing through the rima glottidis.
- Alter the shape and size of the **rima glottidis** by movement of the arytenoids to facilitate respiration and phonation. (The rima glottidis is wide during inspiration and narrow and wedge-shaped during expiration and sound production.)

V. MUSCLES (Figure 8.51; Table 8.9)

VI. INNERVATION (FIGURE 8.52)

A. Recurrent Laryngeal Nerve

- Innervates all of the intrinsic muscles of the larynx except the cricothyroid, which is innervated by the external laryngeal branch of the superior laryngeal branch of the vagus nerve.
- Supplies sensory innervation below the vocal cord.
- Has a terminal portion above the lower border of the cricoid cartilage called the **inferior laryngeal nerve**.

CLINICAL CORRELATES

Lesion of the recurrent laryngeal nerve could be produced during thyroidectomy or cricothyrotomy or by aortic aneurysm and may cause respiratory obstruction, hoarseness, inability to speak, and loss of sensation below the vocal cord.

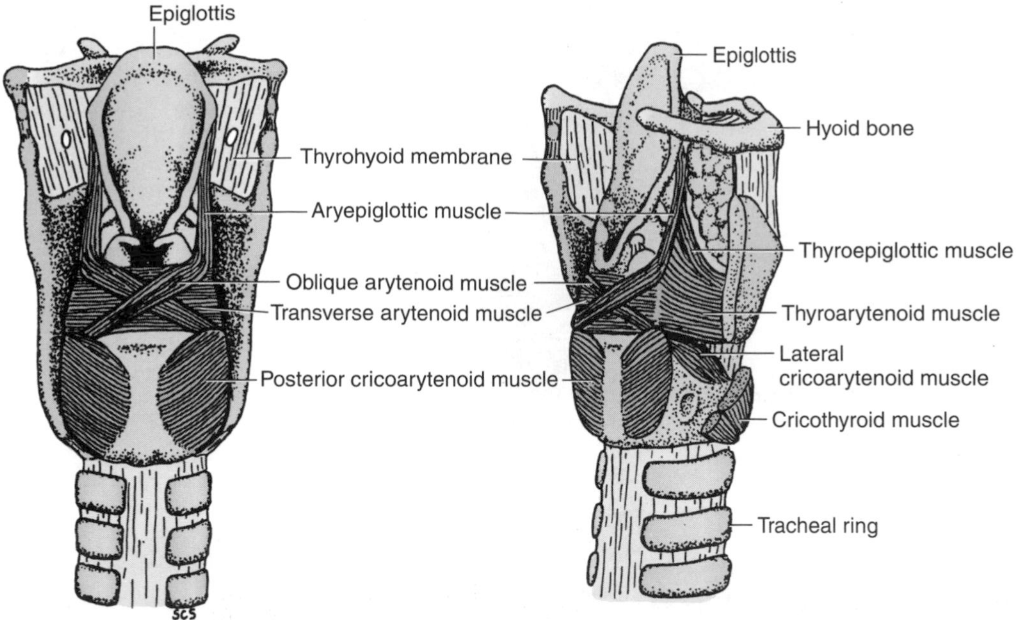

FIGURE 8.51. Muscles of the larynx.

table 8.9 Muscles of the Larynx

Muscle	Origin	Insertion	Nerve	Action on Vocal Cords
Cricothyroid	Arch of cricoid cartilage	Inferior horn and lower lamina of thyroid cartilage	External laryngeal	Tenses; adducts; elongates
Posterior cricoarytenoid*	Posterior surface of lamina of cricoid cartilage	Muscular process of arytenoid cartilage	Recurrent laryngeal	Abducts; opens rima glottidis by rotating arytenoid cartilage laterally
Lateral cricoarytenoid	Arch of cricoid cartilage	Muscular process of arytenoid cartilage	Recurrent laryngeal	Adducts; closes rima glottidis by rotating arytenoid cartilage medially
Transverse arytenoids	Posterior surface of arytenoid cartilage	Opposite arytenoid cartilage	Recurrent laryngeal	Adducts; closes rima glottidis
Oblique arytenoids	Muscular process of arytenoid cartilage	Apex of opposite arytenoids	Recurrent laryngeal	Adducts; closes rima glottidis
Aryepiglottic	Apex of arytenoid cartilage	Side of epiglottic cartilage	Recurrent laryngeal	Adducts
Thyroarytenoid	Inner surface of thyroid lamina	Anterolateral surface of arytenoid cartilage	Recurrent laryngeal	Adducts; relaxes
Thyroepiglottics	Anteromedial surface of lamina of thyroid cartilage	Lateral margin of epiglottic cartilage	Recurrent laryngeal	Adducts
Vocalis	Angle between two laminae of thyroid cartilage	Vocal process of arytenoid cartilage	Recurrent laryngeal	Adducts; tenses (anterior part); relaxes (posterior part); controls pitch

*The posterior cricoarytenoid muscle draws the muscular process of the arytenoid cartilage posteriorly and thereby rotates the vocal process laterally, resulting in opening of the rima glottidis, whereas the lateral cricoarytenoid muscle draws the muscular process anteriorly and thereby rotates the vocal process medially.

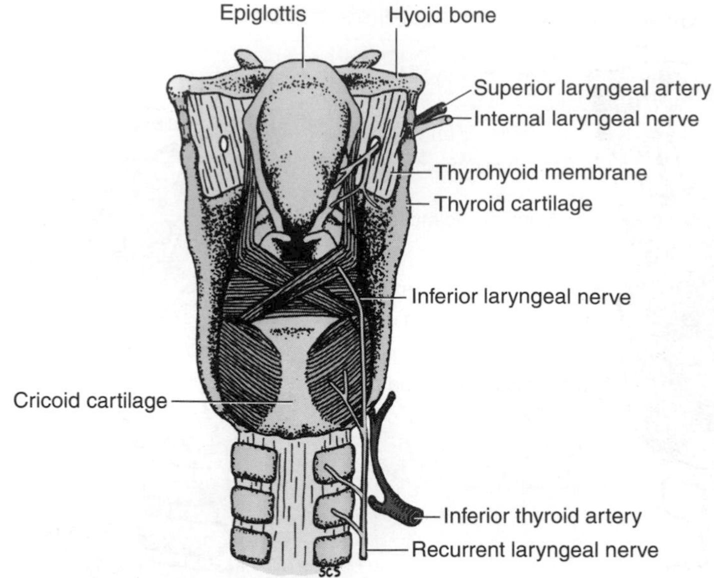

FIGURE 8.52. Nerve supply to the larynx.

B. Superior Laryngeal Nerve

- Is a branch of the vagus nerve and divides into the internal and external laryngeal branches.

C. Internal Laryngeal Nerve

- Innervates the mucous membrane above the vocal cord and taste buds on the epiglottis.
- Is accompanied by the superior laryngeal artery and pierces the thyrohyoid membrane.

CLINICAL CORRELATES

Lesion of the internal laryngeal nerve results in loss of sensation above the vocal cord and loss of taste on the epiglottis.

D. External Laryngeal Nerve

- Innervates the cricothyroid and inferior pharyngeal constrictor (cricopharyngeus part) muscles.
- Is accompanied by the superior thyroid artery.

CLINICAL CORRELATES

Lesion of the external laryngeal nerve may occur during **thyroidectomy** because the nerve accompanies the superior thyroid artery. It causes **paralysis of the cricothyroid muscle**, resulting in paralysis of the laryngeal muscles and thus inability to lengthen the vocal cord and loss of the tension of the vocal cord. Such stresses to the vocal cord cause a fatigued voice and a weak hoarseness.

VII. DEVELOPMENT OF THE LARYNX

- The respiratory diverticulum (laryngotracheal diverticulum) forms as a ventral epithelial outgrowth of the foregut, and its opening becomes the laryngeal orifice.
- The diverticulum elongates in the caudal direction and soon become separated from the foregut by the esophagotracheal septum. The ventral portion forms the larynx, trachea, and lung buds, while the dorsal part forms the esophagus.

- The laryngeal epithelium and glands are derived from **endoderm** of the cranial part of the laryngotracheal tube.
- The laryngeal **cartilages** and the laryngeal **muscles** are derived from **somitomeric mesoderm** of pharyngeal (branchial) arches 4 and 6, and thus, the laryngeal muscles are innervated by branches of the vagus nerve such as the superior laryngeal and recurrent laryngeal nerve, respectively.

EAR

I. EXTERNAL EAR (Figure 8.53)

- Consists of the auricle and the external acoustic meatus and receives sound waves.

A. Auricle

- Consists of cartilage connected to the skull by ligaments and muscles and is covered by skin.
- Funnels sound waves into the external auditory meatus.
- Receives sensory nerves from the auricular branch of the **vagus** and **facial** nerves and the **greater auricular** nerve, auriculotemporal branch of the **trigeminal** nerve, and **lesser occipital** nerves.
- Receives blood from the superficial temporal and posterior auricular arteries.
- Has the following features:

1. Helix
- The slightly curved rim of the auricle.

2. Antihelix
- A broader curved eminence internal to the helix, which divides the auricle into an outer scaphoid fossa and the deeper concha.

3. Concha
- The deep cavity in front of the antihelix.

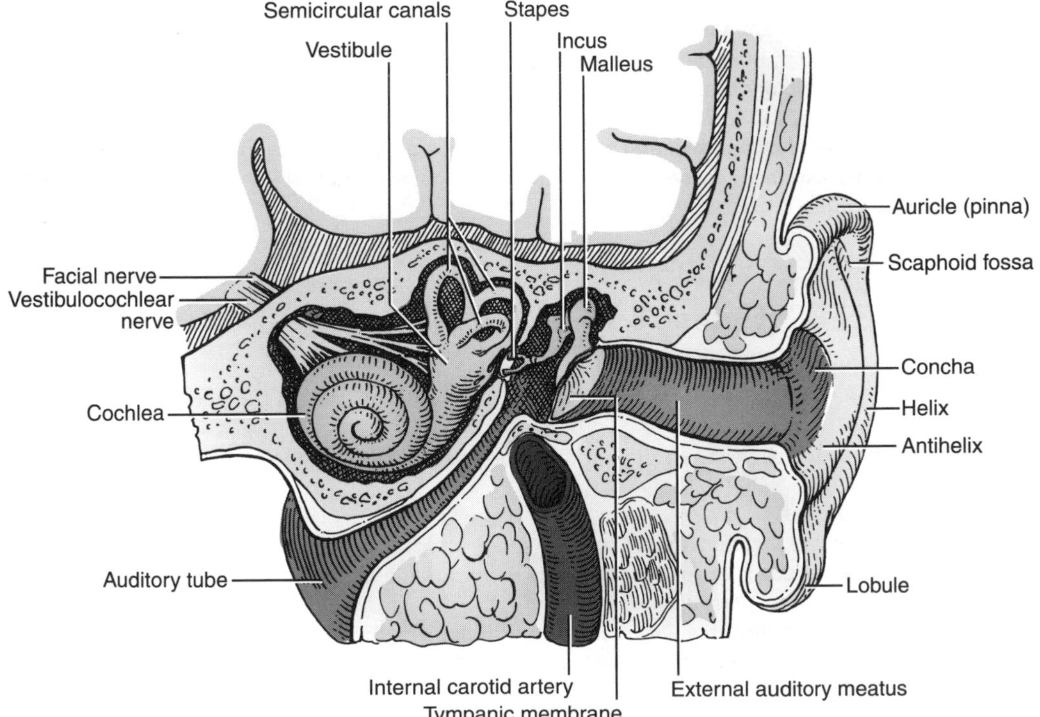

FIGURE 8.53. External, middle, and inner ear.

4. **Tragus**
   - A small projection from the anterior portion of the external ear anterior to the concha
5. **Lobule**
   - A structure made up of areolar tissue and fat but no cartilage.

B. External Acoustic (Auditory) Meatus

- Is approximately 2.5 cm long, extending from the concha to the tympanic membrane.
- Its external one-third is formed by cartilage, and the internal two-thirds is formed by bone. The cartilaginous portion is wider than the bony portion and has numerous **ceruminous glands** that produce earwax.
- Is innervated by the auriculotemporal branch of the **trigeminal** nerve and the auricular branch of the **vagus** nerve, which is joined by a branch of the **facial** nerve and the **glossopharyngeal** nerve.
- Receives blood from the superficial temporal, posterior auricular, and maxillary arteries (a deep auricular branch).

C. Tympanic Membrane (Eardrum)

- Lies obliquely across the end of the meatus sloping medially from posterosuperiorly to anteroinferiorly; thus, the anterior–inferior wall is longer than the posterior–superior wall.
- Consists of **three layers**: an outer (cutaneous), an intermediate (fibrous), and an inner (mucous) layer.
- Has a thickened fibrocartilaginous ring at the greater part of its circumference, which is fixed in the tympanic sulcus at the inner end of the meatus.
- Has a small triangular portion between the anterior and posterior malleolar folds called the **pars flaccida** (deficient ring and lack of fibrous layer). The remainder of the membrane is called the **pars tensa**.
- Contains the **cone of light**, which is a triangular reflection of light seen in the anterior–inferior quadrant.
- Contains the most depressed center point of the concavity, called the **umbo** (Latin for "knob").
- Conducts sound waves to the middle ear.
- Its external (lateral) concave surface is covered by skin and is innervated by the auriculotemporal branch of the **trigeminal** nerve and the auricular branch of the **vagus** nerve. The auricular branch is joined by branches of the **glossopharyngeal** and **facial** nerves. This surface is supplied by the deep auricular artery of the maxillary artery.
- Its internal (medial) surface is covered by mucous membrane, is innervated by the tympanic branch of the **glossopharyngeal** nerve, and serves as an attachment for the handle of the **malleus**. This surface receives blood from the auricular branch of the occipital artery and the anterior tympanic artery.

II. MIDDLE EAR (Figures 8.54 to 8.55)

- Consists of the tympanic cavity with its ossicles and is located within the petrous portion of the temporal bone.
- Transmits the sound waves from air to auditory ossicles and then to the inner ear.

A. Tympanic (Middle Ear) Cavity

- Includes the **tympanic cavity proper** (the space internal to the tympanic membrane) and the **epitympanic recess** (the space superior to the tympanic membrane that contains the head of the malleus and the body of the incus).
- Communicates anteriorly with the nasopharynx via the **auditory (eustachian) tube** and posteriorly with the **mastoid air cells** and the **mastoid antrum** through the **aditus ad antrum**.
- Is traversed by the chorda tympani and lesser petrosal nerve.

1. **Boundaries of the Tympanic Cavity**
   - **Roof**: tegmen tympani.
   - **Floor**: jugular fossa.

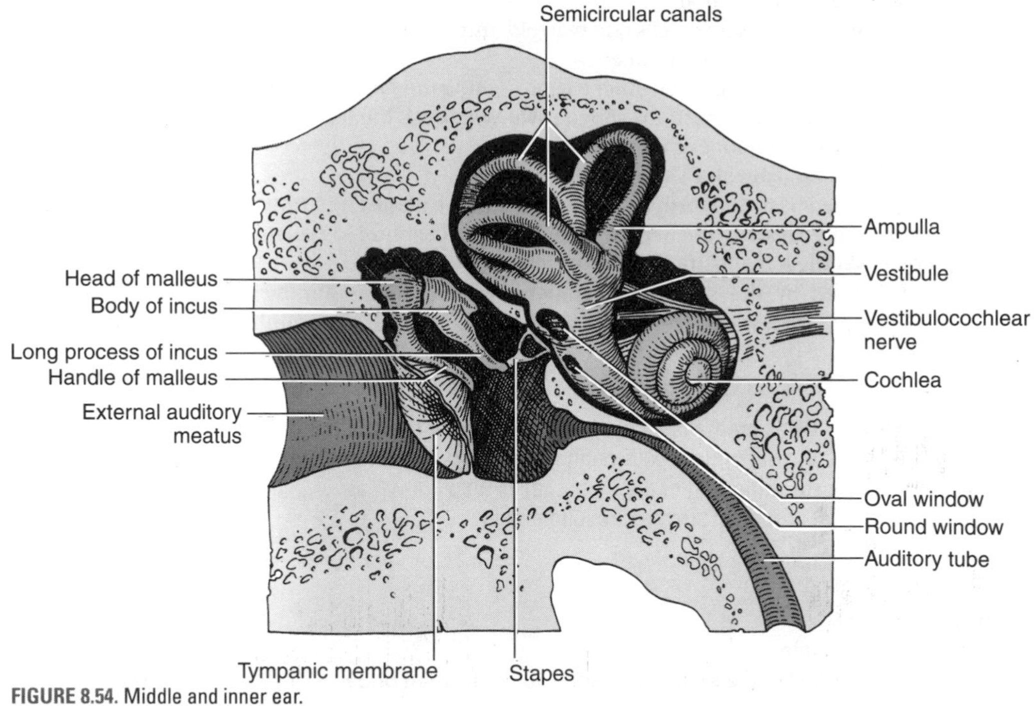

FIGURE 8.54. Middle and inner ear.

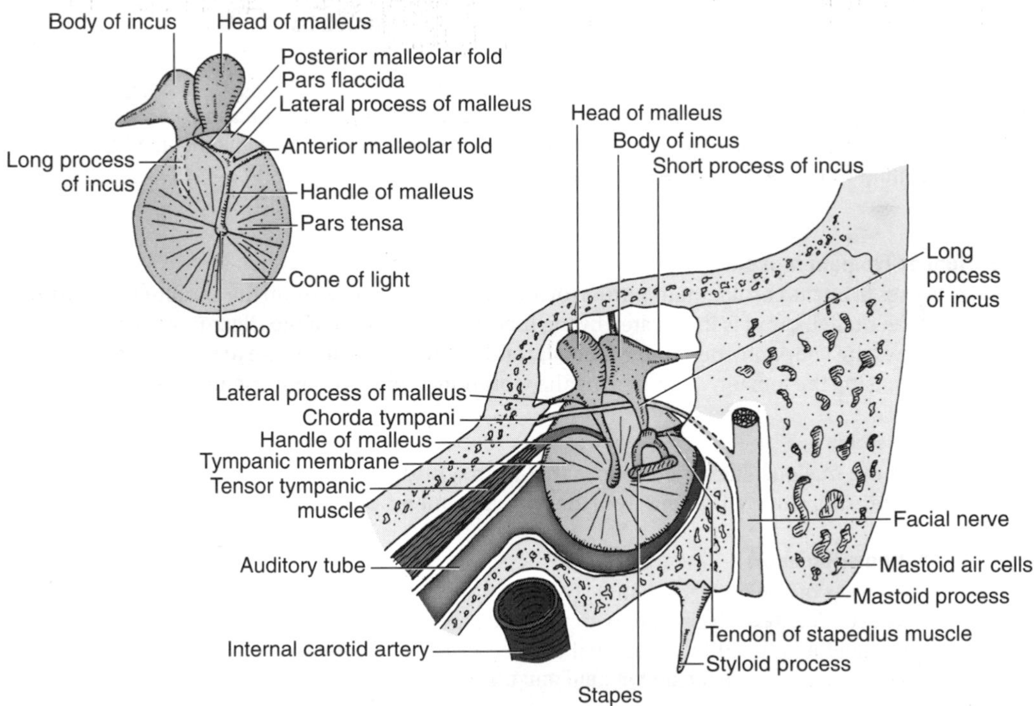

FIGURE 8.55. Ossicles of the middle ear and tympanic membrane.

- **Anterior**: carotid canal.
- **Posterior**: mastoid air cells and mastoid antrum through the aditus ad antrum.
- **Lateral**: tympanic membrane.
- **Medial**: lateral wall of the inner ear, presenting the **promontory** formed by the basal turn of the cochlea, the fenestra vestibuli (**oval window**), the fenestra cochlea (**round window**), and the prominence of the facial canal.

2. **Oval Window (Fenestra Vestibuli)**
   - Is pushed back and forth by the **footplate of the stapes** and **transmits the sonic vibrations** of the ossicles into the perilymph of the scala vestibuli in the inner ear.
3. **Round Window (Fenestra Cochlea or Tympani)**
   - Is closed by the secondary tympanic (mucous) membrane of the middle ear and accommodates the pressure waves transmitted to the perilymph of the scala tympani.

CLINICAL CORRELATES **Otitis media** is a condition of **middle ear infection** that may be spread from the nasopharynx through the auditory tube, causing temporary or permanent deafness. **Otitis externa**, infection of the ear canal, is also known as swimmer's ear, which is usually caused by a bacterial organism such as Pseudomonas.

B. Muscles

1. **Stapedius Muscle**
   - Is the **smallest of the skeletal muscles** in the human body.
   - Arises from the pyramidal eminence, and its tendon emerges from the eminence.
   - Inserts on the neck of the stapes, and is innervated by a branch of the facial nerve.
   - Pulls the head of the stapes posteriorly, thereby tilting the base of the stapes.
   - Prevents (or reduces) excessive oscillation of the stapes and thus protects the inner ear from injury from a loud noise, and its paralysis results in **hyperacusis**.

CLINICAL CORRELATES **Hyperacusis (hyperacusia)** is **excessive acuteness of hearing**, because of paralysis of the stapedius muscle (causing uninhibited movements of the stapes), resulting from a lesion of the facial nerve.

2. **Tensor Tympani Muscle**
   - Arises from the cartilaginous portion of the auditory tube, inserts on the handle (manubrium) of the malleus, and is innervated by the mandibular branch of the trigeminal nerve.
   - Draws the tympanic membrane medially and tightens it (in response to loud noises), thereby increasing the tension and reducing the vibration of the tympanic membrane.

C. Auditory Ossicles

- Include the malleus, incus, and stapes that form a bridge by synovial joints in the middle ear cavity, transmit sonic vibrations from the tympanic membrane to the inner ear, and amplify the force.

1. **Malleus (Hammer)**
   - Consists of a head, neck, handle (manubrium), and anterior and lateral processes.
   - Its rounded **head** articulates with the incus in the epitympanic recess.
   - Its **handle** is fused to the medial surface of the tympanic membrane and serves as an attachment for the **tensor tympani muscle**.
2. **Incus (Anvil)**
   - Consists of a body and two processes (crura). Its **long process** descends vertically, parallel to the handle of the malleus, and articulates with the stapes.
   - Its **short process** extends horizontally backward to the fossa of the incus and provides the attachment for the posterior ligament of the incus.

3. **Stapes (Stirrup)**
   - Consists of a head and neck, two processes (crura), and a base (footplate).
   - Its **neck** provides insertion of the **stapedius muscle**.
   - Has a hole through which the stapedial artery is transmitted in the embryo; this hole is obturated by a thin membrane in the adult.
   - Its base (**footplate**) is attached by the annular ligament to the margin of the **oval window** (fenestra vestibuli). Abnormal ossification between the footplate and the oval window (**otosclerosis**) limits the movement of the stapes, causing deafness.

D. Auditory (Pharyngotympanic or Eustachian) Tube

- Connects the middle ear to the nasopharynx.
- Allows air to enter or leave the middle ear cavity and thus balances the pressure in the middle ear with atmospheric pressure, allowing free movement of the tympanic membrane.
- Has cartilaginous portion that remains closed except during swallowing or yawning.
- Is opened by the simultaneous contraction of the tensor veli palatini and salpingopharyngeus muscles.

E. Sensory Nerve and Blood Supply to the Middle Ear

- Is innervated by the **tympanic** branch of the **glossopharyngeal** nerve, which forms the **tympanic plexus** with **caroticotympanic** nerves from the internal carotid plexus of sympathetic fibers. The tympanic nerve continues beyond the plexus as the **lesser petrosal** nerve, which transmits preganglionic parasympathetic fibers to the otic ganglion.
- Receives blood from the stylomastoid branch of the posterior auricular artery and the anterior tympanic branch of the maxillary artery.

CLINICAL CORRELATES

Otosclerosis is a condition of **abnormal bone formation** around the stapes and the oval window, limiting the movement of the stapes and thus resulting in **progressive conduction deafness**.

Conductive deafness is hearing impairment caused by a **defect of a sound-conducting apparatus** such as the auditory meatus, eardrum, or ossicles.

Neural or sensorineural deafness is hearing impairment because of a lesion of the auditory nerve or the central afferent neural pathway.

III. INNER EAR (Figure 8.54)

- Consists of the **acoustic apparatus**, the cochlea housing the cochlear duct for auditory sense, and the **vestibular apparatus**, the vestibule housing the utricle and saccule, and the semicircular canals housing the semicircular ducts for the sense of balance and position.
- Is the place where vibrations are transduced to specific nerve impulses that are transmitted through the acoustic nerve to the central nervous system.
- Is composed of the bony labyrinth and the membranous labyrinth.

A. Bony Labyrinth

- Consists of three parts: the **vestibule**, the **semicircular canals**, and the **cochlea**, all of which contain the **perilymph**, in which the membranous labyrinth is suspended.
- The **vestibule** is the central part (cavity) of the bony labyrinth and contains two membranous parts, the **utricle** and **saccule**. It communicates with the cochlea anteriorly and the semicircular canals posteriorly.
- The **semicircular canals** (anterior, posterior, and lateral) are arranged in planes at right angles to each other. Each canal forms two-thirds of a circle, has a dilated **ampulla**, and opens into the posterior part of the vestibule.

- The **cochlea** resembles a snail shell, is concerned with hearing, contains a membranous cochlea duct (**scala media**), and opens into the anterior part of the vestibule. The **spiral canal** of the cochlea begins at the vestibule, makes **two-and-a-half turns** around the central bony core, the **modiolus**, and is subdivided into two passages: (a) the upper **scala vestibule**, which begins in the vestibule and receives the **vibrations** transmitted to the perilymph at the **oval window**, and (b) the lower **scala tympani**, which communicates with the scala vestibule through a small opening, the **helicotrema** at the apex of the cochlea and ends at the **round window**, at which the sound pressure waves are dissipated. The screw-shaped modiolus transmits the cochlear nerve and contains the spiral ganglion.

B. Membranous Labyrinth

- Is suspended in perilymph within the bony labyrinth, is filled with **endolymph**, and contains the sensory organs.
- The **utricle** and **saccule** are dilated membranous sacs of the vestibule and house sense organs called **maculae**. The **macula** of the **utricle** detects a horizontal acceleration (orientation), and the **macula** of the **saccule** detects vertical orientation.
- Its **semicircular ducts** consist of anterior (superior), lateral, and posterior ducts, and their dilated ends called **ampullae**, house sensory organs (epithelial areas), the **cristae ampulares**, which detect rotational or angular acceleration of the head. The cristae ampullares contain neuroepithelial cells, the hairs of which project into a gelatinous mass (cupula).
- Its **cochlear duct (scala media)** is wedged between the scala vestibuli and scala tympani and contains endolymph and the spiral **organ of Corti**, with receptor cells (hair cells) for auditory stimuli (the sense of hearing). The cochlear duct is connected with the sacule by a narrow canal, the ductus reunions.

IV. HEARING AND EQUILIBRIUM

A. Hearing

- **Sound waves** entering the external auditory meatus **induce vibration of the tympanic membrane.** These waves, in turn, **vibrate** (stimulate) the **ossicles**, which amplify the intensity of the sound waves. The **vibrations of the stapes** against the oval window **transmit the sound waves to the perilymph** in the scala vestibule and then in the scala tympani through the helicotrema. Sound waves could be **transmitted across** the **vestibular (Reissner) membrane to the endolymph** of the cochlear duct. **Vibrations** or pressure waves of the perilymph and of endolymph **stimulate** oscillatory movements of the **basilar membrane** and hence **hair cells** in the organ of Corti on the basilar membrane, which **convert** (transduce) **sound waves to nerve impulses** that travel via the cochlear nerve to the brain.

B. Equilibrium

- **Sound waves** entering the **vestibular apparatus** include the three semicircular canals, the utricle and the saccule, which **detect** sensations regarding **body position and equilibrium. Sensory hair cells** within the vestibular apparatus transmit information about the position of the head (produced by the **flow of endolymph)** to **the brain** via the vestibular nerve.

CLINICAL CORRELATES **Ménière disease (endolymphatic or labyrinthine hydrops)** is characterized by a **loss of balance (vertigo), tinnitus** (ringing or buzzing in the ears), **progressive hearing loss** resulting from hydrops of the endolymphatic duct or **edema of the labyrinth** (excessive amounts of endolymph that distort the membranous labyrinth) or inflammation of the vestibular division of the vestibulocochlear nerve, and nausea and vomiting.

V. DEVELOPMENT OF THE EAR

A. External Ear

- **Pharyngeal groove 1** forms the external auditory meatus and tympanic membrane.
- **Auricular hillocks** form the auricle.

B. Middle Ear

- **Pharyngeal arch 1** forms the incus, malleus, tensor tympani muscle, and trigeminal nerve.
- **Pharyngeal arch 2** forms the stapes, stapedius muscle, and facial nerve.
- **Pharyngeal pouch 1** forms the auditory tube and middle ear cavity.
- **Pharyngeal membrane 1** forms the tympanic membrane.

C. Internal Ear

- Develops from the otic placodes (thickening of embryonic ectoderm), which invaginate to form the otic or auditory vesicles (otocysts).

1. **Auditory vesicle (otocyst)** is the primordium of the internal ear and is derived from the surface ectoderm.
   - **Utricular portion** forms the utricle, semicircular ducts, and vestibular ganglion of CN VIII.
   - **Saccular portion** forms the saccule, cochlear duct, and spiral ganglion of CN VIII.
   - **Vestibular pouch** forms the semicircular canals, the utricle, and endolymphatic duct.
   - **Cochlear pouch** gives rise to the saccule, which forms a diverticulum that, in turn, forms the cochlear duct.
2. **Otic capsule** develops from the mesenchyme around the otocyst and forms the perilymphatic space, which develops into the scala tympani and scala vestibule. The cartilaginous otic capsule ossifies to form the bony labyrinth.

HIGH-YIELD TOPICS

- The **posterior cervical triangle** is bounded by the trapezius, sternocleidomastoid, and clavicle and is subdivided by the posterior belly of the omohyoid into the occipital and subclavian triangles. It contains the spinal accessory nerve; external jugular vein; cervical plexus; roots and trunks of the brachial plexus; and subclavian, transverse cervical, and suprascapular arteries.
- **Torticollis (wryneck)** is a spasmodic **contraction or shortening of the neck muscles**, producing twisting of the neck with the chin pointing upward and to the opposite side. It is due to injury to the sternocleidomastoid muscle or avulsion of the accessory nerve at the time of birth and unilateral fibrosis in the muscle, which cannot lengthen with the growing neck (congenital torticollis).
- **Eagle's syndrome** is an elongation of the styloid process or excessive calcification of the styloid process or stylohyoid ligament that causes neck, throat, or facial pain and dysphagia (difficulty in swallowing). The pain may occur due to compression of the glossopharyngeal nerve, which winds around the styloid process or stylohyoid ligament as it descends to supply the tongue, pharynx, and neck. Also, the pain may be caused by pressure on the internal and external carotid arteries by a deviated and elongated styloid process. Its treatment is styloidectomy.
- The **anterior cervical triangle** is bounded by the sternocleidomastoid, mandible, and midline of the neck and is subdivided by the digastric anterior and posterior bellies and anterior belly of the omohyoid into the submandibular, carotid, muscular, and submental triangles.
- The **accessory nerve** runs on the levator scapulae, deep to the trapezius, and innervates the trapezius and sternocleidomastoid muscles. **Lesion of the accessory nerve in the neck** denervates the trapezius, leading to atrophy of the muscle. It causes a downward displacement or **drooping of the shoulder**.
- Superficial (cutaneous) branches of the **cervical plexus** include the **great auricular**, **transverse cervical**, **supraclavicular**, and **lesser occipital nerves**. The deep branches of the cervical plexus consist of the **ansa cervicalis**, which supplies the infrahyoid or strap muscles, and the **phrenic** nerve, which runs on the anterior scalene and enters the thorax to supply the diaphragm.

- The posterior belly of the **digastric**and**stylohyoid** muscles are innervated by the facial nerve, whereas the anterior belly of the digastric and mylohyoid muscles are innervated by the trigeminal nerve. The geniohyoid and thyrohyoid muscles are innervated by C1 through the hypoglossal nerve.
- The **trachea** extends from the inferior border of the cricoid cartilage to its bifurcation into the primary bronchi at the level of the sternal angle. It is kept open by a series of **C-shaped** hyaline cartilages.
- The **esophagus** is a muscular tube that connects the pharynx to the stomach. It contains branchiomeric skeletal muscles innervated by special visceral efferent (SVE) fibers from the recurrent laryngeal nerves and smooth muscles innervated by sympathetic nerve fibers from the sympathetic trunk and the esophageal plexus of the vagus nerve.
- The **thyroid gland** is an endocrine gland that secretes the hormones thyroxine and thyrocalcitonin, which regulate metabolic rate. The isthmus overlies the second to the third or fourth tracheal rings.
- The **parathyroid glands** are two superior and two inferior (four to six) small endocrine glands, which secrete PTH for calcium metabolism. If there is no secretion of PTH, fetal tetany is produced.
- **Injury to the upper trunk of the brachial plexus** may be caused by a violent separation of the head from the shoulder such as occurs in a fall from a motorcycle. Due to paralysis of the lateral rotators, the arm is in medial rotation, resulting in **waiter's tip hand**. Upper trunk injury can also result from stretching an infant's neck during a difficult delivery. This is referred to as **birth palsy** or obstetric paralysis.
- The **carotid sheath** contains the common and internal carotid arteries, internal jugular vein, and vagus nerve. It does not contain the sympathetic trunk, which lies posterior to the carotid sheath and is embedded in the prevertebral fascia.
- The **common carotid artery** arises from the brachiocephalic trunk on the right and from the aortic arch on the left. It divides into the internal and external carotid arteries at the level of the upper border of the thyroid cartilage. The internal carotid artery has no named branch in the neck, and the external carotid artery has numerous branches such as the superior thyroid, ascending pharyngeal, occipital, lingual, facial, posterior auricular, maxillary, and superficial temporal arteries. The **carotid body** lies at the bifurcation of the common carotid artery and serves as a chemoreceptor. The **carotid sinus** lies at the origin of the internal carotid artery and functions as a pressoreceptor or baroreceptor. The carotid sinus nerve of the glossopharyngeal nerve and the nerve to the carotid body from the vagus nerve innervate the carotid sinus and carotid body, respectively.
- **Neurovascular compression (thoracic outlet) syndrome** produces symptoms of compression of the brachial plexus and/or the subclavian vessels. It can be caused by **abnormal insertion** of the anterior and middle scalene muscles (scalene syndrome) and by a **cervical rib**, which is a cartilaginous accessory rib attached to vertebra C7. Treatment can be nonsurgical (physical therapy) or surgical by removing the cervical rib and/or releasing the anterior scalene muscle.
- **Subclavian steal syndrome** is a cerebral and brain stem ischemia caused by occlusion in the proximal subclavian artery (proximal to the vertebral artery) resulting in retrograde blood flow in the vertebral artery into the subclavian. The arm can be supplied by the vertebral artery at the expense of the vertebrobasilar circulation. Vertebrobasilar insufficiency and thus brain stem ischemia and strokecan result as**blood flow is stolen**from the carotid, circle of Willis, and basilar circulation and diverted into the subclavian artery. Symptoms are dizziness, ataxia, vertigo, visual disturbance, motor deficit, confusion, aphasia, headache, syncope, arm weakness, and arm claudication with exercise. Stenting of the occlusion or carotid–subclavian bypass can relieve symptoms.
- **Carotid sinus syncope** is a temporary loss of consciousness or fainting caused by diminished cerebral blood flow. It results from hypersensitivity of the carotid sinus, and attacks may be produced by pressure on a sensitive carotid sinus such as taking the carotid pulse near the superior border of the thyroid cartilage.
- **Carotid endarterectomy** is the excision of atherosclerotic thickening of intima of the internal carotid artery for the prevention of stroke in patients with symptoms of obstructive disease of the carotid artery.
- **Temporal (giant cell) arteritis** is granulomatous inflammation with multinucleated giant cells, affecting the medium-sized arteries, especially the temporal artery. Symptoms include severe headache, excruciating pain in the temporal area, temporal artery tenderness, visual impairment,

transient diplopia, jaw claudication, fever, fatigue, and weight loss. Its cause is unknown, but it is diagnosed by a temporal artery biopsy and can be treated with corticosteroids such as prednisone.

- **Central venous line** is an intravenous needle and catheter placed into a large vein such as the internal jugular or subclavian vein to give fluids or medication. A **central line** is inserted in the apex of the triangular interval between the clavicle and the clavicular and sternal heads of the sternocleidomastoid muscle into the **internal jugular vein** through which the catheter is threaded into the superior vena cava (a large central vein in the chest). Air embolism or laceration of the internal jugular vein is a possible complication of catheterization. A **central line** may also be inserted into the retroclavicular portion of the **right subclavian vein**. The lung is vulnerable to injury, and pneumothorax and arterial puncture, causing hemothorax, are potential complications of a subclavian catheterization.
- **Tracheotomy (tracheostomy)** is a procedure to create an opening through the trachea. An incision is made between the third and fourth rings of cartilage to allow entry of a tube into the airway. Tracheotomy is typically an emergent procedure to reestablish airway. It can also be done on a patient who has been on life support with an endotracheal tube for a prolonged period of time to decrease the risk of tracheomalacia.
- **Goiter** is an **enlargement of the thyroid gland**, which is commonly caused by **iodine deficiency** (because iodine is vital to the formation of thyroid hormone), **hyperthyroidism** (overproduction of thyroid hormones), or **hypothyroidism** (which causes the gland to swell in its attempt to produce more hormones). The enlarged gland compresses the trachea, larynx, esophagus, and recurrent laryngeal nerve, causing symptoms of breathing difficulties (dyspnea), loss of speech, cough or wheezing, swallowing difficulties (dysphagia), neck vein distention, and dizziness. The goiter can be treated with radioactive iodine to shrink the gland or with thyroidectomy.
- **Graves disease** is an autoimmune disease in which the immune system overstimulates the thyroid gland, causing **hyperthyroidism** resulting in **goiter** and **exophthalmos** (or **proptosis**). The most common symptoms include insomnia, irritability, weight loss, increased perspiration, muscle weakness, palpitations, nervousness, and hand tremors. **Hashimoto disease** (chronic **thyroiditis**) is an autoimmune disease in which the immune system destroys the thyroid gland, resulting in **hypothyroidism** and goiter.
- **Papillary carcinoma of the thyroid** is a malignancy of the thyroid and is the most common type of thyroid carcinoma, accounting for approximately 70% of all thyroid tumors. The cancer occurs more in females, and its symptoms include a lump on the side of the neck, hoarseness of the voice, and difficulty swallowing. Its treatment is surgical removal of the tumor, and after surgery, most patients are treated with radioactive iodine and should take thyroid hormone for life.
- **Thyroidectomy** is surgical removal of the thyroid gland. During surgery, the thyroid ima artery and inferior thyroid veins are vulnerable to injury. Potential complications may include **hemorrhage** from injury of the anterior jugular veins; **nerve paralysis**, particularly of the recurrent laryngeal nerves; **pneumothorax** resulting from damage of the cervical dome of the pleura; and **esophageal injury** due to its immediate posterior location to the trachea.
- **Inadvertent parathyroidectomy** may occur during thyroidectomy which would result in decreased production of parathyroid hormone (PTH) and lead to low calcium levels, which in turn would lead to muscle spasms (tetany) as well as high levels of phosphorus and low levels of vitamin D.
- **Cricothyrotomy** is an incision through the skin and cricothyroid membrane for insertion of a tracheotomy tube into the trachea for relief of acute respiratory obstruction. When making a skin incision, care must be taken not to injure the anterior jugular veins, which lie near the midline of the neck.
- **Horner syndrome** is caused by thyroid carcinoma, which may cause a lesion of the cervical sympathetic trunk; by Pancoast tumor at the apex of the lungs, which injures the stellate ganglion; or by a penetrating injury to the neck, injuring cervical sympathetic nerves. This syndrome is characterized by the presence of ptosis, miosis, enophthalmos, anhidrosis, and vasodilation. (These are explained in the sections pertaining to the eye. See the section on the orbit.)
- **Stellate ganglion block** is performed under fluoroscopy by inserting the needle at the level of the C6 vertebra to avoid piercing the pleura, although the ganglion lies at the level of the C7 vertebra. The needle of the anesthetic syringe is inserted between the trachea and the carotid sheath through the skin over the anterior tubercle of the transverse process of the C6 vertebra (Chassaignac or carotid

tubercle). Once needle position close to the ganglion is confirmed, the local anesthetic is injected beneath the prevertebral fascia.

- **Retropharyngeal abscess or infection** may spread from the neck into the posterior mediastinum through the retropharyngeal space.
- **Thyroglossal duct cyst** is a cyst in the midline of the neck, resulting from lack of closure of a segment of the embryonic thyroglossal duct through which the thyroid gland descended through the tongue to the root of the neck. It occurs most commonly in the region below the hyoid bone. As the cyst enlarges, it is prone to infection. Occasionally, a **thyroglossal cyst** ruptures spontaneously, producing a sinus as a result of an infection of the cyst.
- **Muscles of facial expression** are innervated by the facial nerve, and the cutaneous sensation of the face is supplied by the trigeminal nerve. The face receives **arterial blood** from the facial artery, which gives rise to the inferior labial, superior labial, and lateral nasal branches and ends as the angular artery. The **facial vein** has the corresponding branches of the facial artery, drains into the internal jugular vein, and communicates with the pterygoid venous plexus by way of the deep facial vein.
- **Danger space** is the space between the anterior (alar part) and posterior layers of prevertebral fascia because of its extension from the base of the skull to the diaphragm, providing a route for the spread of infection.
- **Bell palsy** (facial paralysis) caused by a **lesion of the facial nerve** is marked by characteristic **distortions of the face** such as no wrinkles on the forehead, drooping of the eyebrow, inability to close or blink the eye, sagging corner of the mouth, inability to smile, whistle, or blow. The palsy also causes loss of taste in the anterior portion of the tongue, decreased salivation and lacrimation, deviation of the lower jaw, and hyperacusis.
- **Danger area of the face** is the **area of the face near the nose** drained by the facial veins. Pustules (pimples) or boils or other skin infections, particularly on the side of the nose and upper lip, may spread to the cavernous venous sinus via the facial vein, pterygoid venous plexus, and ophthalmic veins. **Septicemia** (blood infection) is a systemic disease caused by the presence of pathogenic organisms or their **toxins** in the bloodstream and is often associated with severe infections, leading to meningitis and cavernous sinus thrombosis, both of which may cause neurologic damage and may be life-threatening.
- The **scalp** consists of the skin, connective tissue, aponeurosis, loose connective tissue, and pericranium (periosteum); receives sensory innervation from branches of the ophthalmic, maxillary, and mandibular nerves and the lesser, greater, and third occipital nerves; and receives blood from branches of the internal and external carotid arteries. The loose connective tissue layer is known as a dangerous layer and communicates with cranial dural venous sinuses by way of the emissary veins.
- **Scalp hemorrhage** results from laceration of arteries in the dense connective tissue layer that is unable to contract or retract and thus remain open, leading to profuse bleeding. **Deep scalp wounds** gape widely when the epicranial aponeurosis is lacerated in the coronal plane because of the pull of the frontal and occipital bellies of the epicranius muscle in opposite directions. **Scalp infection** localized in the loose connective tissue layer spreads across the calvaria to the intracranial dural venous sinuses through emissary veins, causing **meningitis** or **septicemia**.
- **Trigeminal neuralgia (tic douloureux)** is marked by **paroxysmal pain** along the course of the trigeminal nerve, especially radiating to the maxillary or mandibular area. The common causes of this disorder are aberrant blood vessels, aneurysms, chronic meningeal inflammation, brain tumors compressing on the trigeminal nerve at the base of the brain, and other lesions such as multiple sclerosis. Carbamazepine is regarded as the treatment of choice, but the synergistic combination of carbamazepine and baclofen may provide relief from episodic pain. If medical treatments are not effective, the neuralgia may be alleviated by sectioning the sensory root of the trigeminal nerve in the trigeminal (Meckel) cave in the middle cranial fossa.
- The **infratemporal fossa** contains muscles of mastication, the mandibular nerve and its branches, and the maxillary artery and its branches.
- The **muscles of mastication** are innervated by the mandibular branch of the trigeminal nerve. The lateral pterygoid opens the jaw, and other muscles close the jaw. The mandible can be protruded by the lateral and medial pterygoid muscles, whereas it can be retracted by the temporalis and masseter muscles.

- The **maxillary artery** gives rise to the deep auricular, anterior tympanic, inferior alveolar, deep temporal, middle meningeal, and buccal branches in the infratemporal fossa. The **middle meningeal artery** passes between two roots of the auriculotemporal nerve and enters the cranial cavity through the foramen spinosum. The **inferior alveolar artery** enters the mandibular canal and supplies the lower teeth and chin.
- The **mandibular nerve** gives off inferior alveolar, lingual, buccal, deep temporal, and other muscular branches. The **lingual nerve** is joined by the **chorda tympani**, which carries preganglionic parasympathetic fibers to the submandibular ganglion and taste fibers to the anterior two-thirds of the tongue. The inferior alveolar nerve gives off the mylohyoid nerve, which supplies the anterior belly of the digastric and mylohyoid muscles.
- The **parotid gland** secretes a large amount of watery saliva (which contains enzymes) by parasympathetic stimulation and a small amount of viscus saliva in response to sympathetic stimulation. The saliva enters the vestibule opposite the site of the upper second molar tooth by way of the parotid duct.
- **Frey syndrome** produces **flushing and sweating instead of salivation** in response to taste of food after injury of the **auriculotemporal nerve**, which carries parasympathetic secretomotor fibers to the parotid gland and sympathetic fibers to the sweat glands. When the nerve is severed, the fibers can regenerate along each other's pathways and innervate the wrong gland. It can occur after parotid surgery and may be treated by cutting the tympanic plexus in the middle ear.
- **Rupture of the middle meningeal artery** may be caused by fracture of the squamous part of the temporal bone as it runs through the foramen spinosum and just deep to the inner surface of the temporal bone. It causes **epidural hematoma** with increased intracranial pressure.
- **Mumps (epidemic parotitis)** is a highly contagious viral infection. It can be spread to other people by breathing, coughing, kissing, sneezing, and talking. It irritates the auriculotemporal nerve, causing severe pain as the **parotid capsule is stretched** due to **inflammation** and **swelling of the parotid gland**. Pain is exacerbated by compression from swallowing or chewing. Other symptoms include chills, headache, fever, and sore throat. It may be accompanied by inflammation and swelling of the testes (orchitis) or ovaries, causing **sterility** if it occurs after puberty. If the testes are affected, they become swollen and painful; if the ovaries or pancreas are affected, abdominal pain will result.
- **Dislocation of the temporomandibular joint** occurs anteriorly as the mandible head glides across the articular tubercle during yawning and laughing. A blow to the chin with the mouth closed may drive the head of the mandible posteriorly and superiorly, causing fracture of the bony auditory canal and the floor of the middle cranial fossa.
- **Skull fracture**: Fracture at the **pterion** may rupture the middle meningeal artery, and a depressed fracture may compress the underlying brain. A fracture of the petrous portion of the **temporal bone** may cause blood or CSF to escape from the ear, hearing loss, and facial nerve damage. Fracture of the **anterior cranial fossa** causes anosmia, periorbital bruising (raccoon eyes), and CSF leakage from the nose (rhinorrhea). A blow to the top of the head may fracture the skull base with related CN injury, CSF leakage from a dura-arachnoid tear, and dural sinus thrombosis. **Tripod fracture** is a facial fracture involving the three supports of the malar (cheek or zygomatic) bone, including the zygomatic processes of the temporal, frontal, and maxillary bones.
- The **anterior cranial cavity** contains numerous foramina that transmit nerves, blood vessels, and other structures. These include the foramen cecum (emissary vein to superior sagittal sinus), foramina of cribriform plate (olfactory nerves), posterior ethmoidal foramen (posterior ethmoidal nerve and vessels), and optic canal (optic nerve and ophthalmic artery).
- The **middle cranial fossa** contains the superior orbital fissure (CNs III, IV, V1, VI, and the ophthalmic vein), foramen rotundum (maxillary nerve), foramen ovale (mandibular nerve, accessory meningeal artery, and lesser petrosal nerve), foramen spinosum (middle meningeal vessels and meningeal branch of mandibular nerve), foramen lacerum (upper part: internal carotid artery and plexus), hiatus of canal of lesser petrosal nerve, and hiatus of canal of greater petrosal nerve.
- The **posterior cranial fossa** contains the internal acoustic meatus (facial nerve, vestibulocochlear nerve, and labyrinthine artery), mastoid foramen (emissary vein), jugular foramen (CNs IX, X, XI, and the internal jugular vein), condylar canal (emissary vein), hypoglossal canal (CN XII), and foramen magnum (medulla oblongata, meninges, vertebral arteries, spinal roots of CN XI).
- Most veins of the brain drain into the intracranial dural venous sinuses.

- The **superior sagittal sinus** lies in the midline along the convex border of the falx cerebri between the cerebral hemispheres.
- The **inferior sagittal sinus** lies in the free edge of the falx cerebri and is joined by the great cerebral vein of Galen to form the straight sinus.
- The **superior sagittal, straight, and occipital (in the falx cerebelli) sinuses** join at the confluence, which is drained by the transverse sinuses.
- The **transverse sinus** drains into the sigmoid sinus, which becomes the internal jugular vein.
- The **cavernous sinus** is located on each side of the sella turcica; communicates with the ophthalmic vein, pterygoid venous plexus, and facial vein. The abducens nerve and internal carotid artery are located in the middle of the sinus, while the oculomotor, trochlear, ophthalmic, and maxillary nerves are in the lateral wall.
- **Cavernous sinus thrombosis** is the formation of blood clot within the cavernous sinus and is caused by bacterial infections induced commonly by *Staphylococcus*. The common cause is usually from a spreading infection in the nose, sinuses, ears, or teeth. Cavernous sinus thrombosis may produce headache, **papilledema** (edema of the optic disk or nerve due to increased intracranial pressure), **exophthalmos** or proptosis (protrusion of the eyeball), **diplopia** (double vision), **vision loss** (due to damage of the optic nerve or central artery and vein of the retina), **ophthalmoplegia** (paralysis of the eye movement muscles), chemosis (swelling of the conjunctivae), **sluggish pupillary responses** (due to damage of sympathetic and parasympathetic nerves), **meningitis,** and paralysis of the CNs, which course through the cavernous sinus. It can be treated with high-dose antibiotics, and sometimes surgery is needed to drain the infected sinuses. Corticosteroids may reduce edema and inflammation as adjunctive therapy.
- **Pial hemorrhage** is due to damage to the small vessels of the pia and brain tissue. **Cerebral hemorrhage** resulting from rupture of the thin-walled lenticulostriate artery, a branch of the middle cerebral artery, can produce hemiplegia (paralysis of one side of the body).
- **Subarachnoid hemorrhage** is due to rupture of cerebral arteries and veins that cross the subarachnoid space. It may be caused by rupture of an aneurysm on the circle of Willis or, less commonly, by a hemangioma (proliferation of blood vessels leading to a mass that resembles a neoplasm).
- **Epidural hematoma** is due to rupture of the middle meningeal arteries or veins caused by trauma near the pterion, fracture of the greater wing of the sphenoid, or a torn dural venous sinus. An epidural hematoma may put pressure on the brain.
- **Shingles (herpes zoster)** is a viral disease of the spinal nerves and certain cranial (i.e., trigeminal) ganglia that is caused by the **varicella zoster virus**. It is characterized by an eruption of groups of vesicles because of inflammation of ganglia resulting from activation of virus that has remained latent for years.
- **Chicken pox (varicella)** is caused by the **varicella zoster virus**, which later resides latent in the cranial (i.e., trigeminal) or dorsal root ganglia. It is marked by vesicular eruption of the skin and mucous membranes. It is contagious, and a patient may have a runny or stuffy nose, sneezing, cough, itchy rash, fever, and abdominal pain. Ophthalmic zoster (herpes zoster) can cause serious eye complications if not treated.
- The **optic canal** is formed by two roots of the lesser wing of sphenoid and transmits the optic nerve and ophthalmic artery. The superior orbital fissure is formed by the lesser and greater wings of the sphenoid bone; transmits the oculomotor, trochlear, abducens, and ophthalmic nerves and ophthalmic vein. The inferior orbital fissure lies between the greater wing and maxilla and transmits the infraorbital nerve and vessels.
- **Muscles of eye movement** are the levator palpebrae superioris, inferior oblique, and superior, middle, and inferior rectus muscles, which are innervated by the oculomotor nerve; the lateral rectus muscle is innervated by the abducens nerve; and the superior oblique is innervated by the trochlear nerve.
- The **ophthalmic nerve** divides into the lacrimal, frontal (which divides into the supraorbital and supratrochlear branches), and nasociliary nerves. The nasociliary nerve gives off a sensory communicating branch to the ciliary ganglion and the long ciliary nerve, which contains sympathetic postganglionic fibers for the dilator pupillae muscle. Parasympathetic nerves supply the ciliary muscle and the sphincter pupillae muscle.
- The **ophthalmic artery** arises from the internal carotid artery and supplies structures in the orbit and eyeball. The ophthalmic veins communicate with the cavernous sinus and the pterygoid venous plexus.

- **Corneal blink reflex** is **closure of the eyelids** in response to blowing on the cornea or touching it with a wisp of cotton. It is caused by bilateral contraction of the orbicularis oculi muscles. Its efferent limb (of the reflex arc) is the facial nerve; its afferent limb is the nasociliary nerve of the ophthalmic division of the trigeminal nerve.
- **Fracture of the orbital floor** involving the maxillary sinus commonly occurs as a result of a blunt force to the face. This fracture causes displacement of the eyeball, causing symptoms of **double vision** (diplopia), and also causes an injury to the infraorbital nerve, producing loss of sensation of the skin of the cheek and the gum. This fracture may cause entrapment of the inferior rectus muscle, which may limit upward gaze.
- **Hemianopia (hemianopsia)** is a condition characterized by loss of vision (blindness) in one-half of the visual field of each eye. Blindness may occur as the result of a lesion of the **optic nerve**. Types of hemianopia are (a) **bitemporal (heteronymous) hemianopia**, loss of vision in the temporal visual field of both eyes resulting from a lesion of the optic chiasma such as a pituitary tumor; (b) **right nasal hemianopia**, blindness in the nasal field of vision of the right eye as the result of a **right perichiasmal lesion** such as an aneurysm of the internal carotid artery; and (c) **left homonymous hemianopia**, loss of sight in the left half of the visual field of both eyes resulting from a lesion of the **right optic tract** or **optic radiation**.
- **Papilledema (choked disk)** is an edema of the optic disk or optic nerve, often resulting from increased intracranial pressure and increased CSF pressure or thrombosis of the central vein of the retina, slowing venous return from the retina.
- **Diplopia (double vision)** is caused by **paralysis of one or more extraocular muscles**, resulting from injury of the nerves supplying them.
- **Strabismus (squint eye or crossed eye)** is a condition in which the eyes are not aligned properly and point (look) in different directions. It occurs when the eye deviates medially (**internal strabismus** or esotropia) or deviate laterally (**external strabismus** or exotropia) as a result of weakness or paralysis of extrinsic eye muscle due to damage to the oculomotor or abducens nerve. Its symptoms include misaligned eyes, double vision, and a loss of depth perception. Treatments include eyeglasses, prisms, vision therapy, or eye muscle surgery.
- **Crocodile tears syndrome (Bogorad syndrome)** is **spontaneous lacrimation during eating** caused by a lesion of the facial nerve proximal to the geniculate ganglion. It follows facial paralysis and is due to misdirection of regenerating parasympathetic fibers, which formerly innervated the salivary (submandibular and sublingual) glands, to the lacrimal glands.
- **Accommodation** is the adjustment or adaptation of the eye to focus on a near object. It occurs with contraction of the ciliary muscle, causing a relaxation of the suspensory ligament (ciliary zonular fibers) and an increase in thickness, convexity, and refractive power of the lens. It is mediated by parasympathetic fibers running within the oculomotor nerve. The accommodation reflex also causes the eyes to converge.
- **Argyll–Robertson pupil** is a miotic pupil that responds to accommodation (constricts on near focus) but fails to respond to light. It is caused by a lesion in the midbrain and seen in neurosyphilis (or syphilis) and in diabetes.
- **Pupillary light reflex** is constriction of the pupil in response to light stimulation (direct reflex), and the contralateral pupil also constricts (consensual reflex). It is mediated by parasympathetic nerve fibers in the oculomotor nerve (efferent limb) and its afferent limb is the optic nerve.
- **Horner syndrome** is caused by **injury to cervical sympathetic nerves** and characterized by (a) **miosis**, constriction of the pupil resulting from paralysis of the dilator muscle of the iris; (b) **ptosis**, drooping of an upper eyelid from paralysis of the smooth muscle component (superior tarsal plate) of the levator palpebrae superioris; (c) **enophthalmos**, retraction (backward displacement) of an eyeball into the orbit from paralysis of the orbitalis muscle, which is smooth muscle and bridges the inferior orbital fissure and functions in eyeball protrusion; (d) **anhidrosis**, absence of sweating; and (e) **vasodilation**, increased blood flow in the face and neck (flushing). Common causes of lesions to cervical sympathetics include brain stem stroke, tuberculosis, pulmonary Pancoast tumor, trauma, and injury to carotid arteries. There is no specific treatment that improves or reverses the condition.
- **Anisocoria** is an unequal size of the pupil; **miosis** is a constricted pupil caused by paralysis of the dilator pupillae resulting from a lesion of sympathetic nerve; **mydriasis** is a dilated pupil caused by paralysis of the sphincter pupillae resulting from a lesion of the parasympathetic nerve.

- **Myopia (nearsightedness)** is a condition in which the focus of objects lies in front of the retina, resulting from elongation of the eyeball. **Hyperopia** (farsightedness) is a condition in which the focus of objects lies behind the retina.
- **Retinal detachment** is a separation of the sensory layer from the pigment layer of the retina. It may occur in trauma such as a blow to the head and can be reattached surgically by photocoagulation with a laser beam.
- **Retinitis pigmentosa** is an inherited disorder that causes a **degeneration of photoreceptor cells** in the retina or a progressive retinal atrophy, characterized by **constricted visual fields (tunnel vision** or **loss of peripheral vision),** nyctalopia (night blindness), attenuation (thinning) of the retinal vessels, and pigment infiltration of the inner retinal layers.
- **Macular degeneration** (often called age-related macular degeneration) is a degenerative change in the macula in the center of the retina. A patient with this condition sees the edges of images but has **no central vision** (a **ring of peripheral vision**). It occurs in dry and wet forms. The dry type (nonneovascular) is the most common form; in this type, the **light-sensitive layer** of cells in the macula become **thinned** and causes more gradual loss of vision. The wet type (neovascular) is caused by the **growth of abnormal blood vessels** from the choroid underneath the macula. These abnormal blood vessels tend to hemorrhage or **leak**, resulting in the formation of scar tissue if left untreated. There is no treatment for dry macular degeneration. Laser treatments are effective at preventing or slowing the progress of wet type degeneration by sealing the leaking blood vessels, but no treatment restores vision loss.
- **Diabetic retinopathy** is a degenerative disease of the retina and a leading cause of blindness associated with diabetes mellitus. The background type (the earliest phase) is marked by microaneurysms, intraretinal dotlike hemorrhages, exudates (as a result of **leaky vessels**), cotton-wool spots, and **macular edema**. The proliferative type is characterized by neovascularization (proliferation of new, abnormal vessel growth) of the retina and optic disk, which may project into the vitreous, proliferation of fibrous tissue, vitreous hemorrhage, and retinal detachment. It can be treated with laser photocoagulation to seal off leaking blood vessels and destroy new growth.
- **Glaucoma** is characterized by **increased intraocular pressure** resulting from **impaired drainage of aqueous humor** (which is produced by the ciliary process) into the venous system through the scleral venous sinus (**Schlemm canal**), which is a circular vascular channel at the corneoscleral junction or limbus. The increased pressure causes **impaired retinal blood flow**, producing retinal ischemia or atrophy of the retina; degeneration of the nerve fibers in the retina, particularly at the optic disk; defects in the visual field; and blindness. Glaucoma can be treated by surgical iridectomy or laser iridotomy for drainage of aqueous humor or by use of drugs to inhibit the secretion of aqueous humor.
- **Cataract** is a clouding **(opacity or milky white) of the crystalline eye lens or of its capsule**, which must be removed. It results in little light being transmitted to the retina, causing blurred images and poor vision.
- **Presbyopia** is a condition involving a **reduced ability to focus on near objects**. It is caused by the loss of elasticity of the crystalline lens, occurs in advanced age and is corrected with bifocal lenses.
- The palate consists of the hard palate and soft palate. Muscles of the palate (palatoglossus, palatopharyngeus, muscular uvulae, levator veli palatine, and tensor veli palatine) are innervated by the vagus nerve, except the tensor veli palatini, which is innervated by the trigeminal nerve.

Nerves of the Teeth and Gums

- The maxillary teeth are innervated by the superior alveolar nerve, and the mandibular teeth are innervated by the inferior alveolar nerve.
- The outer (buccal) surface of the maxillary gingiva is innervated by the superior alveolar and infraorbital nerves, whereas the inner (lingual) surface is innervated by the greater palatine and nasopalatine nerves.
- The outer (buccal) surface of the mandibular gingiva is innervated by the buccal and mental nerves, whereas the inner (lingual) surface is innervated by the lingual nerves.
- **Muscles of the tongue** are innervated by the hypoglossal nerve except the palatoglossus, which is innervated by the vagus nerve. The anterior two-thirds of the tongue is innervated by the lingual nerve for general sensation and by chorda tympani of the facial nerve for taste (SVA) sensation. The posterior one-third of the tongue is supplied by the glossopharyngeal nerve for both general and taste sensations.

Innervation of the Tongue

- General somatic efferent motor innervation to muscles of the tongue from the hypoglossal nerve.
- GSA sensation from anterior two-thirds of the tongue from the lingual nerve.
- SVA taste sensation from anterior two-thirds of the tongue from the chorda tympani.
- GVA and SVA sensation from posterior one-third of the tongue from the glossopharyngeal nerve.
- The vallate papillae are located on the anterior two-thirds of the tongue in front of the sulcus terminalis, but they are innervated by the glossopharyngeal nerve.

Salivary Glands

- The submandibular gland has a larger superficial portion, which is separated by the mylohyoid muscle from the smaller deep portion.
- The submandibular (Wharton) duct passes medial to the lingual nerve and then superior to the nerve and opens onto the sublingual caruncle.
- The sublingual gland has numerous small ducts that open on the sublingual fold or into the submandibular duct.
- Both glands receive postganglionic parasympathetic fibers from the submandibular ganglion, which receives preganglionic parasympathetic fibers through the chorda tympani (which also contains taste fibers).
- The lingual artery arises from the external carotid artery near the greater horn of the hyoid bone and passes deep to the hyoglossus muscle, but the lingual and hypoglossal nerves pass superficial to the muscle. The artery has the dorsal lingual, deep lingual, and sublingual branches.
- **Lesion of the vagus nerve** causes deviation of the uvula toward the opposite side of the lesion on phonation because of paralysis of the musculus uvulae, which elevates the uvula.
- **Tongue-tie (ankyloglossia)** is an **abnormal shortness of frenulum linguae**, resulting in limitation of tongue movement and thus a severe speech impediment. It can be corrected surgically by cutting the frenulum.
- **Abscess or infection of the maxillary teeth** irritates the **maxillary nerve**, causing upper **toothache**. It may result in symptoms of **sinusitis**, with pain referred to the distribution of the maxillary nerve.
- **Ludwig angina** is an **infection of the floor of the mouth** (submandibular space) with secondary involvement of the sublingual and submental spaces, usually resulting from a dental infection. Symptoms include painful swelling of the floor of the mouth, elevation of the tongue, dysphagia (difficulty in swallowing), dysphonia (impairment of voice production), edema of the glottis, fever, and rapid breathing.
- **Maxillary sinusitis** mimics the clinical signs of maxillary tooth abscess. Infection may spread from the maxillary sinus to the upper teeth and irritate the nerves to these teeth, causing toothache. Only a thin layer of bone separates the roots of the maxillary teeth from the sinus cavity.
- **Cleft palate** occurs when the palatine shelves fail to fuse with each other or the primary palate. **Cleft lip** occurs when the maxillary prominence and the medial nasal prominence fail to fuse.
- **Pharyngeal tumors** may irritate the glossopharyngeal and vagus nerves. Pain that occurs while swallowing is often referred to the ear, as these nerves also contribute sensory innervation to the external ear.
- **Heimlich maneuver** is designed to expel an obstructing bolus of food from the throat of a choking victim. The obstruction can be dislodged by positioning yourself behind the victim, wrapping your arms around the victim's waist, placing a fist between the navel and costal margin, grasping the fist with the other hand, and forcefully pressing into the abdomen with a quick inward and upward thrust.
- **Adenoid** is hypertrophy or **enlargement of the pharyngeal tonsils** that obstructs passage of air from the nasal cavities through the choanae into the nasopharynx and thus causes **difficulty in nasal breathing** and phonation. Adenoids may block the pharyngeal orifices of the auditory tube, thereby contributing to middle ear infection (otitis media). Children are more prone to otitis media, which may result in deafness, due to short auditory tubes and more active adenoids and infections in the nasopharynx that spread through the auditory tube to the middle ear cavity. Adenoidectomy can prevent otitis media.
- **Palatine tonsillectomy** is the surgical removal of a palatine tonsil. During tonsillectomy, the glossopharyngeal nerve may be injured, causing loss of general sensation and taste sensation of the posterior one-third of the tongue. It may cause severe hemorrhage, which may occur from the branches of the facial, ascending pharyngeal, maxillary, and lingual arteries or paratonsillar veins.
- **Quinsy (peritonsillar abscess)** is a painful **pus-filled inflammation** or abscess of the tonsils and surrounding tissues. It develops as a complication of tonsillitis, primarily in adolescents and

young adults. The soft palate and uvula are edematous and displaced toward the unaffected side. Symptoms include sore throat, fever, dysphasia (impairment of speech), and trismus (motor disturbance of the trigeminal nerve, especially spasm of the masseter muscle with difficulty in opening the mouth). It can be treated with antibiotics, surgical aspiration, or tonsillectomy.

- The **nasal cavity** is divided into a **vestibule**, which is a dilated area inside the nostril lined by skin with hairs to filter incoming air; an **olfactory region**, which is the upper third of the nasal cavity lined with olfactory mucosa; and a **respiratory region**, which is the lower two-thirds of the nasal cavity lined with vascular, glandular respiratory mucosa to warm and humidify air.
- It has a **roof** formed by the body of the sphenoid and sphenoid sinus, a **floor** formed by the hard palate, a **medial wall** formed by the nasal septum (septal cartilage, perpendicular plate of ethmoid, and vomer), and a **lateral wall** formed by the inferior concha and the superior and middle concha of the ethmoid.
- The nasal mucosa receives GSA **innervation** by branches of the ophthalmic and maxillary nerves and receives SVA (olfaction) by the olfactory nerves. It receives **blood** from the sphenopalatine branch of the maxillary artery, anterior ethmoidal branch of the ophthalmic artery, and septal branch of the facial artery.
- **Nasal polyp** is an **inflammatory polyp** that develops from the mucosa of the paranasal sinus, which projects into the nasal cavity and may fill the nasopharynx. The most common cause of nasal polyps is allergic rhinitis. Cortisone or nasal steroid sprays slow polyp growth or will shrink them down temporarily. If medical treatment fails, the polyps are removed by endoscopic sinus surgery (polypectomy).
- **Rhinitis** is an inflammation of the nasal mucous membrane, caused by allergies, and has symptoms of runny nose, nasal itching, nasal congestion, and sneezing.
- **Rhinorrhea (runny nose)** can be caused by tear drainage into the inferior nasal meatus through the nasolacrimal duct. It is also associated with the common cold, hay fever, flu, and allergy, which may cause drainage from the paranasal sinus directly into the nasal cavity.
- **Rhinoplasty** is a type of plastic surgery that changes the shape or size of the nose.
- **Deviation of the nasal septum** may obstruct the nasal airway and block the openings of the paranasal sinuses.
- **Epistaxis** is a **nosebleed.** Anterior nosebleed occurs from nose picking, which tears the veins in the vestibule of the nose. It also occurs from the anterior nasal septum (**Kiesselbach area or plexus**), where branches of the sphenopalatine (from maxillary), greater palatine (from maxillary), anterior ethmoidal (from ophthalmic), and superior labial (from facial) arteries converge. More serious posterior nosebleed results from rupture of the sphenopalatine artery. Epistaxis treatment includes compression of the nostrils (application of direct pressure to the septal area) or surgical packing if necessary.
- **Sneeze** is an **involuntary**, **sudden**, **violent**, and **audible expulsion of air** through the mouth and nose. Branches of the maxillary nerve, which convey general sensation from the nasal cavity and palate, carry the afferent limb of the reflex and the efferent limb is mediated by the vagus nerve.
- **Sphenoidal sinusitis** is an infection in the sphenoid sinus that may come from the nasal cavity or from the nasopharynx, and may erode the sinus walls to reach the cavernous sinuses, pituitary gland, optic nerve, or brain stem. Close relationships of the sphenoid sinus with surrounding structures are clinically important because of potential for injury during pituitary surgery and the possible spread of infection to other structures.
- **Pterygopalatine ganglion** receives parasympathetic preganglionic fibers from the facial nerve through the greater petrosal nerve and the nerve of the pterygoid canal.
- Postganglionic parasympathetic fibers supply the lacrimal gland running through the maxillary, zygomatic, zygomaticotemporal, and lacrimal nerves.
- The ganglion receives branches from the maxillary nerve and then sends branches to the palate and nasal mucosae.

Nerves Associated with the Pterygopalatine Ganglion

- The **greater petrosal nerve** contains preganglionic parasympathetic GVE fibers and GVA and SVA (taste) fibers to the palate.
- The **deep petrosal nerve** contains postganglionic sympathetic GVE fibers.
- The **nerve of the pterygoid canal** contains preganglionic parasympathetic GVE fibers to the lacrimal gland and nasal and palatine mucosae and postganglionic sympathetic GVE fibers and GVA and SVA (taste) fibers to the palate.
- **Lesion of the nerve of the pterygoid canal** results in vasodilation; a lack of secretion of the lacrimal, nasal, and palatine glands, and loss of general and taste sensation of the palate.

- The **larynx** has a **cartilaginous framework**, consisting of the thyroid cartilage (Adam's apple, a laryngeal prominence), cricoid cartilage (signet ring shape), arytenoid cartilages (have vocal process and muscular process and rotate on the cricoid cartilage), epiglottic cartilage (leaf-shaped), and corniculate and cuneiform cartilages.
- The **laryngeal muscles** are innervated by the recurrent laryngeal nerve except the cricothyroid, which is innervated by the external laryngeal branch of the superior laryngeal nerve. Only the **posterior cricoarytenoid muscle abducts** the vocal cord, while all other muscles adduct the vocal cord. The chief adductor is the lateral cricoarytenoid; the chief tensor is the cricothyroid; the chief relaxer is the thyroarytenoid. The lateral cricoarytenoid rotates the vocal process of the arytenoid cartilage medially, closing the rima glottidis, whereas the posterior cricoarytenoid rotates the vocal process laterally, opening the rima glottidis.
- **Sensation** above the vocal cord is supplied by the internal laryngeal branch of the superior laryngeal nerve, whereas the recurrent laryngeal nerve supplies sensation below the vocal cord. SVA (taste) sensation on the epiglottis is supplied by the internal laryngeal nerve.
- The larynx receives **blood** from the superior laryngeal artery of the superior thyroid artery and the inferior laryngeal artery of the inferior thyroid artery.
- **Laryngitis** is an **inflammation of the mucous membrane of the larynx**. It is characterized by dryness and soreness of the throat, hoarseness, cough, and dysphagia.
- **Epiglottitis** is an inflammation or acute mucosal swelling of the epiglottis, which may cause a life-threatening airway obstruction, especially in children.
- **Laryngotomy** is an **operative opening into the larynx** through the cricothyroid membrane (cricothyrotomy), through the thyroid cartilage (thyrotomy), or through the thyrohyoid membrane (superior laryngotomy). It is performed when severe edema or an impacted foreign body calls for rapid admission of air into the larynx and trachea.
- **Laryngeal obstruction (choking)** can be caused by aspirated foreign bodies, which are usually lodged at the rima glottidis. The obstruction can be released by abdominal thrusts to expel air from the lungs and thus dislodge the foods (e.g., the Heimlich maneuver). Other causes include severe allergy, trauma, throat cancer, and retropharyngeal abscess.
- **Valsalva maneuver** is forcible exhalation against a closed airway (a closed glottis, nose, or mouth); the resultant increase in intrathoracic pressure impedes venous return to the heart. When the breath is released, the intrathoracic pressure drops, and the trapped blood is quickly propelled through the heart, producing an increase in heart rate (tachycardia) and blood pressure. This maneuver can transiently increase vagal tone and can help stop an episode of supraventricular tachycardia. It can also be used to open the auditory tube.
- **Lesion of the recurrent laryngeal nerve** could be produced during thyroidectomy or cricothyrotomy or by aortic aneurysm and may cause respiratory obstruction, hoarseness, inability to speak, and loss of sensation below the vocal cord.
- **Lesion of the internal laryngeal nerve** results in loss of sensation above the vocal cord and loss of taste on the epiglottis.
- **Lesion of the external laryngeal nerve** may occur during **thyroidectomy** because the nerve accompanies the superior thyroid artery. It causes **paralysis of the cricothyroid muscle**, resulting in paralysis of the laryngeal muscles and thus inability to lengthen the vocal cord and loss of the tension of the vocal cord. Such stresses to the vocal cord cause a fatigued voice and a weak hoarseness.
- The **external ear** consists of the auricle, which is elastic cartilage covered by skin, and is innervated by the great auricular, auriculotemporal, and lesser occipital nerves. The external acoustic meatus consists of a cartilaginous outer third and bony inner two-thirds. It is innervated by the auriculotemporal branch of the trigeminal nerve and the auricular branches of the facial, vagus, and glossopharyngeal nerves.
- The **tympanic membrane** is covered by skin externally and mucosa internally. The external surface is innervated by the trigeminal, facial, glossopharyngeal, and vagus nerves, and the internal surface is innervated by the glossopharyngeal nerve.
- The **auditory ossicles** are the malleus (hammer), incus (anvil), and stapes (stirrup). The handle of the malleus is attached to the tympanic membrane and receives the tendon of the tensor tympani (which is innervated by the trigeminal nerve). The footplate of the stapes occupies the oval window, and its neck receives insertion of the stapedius (which is innervated by the facial nerve).
- The **chorda tympani** arises from the facial nerve in the facial canal, passes between the handle of the malleus and the long process of the incus, exits through the petrotympanic fissure, and joins

the lingual nerve in the infratemporal fossa, carrying preganglionic parasympathetic fibers to the submandibular ganglion and taste fibers to the anterior two-thirds of the tongue.

- The **cochlea** contains the spiral organ of Corti for hearing, the membranous cochlear duct filled with endolymph, and the scala vestibuli and scala tympani filled with perilymph. The vestibule contains the membranous utricle and saccule filled with endolymph and receptors (maculae) for linear acceleration. The semicircular canals contain sensory receptors (cristae) for angular movements in the ampullae at one end of each canal.
- **Otitis media** is a condition of **middle ear infection** that may be spread from the nasopharynx through the auditory tube, causing temporary or permanent deafness. **Otitis externa**, infection of the ear canal, is also known as swimmer's ear, which is usually caused by a bacterial organism such as *Pseudomonas*.
- **Hyperacusis (hyperacusia)** is **excessive acuteness of hearing**, because of paralysis of the stapedius muscle (causing uninhibited movements of the stapes), resulting from a lesion of the facial nerve.
- **Otosclerosis** is a condition of **abnormal bone formation** around the stapes and the oval window, limiting the movement of the stapes and thus resulting in **progressive conduction deafness**.
- **Conductive deafness** is hearing impairment caused by a **defect of a sound-conducting apparatus** such as the auditory meatus, eardrum, or ossicles.
- **Neural or sensorineural deafness** is hearing impairment because of a lesion of the auditory nerve or the central afferent neural pathway.
- **Ménière disease (endolymphatic or labyrinthine hydrops)** is characterized by a **loss of balance (vertigo)**, nausea and vomiting, **tinnitus** (ringing or buzzing in the ears), **progressive hearing loss** resulting from hydrops of the endolymphatic duct or **edema of the labyrinth** (excessive amounts of endolymph that distort the membranous labyrinth), or inflammation of the vestibular division of the vestibulocochlear nerve.

Head and Neck Muscle Innervation

- All of the **infrahyoid muscles** are innervated by the ansa cervicalis except the thyrohyoid muscle, which is innervated by C1 through the hypoglossal nerve.
- All of the **muscles of facial expression** are innervated by the facial nerve, and all of the **muscles of mastication** are innervated by the trigeminal nerve.
- All of the **tongue muscles** are innervated by the hypoglossal nerve except the palatoglossus muscle, which is innervated by the vagus nerve.
- All of the **palate muscles** are innervated by the vagus nerve except the tensor veli palatini muscle, which is innervated by the trigeminal nerve.
- All of the **pharyngeal muscles** are innervated by the vagus nerve except the stylopharyngeus muscle, which is innervated by the glossopharyngeal nerve.
- All of the **laryngeal muscles** are innervated by the recurrent laryngeal nerve except the cricothyroid muscle, which is innervated by the external laryngeal nerve.
- For the **suprahyoid muscles**, the stylohyoid and digastric posterior belly are innervated by the facial nerve, whereas the mylohyoid and digastric anterior belly are innervated by the trigeminal nerve, and the geniohyoid is innervated by C1 through the hypoglossal nerve.
- In the **neck**, the sternocleidomastoid and trapezius are innervated by the accessory nerve.
- In the **middle ear**, the tensor tympani and stapedius are innervated by the trigeminal and facial nerves, respectively.

Functions of Autonomic Nerves

	Sympathetic Nerve	Parasympathetic Nerve
Eyes	Dilates pupil	Constricts pupil; contracts ciliary muscle to thicken lens
Lacrimal gland	Reduces secretion	Promotes secretion
Nasal mucous gland	Reduces secretion	Promotes secretion
Salivary gland	Reduces secretion and more viscid	Increases secretion and watery
Sweat gland	Stimulates secretion	No effect
Blood vessels	Constricts	No effect

Review Test

Directions: Each of the numbered items or incomplete statements in this section is followed by answers or by completions of the statement. Select the **one**-lettered answer or completion that is **best** in each case.

1. A 38-year-old man has had thyroid surgery to remove his papillary carcinoma. The external laryngeal nerve that accompanies the superior thyroid artery is damaged during the surgery. This injury could result in a severe impairment of function of which of the following?

(A) Relaxing the vocal cords
(B) Rotating the arytenoid cartilages
(C) Tensing the vocal cords
(D) Widening the rima glottidis
(E) Abducting the vocal cords

2. A 27-year-old woman with a goiter comes to the hospital for surgical treatment. The surgeon must ligate the superior laryngeal artery before surgically resecting the goiter, so care must be taken to avoid injury to which of the following nerves?

(A) External laryngeal nerve
(B) Internal laryngeal nerve
(C) Superior laryngeal nerve
(D) Hypoglossal nerve
(E) Vagus nerve

3. A 19-year-old woman complains of numbness of the nasopharynx after surgical removal of the adenoid. A lesion of which of the following nerves would be expected?

(A) Maxillary nerve
(B) Superior cervical ganglion
(C) External laryngeal nerve
(D) Glossopharyngeal nerve
(E) Vagus nerve

4. During surgery on a 56-year-old man for a squamous cell carcinoma of the neck, the surgeon notices profuse bleeding from the deep cervical artery. Which of the following arteries must be ligated immediately to stop bleeding?

(A) Inferior thyroid artery
(B) Transverse cervical artery
(C) Thyrocervical trunk
(D) Costocervical trunk
(E) Ascending cervical artery

5. A 17-year-old boy receives an injury to the phrenic nerve by a knife wound in the neck. The damaged nerve passes by which of the following structures in the neck?

(A) Anterior to the subclavian vein
(B) Posterior to the subclavian artery
(C) Deep to the brachial plexus
(D) Medial to the common carotid artery
(E) Superficial to the anterior scalene muscle

6. A 45-year-old woman is suffering from numbness over the tip of her nose. Which of the following nerves is most likely to be damaged?

(A) Ophthalmic division of the trigeminal nerve
(B) Maxillary division of the trigeminal nerve
(C) Mandibular division of the trigeminal nerve
(D) Facial nerve
(E) Auriculotemporal nerve

7. A 26-year-old singer visits her physician—an ear, nose, and throat (ENT) surgeon—and complains of changes in her voice. A laryngoscopic examination demonstrates a lesion of the superior laryngeal nerve, causing weakness of which of the following muscles?

(A) Inferior pharyngeal constrictor
(B) Middle pharyngeal constrictor
(C) Superior pharyngeal constrictor
(D) Thyroarytenoid
(E) Thyrohyoid

8. A 44-year-old man with "crocodile tears syndrome" has spontaneous lacrimation during eating because of misdirection of regenerating autonomic nerve fibers. Which of the following nerves has been injured?

(A) Facial nerve proximal to the geniculate ganglion
(B) Auriculotemporal nerve
(C) Chorda tympani in the infratemporal fossa
(D) Facial nerve at the stylomastoid foramen
(E) Lacrimal nerve

9. A young girl complains of dryness of the nose and the palate. This would indicate a lesion of which of the following ganglia?

(A) Nodose ganglion
(B) Otic ganglion
(C) Pterygopalatine ganglion
(D) Submandibular ganglion
(E) Ciliary ganglion

10. A 33-year-old woman develops Bell palsy. She must be cautious because this can result in corneal inflammation and subsequent ulceration. This symptom results from which of the following conditions?

(A) Sensory loss of the cornea and conjunctiva
(B) Lack of secretion of the parotid gland
(C) Absence of the corneal blink reflex
(D) Absence of sweating on the face
(E) Inability to constrict the pupil

11. A 39-year-old woman presents to your clinic with complaints of headache and dizziness. She has an infection of a cranial dural sinus. The sinus that lies in the margin of the tentorium cerebelli and runs from the posterior end of the cavernous sinus to the transverse sinus is infected. Which of the following sinuses is affected by inflammation?

(A) Straight sinus
(B) Inferior sagittal sinus
(C) Sphenoparietal sinus
(D) Superior petrosal sinus
(E) Cavernous sinus

12. A 24-year-old man falls from his motorcycle and lands in a creek. Death may result from bilateral severance of which of the following nerves?

(A) Trigeminal nerve
(B) Facial nerve
(C) Vagus nerve
(D) Spinal accessory nerve
(E) Hypoglossal nerve

13. A 25-year-old man is involved in an automobile accident and slams his head into a concrete wall of a bridge. His CT scan reveals that the middle meningeal artery has ruptured but the meninges remain intact. Blood leaking from this artery enters which of the following spaces?

(A) Subarachnoid space
(B) Subdural space
(C) Epidural space
(D) Subpial space
(E) Cranial dural sinuses

14. A 27-year-old paratrooper lands on a pine tree. Consequently, preganglionic parasympathetic nerves leaving the central nervous system are lacerated. Which of the following structures contain cell bodies of the damaged nerve fibers?

(A) Cervical and sacral spinal cord
(B) Cervical and thoracic spinal cord
(C) Brain stem and cervical spinal cord
(D) Thoracic and lumbar spinal cord
(E) Brain stem and sacral spinal cord

15. A 67-year-old woman comes to her physician complaining of visual loss. Her MRI scan shows an enlarged pituitary gland that lies in the sella turcica, immediately posterior and superior to which of the following structures?

(A) Frontal sinus
(B) Maxillary sinus
(C) Ethmoid air cells
(D) Mastoid air cells
(E) Sphenoid sinus

16. After having a tonsillectomy, a 57-year-old man with a long history of chewing tobacco use is unable to detect taste on the posterior one-third of his tongue. Which of the following nerves has most likely been injured?

(A) Internal laryngeal nerve
(B) Lingual nerve
(C) Glossopharyngeal nerve
(D) Greater palatine nerve
(E) Chorda tympani

17. A 14-year-old boy hits his head on the asphalt road after falling off his skateboard. His radiograph reveals damage to the sella turcica. This is probably due to fracture of which of the following bones?

(A) Frontal bone
(B) Ethmoid bone
(C) Temporal bone
(D) Basioccipital bone
(E) Sphenoid bone

18. The nerve accompanying the superior thyroid artery may be damaged during an operation on the thyroid gland. Which of the following functional defects may result from this injury?

(A) Loss of sensation above the vocal cord
(B) Loss of lateral rotation of the arytenoid cartilages
(C) Paralysis of the vocalis muscle
(D) Lack of abduction of the vocal cord
(E) Decreased tension of the vocal cord

19. A 37-year-old patient has an infectious inflammation of the dural venous sinus closest to the pituitary gland and a secondary thrombus formation. Which of the following is the most likely site of infection?

(A) Straight sinus
(B) Cavernous sinus
(C) Superior petrosal sinus
(D) Sigmoid sinus
(E) Confluence of sinuses

20. A young singer at the local music theater visits her physician and complains of vocal difficulties. On examination, she is unable to abduct the vocal cords during quiet breathing. Which of the following muscles is most likely paralyzed?

(A) Vocalis muscle
(B) Cricothyroid muscle
(C) Oblique arytenoid muscle
(D) Posterior cricoarytenoid muscle
(E) Thyroarytenoid muscle

21. A 71-year-old woman often visits an emergency department with swallowing difficulties and subsequent choking while eating food. Which of the following pairs of muscles is most instrumental in preventing food from entering the larynx and trachea during swallowing?

(A) Sternohyoid and sternothyroid muscles
(B) Oblique arytenoid and aryepiglottic muscles
(C) Inferior pharyngeal constrictor and thyrohyoid muscles
(D) Levator veli palatini and tensor veli palatini muscles
(E) Musculus uvulae and geniohyoid muscles

22. A 31-year-old woman complains of headache and dizziness after hitting a kitchen cabinet door with her head. Her MRI scan and venogram show a large blood clot in the great cerebral vein of Galen. The obstructed vein of the brain is a direct tributary of which of the following venous structures?

(A) Emissary veins
(B) Pterygoid venous plexus
(C) Diploic veins
(D) Dural venous sinuses
(E) Internal jugular vein

23. A 41-year-old woman overdoses on some prescription medications that have a common side effect of autonomic nerve stimulation. Which of the following conditions or actions results from stimulation of the parasympathetic fibers to the eyeball?

(A) Enhanced vision for distant objects
(B) Dilation of the pupil
(C) Contraction of capillaries in the iris
(D) Contraction of the ciliary muscle
(E) Flattening of the lens

24. A 53-year-old woman with a severe middle ear infection comes to the hospital. On examination, the physician finds that the infection has injured the tympanic nerve. The damaged nerve:

(A) Is a branch of the facial nerve
(B) Contains postganglionic parasympathetic fibers
(C) Synapses with fibers in the lesser petrosal nerve
(D) Is a branch of the glossopharyngeal nerve
(E) Forms the tympanic plexus in the external auditory meatus

25. A 13-year-old boy competing in a motocross competition falls from his bike and sustains massive head injuries. Which of the following cavities are separated from the middle cranial fossa by a thin layer of bone?

(A) Auditory tube and bony orbit
(B) Middle ear cavity and sphenoid sinus
(C) Sigmoid sinus and frontal sinus
(D) Sphenoid sinus and ethmoid sinus
(E) Maxillary sinus and middle ear cavity

26. A 32-year-old house painter suffers from a head injury after falling off a ladder and has bleeding in his head. During intraoperative testing, the neurosurgeon notes loss of general sensation in the dura of the middle cranial fossa. Which of the following nerves has been affected?

(A) Vagus nerve
(B) Facial nerve
(C) Hypoglossal nerve
(D) Trigeminal nerve
(E) Glossopharyngeal nerve

27. During a carotid endarterectomy of a 57-year-old man who suffered a stroke, the carotid sinus is damaged. A third-year medical student in surgical rotation notices that the injured structure:

(A) Is located at the origin of the external carotid artery
(B) Is innervated by the facial nerve
(C) Functions as a chemoreceptor
(D) Is stimulated by changes in blood pressure
(E) Communicates freely with the cavernous sinus

28. During a game, a 26-year-old baseball player is hit in the head by a baseball, which fractures the optic canal. Which of the following pairs of structures is most likely to be damaged?

(A) Optic nerve and ophthalmic vein
(B) Ophthalmic vein and ophthalmic nerve
(C) Ophthalmic artery and optic nerve
(D) Ophthalmic nerve and optic nerve
(E) Ophthalmic artery and ophthalmic vein

29. A 43-year-old man has new onset of difficulty with speaking. Examination by the ENT resident reveals problems in elevating the hyoid bone and floor of the mouth, secondary to paralysis of the posterior belly of the digastric muscle. Which of the following nerves is most likely involved?

(A) Accessory nerve
(B) Trigeminal nerve
(C) Ansa cervicalis
(D) Facial nerve
(E) Glossopharyngeal nerve

30. The drummer of a local band presents to your clinic with hearing loss. Otoscopic examination reveals loss of contraction of the tensor tympani and the stapedius, which prevents damage to the eardrum and middle ear ossicles. These muscles are most likely controlled by which of the following nerves?

(A) Chorda tympani and tympanic nerve
(B) Trigeminal and facial nerves
(C) Auditory and vagus nerves
(D) Facial and auditory nerves
(E) Trigeminal and accessory nerves

31. The pupil in the eye of a 43-year-old patient remains small even when room lighting is dim. Which of the following nerves would be injured?

(A) Trochlear nerve
(B) Superior cervical ganglion
(C) Oculomotor nerve
(D) Ophthalmic nerve
(E) Abducens nerve

32. A pharyngeal (gag) reflex is the contraction of the pharyngeal constrictor muscles that is elicited by touching the back of a patient's pharynx (e.g., with a tongue depressor). Afferent nerve fibers that innervated the pharyngeal mucosa are branches of which of the following nerves?

(A) Trigeminal nerve
(B) Facial nerve
(C) Glossopharyngeal nerve
(D) Vagus nerve
(E) Hypoglossal nerve

33. A benign tumor in the orbit of a 49-year-old man compresses a structure that runs through both the superior orbital fissure and the common tendinous ring. Which of the following structures is most likely damaged?

(A) Frontal nerve
(B) Lacrimal nerve
(C) Trochlear nerve
(D) Abducens nerve
(E) Ophthalmic vein

34. A 37-year-old man feels a little discomfort when moving his tongue, pharynx, and larynx. Physical examination indicates that the muscles attached to the styloid process are paralyzed. Which of the following groups of cranial nerves are damaged?

(A) Facial, glossopharyngeal, and hypoglossal nerves
(B) Hypoglossal, vagus, and facial nerves
(C) Glossopharyngeal, trigeminal, and vagus nerves
(D) Vagus, spinal accessory, and hypoglossal nerves
(E) Facial, glossopharyngeal, and vagus nerves

35. A high school basketball player experiences a sudden difficulty in breathing and is brought to an emergency department. When a low tracheotomy is performed below the isthmus of the thyroid, which of the following vessels may be encountered?

(A) Inferior thyroid artery
(B) Inferior thyroid vein
(C) Costocervical trunk
(D) Superior thyroid artery
(E) Right brachiocephalic vein

36. A 59-year-old man complains of numbness in the anterior cervical triangle. Therefore, damage has occurred to which of the following nerves?

(A) Phrenic nerve
(B) Greater auricular nerve
(C) Transverse cervical nerve
(D) Supraclavicular nerve
(E) Lesser occipital nerve

37. A 53-year-old man has difficulty with breathing through his nose. On examination, his physician finds that he has swelling of the mucous membranes of the superior nasal meatus. Which opening of the paranasal sinuses is most likely plugged?

(A) Middle ethmoidal sinus
(B) Maxillary sinus
(C) Posterior ethmoidal sinus
(D) Anterior ethmoidal sinus
(E) Frontal sinus

38. A 61-year-old woman is found to have ocular lymphoma invading her optic canal. Which of the following structures would most likely be damaged?

(A) Ophthalmic vein
(B) Ophthalmic nerve
(C) Oculomotor nerve
(D) Trochlear nerve
(E) Ophthalmic artery

39. A 76-year-old man with swallowing difficulties undergoes imaging for a possible mass. The CT scan image at the level of the cricothyroid ligament in his neck should show which of the following structures?

(A) Inferior laryngeal nerves
(B) External carotid arteries
(C) Inferior thyroid veins
(D) Thyrocervical trunks
(E) Internal laryngeal nerves

40. The muscles that are of branchiomeric origin are paralyzed in a 26-year-old patient. A lesion of which of the following nerves would cause muscle dysfunction?

(A) Oculomotor nerve
(B) Trochlear nerve
(C) Trigeminal nerve
(D) Abducens nerve
(E) Hypoglossal nerve

41. During surgery for a malignant parotid tumor in a 69-year-old woman, the main trunk of the facial nerve is lacerated. Which of the following muscles is paralyzed?

(A) Masseter muscle
(B) Stylopharyngeus muscle
(C) Anterior belly of the digastric muscle
(D) Buccinator muscle
(E) Tensor tympani

42. During a gang fight, a 17-year-old boy is punched, and his nasal septum is broken. Which of the following structures would be damaged?

(A) Septal cartilage and nasal bone
(B) Inferior concha and vomer
(C) Vomer and perpendicular plate of ethmoid
(D) Septal cartilage and middle concha
(E) Cribriform plate and frontal bone

43. A 58-year-old woman comes to the hospital and complains of progressive loss of voice, numbness, loss of taste on the back part of her tongue, and difficulty in shrugging her shoulders. Her MRI scan reveals a dural meningioma that compresses the nerves leaving the skull. These nerves leave the skull through which of the following openings?

(A) Foramen spinosum
(B) Foramen rotundum
(C) Internal auditory meatus
(D) Jugular foramen
(E) Foramen lacerum

44. A 21-year-old woman presents to her physician with a swelling on her neck. On examination, she is diagnosed with an infection within the carotid sheath. Which of the following structures would be damaged?

(A) Vagus nerve and middle cervical ganglion
(B) Internal carotid artery and recurrent laryngeal nerve
(C) Internal jugular vein and vagus nerve
(D) Sympathetic trunk and common carotid artery
(E) External carotid artery and ansa cervicalis

45. An angiogram of a 45-year-old man shows an occlusion of the costocervical trunk. This obstruction could produce a marked decrease in the blood flow in which of the following arteries?

(A) Superior thoracic artery
(B) Transverse cervical artery
(C) Ascending cervical artery
(D) Deep cervical artery
(E) Inferior thyroid artery

46. A 57-year-old man comes to the local hospital with fever, headache, nausea, and vomiting. Laboratory tests reveal an infection, and radiologic examination localizes the infection to the cavernous sinus. Which of the following nerves would be unaffected by this condition?

(A) Oculomotor nerves
(B) Abducens nerves
(C) Trochlear nerves
(D) Mandibular nerves
(E) Ophthalmic nerves

47. A 7-year-old girl has difficulty breathing through her nose and is brought to her pediatrician. On examination, she is diagnosed with adenoids. Which of the following tonsils is enlarged?

(A) Palatine tonsil
(B) Pharyngeal tonsil
(C) Tubal tonsil
(D) Lingual tonsil
(E) Eustachian tonsil

48. A 59-year-old woman with pain at the side of her skull comes to the emergency department. An emergent head CT scan shows a large lesion in the internal auditory meatus. This condition may progress and damage which of the following pairs of structures?

(A) Vagus and glossopharyngeal nerves
(B) Internal carotid and vertebral arteries
(C) Internal jugular vein and trigeminal nerve
(D) Facial and vestibulocochlear nerves
(E) Hypoglossal and accessory nerves

49. After ingesting a toxic substance found in her friend's home, a 12-year-old girl is unable to close her lips. Which of the following muscles may be paralyzed?

(A) Levator labii superioris
(B) Zygomaticus minor
(C) Orbicularis oris
(D) Lateral pterygoid
(E) Depressor labii inferioris

50. A 37-year-old man receives a direct blow to his head and is brought to an emergency department. His radiograph shows a fracture of the floor of the middle cranial cavity, causing severance of the greater petrosal nerve. Which of the following conditions could be produced by this injury?

(A) Increased lacrimal gland secretion
(B) Loss of taste sensation in the epiglottis
(C) Dryness in the nose and palate
(D) Decreased parotid gland secretion
(E) Loss of sensation in the pharynx

51. A 65-year-old man with multiple vision problems comes to the local eye clinic. The pupillary light reflex can be eliminated by cutting which of the following nerves?

(A) Short ciliary, ophthalmic, and oculomotor nerves
(B) Long ciliary, optic, and short ciliary nerves
(C) Oculomotor, short ciliary, and optic nerves
(D) Optic and long ciliary nerves and ciliary ganglion
(E) Ophthalmic and optic nerves and ciliary ganglion

52. A 12-year-old boy has difficulty in breathing because he is choking on food. A school nurse performs the Valsalva maneuver to expel air from his lungs and thus dislodge the food. When that fails, she performs a needle cricothyrotomy, which would open into which of the following regions?

(A) Rima glottidis
(B) Laryngeal vestibule
(C) Laryngeal ventricle
(D) Infraglottic cavity
(E) Piriform recess

53. A 59-year-old stroke patient is unable to swallow because of a nerve injury. Which of the following nerves is unaffected?

(A) Hypoglossal nerve
(B) Spinal accessory nerve
(C) Vagus nerve
(D) Facial nerve
(E) Trigeminal nerve

54. A 2-year-boy presents with midfacial and mandibular hypoplasia, cleft palate, deformed external ear, and defect in hearing. Which of the following embryonic structures is most likely developed abnormally?

(A) First pharyngeal arch
(B) Second pharyngeal arch
(C) Third pharyngeal arch
(D) Fourth pharyngeal arch
(E) Sixth pharyngeal arch

55. A 64-year-old woman is unable to open her mouth or jaw because of tetanus resulting from a penetrating wound from a rusty nail. Which of the following muscles would most likely be paralyzed?

(A) Masseter muscle
(B) Medial pterygoid muscle
(C) Lateral pterygoid muscle
(D) Buccinator muscle
(E) Temporalis muscle

56. A 60-year-old man is unable to open his eye because of a rare neuromuscular disease. Which of the following muscles would most likely be paralyzed?

(A) Orbicularis oculi
(B) Orbicularis oris
(C) Frontalis
(D) Levator palpebrae superioris
(E) Superior rectus

57. A 46-year-old man visits the speech therapist complaining of dryness of the mouth. The therapist performs a swallowing study and, on examination, finds that the man has a lack of salivary secretion from the submandibular gland. This indicates a lesion of which of the following nervous structures?

(A) Lingual nerve at its origin
(B) Chorda tympani in the middle ear cavity
(C) Superior cervical ganglion
(D) Lesser petrosal nerve
(E) Auriculotemporal nerve

58. A 51-year-old woman traveling through British Columbia can see the beautiful blue sky with white clouds but is unable to focus on her face in the mirror. Her lack of accommodation results from paralysis of which of the following muscles?

(A) Tarsal muscle
(B) Sphincter pupillae
(C) Dilator pupillae
(D) Ciliary muscles
(E) Orbitalis muscles

59. A 3-year-old girl is admitted to the hospital with pain and hearing defect. An MRI examination reveals that she has developmental defects in the auditory tube and middle ear cavity. Which of the following pharyngeal pouches is most likely developed abnormally?

(A) First pouch
(B) Second pouch
(C) Third pouch
(D) Fourth pouch
(E) Second and fourth pouches

60. A 42-year-old patient has an aneurysm at the junction of the posterior cerebral and posterior communicating arteries that has compressed a nerve. On the affected side, the patient is most likely to exhibit:

(A) Bitemporal hemianopsia
(B) A dilated pupil
(C) A medially deviated eye
(D) A constricted pupil
(E) Anosmia

Questions 61 to 65: Choose the appropriate lettered structure in this radiograph of the lateral view of the head (below).

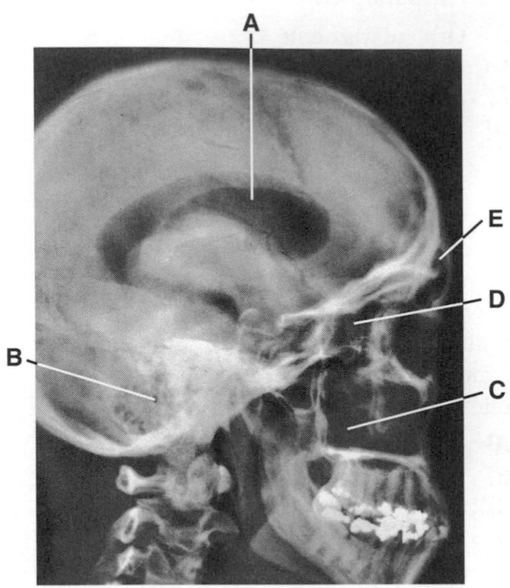

61. Which structure lies lateral to the lateral wall of the nasal cavity and inferior to the floor of the orbit?

62. A middle ear infection may spread into which structure?

63. Which structure has numerous small cavities and lies between the orbit and the nasal cavity?

64. Which structure would spread infection into the anterior part of the middle nasal meatus through the frontonasal duct?

65. CSF is formed by vascular choroid plexus in which structure?

Questions 65 to 70: Choose the appropriate lettered structure in this MRI scan (see Figure below) showing a sagittal section through the head and neck.

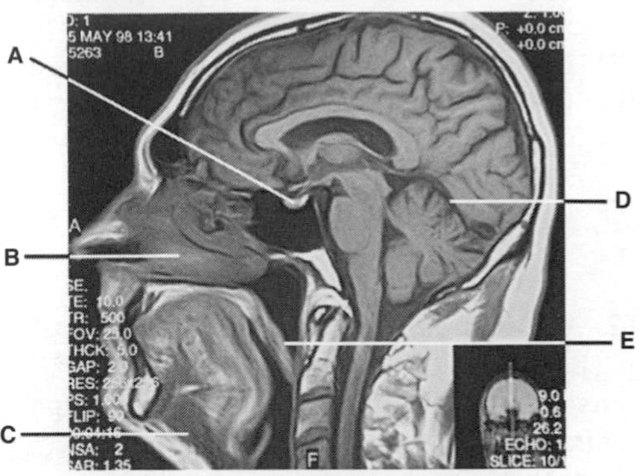

66. When the nerve on the right side is damaged, which structure is deviated to the left side?

67. A lesion of the first cervical spinal nerve would cause functional impairment of which structure?

68. Tears drain through the nasolacrimal duct into the space below which structure?

69. Which structure runs along the line of attachment of the falx cerebri to the tentorium cerebelli?

70. A tumor of which structure can be removed through the transsphenoidal approach following the septum of the nose through the body of the sphenoid?

Questions 71 to 75: Choose the appropriate lettered structure in this MRI scan showing a transaxial section through the head (see Figure below).

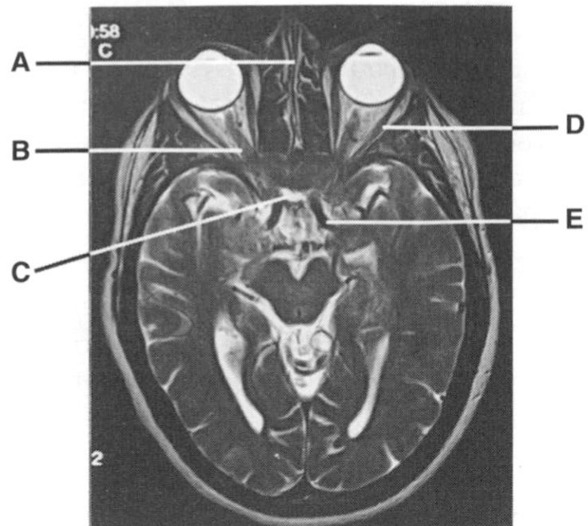

71. Which structure mediates the afferent limb of the pupillary light reflex?

72. Which structure is formed by the perpendicular plate of the ethmoid bone, vomer, and septal cartilage?

73. Which structure may be paralyzed as a result of infection of the cavernous sinus?

74. Which structure pierces the dural roof of the cavernous sinus between the anterior and middle clinoid processes?

75. Which structure may be obliterated by a pituitary tumor?

Questions 76 to 80: Choose the appropriate lettered structure in this angiogram of the cerebral vasculature (see Figure below). Collateral circulations are discounted for the next five questions.

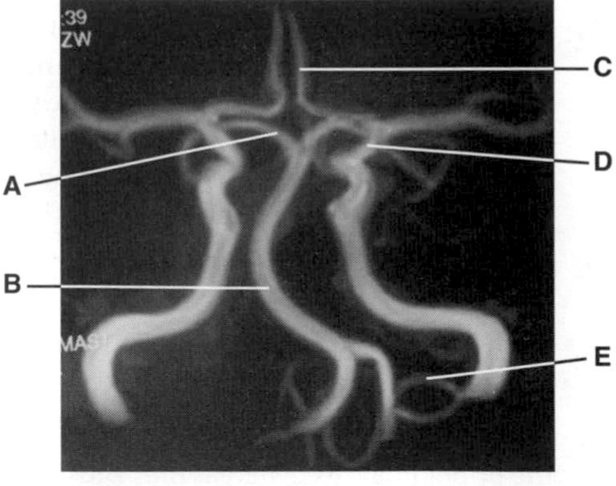

76. Aneurysm of which artery causes a perichiasmal lesion that may cause nasal hemianopia?

77. A large tumor in the foramen magnum may decrease blood flow in which artery?

78. A blockage of which artery may cause ischemia of the midbrain and the temporal and occipital lobes of the cerebrum?

79. Ischemia of the posterior inferior surface of the cerebellum is caused by obstruction of which artery?

80. A lesion of which artery may cause oxygen deficiency to the medial surface of the frontal and parietal lobes of the brain?

Answers and Explanations

1. **The answer is C.** The external laryngeal nerve innervates the cricothyroid muscle (major tensor), which tenses the vocal cord. The anterior part of the vocalis muscle can tense the vocal cord, and its posterior part can relax the vocal cord. The lateral cricoarytenoid muscle rotates the vocal process of the arytenoids cartilage medially, closing the rima glottides. The rima glottidis is opened (widened) by rotating the vocal process of the arytenoid cartilage laterally by the posterior cricoarytenoid muscle. Other laryngeal muscles adduct the vocal cords.

2. **The answer is B.** The internal laryngeal nerve accompanies the superior laryngeal artery, whereas the external laryngeal nerve accompanies the superior thyroid artery. The superior laryngeal, hypoglossal, and vagus nerves are not closely associated with the superior laryngeal artery.

3. **The answer is D.** The glossopharyngeal nerve supplies sensory innervation to the mucosa of the upper pharynx, whereas the vagus nerve supplies sensory innervation to the lower pharynx and larynx. The maxillary nerve supplies sensory innervation to the face below the level of the eye and above the level of the upper lip and the palate and nasal mucosa. The superior cervical ganglion contributes to a formation of the pharyngeal plexus but contains no afferent fibers. The external laryngeal nerve innervates the cricothyroid and inferior pharyngeal constrictor muscles.

4. **The answer is D.** The surgeon should ligate the costocervical trunk because it divides into the deep cervical and superior intercostal arteries. The thyrocervical trunk gives off the suprascapular, transverse cervical, and inferior thyroid artery. The ascending cervical artery is a branch of the inferior thyroid artery.

5. **The answer is E.** The phrenic nerve descends on the superficial surface of the anterior scalene muscle and passes into the thorax posterior to the subclavian vein, anterior to the subclavian artery, and lateral to the common carotid artery. The brachial plexus passes deep to the anterior scalene muscle.

6. **The answer is A.** The skin over the tip of the nose is innervated by the external nasal branch of the nasociliary branch of the ophthalmic division of the trigeminal nerve. The maxillary division of the trigeminal nerve innervates the skin of the face above the upper lip but below the lower eyelid. The mandibular division of the trigeminal nerve supplies the lower part of the face below the lower lip. The facial nerve provides no cutaneous sensation on the face but innervates muscles of facial expression. The auriculotemporal nerve is a branch of the mandibular division of the trigeminal nerve and innervates the skin of the auricle and the scalp.

7. **The answer is A.** The external laryngeal branch of the superior laryngeal nerve supplies the cricothyroid and inferior pharyngeal constrictor muscles. The superior, middle, and inferior pharyngeal constrictors are innervated by the vagus nerve through the pharyngeal plexus. The recurrent (or inferior) laryngeal nerve supplies the thyroarytenoid muscle and the C1 via the hypoglossal nerve supplies the thyrohyoid muscle.

8. **The answer is A.** "Crocodile tears syndrome" (lacrimation during eating) is caused by a lesion of the facial nerve proximal to the geniculate ganglion resulting from misdirection of regenerating parasympathetic fibers, which formerly innervated the salivary glands, to the lacrimal glands. An injury to the auriculotemporal nerve may result in Frey syndrome (sweating while eating), which results from misdirection of regenerating parasympathetic and sympathetic fibers. The chorda tympani carries preganglionic parasympathetic fibers to the submandibular ganglion and taste fibers to the anterior two-thirds of the tongue. The facial nerve innervates the muscles of facial expression. The terminal part of the lacrimal nerve contains postganglionic parasympathetic fibers for lacrimation.

9. **The answer is C.** Postganglionic parasympathetic fibers originating in the pterygopalatine ganglion innervate glands in the palate and nasal mucosa. The postganglionic parasympathetic fibers from the otic ganglion supply the parotid gland, those from the submandibular ganglion supply the submandibular and sublingual glands, and those from the ciliary ganglion supply the ciliary muscle and sphincter pupillae. The nodose (inferior) ganglion of the vagus nerve is a sensory ganglion.

10. **The answer is C.** Bell palsy (facial paralysis) can involve inflammation of the cornea, leading to corneal ulceration, which probably is attributable to an absence of the corneal blink reflex. This is due to paralysis of the orbicularis oculi, which closes the eyelid. Sensory loss of the cornea and conjunctiva is due to injury of the ophthalmic nerve. Lack of secretion of the parotid salivary gland is due to injury of the glossopharyngeal, tympanic, or lesser petrosal nerve. Absence of sweating is due to damage of the sympathetic nerve. Inability to constrict the pupil is due to paralysis of the sphincter pupillae or damage of parasympathetic nerve fibers to the sphincter.

11. **The answer is D.** The superior petrosal sinus runs from the cavernous sinus to the transverse sinus along the attached margin of the tentorium cerebelli. This patient has meningitis (inflammation of the meninges), which causes headache and dizziness. The straight sinus runs along the line of attachment of the falx cerebri to the tentorium cerebelli; the inferior sagittal sinus lies in the free edge of the falx cerebri; the sphenoparietal sinus lies along the posterior edge of the lesser wing of the sphenoid bone; the cavernous sinus lies on each side of the sella turcica and the body of the sphenoid bone.

12. **The answer is C.** Bilateral severance of the vagus nerve (CN X) causes a loss of reflex control of circulation because of an increase in heart rate and blood pressure; poor digestion results because of decreased gastrointestinal motility and secretion; and difficulty in swallowing, speaking, and breathing occurs because of paralysis of laryngeal and pharyngeal muscles. All of these effects may result in death. Bilateral severance of other nerves does not cause death.

13. **The answer is C.** Rupture of the middle meningeal artery in the cranial cavity causes an epidural hemorrhage. Subarachnoid hemorrhage is due to rupture of cerebral arteries and veins. Subdural hematoma is due to rupture of bridging cerebral veins as they pass from the brain surface into one of the venous sinuses. Subpial hemorrhage is due to damage to the small vessels of the pia and brain tissue. Cranial dural sinuses normally contain venous blood.

14. **The answer is E.** Preganglionic neurons of the parasympathetic nervous system are located in the brain stem (cranial outflow) and sacral spinal cord segments S2 to S4 (sacral outflow). Preganglionic sympathetic neurons are located in the thoracic and lumbar spinal cord.

15. **The answer is E.** The pituitary gland lies in the hypophyseal fossa of the sella turcica of the sphenoid bone, which lies immediately posterior and superior to the sphenoid sinus and medial to the cavernous sinus. The frontal sinus lies in the frontal bone; the maxillary sinus lies in the maxilla lateral to the lateral wall of the nasal cavity; the ethmoid sinus (composed of air cells) lies between the orbit and the nasal cavity; and the mastoid air cells lie in the mastoid process of the temporal bone.

16. **The answer is C.** The posterior one-third of the tongue receives both general and taste innervation from the lingual branch of the glossopharyngeal nerve. The internal laryngeal nerve supplies general and taste sensations to the epiglottis. The lingual nerve supplies general sensation to the anterior two-thirds of the tongue. The greater palatine nerve innervates the hard palate and the inner surface of the maxillary gingival. The chorda tympani supplies taste sensation to the anterior two-thirds of the tongue and preganglionic parasympathetic fibers to the submandibular ganglion for supplying the submandibular and sublingual glands.

17. **The answer is E.** The sella turcica is part of the sphenoid bone and lies superior to the sphenoid sinus. Therefore, none of the other bones listed is fractured.

18. **The answer is E.** The superior thyroid artery is accompanied by the external laryngeal nerve, which innervates the cricothyroid muscle. Paralysis of this muscle due to a lesion of the external laryngeal nerve decreases tension of the vocal cord. Loss of sensation above the vocal cord

is due to injury of the internal laryngeal nerve. The posterior cricoarytenoid muscle draws the muscular process of the arytenoid cartilage posteriorly and thereby rotates its vocal process laterally. Paralysis of the vocalis muscle is due to a lesion of the recurrent laryngeal nerve. Lack of abduction of the vocal cord results from paralysis of the posterior cricoarytenoid muscle.

19. **The answer is B.** The dural venous sinus nearest the pituitary gland is the cavernous sinus. Cavernous sinus thrombophlebitis is an infectious inflammation of the sinus that may produce meningitis, papilledema, exophthalmos, and ophthalmoplegia. The other sinuses listed are not closely associated with the pituitary gland.

20. **The answer is D.** The posterior cricoarytenoid muscle is the only muscle that abducts the vocal cords during quiet breathing. All of the other laryngeal muscles adduct the vocal cords.

21. **The answer is B.** The oblique arytenoid and aryepiglottic muscles tilt the arytenoid cartilages and approximate them, assisting in closing of the larynx and preventing food from entering the larynx and trachea during the process of swallowing. The cricopharyngeus fibers of the inferior pharyngeal constrictors act as a sphincter that prevents air from entering the esophagus. Other muscles are not involved in closing or opening the airway.

22. **The answer is D.** The veins of the brain are direct tributaries of the dural venous sinuses. The emissary veins connect the dural venous sinuses with the veins of the scalp; the pterygoid venous plexus communicates with the cavernous sinus through an emissary vein; the diploic veins lie in channels in the diploë of the skull and communicate with the dural sinuses, the veins of the scalp, and the meningeal veins.

23. **The answer is D.** When the parasympathetic fibers to the eyeball are stimulated, the pupil constricts and the ciliary muscle contracts, resulting in a thicker lens and enhanced vision for near objects (accommodation). Dilation of the pupil, contraction of capillaries in the iris, and enhanced ability to see distant objects (flattening of the lens) result from stimulation of sympathetic nerves.

24. **The answer is D.** The tympanic nerve, or Jacobson nerve, is a branch of the glossopharyngeal nerve, contains preganglionic parasympathetic fibers, and forms a tympanic plexus on the medial wall of the middle ear with sympathetic fibers. The tympanic nerve continues beyond the plexus as the lesser petrosal nerve, which transmits preganglionic parasympathetic fibers to the otic ganglion for synapse.

25. **The answer is B.** The middle ear cavity is separated from the middle cranial fossa by the tegmen tympani, a thin plate of the petrous part of the temporal bone. A part of the roof of the sphenoid bone forms the floor of the hypophyseal fossa. The other pairs of sinuses or bony cavities are not separated from the middle cranial cavity.

26. **The answer is D.** The cranial dura in the middle cranial fossa is innervated by the maxillary and mandibular divisions of the trigeminal nerve, the dura in the anterior cranial fossa is innervated by the ophthalmic division of the trigeminal nerve, and the dura in the posterior cranial fossa is innervated by the vagus and hypoglossal (C1 through the hypoglossal) nerves. The facial and glossopharyngeal nerves do not supply the cranial dura.

27. **The answer is D.** The carotid sinus, a spindle-shaped dilatation of the origin of the internal carotid artery, is a pressoreceptor that is stimulated by changes in blood pressure. The carotid sinus is at the origin of the internal carotid artery and is innervated by the carotid sinus branch of the glossopharyngeal nerve and nerve to the carotid body of the vagus nerve. It is not a venous sinus and thus does not communicate with the cavernous sinus. The carotid body functions as a chemoreceptor.

28. **The answer is C.** The optic canal transmits the optic nerve and ophthalmic artery. The ophthalmic nerve and ophthalmic vein enter the orbit through the superior orbital fissure.

29. **The answer is D.** The digastric posterior belly is innervated by the facial nerve, whereas the digastric anterior belly is innervated by the trigeminal nerve. The accessory nerve supplies the sternocleidomastoid and trapezius muscles. The ansa cervicalis innervates the infrahyoid (or strap) muscles. The glossopharyngeal nerve supplies the stylopharyngeus muscle.

30. **The answer is B.** The tensor tympani is innervated by the trigeminal nerve, and the stapedius is innervated by the facial nerve. The other nerves are not involved.

31. **The answer is B.** The superior cervical ganglion is damaged. When the pupil remains small in a dimly lit room, it is an indication that postganglionic sympathetic fibers that originate from the superior cervical ganglion and innervate the dilator pupillae (radial muscles of the iris) are damaged. Other nerves contain no sympathetic fibers, but the oculomotor nerve contains preganglionic parasympathetic fibers.

32. **The answer is C.** The afferent limb of the pharyngeal (gag) reflex is a pharyngeal branch of the glossopharyngeal nerve, whereas the vagus nerve mediates the efferent limb. The trigeminal, facial, and hypoglossal nerves are not involved in the gag reflex.

33. **The answer is D.** The abducens nerve enters the orbit through the superior orbital fissure and the common tendinous ring. The trochlear, lacrimal, and frontal nerves and the ophthalmic vein enter the orbit through the superior orbital fissure outside the common tendinous ring.

34. **The answer is A.** The styloid process provides attachments for the stylohyoid, styloglossus, and stylopharyngeus muscles. The stylohyoid muscle is innervated by the facial nerve, the styloglossus muscle is innervated by the hypoglossal nerve, and the stylopharyngeus muscle is innervated by the glossopharyngeal nerve. No other muscles are attached to the styloid process.

35. **The answer is B.** A low tracheotomy is a surgical incision of the trachea through the neck and below the isthmus of the thyroid gland. The inferior thyroid veins drain the thyroid gland, descend in front of the trachea, and enter the brachiocephalic veins. Consequently, these veins are closely associated with the isthmus of the thyroid gland. Other blood vessels are not closely related with the front of the trachea and the isthmus of the thyroid gland.

36. **The answer is C.** The transverse cervical nerve turns around the posterior border of the sternocleidomastoid and innervates the skin of the anterior cervical triangle. The phrenic nerve, a branch of the cervical plexus, contains motor and sensory fibers but no cutaneous nerve fibers. The greater auricular nerve innervates the skin behind the auricle and on the parotid gland. The supraclavicular nerve innervates the skin over the clavicle and the shoulder. The lesser occipital nerve innervates the scalp behind the auricle.

37. **The answer is C.** The posterior ethmoidal sinus opens into the superior nasal meatus. The maxillary, frontal, and anterior and middle ethmoidal sinuses drain into the middle nasal meatus.

38. **The answer is E.** The optic canal transmits the ophthalmic artery and optic nerve. The ophthalmic nerve, ophthalmic vein, and oculomotor and trochlear nerves enter the orbit through the superior orbital fissure.

39. **The answer is A.** A CT scan through the cricothyroid ligament shows the inferior laryngeal nerves, which are the terminal portion of the recurrent laryngeal nerves above the lower border of the cricoid cartilage. The external carotid arteries and the internal laryngeal nerves lie above the cricothyroid ligament, and the inferior thyroid veins and the thyrocervical trunks lie below the ligament.

40. **The answer is C.** SVE nerve fibers originate from the first branchial arch (trigeminal), the second arch (facial), the third arch (glossopharyngeal), and the fourth and sixth arches (vagus). Nerves that supply the muscles of the eyeball (oculomotor, trochlear, and abducens) and tongue (hypoglossal) are not of branchiomeric origin.

41. **The answer is D.** The buccinator muscle is innervated by the facial nerve. The masseter, anterior belly of the digastric, and tensor tympani muscles are innervated by the mandibular division of the trigeminal nerve. The stylopharyngeus muscle is innervated by the glossopharyngeal nerve.

42. **The answer is C.** The nasal septum is formed primarily by the vomer, the perpendicular plate of ethmoid bone, and the septal cartilage. The superior, middle, and inferior conchae form the lateral wall of the nasal cavity. The ethmoid (cribriform plate), nasal, frontal, and sphenoid (body) bones form the roof. The floor is formed by the palatine process of the maxilla and the horizontal plate of the palatine bone.

43. **The answer is D.** A loss of voice is due to an injury to the recurrent laryngeal nerve of the vagus nerve; numbness and loss of taste on the posterior part of the tongue are due to a lesion of the glossopharyngeal nerve; an inability to shrug the shoulder is due to damage of the accessory nerve. These three CNs exit the skull through the jugular foramen. The foramen spinosum transmits the middle meningeal artery. The foramen rotundum transmits the maxillary division of the trigeminal nerve. The internal auditory meatus transmits the facial and vestibulocochlear nerves. The foramen lacerum transmits nothing, but its upper part is traversed by the internal carotid artery with sympathetic nerve plexus.

44. **The answer is C.** The carotid sheath contains the internal jugular vein, vagus nerve, and common and internal carotid arteries. The recurrent laryngeal nerve lies in a groove between the trachea and esophagus. The sympathetic trunk, with superior and middle cervical ganglia, lies behind the carotid sheath. The external carotid artery is not contained within the carotid sheath. The ansa cervicalis lies superficial to or within the carotid sheath.

45. **The answer is D.** The costocervical trunk gives rise to the deep cervical and superior intercostal arteries. The superior thoracic artery arises from the axillary artery. The transverse cervical, inferior thyroid, and suprascapular arteries arise from the thyrocervical trunk. The ascending cervical artery arises from the inferior thyroid artery.

46. **The answer is D.** The mandibular division of the trigeminal nerve does not lie in the wall of the cavernous sinus, whereas the oculomotor, abducens, trochlear, and ophthalmic nerves do.

47. **The answer is B.** The enlarged pharyngeal tonsil is called an adenoid. An adenoid obstructs passage of air from the nasal cavities through the choanae into the nasopharynx, thus causing difficulty in nasal breathing and phonation. The tubal tonsil is also called the eustachian tonsil. The palatine tonsil is called the faucial tonsil. The submerged tonsil is a palatine tonsil that is shrunken and atrophied and is partly or entirely hidden by the palatoglossal arch.

48. **The answer is D.** The internal auditory meatus transmits the facial and vestibulocochlear nerves. The jugular foramen transmits the glossopharyngeal, vagus, and accessory nerves and the internal jugular vein. The ophthalmic, maxillary, and mandibular divisions of the trigeminal nerve run through the superior orbital fissure, foramen rotundum, and foramen ovale, respectively. The hypoglossal nerve runs through the hypoglossal canal.

49. **The answer is C.** The lips are closed by the orbicularis oris muscles. The lips are opened by the levator labii superioris, zygomaticus minor, and depressor labii inferioris muscles. The lateral pterygoid muscle can open the mouth by depressing the lower jaw.

50. **The answer is C.** The greater petrosal nerve carries parasympathetic (preganglionic) fibers, which are secretomotor fibers, to the lacrimal glands and mucous glands in the nasal cavity and palate; carries taste fibers from the palate; and carries GVA fibers from the nasal cavity, palate, and roof of the oral cavity but not from the pharynx and larynx. Therefore, a lesion of the greater petrosal nerve causes dryness in the nose and palate and decreased lacrimal secretion. Decreased parotid gland secretion is due to a lesion of the lesser petrosal nerve. Taste sensation in the epiglottis is carried by the internal laryngeal branch of the superior laryngeal nerve. General visceral sensation in the pharynx is carried by the glossopharyngeal nerve.

51. **The answer is C.** The efferent limbs of the reflex are involved in the pupillary light reflex (i.e., constriction of the pupil in response to illumination of the retina) and are composed of parasympathetic preganglionic fibers in the oculomotor nerve, parasympathetic fibers and ganglionic cells in the ciliary ganglion, and parasympathetic postganglionic fibers in the short ciliary nerves. The afferent limbs of this reflex are optic nerve fibers. The long ciliary nerves contain postganglionic sympathetic fibers. The ophthalmic nerve contains GSA fibers.

52. **The answer is D.** The infraglottic cavity extends from the rima glottidis to the lower border of the cricoid cartilage. The rima glottidis is the space between the vocal folds and arytenoid cartilages. The vestibule extends from the laryngeal inlet to the vestibular folds. The ventricle extends between the vestibular fold and the vocal fold. The piriform recess is a pear-shaped fossa in the wall of the laryngopharynx lateral to the arytenoid cartilage.

53. **The answer is B.** The spinal accessory nerve supplies the sternocleidomastoid and trapezius muscles, which are not involved in the act of swallowing. Swallowing involves movements of the tongue to push the food into the oropharynx, elevation of the soft palate to close the entrance of the nasopharynx, elevation of the hyoid bone and the larynx to close the opening into the larynx, and contraction of the pharyngeal constrictors to move the food through the pharynx. The hypoglossal nerve supplies all of the tongue muscles except the palatoglossus, which is innervated by the vagus nerve. The vagus nerve innervates the muscles of the palate, larynx, and pharynx. The mandibular division of the trigeminal nerve supplies the suprahyoid muscles (e.g., the anterior belly of the digastric and the mylohyoid muscles).

54. **The answer is A.** The patient's abnormal appearance results from abnormal development of the first pharyngeal arch because the first pharyngeal arch develops into muscles of mastication, mylohyoid, digastric anterior belly, tensor veli palatini, tensor tympani, maxilla, mandible, malleus, incus, zygomatic bone, temporal bone, palatine bone, vomer, and sphenomandibular ligament.

55. **The answer is C.** The lateral pterygoid muscle opens the mouth by depressing the jaw. The masseter, medial pterygoid, and temporalis muscles close the jaw. The buccinator muscle is a muscle of facial expression.

56. **The answer is D.** The levator palpebrae superioris muscle opens the eye by elevating the upper eyelid. The orbicularis oculi closes the eye, the orbicularis oris closes the lips, the frontalis elevates the eyebrow, and the superior rectus elevates the eyeball.

57. **The answer is B.** The chorda tympani nerve contains preganglionic parasympathetic fibers responsible for secretion of the submandibular gland. The lingual nerve at its origin is not yet joined by the chorda tympani. The superior cervical ganglion provides sympathetic fibers, which supply blood vessels in the submandibular gland. The lesser petrosal nerve contains preganglionic parasympathetic fibers that synapse in the otic ganglion. The auriculotemporal nerve contains postganglionic parasympathetic fibers, which are responsible for secretion of the parotid gland.

58. **The answer is D.** Near focus (accomodation) occurs with contraction of the ciliary muscles and is mediated by parasympathetic fibers running within the oculomotor nerve. The levator palpebrae superioris inserts on the tarsal smooth muscle plate in the upper eyelid and skin of the upper eyelid and opens the eye by elevating the upper eyelid. The sphincter pupillae and dilator pupillae constrict and dilate the pupil, respectively. The orbitalis muscle is a smooth muscle that bridges the inferior orbital fissure and protrudes the eye.

59. **The answer is A.** The first pharyngeal pouch gives rise to the auditory tube and middle ear cavity. The second pouch forms the palatine tonsils. The third pouch gives rise to the inferior parathyroid gland and thymus. The fourth pouch develops into the superior parathyroid gland and ultimobranchial body of the thyroid.

60. **The answer is B.** An aneurysm at the junction of the posterior communicating and posterior cerebral arteries compresses parasympathetic nerve fibers of the oculomotor nerve, causing a dilated pupil. Bitemporal hemianopsia is caused by the pituitary tumor that compresses the optic chiasma. A medially deviated eye (internal strabismus) is caused by a paralysis of the lateral rectus due to an injury to the abducens nerve. A constricted pupil is caused by a damage of the cervical sympathetic nerve fibers to the dilator muscle of the pupil. An anosmia is caused by an injury to the olfactory nerves due to a fracture of the cribriform plate.

61. **The answer is C.** The maxillary sinus lies lateral to the lateral wall of the nasal cavity and inferior to the floor of the orbit.

62. **The answer is B.** Mastoid air cells communicate with the middle ear cavity through the antrum and aditus.

63. **The answer is D.** The ethmoid sinus has numerous small cavities and lies between the orbit and the nasal cavity.

64. **The answer is E.** The frontal sinus drains into the anterior part of the middle nasal meatus via the frontonasal duct or infundibulum.

65. **The answer is A.** CSF is formed by vascular choroid plexus in the ventricles in the brain; the letter "A" indicates the lateral ventricle.

66. **The answer is E.** The musculus uvulae is innervated by the vagus nerve. A lesion of the right vagus nerve causes deviation of the uvula to the left side.

67. **The answer is C.** The geniohyoid muscle is innervated by the first cervical nerve through the hypoglossal nerve.

68. **The answer is B.** The inferior nasal meatus below the inferior concha receives the nasolacrimal duct.

69. **The answer is D.** The straight sinus runs along the line of the attachment of the falx cerebri to the tentorium cerebelli, which supports the occipital lobe of the cerebrum and covers the cerebellum.

70. **The answer is A.** The pituitary gland can be reached through the transsphenoidal approach following the septum of the nose through the body of the sphenoid.

71. **The answer is B.** The optic nerve mediates the afferent limb of the pupillary light reflex, whereas the efferent limb is mediated by the facial nerve.

72. **The answer is A.** The nasal septum is formed primarily by the perpendicular plate of the ethmoid bone, vomer, and septal cartilage.

73. **The answer is D.** The lateral rectus is innervated by the abducens nerve, which runs through the cavernous sinus.

74. **The answer is E.** The internal carotid artery pierces the dural roof of the cavernous sinus between the anterior and middle clinoid processes.

75. **The answer is C.** The suprasellar cistern can be obliterated by a pituitary tumor.

76. **The answer is D.** Nasal hemianopia is blindness in the nasal field of vision of the eye because of a perichiasmal lesion such as an aneurysm of the internal carotid artery.

77. **The answer is B.** The basilar artery is formed by the union of the two vertebral arteries at the lower border of the pons. A large tumor in the foramen magnum compresses the vertebral arteries, resulting in decreased blood flow in the basilar artery.

78. **The answer is A.** The posterior cerebral artery provides the blood supply to the midbrain and the temporal and occipital lobes of the cerebrum.

79. **The answer is E.** The posterior inferior cerebellar artery supplies the posterior inferior surface of the cerebellum.

80. **The answer is C.** The anterior cerebral artery supplies the medial surface of the frontal and parietal lobes of the cerebrum.

chapter **9**

Cranial and Autonomic Nerves

I. CRANIAL NERVES (Figure 9.1; Tables 9.1 to 9.3)

- Are 12 pairs of nerves that leave the CNS to pass through the bones of the skull. Most cranial nerves are connected to the brain stem, and all but one (vagus nerve, CN X) are distributed only in the head and the neck.
- Most cranial nerves emerge either from the ventral aspect of the brainstem (CN III, VI, XII) or laterally (CN V, VII, VIII, IX, X, XI). The only nerve to leave the dorsal surface of the brain stem is the trochlear nerve (CN IV), which arises from the dorsal aspect of the midbrain.
- Functional components in the cranial nerves.
- Most cranial nerves have only one function. Only two cranial nerves have two functions (CN III and CN V), and three cranial nerves have more than two functions (CN VII, IX, X). The three cranial nerves with more than two functions will be found to have the same five functions and can be described in a very similar way.

A. Olfactory Nerves (CN I) (Figure 9.1)

- Consist of approximately 20 bundles of unmyelinated afferent fibers (special visceral afferent [SVA]) that arise from neurons in the olfactory area, the upper one-third of the nasal mucosa, and mediate the sense of smell (olfaction).
- They pass through the foramina in the **cribriform plate** of the ethmoid bone and synapse in the **olfactory bulb**.

CLINICAL CORRELATES **Lesion of the olfactory nerve** may occur as a result of ethmoidal bone fracture and cause **anosmia**, or loss of olfactory sensation. Many people with anosmia may complain of loss or alteration of taste since these senses are connected. Also, one may have a runny nose from CSF loss from fracture of the ethmoid bone.

B. Optic Nerve (CN II) (Figure 9.1)

- Is formed by the axons of **ganglion cells of the retina**, which converge at the optic disk.
- These fibers of the optic nerve are covered by a membrane continuous with the dura, and the myelin of the optic nerves is formed by oligodendroglia, just like CNS tracts.
- These nerves carry afferent fibers for vision (special somatic afferent [SSA]) from the retina to brain.

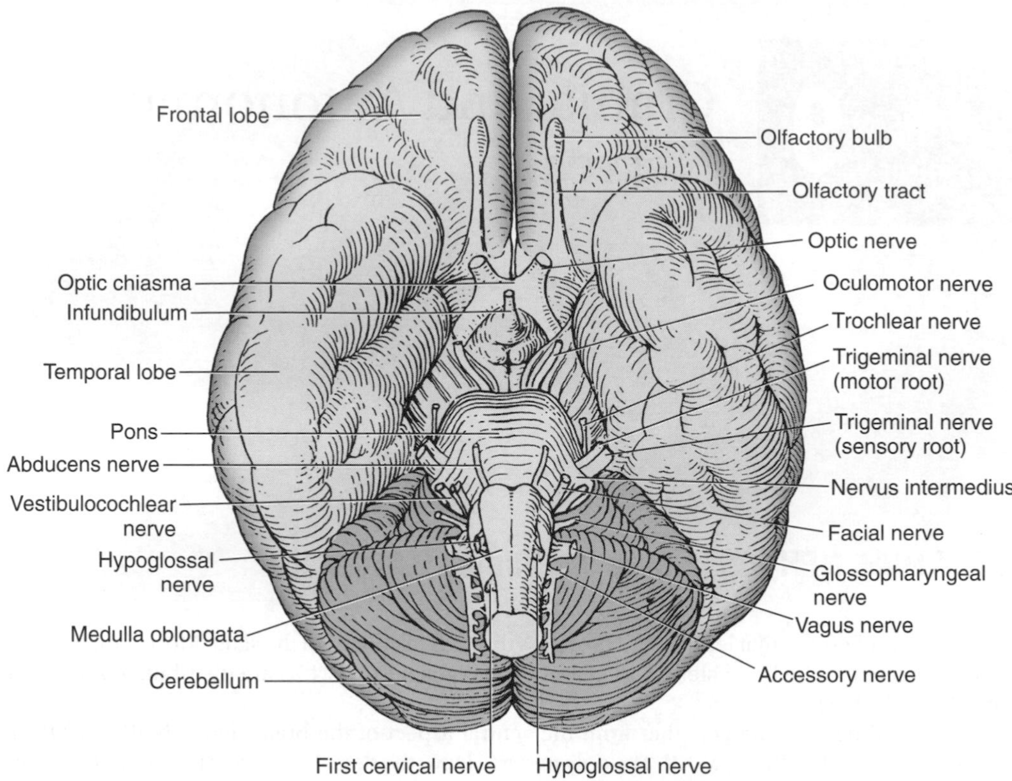

FIGURE 9.1. Cranial nerves on the base of the brain.

table 9.1 Cranial Nerves

Nerve	Cranial Exit	Cell Bodies	Components	Chief Functions
CN I: Olfactory	Cribriform plate	Nasal mucosa	SVA	Smell
CN II: Optic	Optic canal	Ganglion cells of retina	SSA	Vision
CN III: Oculomotor	Superior orbital fissure	Nucleus CN III (midbrain)	GSE	Eye movements (superior, inferior, and medial recti, inferior oblique, and levator palpebrae superioris Müller muscle)
		Edinger–Westphal nucleus (midbrain)	GVE	Constriction of pupil (sphincter pupillae muscle) and accommodation (ciliary muscle)
CN IV: Trochlear	Superior orbital fissure	Nucleus CN IV (midbrain)	GSE	Eye movements (superior oblique muscle)
CN V: Trigeminal	Superior orbital fissure; foramen rotundum and foramen ovale	Motor nucleus CN V (pons)	SVE	Muscles of mastication, mylohyoid, anterior belly of digastric, tensor veli palatini, and tensor tympani muscles
		Trigeminal ganglion	GSA	Sensation on head (skin and mucous membranes of face and head)
CN VI: Abducens	Superior orbital fissure	Nucleus CN VI (pons)	GSE	Eye movement (lateral rectus muscle)
CN VII: Facial	Stylomastoid foramen	Motor nucleus CN VII (pons)	SVE	Muscle of facial expression, posterior belly of digastric, stylohyoid, and stapedius muscles
		Superior salivatory nucleus (pons)	GVE	Lacrimal and salivary secretion
		Geniculate ganglion	SVA	Taste from anterior two-thirds of tongue and palate

table 9.1 Cranial Nerves *(continued)*

Nerve	Cranial Exit	Cell Bodies	Components	Chief Functions
		Geniculate ganglion	GVA	Sensation from palate
		Geniculate ganglion	GSA	Auricle and external acoustic meatus
CN VIII: Vestibulocochlear	Does not leave skull	Vestibular ganglion	SSA	Equilibrium
		Spiral ganglion	SSA	Hearing
CN IX: Glossopharyngeal	Jugular foramen	Nucleus ambiguus (medulla)	SVE	Elevation of pharynx (stylopharyngeus muscle)
		Inferior salivary nucleus (medulla)	GVE	Secretion of saliva (parotid gland)
		Inferior ganglion	GVA	Carotid sinus and body, tongue, pharynx, and middle ear
		Inferior ganglion	SVA	Taste from posterior one-third of tongue
		Superior ganglion	GSA	External ear
CN X: Vagus	Jugular foramen	Nucleus ambiguus (medulla)	SVE	Muscles of pharynx, larynx, and palate
		Dorsal nucleus (medulla)	GVE	Smooth muscles and glands in thoracic and abdominal viscera
		Inferior ganglion	GVA	Sensation in lower pharynx, larynx, trachea, and other viscerae
		Inferior ganglion	SVA	Taste on epiglottis
		Superior ganglion	GSA	Auricle and external acoustic meatus
CN XI: Accessory	Jugular foramen	Spinal cord (cervical)	SVE, GSE, or mixed	Sternocleidomastoid and trapezius muscles
CN XII: Hypoglossal	Hypoglossal canal	Nucleus CN XII (medulla)	GSE	Muscles of movements of tongue

GSA, general somatic afferent; GSE, general somatic efferent; GVA, general visceral afferent; GVE, general visceral efferent; SSA, special somatic afferent; SVA, special visceral afferent; SVE, special visceral efferent.

table 9.2 Functional Components in the Cranial Nerves

Functional Component	Type of Information Carried	Present in These Cranial Nerves
GSA	Pain, temperature, touch, proprioception	CN V, CN VII, CN IX, CN X
GSE	Motor to skeletal muscle of the eye and tongue	CN III, CN IV, CN VI, CN XII
GVA	Sensory from visceral organs	CN VII, CN IX, CN X
GVE	Autonomic motor fibers to smooth muscle, cardiac muscle, glands	CN III, CN VII, CN IX, CN X
SSA	Vision, hearing, equilibrium	CN II, CN VIII
SVA	Smell and taste	CN I, CN VII, CN IX, CN X
SVE or branchial efferent	Motor to skeletal muscles for mastication, facial expression, movement of the pharynx and larynx	CN V, CN VII, CN IX, CN X, CN XI (SVE, GSE, or mixed)

GSA, general somatic afferent; GSE, general somatic efferent; GVA, general visceral afferent; GVE, general visceral efferent; SSA, special somatic afferent; SVA, special visceral afferent; SVE, special visceral efferent.

- CN II leaves the middle cranial fossa to enter the orbit through the optic canal. The **optic chiasma** contains fibers from the nasal retina that cross over to the opposite side of the brain. The fibers from the temporal retina pass ipsilaterally through the chiasma.
- Mediates the afferent limb of the **pupillary light reflex**, whereas parasympathetic fibers in the oculomotor nerve mediate the efferent limb.

table 9.3 Lesion of Cranial Nerves

Nerve	Effects of Nerve Injury	Lesion Site and Cause
CN I: Olfactory nerve	Loss of smell (anosmia)	Fracture of cribriform plate
CN II: Optic nerve	Blindness; loss of afferent limb of pupillary light reflex	Fracture of orbit; lesion of optic pathway
CN III: Oculomotor nerve	Dilated pupil; ptosis; loss of accommodation and efferent limb of pupillary reflex; diplopia (double vision); external strabismus; downward and lateral gage deviation	Cavernous sinus thrombosis; midbrain lesion; aneurysm of posterior cerebral and superior cerebellar arteries
CN IV: Trochlear nerve	Inability to turn eye inferolaterally; trouble going downstairs	Cavernous sinus thrombosis; fracture of orbit; severe head injury
CN V: Trigeminal nerve	Sensory loss on face; loss of mastication; jaw deviation toward lesion side; loss of afferent limb of corneal and sneeze reflexes	Lesion of pons; fracture or tumor in region of trigeminal ganglion
CN VI: Abducens nerve	Diplopia; inability to abduct eye; internal strabismus	Cavernous sinus thrombosis; brain stem lesion; fracture of orbit
CN VII: Facial nerve	Facial paralysis (Bell palsy); loss of efferent limb of corneal reflex; loss of taste to anterior two-thirds of tongue; loss of secretion of lacrimal, submandibular, sublingual, nasal and palatine glands	Lesion of pons; Injury to internal auditory meatus; laceration in parotid region; fracture of temporal bone; inflammation in facial canal
CN VIII: Vestibulocochlear nerve	Loss of hearing and balance	Tumor in internal auditory meatus and at cerebellopontine angle
CN IX: Glossopharyngeal nerve	Loss of taste to posterior one-third of tongue; loss of receptors in carotid body and sinus; loss of parotid gland secretion; paralysis of stylopharyngeus muscle; loss of afferent limb of gag reflex	Brain stem lesion; penetrating neck injury
CN X: Vagus nerve	Deviation of uvula toward normal side; vocal cord paralysis; paralysis of palate, pharynx, and larynx; loss of receptors in aortic body and arch; loss of efferent limbs of gag and sneeze reflexes and both limbs of cough reflex	Brain stem lesion; penetrating neck injury; skull base fracture
CN XI: Accessary nerve	Inability to shrug shoulder; difficulty in turning head to opposite side	Penetrating injury to posterior cervical triangle; skull base fracture
CN XII: Hypoglossal nerve	Loss of tongue movements; tongue deviation toward lesion side	Deep laceration of neck and basal skull fracture
Sympathetics to head	Horner syndrome: constricted pupil (miosis); ptosis; enophthaloms; anhidrosis; vasodilation (flushing face)	Lesion of cervical sympathetic nerves; deep laceration of neck

CLINICAL CORRELATES

Lesion of the optic nerve (optic neuritis) may be caused by inflammatory, degenerative, demyelinating, or toxic disorders and may result in **blindness** or diminished visual acuity and **no pupillary light reflex** in the effected eye. A lesion of the **optic chiasma** due to a pituitary tumor produces bitemporal hemianopsia or tunnel vision. A lesion of the **optic tract** produces a loss of the opposite visual field, a contralateral homonymous hemianopsia.

C. Oculomotor Nerve (CN III) (Figure 9.2)

- Enters the orbit through the superior orbital fissure within the tendinous ring.
- Supplies efferent fibers (general somatic efferent [GSE]) for contraction of the extraocular muscles (i.e., medial, superior, and inferior recti; inferior oblique; and levator palpebrae superioris).
- It also contains preganglionic parasympathetic fibers from neuronal cell bodies located in the Edinger–Westphal nucleus that supply the ciliary ganglion. Postganglionic fibers derived from the ciliary ganglion run in the **short ciliary nerves** to supply the **sphincter pupillae** (miosis) and the **ciliary smooth muscle** (accommodation/near vision).
- These parasympathetic fibers mediate the efferent limb of the pupillary light reflex.

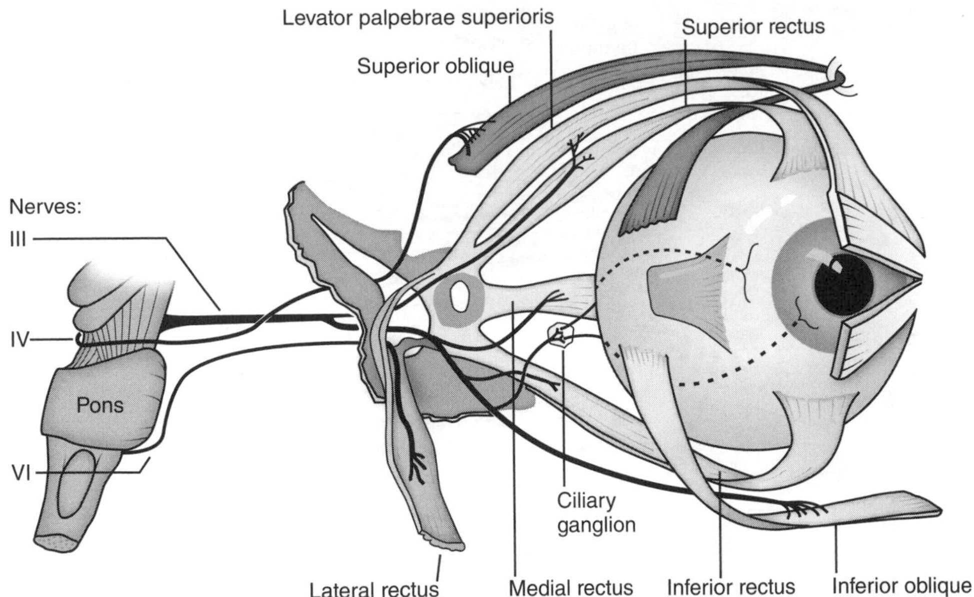

FIGURE 9.2. Distribution of the oculomotor, trochlear, and abducens nerves.

CLINICAL CORRELATES **Lesion of oculomotor nerve** causes paralysis of the levator palpebrae superioris (**ptosis**), paralysis of the medial rectus (**external strabismus**), paralysis of sphincter pupillae, resulting in **dilation of the pupil** (mydriasis is the result of unopposed sympathetic supply to the dilator papillae muscles), and paralysis of ciliary muscles, resulting in **loss of accommodation** (near vision) because of damage to the preganglionic parasympathetic fibers. Lesion also causes **loss of pupillary light reflex** because of damage to parasympathetic fibers that mediate the efferent limb of the pupillary light reflex.

D. Trochlear Nerve (CN IV) (Figure 9.2)

- Passes through the lateral wall of the cavernous sinus in the middle cranial fossa and enters the orbit by passing through the superior orbital fissure.
- Motor fibers (GSE) supply the superior oblique muscle.
- This is the **smallest** of all **cranial nerves** and the only CN that emerges from the dorsal aspect of the brain stem.

CLINICAL CORRELATES **Lesion of the trochlear nerve** causes paralysis of the superior oblique muscle of the eye, which causes diplopia (double vision) and inability to look inferolaterally. Injuries are seen with severe head injuries or meningitis because of its long intracranial course.

E. Trigeminal Nerve (CN V) (Figures 9.3 to 9.4)

- Develops in association with the first branchial arch and supplies motor fibers (SVE) to the muscles of mastication, as well as the mylohyoid, anterior belly of the digastric muscle, and tensor tympani and tensor veli palatini.
- This is a major sensory nerve (general somatic afferent [GSA]) supplying fibers to the face, scalp, auricle, external auditory meatus, nose, paranasal sinuses, mouth (except the posterior one-third of the tongue), parts of the nasopharynx, auditory tube, and cranial dura mater.
- The ganglion (**semilunar or trigeminal ganglion**) consists of cell bodies of sensory fibers that distribute along three nerve paths designated V1, V2, and V3 (see Ophthalmic Division (V1), Maxillary Division (V2), and Mandibular Division (V3)). The trigeminal ganglion occupies the

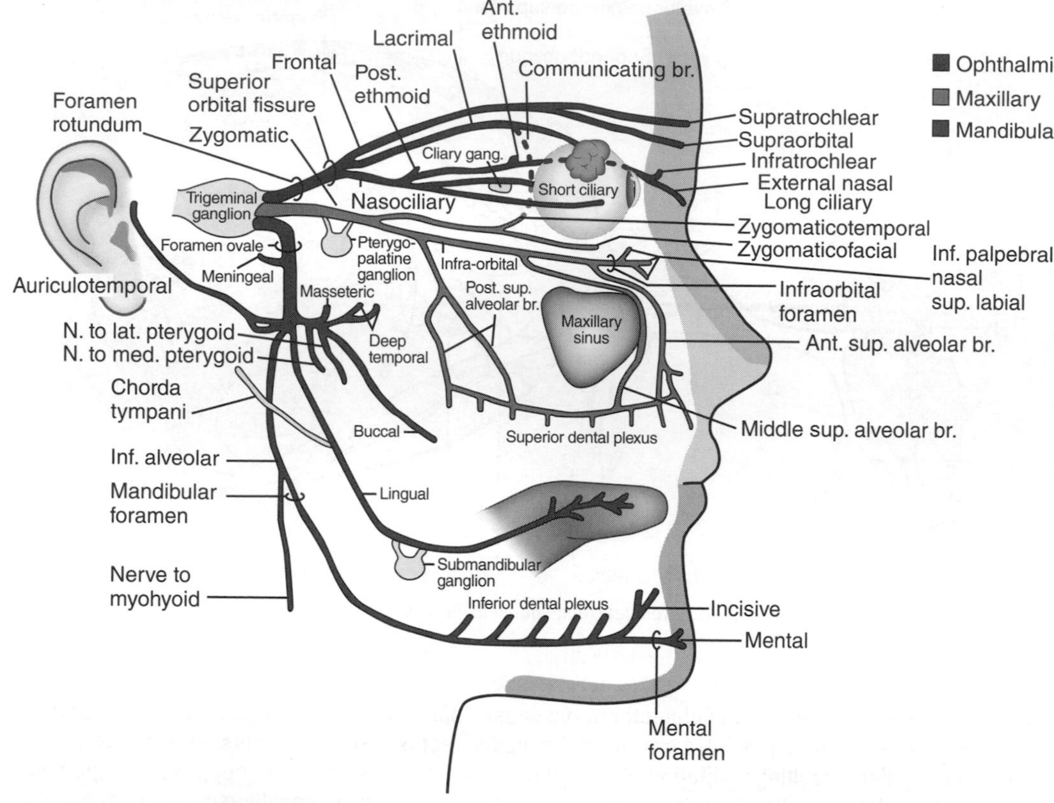

FIGURE 9.3. Branches of the trigeminal nerve.

trigeminal impression at the apex of the petrous portion of the temporal bone in the middle cranial fossa. The ganglion itself is housed in a pouch webbed with arachnoid between two layers of dura (**Meckel cave**).

1. Ophthalmic Division (V1) (See Orbit: II. A, Chapter 8)

- Runs in the dura of the lateral wall of the cavernous sinus and enters the orbit through the **supraorbital fissure.**
- Provides sensory innervation to the eyeball, tip of the nose, and skin of the face above the eye.
- Mediates the **afferent limb of the corneal reflex** by way of the nasociliary branch, whereas the facial nerve mediates the efferent limb.
- Major branches of the ophthalmic division (V1) include the following:
  1. **Lacrimal nerve** supplies sensation to the lacrimal gland, the conjunctiva, and the skin of the upper lateral eyelid.
  2. **Frontal nerve** divides into the supraorbital and supratrochlear nerve and supplies the scalp, forehead, frontal sinus, and upper central eyelid.
  3. **Nasociliary nerve** gives rise to a number of branches:
     - A communicating branch to the ciliary ganglion.
     - Short ciliary nerves, which carry postganglionic parasympathetic and sympathetic and afferent fibers.
     - Long ciliary nerves, which carry postganglionic sympathetic fibers to the dilator pupillae and afferent fibers from the iris and cornea.
     - Posterior ethmoidal nerve, which supplies the sphenoidal and posterior ethmoidal sinuses.
     - Anterior ethmoidal nerve, which supplies the anterior ethmoidal air cells and divides into the internal and external nasal branches.
     - Infratrochlear nerve, which innervates the eyelids, conjunctiva, skin of the nose, and lacrimal sac.
  4. **Meningeal branch** supplies dura in the anterior cranial fossa.

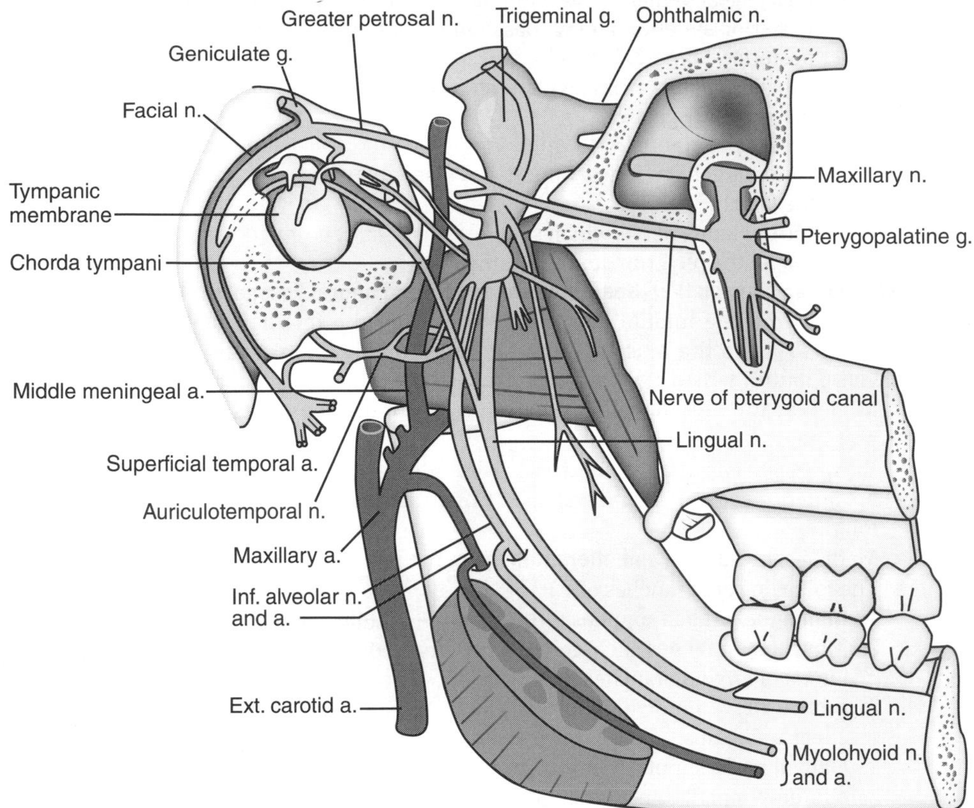

FIGURE 9.4. Trigeminal and facial nerves, and otic and pterygopalatine ganglia viewed from the medial side.

2. **Maxillary Division (V2) (See Pterygopalatine Fossa: II. A, Chapter 8)**

- Passes through the lateral wall of the cavernous sinus of the middle cranial fossa and through the **foramen rotundum** to enter the pterygopalatine fossa (at the back of the orbit).
- Sensory fibers (GSA) provide innervation to the face below the eyes and to the upper lip), palate, paranasal sinuses, and maxillary teeth.
- The cell bodies for these sensory fibers are in the trigeminal ganglion in the middle cranial fossa.
- These sensory fibers mediate the **afferent limb of the sneeze reflex** (irritation of the nasal mucosa), and the vagus nerve mediates the efferent limb.
- Major branches of this complex nerve include the following:
  1. **Meningeal branch** innervates the dura mater of the middle cranial fossa.
  2. **Pterygopalatine (communicating) nerve** connects sensory fibers that pass through the pterygopalatine ganglion and join branches off the ganglion.
  3. **Posterior–superior alveolar nerve** leaves the pterygopalatine fossa to innervate the cheeks, gums, molar teeth, as well as the maxillary sinus.
  4. **Zygomatic nerve** courses through the zygomatic bone in the maxillary sinus and divides into the zygomaticofacial and zygomaticotemporal nerves. The latter carries postganglionic parasympathetic fibers destined for the lacrimal nerve to stimulate lacrimal secretion.
  5. **Infraorbital nerve** is the anterior continuation of the maxillary nerve and gives rise to the middle and anterior–superior alveolar nerves that supply the maxillary sinus, teeth, and gums. It then emerges through the infraorbital foramen and divides in the face into the inferior palpebral, lateral nasal, and superior labial branches.
  6. **Branches of the maxillary division that pass through the pterygopalatine ganglion** without synapsing include the following:
     - Orbitalbranches, whichsupplythe orbit and posterior ethmoidal and sphenoidal sinuses.

- Pharyngeal branch, which supplies the roof of the pharynx and sphenoidal sinus.
- Posterior-superior lateral nasal branches, which innervate the nasal septum, posterior ethmoidal air cells, and superior and middle conchae.
- Greater palatine nerve, which innervates the hard palate and the inner surface of the maxillary gingiva.
- Lesser palatine nerve, which innervates the soft palate and palatine tonsil and contains general sensory fibers and taste fibers (from the greater petrosal branch of the facial).
- Nasopalatine nerve, which supplies the nasal septum, the hard palate, incisors, the skin of the phyltrum,and the gums.

3. Mandibular Division (V3) (See Temporal and Infratemporal Fossae: III. A, Chapter 8)

- Passes from the middle cranial fossa through the **foramen ovale** to supply motor fibers (SVE) to the muscles from the first branchial arch, which include the tensor veli palatini, tensor tympani, anterior belly of the digastric, and mylohyoid muscle as well as the muscles of mastication (temporalis, masseter, and lateral and medial pterygoid).
- Provides sensory innervation (GSA) to the lower part of the face, including the lower lip, anterior ear and chin as well as the mandibular teeth, and anterior two-thirds of the tongue.
- Mediates the afferent and **efferent limbs of the jaw jerk reflex**.
- The following are branches of V3:
  1. **Meningeal branch** supplies the dura in the middle cranial fossa.
  2. **Muscular branches** include the masseteric, deep temporal, medial pterygoid, and lateral pterygoid branches.
  3. **Buccal nerve** innervates skin on the buccinator and the mucous membrane of the cheek and gums.
  4. **Lingual nerve** supplies general sensation to the anterior two-thirds of the tongue. The chorda tympani joins the lingual nerve in the infratemporal fossa. The functions of chorda tympani are covered under the CN VII section.
  5. **Inferior alveolar nerve** gives rise to several important branches:
     - Mylohyoid nerve, which innervates the mylohyoid and anterior belly of the digastric muscles.
     - Inferior dental branch, which innervates the lower teeth.
     - Mental nerve, which innervates the skin over the chin.
     - Incisive branch, which innervates the mandibular canine and incisors.

CLINICAL CORRELATES

Lesion of the trigeminal nerve causes sensory loss on the face and weakness of the muscles of mastication that manifests as a deviation of the mandible toward the side of the lesion. Lesion of the **lingual nerve** near the neck of the third molar causes loss of general sensation and taste to the anterior two-thirds of the tongue as well as salivary secretion from submandibular and sublingual glands (due to loss of preganglionic parasympathetic fibers from the chorda tympani branch of CN VII). Lesion of the **ophthalmic division** cannot mediate the afferent limb of the corneal reflex by way of the nasociliary branch (the facial nerve mediates the efferent limb). Lesion of the **maxillary division** cannot mediate the afferent limb of the sneeze reflex (vagus nerve mediates the efferent limb). Lesion of the **mandibular division** would be associated with loss of both the afferent and efferent limbs of the jaw jerk reflex.

Trigeminal neuralgia (tic douloureux) is marked by **paroxysmal pain** along the course of the trigeminal nerve, especially radiating to the maxillary or mandibular area. The common causes of this disorder are aberrant blood vessels, aneurysms, chronic meningeal inflammation, brain tumors compressing on the trigeminal nerve at the base of the brain, and other lesions such as multiple sclerosis. If medical treatments are not effective, the neuralgia may be alleviated by sectioning the sensory root of the trigeminal nerve in the trigeminal (Meckel) cave in the middle cranial fossa.

F. **Abducens Nerve (CN VI) (Figure 9.2)**
- Leaves the brain at the pontomedullary junction and then pierces the dura on the dorsum sellae of the sphenoid bone.
- Passes through the cavernous sinus and enters the orbit through the supraorbital fissure to supply motor fibers (GSE) to the lateral rectus.

CLINICAL CORRELATES **Lesion of the abducens nerve** causes weakness/paralysis of the lateral gaze due to loss of the rectus muscle of the eye. The patient will present with a **medial deviation** of the affected eye (**internal strabismus**) or diplopia on lateral. It may result from a sepsis or thrombosis in the cavernous sinus. If the opposite side of the body is affected, there is a brain stem tumor or midline pontine stroke.

G. **Facial Nerve (CN VII) (Figures 9.4, 9.5 and 9.7)**
- Leaves the pons at the pontocerebellar angle as a large root, which carries motor fibers (SVE) to innervate the muscles of facial expression, and a smaller root, termed the nervus intermedius, which contains taste fibers (SVA) from the anterior two-thirds of the tongue. In addition, it contains preganglionic parasympathetic fibers (GVE) for the lacrimal, submandibular, sublingual, nasal, and palatine glands and visceral afferent fibers from the palate and nasal mucosa. A small number of fibers carry general sensory fibers from the external acoustic meatus and the auricle.
- Is the nerve of the second branchial arch.
- Enters the **internal acoustic meatus**, the **facial canal** in the temporal bone, and the main trunk emerges from the **stylomastoid foramen** to form terminal branches.
- All sensory cell bodies for the facial nerve reside in the **geniculate ganglion**, which lies at the external bend or genu (Latin for "knee") within the petrous portion of the temporal bone.
- Mediates the closure of the orbicularis oculi, which is the efferent limb of the **corneal (blink) reflex**.
- Lesion produces Bell's palsy (facial paralysis), which will affect all muscles of facial expression on the side of the lesion.
- Gives rise to the following branches:

1. **Greater Petrosal Nerve**
   - Contains preganglionic parasympathetic fibers destined for the pterygopalatine ganglion and joins the deep **petrosal nerve** (containing postganglionic sympathetic fibers) to form the **nerve of the pterygoid canal** (Vidian nerve).
   - Carries taste sensation (from anterior two-thirds of tongue) and visceral afferent fibers from the palate.
2. **Communicating Branch**
   - Joins the lesser petrosal nerve.
3. **Stapedial Nerve**
   - Supplies motor fibers to the stapedius, which helps attenuate loud sound.
4. **Chorda Tympani**
   - Arises in the descending part of the facial canal and crosses the tympanic membrane, passing between the handle of the malleus and the long process of the incus.
   - Exits the skull through the **petrotympanic fissure** and joins the lingual nerve in the infratemporal fossa.
   - Contains preganglionic parasympathetic fibers (GVE) that synapse on postganglionic cell bodies in the **submandibular ganglion**. Their postganglionic fibers innervate the submandibular, sublingual, and lingual glands.
   - Also contains taste fibers (SVA) from the anterior two-thirds of the tongue (ectodermal tongue), with cell bodies located in the geniculate ganglion.
   - May communicate with the otic ganglion below the base of the skull.
5. **Muscular Branches**
   - Supply motor fibers (SVE) to the stylohyoid and the posterior belly of the digastric muscle.
6. **Fine Communicating Branch**
   - Joins the auricular branch of the vagus nerve and the glossopharyngeal nerve to supply GSA fibers to the external ear.

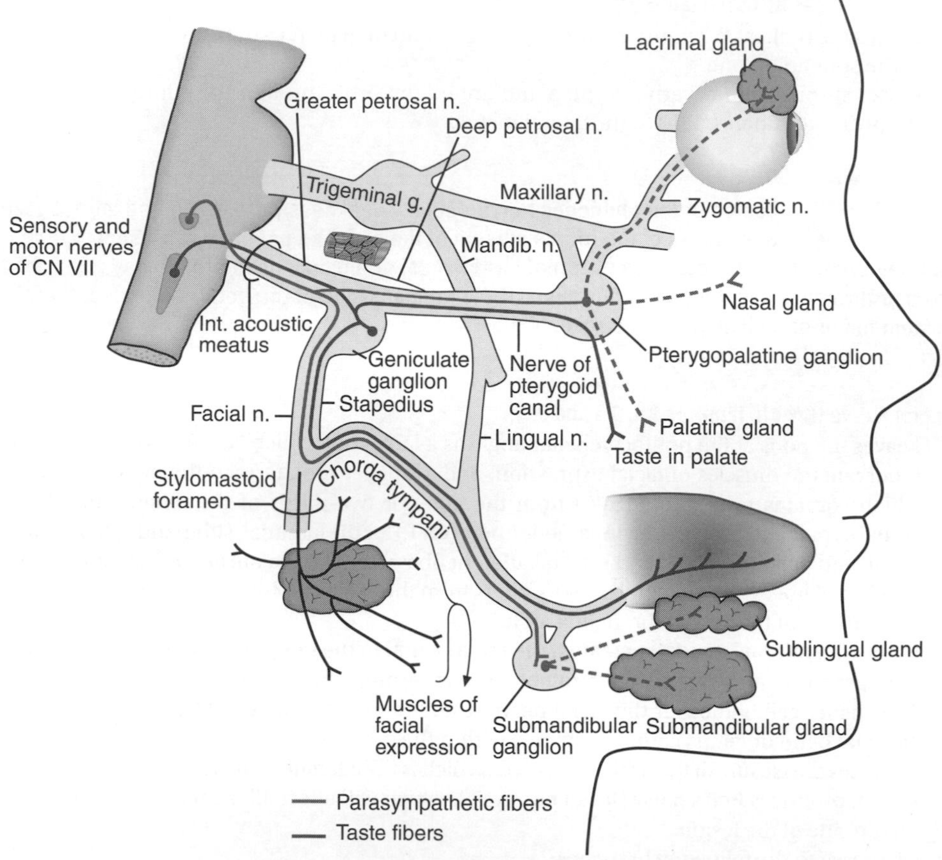

FIGURE 9.5. Distribution of the facial nerve.

7. **Posterior Auricular Nerve**
   - Runs behind the auricle with the posterior auricular artery.
   - Supplies SVE fibers to the muscles of the auricle and the occipitalis muscle.
8. **Terminal Branches**
   - Arise in the parotid gland and radiate onto the face as the temporal, zygomatic, buccal, marginal mandibular, and cervical branches.
   - Supply motor fibers (SVE) to the muscles of facial expression.

CLINICAL CORRELATES

Lesion of the facial nerve causes **Bell's palsy**, which is marked by characteristic **distortion of the face** such as no wrinkles on the forehead, drooping of the eyebrow, inability to close or blink the eye, sagging corner of the mouth, and inability to smile, whistle, or blow. The palsy also causes loss of taste in the anterior two-thirds of the tongue, decreased salivary secretion and lacrimation, painful sensitivity to sounds, and deviation of the lower jaw. Facial paralysis may be caused by a lesion of the facial nerve, a stroke, or a brain tumor. A **central lesion** of the facial nerve results in paralysis of muscles in the lower face on the contralateral (opposite) side; consequently, forehead wrinkle is not impaired. Therefore, the patient with **peripheral facial palsy** shows **no wrinkles** on the affected side, but the patient with a **stroke** or a **brain tumor** shows **wrinkles on both sides**. The definite cause of Bell palsy is unknown, but it may be caused by herpes simplex (viral) infection. Its treatment includes a course of steroid treatment – 60 to 80 mg of prednisone (anti-inflammatory drug) daily during the first 5 days, followed by tapering doses over the next 5 days, which may help reduce paralysis and expedite recovery by reducing inflammation and swelling and relieving pressure on the facial nerve for some patients. Treatment also includes antiviral drugs, such as acyclovir alone or in combination with prednisone. The patient is advised to protect the eyes from drying out with artificial tears and eye patches. Recovery is likely to take a few weeks to months.

H. Vestibulocochlear (Acoustic or Auditory) Nerve (CN VIII) (Figure 9.1)

- Leaves the pontocerebellar angle laterally and enters the internal acoustic meatus (with the facial nerve) and remains within the temporal bone to supply sensory fibers to the sensory cells of the inner ear.
- The **cochlear portion** (for hearing) derives from bipolar neurons in the spiral (cochlear) ganglion that innervate the hair cells of the cochlea (organ of Corti).
- The **vestibular portion** (for equilibrium) arises from bipolar neurons in the vestibular ganglion that innervate sensory cells of the ampullae of the semicircular ducts as well as the utricle and saccule.

CLINICAL CORRELATES **Lesion of the vestibulocochlear nerve** causes loss of hearing or vestibular sense. The most common loss of hearing is the loss of hair cells of the cochlea (organ of Corti) that occurs for high tones with advanced age (**presbycusis**). Disruptions of the ampullae of the semicircular ducts, and the utricle and saccule would result in **vertigo** (dizziness, loss of **balance**). Other problems with the labyrinth may cause **tinnitus** (ringing or buzzing in ears).

I. Glossopharyngeal Nerve (CN IX) (Figures 9.1 and 9.7)

- Is the nerve of the third branchial arch and contains SVE, SVA (taste), GVE, general visceral afferent (GVA), and GSA fibers.
- Leaves the postolivary sulcus of the lateral medulla to pass through the **jugular foramen** and gives rise to the following branches:

1. Tympanic Nerve

- Forms the **tympanic plexus** on the medial wall of the middle ear with sympathetic fibers from the internal carotid plexus (caroticotympanic nerves) and a branch from the geniculate ganglion of the facial nerve.
- Conveys visceral sensory fibers to the tympanic cavity, the mastoid antrum and air cells, and the auditory tube.
- Continues beyond the plexus as the **lesser petrosal nerve** in the floor of the middle cranial fossa and leaves through the foramen ovale to bring preganglionic parasympathetic fibers to the otic ganglion. Postganglionic parasympathetic fibers leave the otic ganglion to innervate the parotid gland.

2. Communicating Branch

- Joins the auricular branch of the vagus nerve and provides general sensation and pain fibers to the ear.

3. Pharyngeal Branch

- Supplies visceral sensory fibers to the posterior tongue and pharyngeal wall, including the tonsillar bed. It joins with the pharyngeal branch of the vagus nerve and branches from the sympathetic trunk to form the pharyngeal plexus on the middle constrictor muscle.
- Sensory fibers mediate the afferent limb of the gag (pharyngeal) reflex. The vagus nerve mediates the efferent limb.

4. Carotid Sinus Branch

- Supplies baroreceptive and chomoreceptive fibers (GVA) to the carotid sinus and the carotid body (respectively).
- Mediates the afferent limbs of the carotid sinus and body reflexes that can cause a drop in heart rate and blood pressure with carotid massage. The vagus nerve mediates the efferent limb.

5. Tonsillar Branches

- Supplies sensory fibers to the palatine tonsil and the soft palate.

6. Motor Branch

- Supplies motor fibers (SVE) to the stylopharyngeus.

7. Lingual Branch

- Supplies taste and visceral afferent fibers to the posterior one-third of the tongue and the vallate papillae (endodermal tongue behind the terminal sulcus).

CLINICAL CORRELATES **Lesion of the glossopharyngeal nerve** causes loss of motor fibers to the **stylopharyngeus** muscle; **loss of taste on the posterior one-third** of the tongue and vallate papillae; **loss of parasympathetic supply to the parotid** via fibers to the otic ganglion; loss of visceral afferents fibers to the pharynx, the carotid body and sinus, posterior one-third of the tongue, tympanic cavity, the mastoid antrum and air cells, and the auditory tube; and loss of general sensory fibers to the external ear. Lesions result in loss of the **afferent limb of the gag** (pharyngeal) reflex. Pharyngitis can lead to glossopharyngeal neuralgia, which manifests as sore throat and horrible ear pain without corresponding ear infection.

J. Vagus Nerve (CN X) (Figures 9.1, 9.3 and 9.7)

- Is the nerve of the fourth and sixth branchial arches.
- Passes out of the postolivary sulcus to exit the posterior cranial fossa through the jugular foramen.
- Provides motor innervation (SVE) to all muscles of the larynx, pharynx (except the stylopharyngeus), and palate (except the tensor veli palatini).
- Also provides parasympathetic preganglionic innervation (GVE) to smooth muscles and glands of the pharynx, esophagus, and gastrointestinal track (from the stomach to the transverse colon) as well as for the cardiac muscle of the heart; and visceral afferent fibers (GVA) from all mucous membranes in the lower pharynx, larynx, trachea, bronchus, esophagus, and thoracic and abdominal visceral organs (except for the descending colon, sigmoid colon, rectum, and other pelvic organs).
- Mediates the afferent and efferent limbs of the **cough reflex** (caused by irritation of the bronchial mucosa) and the efferent limbs of the **gag (pharyngeal) reflex** and **sneeze reflex.**
- During phonation, a lesion is revealed by the loss of palate elevation and the uvula deviates toward the intact side, away from the side of the lesion.
- Gives rise to the following branches:

1. Meningeal Branch

- Arises from the superior ganglion and supplies the dura mater of the posterior cranial fossa.

2. Auricular Branch

- Is joined by a branch from the glossopharyngeal nerve and the facial nerve and supplies general sensory fibers to the external acoustic meatus.

3. Pharyngeal Branch

- Supplies motor fibers to all the skeletal muscles of the pharynx, except the stylopharyngeus, by way of the pharyngeal plexus and all muscles of the palate except the tensor veli palatini.
- Gives rise to the **nerve to the carotid body**, which supplies visceral fibers to the carotid body and the carotid sinus.

4. Superior, Middle, and Inferior Cardiac Branches

- Carry parasympathetic supply toward, and visceral afferent fibers back from, the cardiac plexuses.

5. Superior Laryngeal Nerve

- Divides into internal and external branches:

a. Internal Laryngeal Nerve

- Provides general sensory fibers to the larynx above the vocal cord, lower pharynx, and epiglottis.
- Supplies taste fibers to the taste buds on the root of the tongue near and on the epiglottis.

b. External Laryngeal Nerve

- Supplies motor fibers to the cricothyroid and inferior pharyngeal constrictor muscles.

6. Recurrent Laryngeal Nerve

- Hooks around the subclavian artery on the right and around the arch of the aorta lateral to the ligamentum arteriosum on the left.
- Ascends in the groove between the trachea and the esophagus.

- Provides general sensory fibers to the larynx below the vocal cord and motor fibers to all muscles of the larynx except the cricothyroid muscle.
- Becomes the **inferior laryngeal nerve** at the lower border of the cricoid cartilage.

CLINICAL CORRELATES **Lesion of the vagus nerve** causes **dysphagia** (difficulty in swallowing) resulting from lesion of pharyngeal branches; numbness of the upper part of the larynx and paralysis of cricothyroid muscle resulting from lesion of the superior laryngeal nerve; and hoarseness, **dysphonia** (difficulty in speaking), **aphonia** (loss of voice), and numbness of the lower part of the larynx resulting from lesion of the recurrent laryngeal nerve. Lesion results in **deviation of the uvula toward the uninjured side** on phonation. Lesion cannot mediate the afferent and efferent limbs of the **cough reflex** and the efferent limbs of the **gag (pharyngeal) reflex** and **sneeze reflex**. In addition, lesion causes loss of motor fibers to muscles of the larynx, pharynx (except the stylopharyngeus), and palate (except the tensor veli palatini); **loss of taste on the epiglottis**; and loss of parasympathetic supply to the thorax and abdomen as well as some visceral afferents.

K. Accessory Nerve (CN XI) (Figure 9.1)

- The spinal root leaves the upper cervical spinal cord laterally to pass into the posterior cranial fossa through the foramen magnum before it passes out of the skull through the jugular foramen.
- Provides motor fibers to the sternocleidomastoid and trapezius muscles.
- The cranial portion contains motor fibers that exit the medulla and pass through the jugular foramen where they join the vagus nerve as the recurrent laryngeal nerve to supply muscles of the pharynx and larynx.

CLINICAL CORRELATES **Lesion of the spinal accessory nerve** causes loss of motor fibers to the sternocleidomastoid and trapezius muscles. The arm cannot be abducted beyond the horizontal position as a result of an inability to rotate the scapula. Lesion also causes **torticollis** because of paralysis of the sternocleidomastoid and shoulder drop from paralysis of the trapezius.

L. Hypoglossal Nerve (CN XII) (Figures 9.1 and 9.3)

- Passes out of the medulla ventrally in the preolivary sulcus and passes through the **hypoglossal canal**.
- Loops around the occipital artery and the carotid bifurcation to pass between the carotids and internal jugular vessels. It runs deep to the digastric posterior belly and stylohyoid muscles to enter the submandibular triangle.
- It enters the mouth by passing above the greater horn of the hyoid bone between the middle pharyngeal constrictor and the mylohyoid muscle.
- Supplies motor fibers to all of the intrinsic and extrinsic muscles of the tongue except the palatoglossus (which is supplied by the vagus nerve).
- Carries sensory fibers from C1 to supply the cranial dura mater through the meningeal branch, but the fibers are not components of the hypoglossal nerve.
- Not strictly part of the hypoglossal nerve, it also carries motor fibers from C1 to supply the upper root of the ansa cervicalis and the nerve to both the thyrohyoid and geniohyoid muscles.
- Lesion causes deviation of the tongue toward the injured side on protrusion.

CLINICAL CORRELATES **Lesion of the hypoglossal nerve** causes loss of motor fibers to all of the intrinsic and extrinsic muscles of the tongue except the palatoglossus, which is supplied by the vagus nerve. Lesion causes **deviation of the tongue toward the injured side** on protrusion. Hence, a mnemonic to remember the deviation side is *"you lick your wounds."*

M. Structures Derived from Pharyngeal (Branchial) Arch

Arch	Nerve	Muscles	Skeletal Structures
First (mandibular)	CN V	Muscles of mastication, mylohyoid, digastric anterior belly, tensor tympani	Meckel cartiage: malleus, incus, sphenomandibular ligament
Second (hyoid)	CN VII	Muscles of facial expression, mylohyoid, digastric posterior belly, stylohyoid, stapedius	Stapes, stylohyoid process, lesser horn and upper body of hyoid bone, stylohyoid ligament
Third	CN IX	Stylopharyngeus	Greater horn and lower body of hyoid bone
Fourth	CN X (superior laryngeal nerve)	Muscles of pharynx except tensor veli palatini, muscles of pharynx except stylopharyngeus, crycothyroid	Thyroid and cricoid cartilages
Sixth	CN X (recurrent laryngeal nerve)	Intrinsic muscles of larynx except crycothyroid	Arytenoid, corniculate, and cuneiform cartilages

N. Cranial Nerve Examination

CN I	Smell tested by placing stimuli under one nostril at a time and occluding the other nostril.
CN II	**Visual acuity** is tested by asking to read progressively smaller prints on the near card or Snellen charts (tested with Snellen charts); **color vision** is tested with Ishihara color plate; **visual fields** by having the patient count presented fingers in each of the four quadrants of the tested eye, with the opposite covered; and afferent limb of **pupillary light reflex** by shinning a penlight into one eye and check the pupils on both sides for direct or consensual response.
CNs III, IV, and VI	Extra and intraocular muscles are tested by examining smoothness of eye movements, checking for ptosis, presence of pupillary light reflex, and the accommodation reflex. The accommodation reflex includes eye convergence and pupil constriction. The efferent component of the pupillary reflex is via CN III.
CN V	Sensory is tested by lightly touching the forehead (V1); by touching the cheeks (V2); and by touching the chin; motor (V3) is tested by clenching teeth together, opening mouth, and protruding jaw; corneal reflex) by lightly touching the cornea with the cotton wool (sensation V1) and observing the eye closing (motor with CN VII).
CN VII	Motor by checking wrinkles in forehead, raise eyebrows, smile, puff out cheeks and conducting corneal reflex (with CN V), and testing for taste.
CN VIII	Grossly tested with whisper test and then localization of hearing loss tested by conducting Rinne and Weber tests using a tuning fork; vestibular functions are tested by observing vertigo (Hallpike test) or disturbance of equilibrium (Romberg test).
CN IX	Tested with the gag reflex or by touching the pharynx (sensory IX) with a tongue depressor and the palate elevates (motor IX).
CN X	Tested by observing the symmetrical elevation of the uvula as the patient says "aah."
CN XI	Shrug shoulder and turn head from side to side.
CN XII	Examine symmetry of the tongue or any deviation when protruding the tongue.

II. AUTONOMIC NERVES OF THE HEAD (Figures 9.5 to 9.6; Table 9.4)

A. Sympathetics of the Head and Neck

- The **cervical portion of the sympathetic trunk** contains three sympathetic ganglia that are interconnected: the **superior**, **middle**, and **inferior cervical ganglia**. The **superior cervical ganglion** is at the level of the C1 and C2 vertebrae. The **middle cervical ganglion** lies at the level of the cricoid cartilage. The **inferior cervical ganglion** is usually fused with the first thoracic ganglion to form the **stellate ganglion**. Each cervical ganglion receives preganglionic nerve fibers from the upper thoracic spinal nerves. Postganglionic neurons send fibers to the head and neck visceral organs as well as cardiac nerves to the thorax.
- **Inferior cervical ganglion** provides postganglionic fibers through the **inferior cardiac nerve** to the **cardiopulmonary plexus** (heart/lungs) and other fibers to the inferior segments of the brachial plexus. Some fibers interconnect the inferior cervical ganglion and the first thoracic ganglion by coursing around the subclavian artery (**ansa subclavius**).

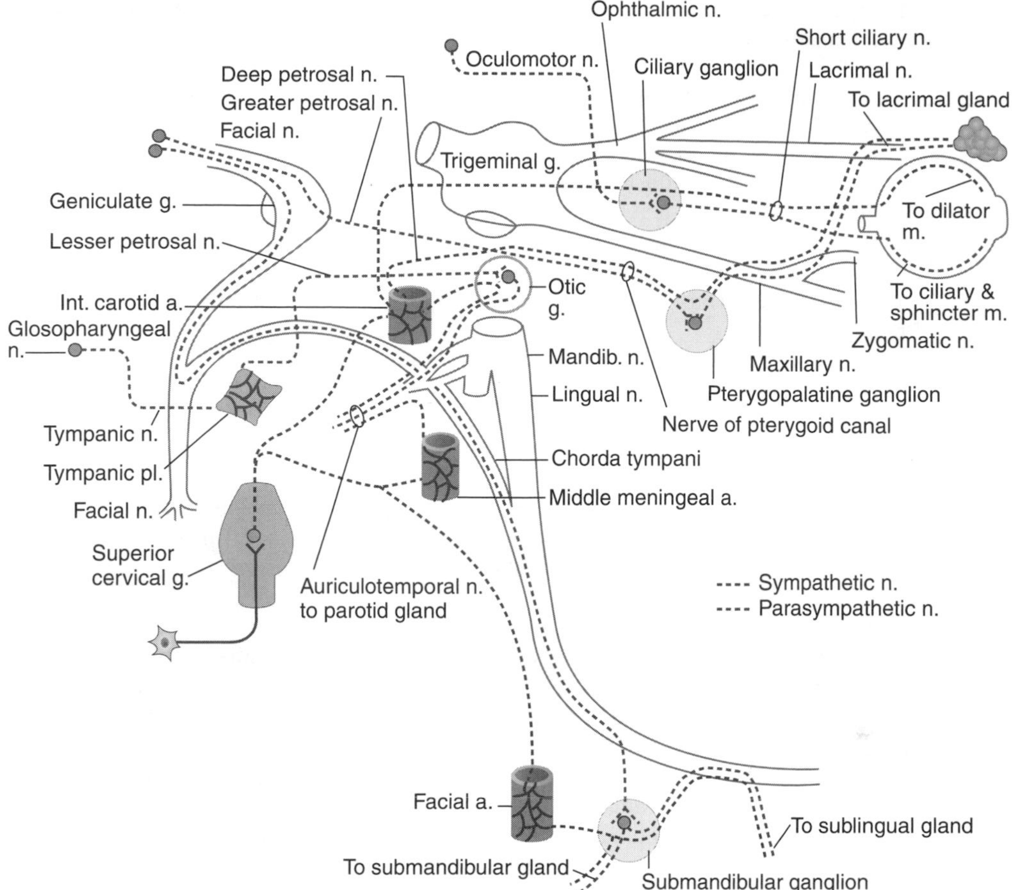

FIGURE 9.6. Autonomics of the head and neck including four parasympathetic ganglia. Note that (1) parasympathetic preganglionic nerve fibers run in the oculomotor nerve, synapse in the ciliary ganglion, and postganglionc fibers run in the short ciliary nerve to supply the ciliary and sphincter muscles; (2) parasympathetic preganglionic nerve fibers run through the facial nerve, greater petrosal nerve, nerve of pteryfoid canal, synapse in the pterygopalatine ganglion, and postganglionic fibers run in the maxillary, zygomatic, zygomaticotemporal, and lacrimal nerves to supply the lacrimal gland; (3) another parasympathetic preganglionic nerve fibers run in the facial nerve, chorda tympani, lingual nerve, synapse in the submandibular ganglion, and postganglionic fibers supply submandibular, sublingual, and lingual glands; (4) parasympathetic preganglionic nerve fibers run in the glossopharyngeal nerve, tympanic plexus, lesser petrosal nerve, synapse in the otic ganglion, and postganglionic fibers run in the auriculotemporal nerve to supply the parotid gland. For sympathetic nerve, preganglionic sympathetic nerve fibers arise from the upper thoracic sympathetic chain ganglia, synapse in the superior cervical ganglion, and postganglionic fibers run along the blood vessel, accompanying parasympathetic fibers to supply blood vessels, sweat glands, and other tissues.

table 9.4 Parasympathetic Ganglia and Associated Autonomic Nerves

Ganglion	Location	Parasympathetic Fibers	Sympathetic Fibers	Chief Distribution
Ciliary	Lateral to optic nerve	Oculomotor nerve and its inferior division	Internal carotid plexus	Ciliary muscle and sphincter pupillae (parasympathetic); dilator pupillae and tarsal muscles (sympathetic)
Pterygopalatine	In pterygopalatine fossa	Facial nerve, greater petrosal nerve, and nerve of pterygoid canal	Internal carotid plexus	Lacrimal gland and glands in palate and nose
Submandibular	On hyoglossus	Facial nerve, chorda tympani, and lingual nerve	Plexus on facial artery	Submandibular and sublingual glands
Otic	Below foramen ovale	Glossopharyngeal nerve, its tympanic branch, and lesser petrosal nerve	Plexus on middle meningeal artery	Parotid gland

- **Middle cervical ganglion** provides postganglionic fibers through the **middle cardiac nerve** to the **cardiopulmonary plexus** (heart/lungs) and other fibers that supply the upper segments of the brachial plexus and the lower segments of the cervical plexus.
- **Superior cervical ganglion** provides postganglionic fibers through the **superior cardiac nerve** to the **cardiopulmonary plexus** (heart/lungs) and other fibers supply the upper segments of the cervical plexus. In addition, sympathetic postganglionic fibers for the head travel through two routes to all destinations in the head: through the **carotid plexus** and the **deep petrosal nerve**.

1. Carotid Plexus

- These are postganglionic fibers that arise from neurons chiefly located in the superior cervical ganglion, and they distribute on the surface of either the internal or external carotid arteries. Thus, there is an internal carotid plexus and an external carotid plexus.

2. Deep Petrosal Nerve

- Arises from the plexus on the internal carotid plexus.
- Contains **postganglionic sympathetic** fibers with cell bodies located in the superior cervical ganglion.
- These fibers ascend through foramen lacerum to join the greater petrosal nerve and become the nerve of the pterygoid canal.
- These sympathetic fibers pass through the pterygopalatine ganglion without synapsing, and then join the postganglionic parasympathetic fibers in supplying the lacrimal gland, the nasal glands, and glands of the palate.

B. Parasympathetics of the Head

- Four **cranial nerves** contain parasympathetic preganglionic nerve fibers. The head contains **four parasympathetic ganglia**. The first three cranial nerves provide the parasympathetic supply for the entire head, while the vagus is involved mostly with the pharynx, thorax, and abdomen. The trigeminal nerve does not have parasympathetic fibers as it leaves the middle cranial fossa. However, the distal branches of each division of the trigeminal acts like a scaffold to carry autonomic supply throughout the head.
- In the eye, smooth muscle of the ciliary apparatus and the sphincter pupillae are supplied by the **oculomotor nerve.** The **parasympathetic preganglinic nerve** fibers travel from neurons located in the Edinger–Westphal nucleus of the midbrain (mesencephalon). They travel along the inferior division of the oculomotor nerve and enter the **ciliary ganglion** where they synapse. Postganglionic fibers distribute with the short ciliary nerve branches of the trigeminal nerve and supply the **ciliary muscle** and **spincter pupillae**.
- The major parasympathetic nerve of the head is the **facial nerve** and it supplies all secretory elements from the lacrimal glands to the hyoid bone with only one exception (the parotid gland). The **facial nerve** carries parasympathetic preganglionic fibers along two different paths. The first is associated with the maxillary prominence of the first branchial arch. The greater petrosal nerve gives rise to the parasympathetic portion of the nerve of the pterygoid canal (Vidian nerve). These fibers enter the **pterygopalatine ganglion** where they synapse. Postganglionic nerve fibers distribute through the branches of CN V2 to the **lacrimal gland** as well as to the nasal and palatine glands. The second pathway supplies structures associated with the mandibular prominence of the first branchial arch. These parasympathetic preganglionic nerve fibers branch from the facial nerve as the chorda tympani nerve. The chorda tympani joins the lingual nerve before the fibers synapse in the **submandibular ganglion**. Postganglionic nerve fibers supply the submandibular, sublingual, and lingual glands by traveling with sensory fibers of the lingual nerve.
- The **glossopharyngeal nerve** carries parasympathetic preganglionic nerve fibers destined to supply the otic ganglion and then the parotid gland. The preganglionic fibers run in the tympanic nerve, courses through the tympanic plexus and into the middle cranial fossa as the lesser petrosal nerve. The lesser petrosal nerve leaves the skull and preganglionic fibers synapse in the **otic ganglion**. Postganglionic nerve fibers join the auriculotemporal nerve and supply the **parotid gland** for salivary secretion.
- The **vagus nerve** conveys parasympathetic preganglionic nerve fibers that enter the **terminal ganglia** near or in the organs where they synapse. Postganglionic nerve fibers supply cardiac muscle, **smooth muscle**, and **glands** in the pharynx, larynx, trachea, and in thoracic and abdominal viscera.

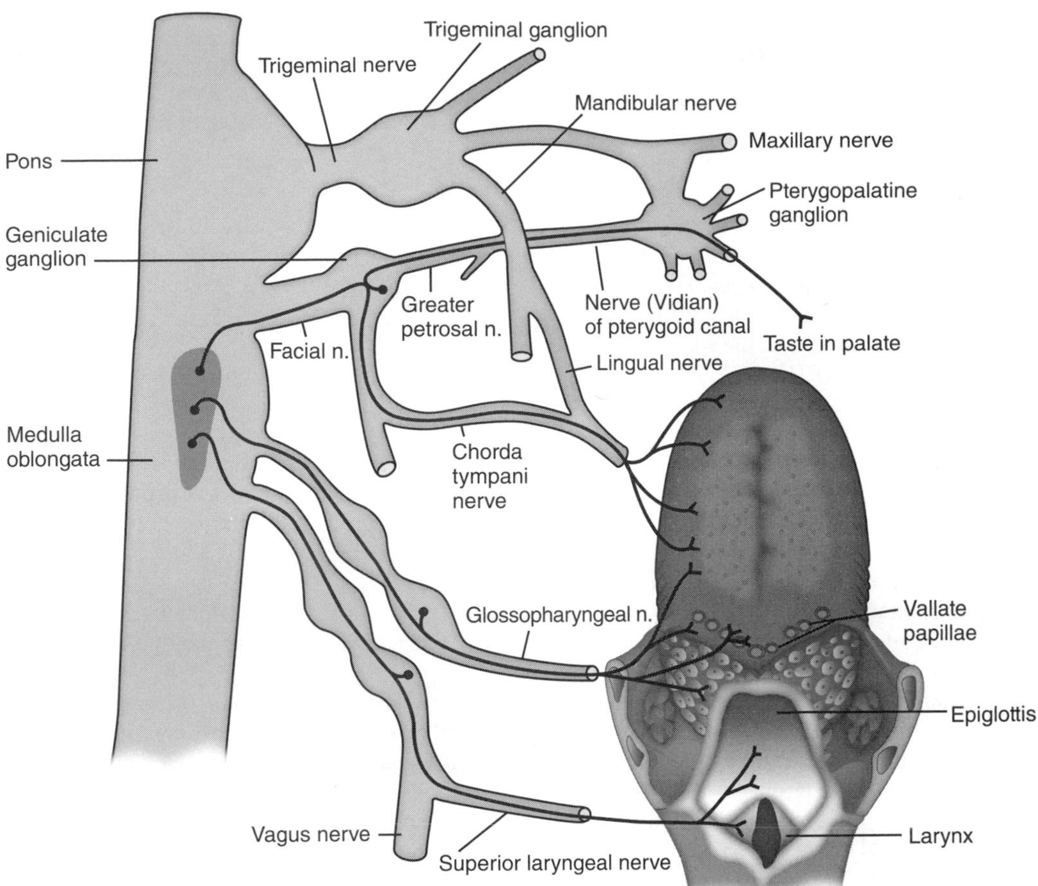

FIGURE 9.7. Cranial nerves that carry sensory fibers for taste (CN VII, IX, and X).

- The **trigeminal nerve** carries **no parasympathetic preganglionic nerve fibers**, but its branches provide pathways for parasympathetic nerve fibers to reach the target organs: (1) postganglionic parasympathetic fibers from the ciliary ganglion run in the **short cilliary nerve** and supply the ciliary muscle and sphincter pupillae; (2) postganglionic parasympathetic fibers from the pterygopalatine ganglion run in the **maxillary, zygomatic, zygomaticotemporal, and lacrimal nerve**, and supply the lacrimal gland; (3) postganglionic parasympathetic fibers from the otic ganglion run in the **auriculotemporal nerve** and supply the parotid gland; and (4) the **lingual nerve** joined by the chorda tympani in the infratemporal fossa carries preganglionic parasympathetic fibers, which synapse in the submandibular ganglion, and postganglionic fibers supply the submandibular gland and then may rejoin the lingual nerve to supply the sublingual and lingual glands.

CLINICAL CORRELATES

Horner syndrome is caused by **lesion of cervical sympathetic nerves** and characterized by (a) **miosis** (constriction of the pupil); (b) **ptosis** (drooping of the upper eyelid); (c) **enophthalmos** (retraction of the eyeball); (d) **anhidrosis** (absence of sweating); and (e) **vasodilation** (increased blood flow in the face and neck [flushing]). **Crocodile tears syndrome** is spontaneous lacrimation during eating, caused by a lesion of the facial nerve proximal to the geniculate ganglion. It is due to misdirection of regenerating parasympathetic fibers, which formerly innervated the salivary (submandibular and sublingual) glands and now stimulate the lacrimal glands. **Frey syndrome** is seen after parotidectomy as uncontrolled sweating over the angle of the mandible during eating. This occurs due to misdirection of regenerating parasympathetic fibers from the otic ganglion that wrongly innervate sweat glands.

HIGH-YIELD TOPICS

Cranial Nerves

- **Olfactory** nerve (SVA, smell).
- **Optic** nerve (SSA, vision).
- **Oculomotor** nerve carries parasympathetic (GVE) nerve fibers that supply the ciliary muscle (accommodation) and sphincter pupillae (constriction of the pupil) and mediate the efferent limb of the pupillary light reflex. It supplies all of the extraocular eye muscles except for the superior oblique and lateral rectus muscles.
- **Trochlear nerve** (GSE, the superior oblique muscle of the eye).
- **Trigeminal** nerve (GSA, skin on face; SVE, muscles of mastication and tensor veli palatini, tensor tympani, mylohyoid, and digastric anterior belly muscles).
- **Abducens** nerve (GSE, the lateral rectus muscle of the eye).
- **Facial** nerve (SVE, muscles of facial expression; SVA, taste on anterior two-thirds of tongue and palate; GVE, parasympathetic nerve to submandibular ganglion and gland, and to pterygopalatine ganglion and lacrimal, nasal, and palatine glands; GVA, nasal and palate mucosae; GSA, external ear).
- **Vestibulocochlear** nerve (SSA, hearing and balance).
- **Glossopharyngeal** nerve (SVE, stylopharyngeus muscle; SVA, taste on posterior one-third of tongue and vallate papillae; GVE, parasympathetic nerve to otic ganglion [parotid gland]; GVA, posterior one-third of tongue; GSA, external ear).
- **Vagus** nerve (SVE, muscles of palate, pharynx, and larynx; SVA, taste on epiglottis; GVE, parasympathetic nerve to smooth muscles, glands, and cardiac muscle in the thorax and abdomen; GVA, mucous membrane of the pharynx, larynx, middle ear cavity, and thoracic and abdominal viscerae; GSA, external ear).
- **Accessory** nerve (SVE, GSE, or mixed) to the trapezius and sternocleidomastoid muscles.
- **Hypoglossal** nerve (GSE, muscles of tongue movement).

Nerves and Muscles of Pharyngeal (Branchial) Arch (See Table under I. M.)

- The nerve of the **first arch,** the **trigeminal nerve** (mandibular branch), innervates muscles of mastication and mylohyoid, digastric anterior belly, and tensor tympani muscles.
- The nerve of the **second arch,** the **facial nerve**, innervates muscles of facial expression and the digastric posterior belly, stylohyoid, and stapedius muscles.
- The nerve of the **third arch**, the **glossopharyngeal nerve**, innervates the stylopharyngeus muscle.
- The nerve of the **fourth arch**, the **vagus nerve (superior laryngeal branch)**, innervates the muscles of the soft palate (except tensor veli palatini), crycothyroid, and muscles of the pharynx (except stylopharyngeus).
- The nerve of the **sixth arch**, the **vagus (recurrent laryngeal nerve)**, innervates the intrinsic muscles of the larynx (except the cricothyroid).

Muscle Innervation and Nerve Lesion

- **Muscles of the eye movement** are innervated by the oculomotor, trochlear, and abducens nerves. Formula to remember innervation of extraocular eye muscles is SO4, LR6, AO3 (**S**uperior **O**blique - CN4; **L**ateral **R**ectus - CN6; **A**ll **O**ther eye movement muscles - CN3).
- **Short ciliary nerve** carries postganglionic parasympathetic nerve fibers to the sphincter pupillae and ciliary muscle and postganglionic sympathetic fibers to the dilator pupillae. The **long ciliary nerve** also carries postganglionic sympathetic fibers.
- **Diplopia (double vision)** is caused by paralysis of one or more extraocular muscles resulting from injury of the nerves supplying them.
- **Lesion of the auriculotemporal nerve** damages postganglionic parasympathetic secretomotor fibers to the parotid gland and postganglionic sympathetic fibers to the sweat glands. When nerve is severed, the fibers can regenerate along each other's pathways and innervate the wrong gland, resulting in **Frey syndrome**, which produces flushing and sweating instead of salivation in response to taste of food.

- **Innervation of the tongue: GSE motor** – by CN XII; **GSA sensory** – anterior two-thirds by CN V3 and posterior one-third by CN IX; **SVA taste** – anterior two-thirds by CN VII, posterior one-third by CN IX, and epiglottis by CN X.
- **Lesion of the chorda tympani** results in loss of salivary secretion from the submandibular and sublingual glands and loss of taste from the anterior two-thirds of the tongue.
- **Bell palsy** (facial paralysis) caused by a **lesion of the facial nerve** is marked by characteristic **distortions of the face**, such as no wrinkles on the forehead, drooping of the eyebrow, inability to close or blink the eye, sagging corner of the mouth, and inability to smile, whistle, or blow. The palsy also causes loss of taste in the anterior portion of the tongue, decreased salivation and lacrimation, deviation of the lower jaw, and hyperacusis.
- **Crocodile tears syndrome** is spontaneous lacrimation during eating, caused by a lesion of the facial nerve proximal to the geniculate ganglion. It is due to misdirection of regenerating parasympathetic fibers, which formerly innervated the salivary (submandibular and sublingual) glands, to the lacrimal glands.
- **Recurrent laryngeal nerve** innervates the laryngeal muscles, and it should be identified and preserved during thyroid surgery. Its lesion could be produced during thyroidectomy or cricothyrotomy or by aortic aneurysm and may cause respiratory obstruction, hoarseness, inability to speak, and loss of sensation below the vocal cord.
- **Innervation of the nasal cavity: SVA olfaction** – by CN I; **GVA sensory** – by CN VII; **GVE secretomotor** to glands – by CN VII (parasympathetic nerve).
- **Nerve of the pterygoid canal** (Vidian nerve) is formed by the union of the greater petrosal (preganglionc parasympathetic) and deep petrosal (postganglionic sympathetic) nerves, and also carries SVA taste fibers from the palate and GVA sensory fibers from the palate and nasal mucosae. Its **lesion** results in vasodilation; a lack of secretion of the lacrimal, nasal, and palatine glands; and a loss of general and taste sensation of the palate.

Reflex ARCS

- Optic nerve mediates the afferent limb of the **pupillary light reflex**, whereas parasympathetic fibers in the oculomotor nerve mediate the efferent limb.
- Ophthalmic nerve mediates the afferent limb of the **corneal (blink) reflex** by way of the nasociliary branch, whereas the facial nerve mediates the efferent limb.
- Maxillary nerve mediates the afferent limb of the **sneeze reflex** (irritation of the nasal mucosa), and the vagus nerve mediates the efferent limb.
- Mandibular nerve mediates the afferent and efferent limbs of the **jaw jerk reflex**.
- Facial nerve mediates the efferent limb of the **corneal reflex**.
- Glossopharyngeal nerve (pharyngeal branch) mediates the afferent limb of the **gag (pharyngeal) reflex**, and the vagus nerve mediates the efferent limb of it.
- Vagus nerve mediates the afferent and efferent limbs of the **cough reflex** (irritation of the bronchial mucosa), and the efferent limbs of the gag and sneeze reflexes.

Cranial Nerves Carrying Taste Sensation

- SVA fibers for taste sensation from anterior two-thirds of the tongue run in the chorda tympani of the **facial nerve**.
- SVA fibers for taste sensation from posterior one-third of the tongue run in the **glossopharyngeal nerve**.
- Taste sensation from the palate is supplied by the **facial nerve** through its greater petrosal branch, which sends fibers into the palatine nerves.
- Taste sensation from the epiglottis is carried by the internal laryngeal branch of the superior laryngeal nerve, which is a branch of the **vagus nerve**.

Cranial Nerves Innervate Skeletal Muscles of the Head and Neck

- Oculomotor nerve (CN III): innervates all of the muscles of eye movement except the superior oblique and lateral rectus muscles.
- Trochlear nerve (CN IV): innervates the superior oblique muscle.
- Trigeminal nerve, mandibular division (CN V3): innervates the muscles of mastication, digastric anterior belly, mylohyoid, tensor belly palatini, and tensor tympani muscles.

- Abducens nerve (CN VI): innervates the lateral rectus muscle.
- Facial nerve (CN VII): innervates the muscles of facial expression, stylohyoid, digastric posterior belly, and stapedius muscles.
- Glossopharyngeal nerve CN IX): innervates the stylopharyngeus muscle.
- Vagus nerve (CN X): innervates all of the palate muscles except the tensor belly palatine muscle, all of the pharyngeal muscles except the stylopharyngeus muscle, and all of the laryngeal muscles.
- Accessory nerve (CN XI): innervates the trapezius and sternocleidomastoid muscles.
- Hypoglossal nerve (XII): innervates all of the tongue muscles except the palatoglossus muscle.

Functions of Autonomic Nerves

	Sympathetic Nerve	Parasympathetic Nerve
Eyes	Dilates pupil	Constricts pupil; contracts ciliary muscle to thicken lens
Lacrimal gland	Reduces secretion	Promotes secretion
Nasal mucous gland	Reduces secretion	Promotes secretion
Salivary gland	Reduces secretion and more viscid	Increases secretion and watery
Sweat gland	Stimulates secretion	No effect
Blood vessels	Constricts	No effect

Review Test

Directions: Each of the numbered items or incomplete statements in this section is followed by answers or by completions of the statement. Select the **one**-lettered answer or completion that is **best** in each case.

1. A 27-year-old man came to his physician with drooping of the upper eyelid (ptosis), a dilated pupil, and a difficulty in focusing on close objects. Furthermore, he has an internal strabismus (medial deviation of the eye) and inability to look inferiorly when the eye is adducted. Which of the following is the most likely cause?

(A) Lesion in the medulla
(B) Tumor in the optic canal
(C) Thrombosis in the cavernous sinus
(D) Lesion of the olfactory nerve
(E) Fracture of the foramen spinosum

2. A 16-year-old boy presents with double vision. Further examination reveals that he has difficulty in turning his eye inferolaterally and trouble going downstairs. Which of the following nerves is most likely damaged?

(A) Oculomotor nerve
(B) Optic nerve
(C) Ophthalmic nerve
(D) Trochlear nerve
(E) Abducens nerve

3. A 31-year-old man with a penetrating injury to the posterior triangle of the neck is unable to shrug his shoulder and turn the head to the opposite side. Which of the following nerves is most likely damaged?

(A) Trigeminal nerve
(B) Facial nerve
(C) Glossopharyngeal nerve
(D) Accessory nerve
(E) Hypoglossal nerve

4. A 23-year-old woman suffers from a fracture of the jugular foramen by car accident. Which of the following nerves is/are most likely damaged?

(A) Cranial nerve V2
(B) Cranial nerve VI
(C) Cranial nerves VII and VIII
(D) Cranial nerves IX, X, and XI
(E) Cranial nerve XII

5. A 17-year-old boy is involved in a gang fight and receives a penetrating injury to the neck. Which of the following conditions is most likely exhibited by this misadventure?

(A) Internal strabismus
(B) Trouble going down the stairs
(C) Constricted pupil
(D) Inability close the eye
(E) Deviation of tongue toward lesion side

6. A 28-year-old woman comes to her family physician and complains of difficulty in swallowing. Further examination reveals that she has no taste sensation of the posterior one-third of her tongue and a lack of secretion of the parotid gland. Which of the following would most likely cause this condition?

(A) Fracture of the mandibular canal
(B) Section of the zygomatic nerve
(C) Glossopharyngeal nerve injury
(D) Tumor in the pituitary gland
(E) Lesion of the hypoglossal nerve

7. A 34-year-old man in a bar fight suffers a knife wound that severs the abducens nerve proximal to its entrance into the orbit. Which of the following conditions results from this injury?

(A) Ptosis of the upper eyelid
(B) Loss of the ability to dilate the pupil
(C) External strabismus (lateral deviation)
(D) Loss of visual accommodation
(E) Internal strabismus (medial deviation)

8. Following radical resection of a primary tongue tumor, a 72-year-old patient has lost general sensation on the anterior two-thirds of the tongue. This is probably due to injury to branches of which of the following nerves?

(A) Trigeminal nerve
(B) Facial nerve
(C) Glossopharyngeal nerve
(D) Vagus nerve
(E) Hypoglossal nerve

9. A 53-year-old woman is diagnosed as having a pituitary tumor. If the tumor is large enough, she could exhibit which of the following disorders?

(A) Blindness
(B) Bitemporal (heteronymous) hemianopia
(C) Right nasal hemianopia
(D) Left homonymous hemianopia
(E) Binasal hemianopia

10. A patient can move his eyeballs normally and see distant objects clearly but cannot focus on near objects. This condition may indicate damage to which of the following structures?

(A) Ciliary ganglion and oculomotor nerve
(B) Oculomotor nerve and long ciliary nerve
(C) Short ciliary nerves and ciliary ganglion
(D) Superior cervical ganglion and long ciliary nerve
(E) Oculomotor, trochlear, and abducens nerves

11. A 32-year-old woman has hoarseness in her voice, and her uvula is deviated to the left on phonation. Which of the following nerve is most likely damaged?

(A) Right trigeminal nerve
(B) Left trigeminal nerve
(C) Right vagus nerve
(D) Left vagus nerve
(E) Left glosopharyngeal nerve

12. Following a penetrated injury in the submandibular triangle, the tongue of a 45-year-old patient deviates to the left on protrusion. Which of the following nerves is injured?

(A) Right lingual nerve
(B) Left lingual nerve
(C) Right hypoglossal nerve
(D) Left hypoglossal nerve
(E) Left glossopharyngeal nerve

13. A 47-year-old man cannot move his eyeball laterally. Which of the following conditions would cause such a clinical sign?

(A) Tumor of the pituitary gland
(B) Occlusion of the posterior cerebral artery
(C) Infection in the maxillary sinus
(D) Infection in the cavernous sinus
(E) Tumor in the anterior cranial fossa

14. A young boy with a tooth abscess from a longstanding infection suffers damage of the lingual nerve as it enters the oral cavity. Which of the following structures contain cell bodies of injured nerve fibers?

(A) Geniculate and otic ganglia
(B) Trigeminal and submandibular ganglia
(C) Trigeminal and dorsal root ganglia
(D) Geniculate and trigeminal ganglia
(E) Geniculate and pterygopalatine ganglia

15. A knife wound has severed the oculomotor nerve in a 45-year-old man. Which of the following conditions will occur because of this injury?

(A) Constricted pupil
(B) Abduction of the eyeball
(C) Complete ptosis
(D) Impaired lacrimal secretion
(E) Paralysis of the ciliary muscle

16. A 20-year-old guard at the gate of the Royal King's palace blinks his eyes when a strong wind hits the cornea of his eye. The afferent fibers of the corneal reflex arc are carried by which of the following nerves?

(A) Optic nerve
(B) Lacrimal nerve
(C) Nasociliary nerve
(D) Zygomatic nerve
(E) Oculomotor nerve

17. A 71-year-old man suffers from a known benign tumor in the pterygoid canal. Which of the following nerve fibers could be injured by this condition?

(A) Postganglionic parasympathetic fibers
(B) Taste fibers from the epiglottis
(C) General somatic afferent (GSA) fibers
(D) Preganglionic sympathetic fibers
(E) General visceral afferent (GVA) fibers

18. A 22-year-old patient has dryness of the corneal surface of his eye because of a lack of tears. Which of the following nerves may be damaged?

(A) Proximal portion of the lacrimal nerve
(B) Zygomatic branch of the facial nerve
(C) Lesser petrosal nerve
(D) Greater petrosal nerve
(E) Deep petrosal nerve

19. A 31-year-old hockey player is hit in the head by a puck. His radiogram shows a fracture of the foramen rotundum. Which of the following nerves would be damaged by this event?

(A) Ophthalmic nerve
(B) Mandibular nerve
(C) Maxillary nerve
(D) Optic nerve
(E) Trochlear nerve

20. Muscles derived from the second (hyoid) pharyngeal arch are innervated by which of the following cranial nerves?

(A) Trigeminal nerve
(B) Facial nerve
(C) Glossopharyngeal nerve
(D) Vagus nerve
(E) Accessory nerve

Answers and Explanations

1. **The Answer is C.** Thrombosis in the cavernous sinus might damage all three CNs (III, IV, VI): lesion of CN III causes ptosis, a dilated pupil, and loss of accommodation; lesion of CN IV causes inability to look inferiorly when adducted; and lesion of CN VI causes the eyeball deviates medially (internal strabismus). Lesion in the medulla may damage CNs IX, X, and XII. Tumor in the optic canal injures the optic nerve and ophthalmic artery. Lesion of the olfactory nerve causes anosmia (loss of smell). Fracture of the foramen spinosum damages the middle meningeal artery.

2. **The Answer is D.** If the trochlear nerve is injured, the patient is unable to turn the eyeball inferolaterally and has trouble going downstairs due to paralysis of the superior oblique muscle. Lesion of the oculomotor nerve causes ptosis due to paralysis of the levator palpebrae superioris, dilation of the pupil due to paralysis of the sphincter pupillae, loss of accommodation due to paralysis of ciliary muscles, and loss of pupillary light reflex due to loss of the efferent limb of the pupillary light reflex. Lesion of the optic nerve causes blindness. Lesion of the ophthalmic nerve causes loss of cutaneous sensation on the face above the upper eyelid. Lesion of the abducens nerve causes internal strabismus in which the eyeball turns medially.

3. **The Answer is D.** Accessory nerve passes through the posterior cervical triangle and is responsible for shrugging the shoulder and turn the head to the opposite side. The trigeminal nerve carries sensory fibers for the face and motor fibers for the muscles of mastication. The facial nerve carries motor fibers to the muscles of facial expression, secretomotor fibers to lacrimal, submandibular, sublingual, and nasal glands, and taste fibers from the anterior two-thirds of the tongue. The glossopharyngeal nerve conveys motor fibers to the stylopharyngeus muscle and taste fibers from the posterior one-third of the tongue. The hypoglossal nerve carries motor fibers for the muscles of tongue movement.

4. **The Answer is D.** The jugular foramen transmits cranial nerves, IX, X, and XI, along with the internal jugular vein. The cranial nerve V2 runs through the foramen rotundum. The cranial nerve VI passes through the superior orbital fissure. The cranial nerves VII and VIII courses through the internal auditory meatus. The cranial nerve XII passes through the hypoglossal canal.

5. **The Answer is C.** Lesion of sympathetic nerves in the cervical region results in a constricted pupil due to paralysis of the dilator pupillae. Internal strabismus is caused by a lesion of the abducens nerve. Lesion of the trochlear nerve results in difficulty going downstairs. Inability to close the eye is due to a lesion of the facial nerve. Lesion of the hypoglossal nerve causes deviation of the tongue toward the lesion side.

6. **The Answer is C.** Injury to the glossopharyngeal nerve causes paralysis of the stylopharoyngeus muscle, which is involved in swallowing, no general and taste sensation of the posterior one-third of the tongue, a lack of salivary secretion from the parotid gland due to parasympathetic nerve injury, and no visceral sensation from the carotid sinus and body. Lesion of the inferior alveolar nerve in the mandibular canal results in a lack of sensation to the canine and incisor teeth and the skin over the chin. Section of the zygomatic nerve causes a lack of lacrimal secretion because it carries postganglionic parasympathetic fibers from the pterygopalatine ganglion for lacrimal secretion. Tumor in the pituitary gland may damage the optic chiasma, resulting in the bitemporal hemianopia. Lesion of the hypoglossal nerve causes deviation of the tongue toward the injured side on protrusion.

7. **The answer is E.** The abducens nerve (CN VI) innervates the lateral rectus muscle, which abducts the eyeball. A lesion of the abducens nerve results in internal strabismus (medial deviation) and diplopia (double vision). Ptosis of the upper eyelid is caused by lesions of the oculomotor nerve or sympathetic nerve to the levator palpebrae superioris. Inability to dilate the

pupil is caused by a lesion of the sympathetic nerve to the dilator pupillae. External strabismus (lateral deviation) is caused by paralysis of the medial rectus muscle, which is innervated by the oculomotor nerve. Loss of visual accommodation is due to a lesion of parasympathetic nerve fibers to the ciliary muscle.

8. **The answer is A.** The anterior two-thirds of the tongue is innervated by the lingual nerve, a branch of the mandibular division of the trigeminal nerve (CN V). The posterior one-third of the tongue is innervated by the glossopharyngeal nerve (CN IX) for general and taste sensations. The facial nerve supplies taste fibers to the tongue through the chorda tympani but does not supply general sensation. The vagus nerve supplies general sensation and taste sensation to the epiglottis by way of the internal laryngeal branch. The hypoglossal nerve innervates the tongue muscles.

9. **The answer is B.** Lesion of the optic chiasma by a pituitary tumor results in bitemporal hemianopia resulting from loss in the nasal field of vision of both eyes. Lesion of the optic nerve causes blindness. A right perichiasmal lesion by an aneurysm of the internal carotid artery leads to right nasal hemianopia because of loss of vision in the nasal field of the right eye. Lesion of the right optic tract or optic radiation causes left homonymous hemianopia resulting from loss of the left half of the visual fields of both eyes. Aneurysms of both internal carotid arteries cause right and left perichiasmal lesions, leading to binasal hemianopia (loss of vision in the nasal fields of both eyes).

10. **The answer is C.** Damage to the parasympathetic ciliary ganglion and parasympathetic fibers in the short ciliary nerve impairs the ability to focus on close objects (accommodation). Because the patient can move his eyeballs normally, the oculomotor nerve is not damaged even if this nerve contains preganglionic parasympathetic fibers. The patient is able to see distant objects clearly because the long ciliary nerve also carries sympathetic fibers to the dilator pupillae. The ability to move the eyeball normally indicates that the oculomotor, trochlear, and abducens nerves are intact.

11. **The answer is C.** The vagus nerve innervates the musculus uvulae. A lesion of the vagus nerve causes deviation of the uvula toward the opposite side of the injury. Because her uvula deviates to the left on phonation, the right vagus nerve is damaged. Hoarseness is caused by a paralysis of the laryngeal muscles resulting from damage to skeletal motor fibers in the recurrent laryngeal branch of the vagus nerve.

12. **The answer is D.** A lesion of the hypoglossal nerve causes deviation of the tongue toward the injured side on protrusion. The lingual and glossopharyngeal nerves do not supply the tongue muscles.

13. **The answer is D.** The abducens nerve, which innervates the lateral rectus muscle, runs through the middle of the cavernous sinus. The other conditions listed do not injure the abducens nerve. A tumor in the pituitary gland may injure the optic chiasma, causing bitemporal hemianopsia.

14. **The answer is D.** The lingual nerve is joined by the chorda tympani in the infratemporal fossa. Therefore, the lingual nerve contains GSA fibers whose cell bodies are located in the trigeminal ganglion and SSA or taste fibers that have cell bodies located in the geniculate ganglion. In addition, the lingual nerve carries parasympathetic preganglionic GVE fibers that originated from the chorda tympani; the cell bodies are located in the superior salivatory nucleus in the pons. The chorda tympani and lingual nerves contain no fibers from the otic, submandibular, pterygopalatine, or dorsal root ganglia.

15. **The answer is E.** The oculomotor nerve carries parasympathetic fibers to the ciliary and sphincter pupillae ciliary muscles; thus, a lesion of the oculomotor nerve leads to ciliary muscle paralysis and a dilated pupil. The abducens nerve supplies the lateral rectus, which is an abductor of the eye. The levator palpebrae superioris inserts on the tarsal plate in the upper eyelid, which is innervated by sympathetic fibers. Thus, a lesion of the oculomotor nerve does not cause complete ptosis. The secretomotor fibers for lacrimal secretion come through the pterygopalatine ganglion. Thus, severance of the oculomotor nerve has no effect on lacrimal secretion.

16. **The answer is C.** The afferent limb of the corneal reflex arc is the nasociliary nerve, and its efferent limb is the facial nerve. The other nerves are not involved in the reflex arc. The opening of the eye is conducted by the oculomotor nerve, but it is not a part of the corneal reflex.

17. **The answer is E.** The nerve of the pterygoid canal (Vidian nerve) contains taste SVA fibers from the palate, GVA fibers, postganglionic sympathetic fibers, and preganglionic parasympathetic fibers.

18. **The answer is D.** The secretomotor fibers to the lacrimal gland are parasympathetic fibers that run in the facial, greater petrosal, Vidian (nerve of the pterygoid canal), maxillary, zygomatic (of maxillary), zygomaticotemporal, and lacrimal (terminal portion) nerves. The lesser petrosal nerve carries secretomotor (preganglionic parasympathetic) fibers to the parotid gland. The deep petrosal nerve contains postganglionic sympathetic fibers. The zygomatic branch of the facial nerve supplies the facial muscles.

19. **The answer is C.** The maxillary nerve runs through the foramen rotundum; the ophthalmic nerve runs through the supraorbital fissure; the mandibular nerve passes through the foramen ovale; the optic nerve runs through the optic canal; and the trochlear nerve passes through the superior orbital fissure.

20. **The answer is B.** Muscles derived from the second (hyoid) pharyngeal arch are innervated by the facial nerve. Muscles derived from the first (mandibular) pharyngeal arch are innervated by the mandibular division of the trigeminal nerve. A muscle derived from the third pharyngeal arch is innervated by the glossopharyngeal nerve. Muscles derived from the fourth and sixth pharyngeal arches are innervated by the vagus nerve. Muscles of myotome origin that shrug shoulder and turn head are innervated by the accessory nerve.

Comprehensive Examination

Directions: Each of the numbered items or incomplete statements in this section is followed by answers or by completions of the statement. Select the **one**-lettered answer or completion that is **best** in each case.

1. A young man is brought to the emergency department after being mugged. He was stabbed in the shoulder after refusing to give his wallet to his assailant. If the stab wound lacerates the posterior humeral circumflex artery passing through the quadrangular space on the shoulder region, which of the following nerves might be injured?

(A) Radial nerve
(B) Axillary nerve
(C) Thoracodorsal nerve
(D) Suprascapular nerve
(E) Accessory nerve

2. A victim of an automobile accident is unable to abduct her left arm. This indicates damage to which of the following parts of the brachial plexus?

(A) Middle trunk and posterior cord
(B) Middle trunk and lateral cord
(C) Lower trunk and lateral cord
(D) Upper trunk and posterior cord
(E) Lower trunk and medial cord

3. A biomedical engineer would like to reconstruct the arm of a boy who underwent amputation to treat a life-threatening infection. In designing the prosthetic arm, the engineer will need to know that which of the following muscles flexes the elbow and is innervated by the radial nerve:

(A) Flexor digitorum longus
(B) Brachioradialis
(C) Brachialis
(D) Extensor digitorum longus
(E) Biceps brachii

4. Young Johnny was playing on the playground at school when he fell and struck his arm against the swing set. He ran to the school nurse, complaining of which of the following conditions as a result of injuring the radial nerve in the spiral groove of the humerus?

(A) Numbness over the medial side of the forearm
(B) Inability to oppose the thumb
(C) Weakness in pronating the forearm
(D) Weakness in abducting the arm
(E) Inability to extend the hand

5. An indoor soccer player runs into another player while running after the ball. She falls to the ground and fractures the medial epicondyle of the humerus. Which of the following symptoms might she present with when seeing the physician in the emergency department?

(A) Impaired abduction of the hand
(B) Carpal tunnel syndrome
(C) Wrist drop
(D) Thenar atrophy
(E) Inability to sweat on the medial part of the hand

6. After winning a boxing match, a 24-year-old man is unable to abduct his fingers. Which of the following nerves is injured?

(A) Ulnar nerve
(B) Median nerve
(C) Radial nerve
(D) Musculocutaneous nerve
(E) Axillary nerve

7. A 42-year-old woman presents to an outpatient clinic with a 6-month history of numbness and tingling on the palmar aspect of her lateral three and one-half fingers, loss of pronation, and flattening of the thenar eminence. Injury to which of the following nerves could cause such a condition?

(A) Axillary nerve
(B) Musculocutaneous nerve
(C) Median nerve
(D) Radial nerve
(E) Ulnar nerve

8. A ballet dancer falls to the floor and hurts herself during a practice session before opening night. She sustains an injury to the thoracodorsal nerve that would probably affect the strength of which of the following movements?

(A) Adduction of the scapula
(B) Elevation of the scapula
(C) Abduction of the arm
(D) Extension of the arm
(E) Lateral rotation of the arm

9. A 23-year-old man falls from a ladder and injures his arm. On examination, he feels numbness and has no sweating on the lateral side of his forearm, suggesting damage to the lateral antebrachial cutaneous nerve. The cell bodies of injured nerve fibers involved in sweating are located in which of the following structures?

(A) Collateral ganglia
(B) Dorsal root ganglia
(C) Sympathetic chain ganglia
(D) Lateral horn of spinal cord
(E) Anterior horn of spinal cord

10. There are only 30 minutes left before the concert starts. The pianist, accidentally cuts herself over the palmar surface of her wrist and notices that she is unable to pick up a piece of music between her index and middle fingers. Which of the following nerves is most likely damaged?

(A) Radial nerve
(B) Axillary nerve
(C) Ulnar nerve
(D) Median nerve
(E) Anterior interosseous nerve

11. A 29-year-old carpenter receives a crush injury to his metacarpophalangeal joint of the fourth digit (ring finger) while remodeling his neighbor's porch. Which of the following pairs of nerves innervates the muscle that moves the injured joint?

(A) Median and ulnar nerves
(B) Radial and median nerves
(C) Musculocutaneous and ulnar nerves
(D) Ulnar and radial nerves
(E) Radial and axillary nerves

12. A 21-year-old man celebrating his birthday gets a little carried away with his friends and starts a bar fight. He is stabbed with a knife that severs the roots of C5 and C6 of the brachial plexus. Which of the following muscles is likely to be paralyzed?

(A) Infraspinatus
(B) Flexor carpi ulnaris
(C) Palmar interossei
(D) Adductor pollicis
(E) Palmaris brevis

13. The secretary of a rather verbose academic physician in internal medicine complains of numbness and tingling in her hands and fingers. She is constantly typing long patient visit dictations and now has carpal tunnel syndrome, which is due to compression of which of the following structures?

(A) Ulnar artery
(B) Ulnar nerve
(C) Median nerve
(D) Flexor carpi radialis tendon
(E) Palmaris longus tendon

14. While playing in a Super Bowl game, a 26-year-old professional football player is tackled, and his anterior cruciate ligament is torn. If not injured, the anterior cruciate ligament of the knee joint:

(A) Becomes taut during flexion of the leg
(B) Resists posterior displacement of the femur on the tibia
(C) Inserts into the medial femoral condyle
(D) Helps prevent hyperflexion of the knee joint
(E) Is lax when the knee is extended

15. A man interviewing for a new administrative position as hospital chief executive officer notices difficulty walking after sitting with his leg crossed for 2 hours. He was nervous during the interview but even more so now that he is attempting to stand to follow two board members for a tour of the hospital. Which of the following actions is most seriously affected by compression and temporary paralysis of the deep peroneal nerve?

(A) Plantar flexion of the foot
(B) Dorsiflexion of the foot
(C) Abduction of the toes
(D) Adduction of the toes
(E) Inversion of the foot

16. Deep venous thrombosis is a common complication from sitting in one position for a prolonged duration, such as during a long car trip or a long plane flight. The first vascular channels likely to be obstructed or occluded by an embolus from the deep veins of a lower limb are the:

(A) Tributaries of the renal veins
(B) Branches of the coronary arteries
(C) Sinusoids of the liver
(D) Tributaries of the pulmonary veins
(E) Branches of the pulmonary arteries

17. During recruitment by the local representative for the Marines, a young college student presents with the condition known as flat foot. His foot is displaced laterally and everted, and the head of the talus is no longer supported. Which of the following ligaments probably is stretched?

(A) Plantar calcaneonavicular (spring)
(B) Calcaneofibular
(C) Anterior talofibular
(D) Plantar calcaneocuboid (short plantar)
(E) Anterior tibiotalar

18. During a sports medicine physical by a local family physician, a young woman is tested for stability of her joints before tryouts for the high school team. Which of the following ligaments is important in preventing forward displacement of the femur on the tibia when the weight-bearing knee is flexed?

(A) Medial meniscus
(B) Tibial collateral ligament
(C) Fibular collateral ligament
(D) Posterior cruciate ligament
(E) Anterior cruciate ligament

19. A 21-year-old man falls from the attic and is brought to the emergency department. Examination and x-rays reveal that the lateral longitudinal arch of his foot is flattened. Which of the following bones is displaced?

(A) Talus
(B) Medial three metatarsals
(C) Navicular
(D) Cuneiform
(E) Cuboid

20. A 72-year-old woman with Parkinson's disease fell down in the bathtub at her home and suffered a dislocation of the hip joint that may result in vascular necrosis of the femoral head and neck because of injuries to the arteries. Which of the following arteries might remain intact?

(A) Lateral femoral circumflex artery
(B) Medial femoral circumflex artery
(C) Obturator artery
(D) Inferior gluteal artery
(E) Deep iliac circumflex artery

21. A 78-year-old woman undergoes knee surgery because her lateral meniscus is torn. Before injury, the normal lateral meniscus of the knee joint:

(A) Is C-shaped or forms a semicircle
(B) Is attached to the fibular collateral ligament
(C) Is larger than the medial meniscus
(D) Lies outside the synovial cavity
(E) Is more frequently torn in injuries than the medial meniscus

22. A 17-year-old boy is involved in a group fight, and a stab wound lacerates a ventral root of his thoracic spinal nerve. Cell bodies of the injured nerve fibers are located in which of the following nervous structures?

(A) Dorsal root ganglia and sympathetic trunk
(B) Lateral horn of spinal cord and dorsal root ganglia
(C) Anterior horn and lateral horn of spinal cord
(D) Sympathetic trunk and lateral horn of spinal cord
(E) Anterior horn of spinal cord and sympathetic trunk

23. A race car driver is brought to the city trauma center after a high-speed crash in which his car spun out of control and struck a concrete embankment. He has blunt trauma to his chest and undergoes extensive vascular studies to determine which blood vessels are still intact. The interventional radiologist recalls that one of the following veins drains directly into the superior vena cava. Which vein would this be?

(A) Internal thoracic vein
(B) Azygos vein
(C) Hemiazygos vein
(D) Right superior intercostal vein
(E) Left superior intercostal vein

24. A 58-year-old stockbroker is brought to the cardiac catheterization laboratory emergently after evaluation in the emergency department has determined that he is suffering from an acute myocardial infarction. During the catheterization, he is found to have inadequate blood flow in the artery that runs along the great cardiac vein in the anterior interventricular sulcus of the heart. This is most likely an acute occlusion of the:

(A) Circumflex branch of the left coronary artery
(B) Marginal branch of the right coronary artery
(C) Left coronary artery
(D) Right coronary artery
(E) Posterior interventricular artery

25. A retired teacher suffers from a massive heart attack while playing golf and dies in the intensive care unit. Autopsy reveals the cause of death as severely diminished blood flow in the coronary arteries. This most likely resulted from embolization of an atherosclerotic plaque at the origin of which of the following vascular structures?

(A) Pulmonary trunk
(B) Ascending aorta
(C) Coronary sinus
(D) Descending aorta
(E) Aortic arch

26. A 21-year-old woman comes to the emergency department with acute chest pain and shortness of breath. Her chest x-ray shows opacification of one of her lungs. She undergoes thoracentesis, which reveals that she has a chylothorax resulting from rupture of the thoracic duct. Lymphatic drainage remains normal in which of the following areas?

(A) Left thorax
(B) Right thorax
(C) Left abdomen
(D) Right pelvis
(E) Left lower limb

27. An elderly man is choking on his food at a restaurant, and attempts by other patrons to dislodge the food bolus using the Heimlich procedure have failed. A retired anesthesiologist rushes to his table and prepares for emergent tracheotomy. She locates the manubrium of the sternum and recalls that it is free from articulation with which of the following structures?

(A) Body of the sternum
(B) First rib
(C) Second rib
(D) Third rib
(E) Clavicle

28. A stab wound penetrates the posterior thoracic wall near vertebra of a 24-year-old man. Examination at the emergency department indicates a lesion of gray rami communicantes. Which of the following nerve fibers would most likely be damaged?

(A) General somatic afferent (GSA) fibers
(B) Postganglionic parasympathetic fibers
(C) Preganglionic sympathetic fibers
(D) Postganglionic sympathetic fibers
(E) General visceral afferent (GVA) fibers

29. A 31-year-old NHL hockey player complains of numbness in the area of his umbilicus after the national championship game. Which of the following structures that carries GSA fibers was injured during the hockey game?

(A) Sympathetic trunk
(B) Dorsal root
(C) Greater splanchnic nerve
(D) Gray rami communicantes
(E) White rami communicantes

30. A 75-year-old veteran suffers a heart attack and is found in his home unconscious. He is in ventricular tachycardia and is shocked into normal sinus rhythm. He undergoes emergent catheterization and is found to have thrombosis in the coronary sinus. Which of the following cardiac veins might remain normal in diameter by catheterization study by the cardiologist?

(A) Great cardiac vein
(B) Middle cardiac vein
(C) Anterior cardiac vein
(D) Small cardiac vein
(E) Oblique cardiac vein

31. A 35-year-old man is suffering from an infected mediastinum (mediastinitis) after neck and chest injuries resulting from a head-on automobile collision. He has been intubated since the accident and on broad-spectrum intravenous antibiotics since admission; however, the infection continues to progress throughout the mediastinum. Which of the following structures is free from infection?

(A) Thymus gland
(B) Esophagus
(C) Trachea
(D) Lungs
(E) Heart

32. A 42-year-old man who has a rare neurological disorder comes to the emergency department. On examination, he is unable to protrude his tongue. Which of the following muscles is paralyzed?

(A) Hyoglossus
(B) Genioglossus
(C) Styloglossus
(D) Palatoglossus
(E) Geniohyoid

33. A new biotech company is interested in developing a new mechanical heart with a superficial implantable and rechargeable battery for easy access. During the design phase, the physician hired from the local academic hospital is asked about which structure carries or comes in contact with oxygenated blood. Which of the following answers is correct?

(A) Pectinate muscle
(B) Crista terminalis
(C) Septomarginal trabecula
(D) Pulmonary vein
(E) Pulmonary artery

34. A 62-year-old man is diagnosed with a Pancoast tumor that invades the inferior trunk of the brachial plexus. Which of the following muscle actions most likely resulted from injury to the brachial plexus?

(A) Lateral rotation of the arm
(B) Extension of the ring finger
(C) Abduction of the index finger
(D) Flexion of the forearm
(E) Pronation of the forearm

35. A 67-year-old woman complains of increasing urinary frequency and a heaviness in her pelvic area. On examination, her uterine cervix is visible at the vaginal opening. Which of the following conditions causes this symptom?

(A) Tear of the transversalis fascia
(B) Weakness of the ovarian ligament
(C) Relaxation of the cardinal ligament
(D) Weakness of the arcuate pubic ligament
(E) Paralysis of the piriformis muscle

36. Weight lifters in competition are often concerned about muscle tone and complications with hernias. In particular, the most common hernia in this case is an indirect inguinal hernia, which appears:

(A) Lateral to the inferior epigastric artery
(B) Between the inferior epigastric and obliterated umbilical arteries
(C) Medial to the obliterated umbilical artery
(D) Between the median and medial umbilical folds
(E) Between the linea alba and linea semilunaris

37. A 32-year-old man is involved in a car accident and suffers from a crushed internal injury in his abdomen. Examination reveals a lesion of parasympathetic fibers in the vagus nerve, which interferes with glandular secretory or smooth muscle functions in which of the following organs?

(A) Bladder
(B) Transverse colon
(C) Sigmoid colon
(D) Prostate gland
(E) Rectum

38. Pancreatic cancer has one of the highest mortality rates of all cancers because of the lack of symptoms until an advanced stage of disease. The one exception is the cancer that is slow growing and located in the head of the pancreas. This may present in an early stage by causing compression of which of the following structures?

(A) Duodenojejunal junction
(B) Gastroduodenal artery
(C) Bile duct
(D) Inferior mesenteric artery
(E) Common hepatic duct

39. An elderly man with a known large abdominal aortic aneurysm presents to the emergency department with acute severe and diffuse pain in his abdomen. The physician performing the evaluation considers mesenteric ischemia, a life-threatening disease, as a possible etiology. Which of the following organs may be spared from ischemia in the presence of an occlusive lesion in the celiac trunk?

(A) Liver
(B) Spleen
(C) Pancreas
(D) Gallbladder
(E) Stomach

40. A young woman with cryptogenic cirrhosis presents to the university hospital for an evaluation as a possible candidate for liver transplant. She has late-stage cirrhosis, and her liver-spleen scan shows a high degree of portal hypertension. The portal venous system includes which of the following veins?

(A) Left suprarenal vein
(B) Inferior epigastric vein
(C) Superior rectal vein
(D) Azygos vein
(E) Hepatic vein

41. A 2-month-old boy is admitted to the hospital with diarrhea, vomiting, and difficulty in bowel movements. A computed tomography (CT) scan of his abdomen reveals a distinctly dilated lower colon and is diagnosed as having Hirschsprung's disease. Which of the following is the most likely embryonic mechanism responsible for development of this congenital megacolon?

(A) Malrotation of the hindgut
(B) Abnormal formation of the urorectal septum
(C) Failure of neural crest cell migration into the hindgut
(D) Absence of visceral afferent cells in the myenteric plexus
(E) Failure of partitioning of the cloaca

42. A 29-year-old farmer falls on tractor blades and injures his groin. Several days later, he comes to the emergency department and examination by the physician reveals that the urogenital diaphragm and bulbourethral glands are infected. The infected deep perineal space:

(A) Is formed superiorly by the perineal membrane
(B) Is formed inferiorly by Colles fascia
(C) Contains a segment of the dorsal nerve of the penis
(D) Contains superficial transverse perineal muscles
(E) Contains the greater vestibular glands

43. A 2-day-old baby is admitted to the hospital with vomiting, fever, and rectal bleeding. Physical and CT scan examinations reveal small bowel obstruction and are diagnosed as having Meckel's diverticulum. Which portion of the gastrointestinal tract is most likely involved in the development of the diverticulum that may be connected to the inner surface of the umbilicus by a fibrous cord?

(A) Stomach
(B) Jejunum
(C) Ileum
(D) Appendix
(E) Sigmoid colon

44. A 59-year-old woman has a large pelvic tumor that compresses the inferior hypogastric (pelvic) plexus. Parasympathetic nerve fibers in this plexus come from which of the following nerves?

(A) Lumbar splanchnic nerves
(B) Pelvic splanchnic nerves
(C) Sacral sympathetic chain ganglia
(D) Vagus nerve
(E) Sacral splanchnic nerves

45. Because of a lesion, the parasympathetic nerve fibers are unable to induce a contraction of the detrusor muscle and relaxation of the internal sphincter. The injured parasympathetic fibers that supply the urinary bladder are derived from which of following nerves?

(A) Vagus nerve
(B) Pelvic splanchnic nerve
(C) Sacral splanchnic nerve
(D) Lesser splanchnic nerve
(E) Greater splanchnic nerve

46. At a local hospital tumor board, a gynecologic oncologist discusses the next case for the multidisciplinary team. He explains the rationale for using chemotherapy and radiation after surgical resection because carcinoma of the uterus can spread directly to the labium majus through lymphatics that follow the:

(A) Ovarian ligament
(B) Suspensory ligament of the ovary
(C) Round ligament of the uterus
(D) Uterosacral ligaments
(E) Pubocervical ligaments

47. A young couple is seeing a sex therapist for the first time to determine the cause of some of their recent difficulties. The husband tells the therapist that he no longer has sensation in his scrotum after a race car accident. Which of the following nerves carries undamaged sensory nerve fibers?

(A) Ilioinguinal nerve
(B) Genitofemoral nerve
(C) Iliohypogastric nerve
(D) Perineal branch of the pudendal nerve
(E) Perineal branch of the posterior femoral cutaneous nerve

48. A patient has a damaged pelvic outlet as the result of an automobile accident. Following this accident, which of the following structures is still intact?

(A) Sacrotuberous ligament
(B) Inferior pubic ramus
(C) Pubic crest
(D) Ischial tuberosity
(E) Coccyx

49. A forensic pathologist is examining the pelvic bone of a murder victim to identify the sex of the victim. Which of the following characteristics is that of a female pelvis?

(A) Oval-shaped pelvic inlet
(B) Smaller pelvic outlet
(C) Lesser pubic angle
(D) Narrower and longer sacrum
(E) Narrower and deeper pelvic cavity

50. A 26-year-old woman experiences severe back pain from an automobile accident. A CT scan reveals that the L5 vertebral foramen is completely obliterated by a collapsed L5 laminae and pedicles. In this injury, which of the following structures is crushed?

(A) Vertebral artery
(B) Spinal cord
(C) Filum terminale externus (filum of the dura)
(D) Denticulate ligament
(E) Cauda equina

51. A performer at the traveling circus for the state fair has injured her shoulder during a routine. When she fell off the trapeze, she struck the ground on her back, and most of the blunt force was directed toward her shoulders. A crush injury of the suboccipital nerve would result in paralysis of which of the following muscles?

(A) Splenius capitis
(B) Trapezius
(C) Rectus capitis posterior major
(D) Levator scapulae
(E) Iliocostalis

52. A neonate is brought to the pediatrician with headaches, fevers, and change in mental status, mostly manifesting as lethargy and lack of appetite. The baby is admitted emergently to rule out meningitis and is to undergo a diagnostic lumbar puncture. When withdrawing cerebrospinal fluid (CSF), the needle may penetrate which of the following pairs of structures?

(A) Dura mater and denticulate ligament
(B) Arachnoid mater and pia mater
(C) Dura mater and arachnoid mater
(D) Annulus fibrosus and pia mater
(E) Arachnoid mater and nucleus pulposus

53. Mrs. Jones was riding in the front seat of her son's van when the vehicle abruptly stopped. Unfortunately, she was not wearing her seatbelt and was thrown forward. As a result of the accident, the transverse processes of her cervical vertebrae were crushed against the dashboard of the van. Which of the following muscles might be paralyzed?

(A) Trapezius
(B) Latissimus dorsi
(C) Rhomboid major
(D) Levator scapulae
(E) Serratus posterior superior

54. A middle-aged woman is receiving a shiatsu massage when her therapist notices that the client has numbness in her neck. A lack of sensation of the skin over the anterior triangle of the neck may be due to injury to which of the following nerves?

(A) Great auricular nerve
(B) Transverse cervical nerve
(C) Superior ramus of the ansa cervicalis
(D) Inferior ramus of the ansa cervicalis
(E) Superior laryngeal nerve

55. A young man presents to your clinic with a 3-month history of an enlarging mass in his right neck. He undergoes a CT scan that reveals a fluid-filled mass where the common carotid artery bifurcates. Which of the following is another structure that would be located at this level?

(A) Thyroid isthmus
(B) Cricoid cartilage
(C) Sternal angle
(D) Superior border of the thyroid cartilage
(E) Jugular notch

56. An ultimate fighter is brought into the locker room after being knocked out by his opponent. He has suffered severe trauma to the articular disk and capsule of the temporomandibular joint. This could result in paralysis of which of the following muscles?

(A) Masseter
(B) Temporalis
(C) Medial pterygoid
(D) Lateral pterygoid
(E) Buccinator

57. A 25-year-old woman is suffering from facial paralysis and exhibits ptosis (drooping of the upper eyelid). Injury to which of the following nerves would result in ptosis?

(A) Trochlear nerve
(B) Abducens nerve
(C) Oculomotor nerve
(D) Ophthalmic nerve
(E) Facial nerve

58. A 67-year-old man is known to have an infection in the superior petrosal sinus. The infected sinus lies in the margin of which of the following structures?

(A) Tentorium cerebelli
(B) Falx cerebri
(C) Falx cerebelli
(D) Diaphragma sellae
(E) Straight sinus

59. A 59-year-old man has pus in the loose connective tissue layer of the scalp, and consequently, his superior sagittal sinus is infected. The arachnoid granulations in the infected sinus:

(A) Absorb CSF into the dural venous sinuses
(B) Are storage areas for CSF
(C) Produce CSF
(D) Allow CSF to return to the ventricles of the brain
(E) Filter venous blood into CSF

60. While speaking at a charity program, an elderly woman suddenly collapses to the ground. She is diagnosed as having a massive stroke, but it is unclear where the vascular lesion is located. She undergoes a cerebral arteriogram. Normally, the great cerebral vein of Galen drains directly into which of the following sinuses?

(A) Superior sagittal sinus
(B) Inferior sagittal sinus
(C) Cavernous sinus
(D) Transverse sinus
(E) Straight sinus

61. While resecting a tumor in the palate, the surgical intern removes the mass but finds that it is deeply invasive into the tendon that loops around the pterygoid hamulus. Which of the following muscles would most likely be paralyzed?

(A) Tensor tympani
(B) Tensor veli palatini
(C) Levator veli palatini
(D) Superior pharyngeal constrictor
(E) Stylohyoid

62. During a domestic incident, a 28-year-old woman receives a vertical stab wound that lacerates the pterygomandibular raphe. As a result, which of the following muscles would be paralyzed?

(A) Superior and middle pharyngeal constrictors
(B) Middle and inferior pharyngeal constrictors
(C) Superior pharyngeal constrictor and buccinator muscles
(D) Medial and lateral pterygoid muscles
(E) Tensor veli palatini and levator veli palatini

63. A 31-year-old football player with a head injury is brought to a local emergency department. Physical examination, radiogram, and a magnetic resonance imaging scan indicate a lesion of the trigeminal nerve. Which of the following muscles is most likely paralyzed?

(A) Geniohyoid
(B) Palatoglossus
(C) Cricothyroid
(D) Tensor veli palatini
(E) Levator veli palatini

64. The muscle that indents the submandibular gland and divides it into superficial and deep parts is paralyzed because of compression by a large salivary glandular tumor. Which of the following muscles is involved?

(A) Hyoglossus
(B) Digastric posterior belly
(C) Styloglossus
(D) Stylohyoid
(E) Mylohyoid

65. A young homeless child presents to the emergency department with high fever and low blood pressure. He had strep throat 2 weeks ago when seen in the free clinic; however, his parents did not give him his antibiotic medication. He now has an abscess in the auditory tube that is blocking communication between the nasopharynx and which of the following structures?

(A) Vestibule of the inner ear
(B) Middle ear
(C) Semicircular canals
(D) External ear
(E) Inner ear

66. A man with a neuromuscular autoimmune disease has another attack at home. His wife calls the doctor's office because he is unable to speak. Once at the office, he is unable to open his jaw because of paralysis of which of the following muscles?

(A) Medial pterygoid
(B) Masseter
(C) Temporalis
(D) Lateral pterygoid
(E) Buccinator

67. A 29-year-old baseball player whose head is hit by a ball is brought to an emergency department. Physical examination and radiogram reveal fracture of the temporal bone and damage to the lesser petrosal nerve. Which of the following conditions could occur as a result of injury to the lesser petrosal nerve?

(A) Lack of lacrimal secretion
(B) Lack of submandibular gland secretion
(C) Lack of parotid gland secretion
(D) Constriction of the pupil
(E) Ptosis of the upper eyelid

68. A 26-year-old woman with the flu comes to an outpatient clinic. On examination, a physician diagnoses her with sinus and palate infection, and her uvula deviates to the left side on phonation. Which of the following nerves is injured?

(A) Left hypoglossal nerve
(B) Right hypoglossal nerve
(C) Left vagus nerve
(D) Right vagus nerve
(E) Left trigeminal nerve

69. During a palatine tonsillectomy, a surgeon must ligate arteries to avoid bleeding within the surgical field. Which of the following arteries can be spared?

(A) Lesser palatine artery
(B) Facial artery
(C) Lingual artery
(D) Superior thyroid artery
(E) Ascending pharyngeal artery

70. A young child is evaluated by his pediatrician for chronic nosebleeds. He is referred to an allergist when it is determined that his nasal cavity is chronically dry because of a lack of glandular secretions. A possible etiology may be a lesion of which of the following structures?

(A) Superior cervical ganglion
(B) Lesser petrosal nerve
(C) Facial nerve in the facial canal
(D) Greater petrosal nerve
(E) Deep petrosal nerve

Questions 71 to 72

A 12-year-old girl suffers from a type of neural tube defect called tethered cord syndrome, a congenital anomaly that results from defective closure of the neural tube. This syndrome is characterized by an abnormally low conus medullaris, which is tethered by a short, thickened filum terminale, leading to progressive neurologic defects in the legs and feet.

71. Which of the following defects is commonly associated with the tethered cord syndrome?

(A) Spina bifida occulta
(B) Kyphosis
(C) Meningomyelocele
(D) Herniated disk
(E) Scoliosis

72. This girl has strong muscle function of the flexors of the thigh, but she has weakness of the extensors (hamstrings). A lesion has occurred at which of the following spinal cord levels?

(A) T12
(B) L1
(C) L3
(D) L5
(E) S5

73. A 36-year-old plumber slips and breaks a porcelain sink, cutting an anterior aspect of his wrist deeply on a sharp edge. On arrival to the emergency department, he can adduct his thumb but not oppose it. Which of the following structures has been severed?

(A) Radial nerve
(B) Median nerve
(C) Ulnar nerve
(D) Anterior interosseous nerve
(E) Posterior interosseous nerve

74. A 21-year-old soccer player is tackled via a high-impact sweeping injury about the right knee, causing a posterior knee dislocation. Soon after, he is unable to plantar flex his right ankle or flex his toes. He also experiences loss of sensation on the sole of his right foot. Which of the following nerves is most likely injured?

(A) Saphenous nerve
(B) Tibial nerve
(C) Deep peroneal nerve
(D) Superficial peroneal nerve
(E) Common peroneal nerve

75. A 56-year-old man with a one pack/day history of cigarette smoking is found to have a malignant squamous cell carcinoma located in the superior sulcus of Pancoast (superior apex of the lung). Shortly after the diagnosis is known, the patient develops symptoms that consist of shoulder pain along with ptosis, miosis, enophthalmos, and anhidrosis. Which of the following nerves is most likely compressed by the tumor mass?

(A) Phrenic nerve
(B) Vagus nerve
(C) Cervical sympathetic trunk
(D) Ansa cervicalis
(E) Recurrent laryngeal nerve

76. A 57-year-old woman presents with increasing numbness of the fourth and fifth digits on her right hand. On examination, it is noticed that she has a wasted hypothenar eminence, inability to abduct the thumb, and a characteristic claw hand. Which of the following nerves has most likely been injured?

(A) Axillary nerve
(B) Anterior interosseous nerve
(C) Radial nerve
(D) Ulnar nerve
(E) Median nerve

77. A 47-year-old woman has had a lumpectomy and axillary dissection to check for metastasis. She has come in for her follow-up appointment, and her physician notices on her physical examination that the medial part of her scapula protrudes from her back and that she is not able to raise her arm above the horizontal level. Which of the following nerves has been damaged during her surgery?

(A) Median nerve
(B) Ulnar nerve
(C) Thoracodorsal nerve
(D) Long thoracic nerve
(E) Radial nerve

78. A 31-year-old carpenter cuts his left arm with a utility knife and is brought to a local emergency department. He complains of numbness on the medial side of his arm. Which of the following nerves is most likely injured?

(A) Axillary nerve
(B) Musculocutaneous nerve
(C) Medial brachial cutaneous nerve
(D) Medial antebrachial cutaneous nerve
(E) Radial nerve

79. A 54-year-old high school teacher has been diagnosed with coronary artery disease and is to undergo coronary bypass surgery. During the surgery, the thoracic surgeon decides to use the internal thoracic artery for one of the bypasses. Which of the following arteries gives rise to the internal thoracic artery?

(A) Axillary artery
(B) Superior epigastric artery
(C) Costocervical trunk
(D) Subclavian artery
(E) Ascending aorta

80. A 34-year-old singer has been diagnosed with thyroid cancer and consequently has a thyroidectomy. He has been hoarse ever since the surgery 8 weeks ago. It has been suspected that a nerve was injured during the operation. Which of the following nerves is most likely damaged?

(A) External laryngeal nerve
(B) Internal laryngeal nerve
(C) Recurrent laryngeal nerve
(D) Hypoglossal nerve
(E) Glossopharyngeal nerve

81. A 24-year-old woman presents with an asymptomatic fluid-filled cyst on the midline of the neck. She is diagnosed with a thyroglossal duct cyst. Which organ migrates through the thyroglossal duct during embryological development?

(A) Inferior parathyroid glands
(B) Submandibular glands
(C) Thyroid gland
(D) Thymus
(E) Tongue

82. Otitis media is an infection in the middle ear cavity. From which embryological structure does the middle ear cavity form?

(A) Pharyngeal groove 1
(B) Pharyngeal pouch 1
(C) Auricular hillocks
(D) Pharyngeal membrane 1
(E) Pharyngeal pouch 2

Questions 83 to 87

Choose the appropriate lettered structure in the radiograph of the bones of the hand (see Figure below).

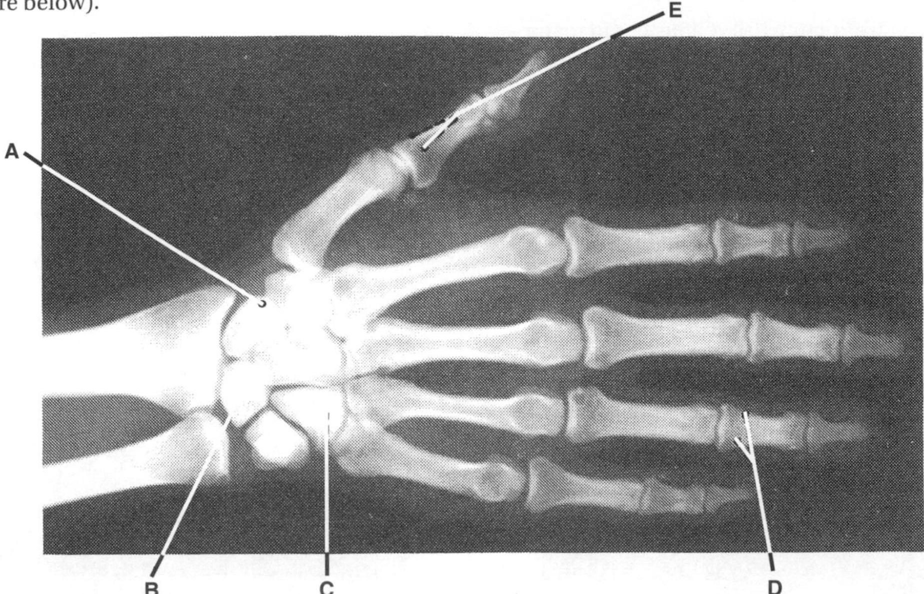

83. Which bone articulates with the radius and triquetrum?

84. Fracture of which bone may cause paralysis of the flexor digiti minimi and opponens digiti minimi muscles?

85. Which is the site of attachment of the muscles that form the thenar eminence?

86. Which is the site of tendinous attachment of the flexor digitorum superficialis?

87. Fracture of which bone may cause a deep tenderness in the anatomic snuffbox?

Questions 88 to 92

Choose the appropriate lettered structure in the CT scan of the abdomen (see Figure below).

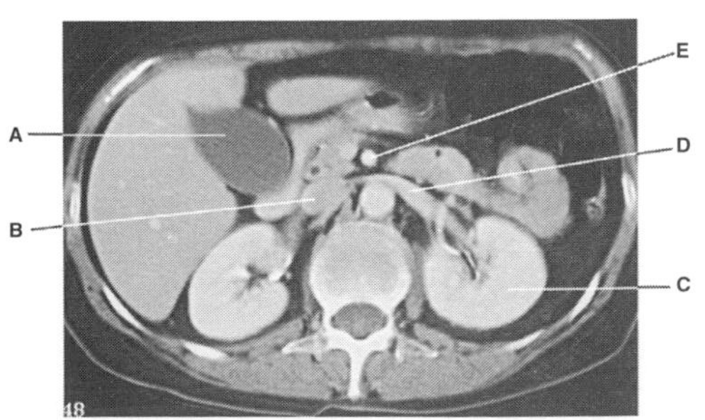

88. Thrombosis in which vessel causes a dilation of the left testicular vein?

89. Which structure concentrates and stores bile?

90. Laceration of which structure decreases blood flow in the middle colic artery?

91. Which structure produces and excretes urine?

92. Thrombosis in which vessel causes a dilation of the right suprarenal vein?

Questions 93 to 97

Choose the appropriate lettered structure in the CT scan of the female pelvis (see Figure below).

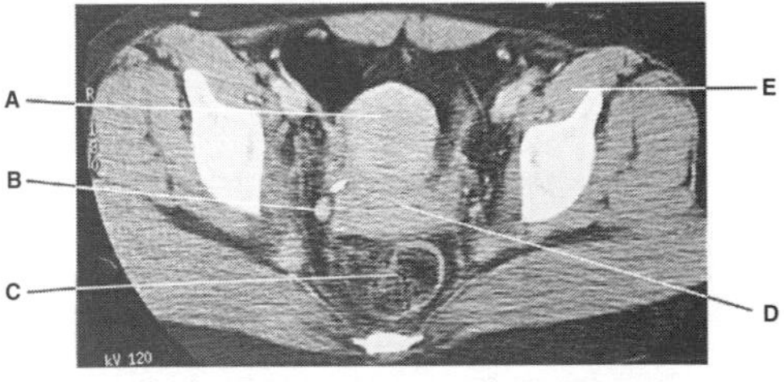

93. Which structure is a common site of uterine cancer?

94. Which structure descends retroperitoneally on the psoas muscle and runs under the uterine artery?

95. Which structure has venous blood that returns to the portal and caval (systemic) venous systems?

96. Stimulation of parasympathetic nerve causes a contraction of the detrusor muscle in which structure?

97. When the lesser trochanter is fractured, which structure is paralyzed?

Questions 98 to 100

Choose the appropriate lettered structure in the CT scan of the male pelvis (see Figure below).

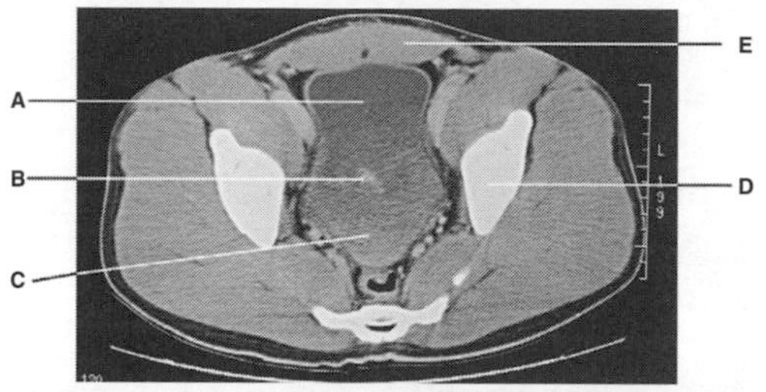

98. Which structure forms a medial boundary of the inguinal triangle?

99. Rupture of which structure impairs secretion of a fluid that produces the characteristic odor of semen?

100. Which structure receives the ejaculatory duct?

Questions 101 to 102

Choose the appropriate lettered structure in the radiograph of the head (see Figure below).

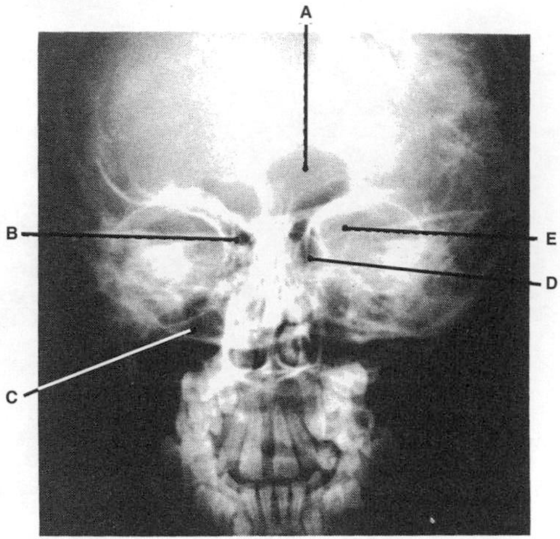

101. Which sinus opens into the hiatus semilunaris of the middle nasal meatus by way of the frontonasal duct or infundibulum?

102. Meningioma in which structure compresses the ophthalmic vein and trochlear nerve?

Answers and Explanations

1. **The answer is B.** The axillary nerve runs posteriorly to the humerus, accompanying the posterior humeral circumflex artery through the quadrangular space and innervating the teres minor and deltoid muscles. None of the other nerves pass through the quadrangular space.

2. **The answer is D.** Both the upper trunk and posterior cord of the brachial plexus are damaged. The abductors of the arm are the deltoid and supraspinatus muscles. The deltoid is innervated by the axillary nerve, which arises from the posterior cord of the brachial plexus. The supraspinatus is innervated by the suprascapular nerve, which arises from the upper trunk of the brachial plexus. The middle and lower trunks give rise to no branches. The lateral and medial cords supply no abductors of the arm.

3. **The answer is B.** The brachioradialis is innervated by the radial nerve and functions to flex the elbow. The flexor digitorum longus and extensor digitorum longus do not act in the elbow. The biceps brachii and brachialis muscles flex the elbow and are innervated by the musculocutaneous nerve.

4. **The answer is E.** The radial nerve innervates the extensor muscles of the hand; hence, Johnny could not extend his hand because of an injury to the radial nerve. Numbness would occur on the posterior aspects of the arm and forearm because of an injury to the radial nerve. The skin on the medial side of the forearm is innervated by the medial antebrachial cutaneous nerve; thus, numbness over the medial side of the forearm would not occur. The opponens pollicis, pronator teres, and pronator quadratus muscles are innervated by the median nerve. Therefore, inability to oppose the thumb or weakness in pronating the forearm would not occur. The abductors of the arm (deltoid and supraspinatus muscles) are innervated by the axillary nerve and upper trunk of the brachial plexus, respectively.

5. **The answer is E.** Fracture of the medial epicondyle of the humerus might injure the ulnar nerve, which supplies the skin of the medial side of the hand; thus, a lesion of the ulnar nerve would cause no cutaneous sensation and lack of sweating in that area. The muscles involved in abduction of the hand are the flexor carpi radialis and the extensor carpi radialis longus and brevis, which are innervated by the median and radial nerves, respectively. Carpal tunnel syndrome and thenar atrophy result from a lesion of the median nerve, whereas wrist drop results from a lesion of the radial nerve.

6. **The answer is A.** The ulnar nerve innervates the dorsal interossei, which are the only abductors of the fingers. The little finger is abducted by the abductor digiti minimi, which is innervated by the ulnar nerve. The thumb is abducted by the abductor pollicis brevis and longus, which are innervated by the median and radial nerves, respectively. The musculocutaneous and axillary nerves do not supply the hand muscles.

7. **The answer is C.** The median nerve supplies the skin on the palmar aspect of the lateral three and one-half fingers and the dorsal side of the index finger, middle finger, and one-half of the ring finger. The median nerve innervates the pronator teres and pronator quadratus muscles and the thenar muscles. The axillary and musculocutaneous nerves do not supply the skin or muscles of the hand. The radial nerve does not innervate muscles of the hand but innervates the skin of the radial side of the hand and the radial two and one-half digits over the proximal phalanx. The ulnar nerve innervates not only the palmaris brevis, hypothenar muscles, adductor pollicis, dorsal and palmar interosseous, and medial two lumbrical muscles but also the skin over the palmar and dorsal surfaces of the medial one-third of the hand and the skin of the little finger and the medial side of the ring finger.

8. **The answer is D.** The thoracodorsal nerve innervates the latissimus dorsi, which adducts, extends, and medially rotates the arm. The arm is abducted by the supraspinatus and laterally

rotated by the infraspinatus, teres minor, and deltoid (posterior part) muscles. The scapula is elevated by the trapezium and levator scapulae muscles and adducted by the rhomboid and trapezius muscles.

9. **The answer is C.** The lateral antebrachial cutaneous nerve contains sympathetic postganglionic general visceral efferent (GVE) fibers, which have cell bodies located in the sympathetic chain ganglia, and general somatic afferent (GSA) fibers, which have cell bodies located in the dorsal root ganglia. Sympathetic nerve fibers are involved in sweating, whereas GSA fibers are involved in numbness and tingling in the skin.

10. **The answer is C.** This pianist is unable to pick up a music piece between the index and middle fingers because she cannot adduct her index finger and abduct the middle finger. The adductor of the index finger is the palmar interosseous muscle, which is innervated by the ulnar nerve. Abductors of the middle finger are dorsal interosseous muscles, which are innervated by the ulnar nerve. The other nerves do not innervate adductors or abductors of the fingers.

11. **The answer is D.** The metacarpophalangeal joint of the ring finger is extended by the extensor digitorum, which is innervated by the radial nerve. This joint is flexed by the lumbrical and interossei muscles, abducted by the dorsal interosseous, and adducted by the palmar interosseous. The medial two lumbricales and both the dorsal and palmar interossei are innervated by the ulnar nerve. The median, musculocutaneous, and axillary nerves are not involved in movement of the metacarpophalangeal joint of the ring finger.

12. **The answer is A.** In Erb–Duchenne paralysis (or upper trunk injury), the nerve fibers in the roots of C5 and C6 of the brachial plexus are damaged. The infraspinatus, a lateral rotator muscle, is innervated by the suprascapular nerve (C5 and C6). All the other muscles, including the flexor carpi ulnaris, palmar interossei, adductor pollicis, and palmaris brevis muscles, are innervated by the ulnar nerve (C8 and T1).

13. **The answer is C.** In carpal tunnel syndrome, structures entering the palm deep to the flexor retinaculum are compressed; these include the median nerve and the tendons of the flexor pollicis longus, flexor digitorum profundus, and flexor digitorum superficialis muscles. The flexor carpi radialis runs lateral to the carpal tunnel and inserts on the bases of the second and third metacarpals. Structures entering the palm superficial to the flexor retinaculum include the ulnar nerve, ulnar artery, and palmaris longus tendon (which inserts on the palmar aponeurosis).

14. **The answer is B.** The anterior cruciate ligament of the knee joint prevents posterior displacement of the femur on the tibia and limits hyperextension of the knee joint. This ligament becomes taut when the knee is extended and lax when the knee is flexed. It inserts into the lateral femoral condyle posteriorly within the intercondylar notch.

15. **The answer is B.** The deep peroneal nerve innervates the dorsiflexors of the foot, which include the tibialis anterior, extensor hallucis longus, extensor digitorum longus, and peroneus tertius muscles. The plantar flexors include the triceps surae, tibialis posterior, flexor digitorum longus, and flexor hallucis longus, which are innervated by the tibial nerve, and peroneus longus and brevis, which are innervated by the superficial peroneal nerve. The toes are abducted and adducted by dorsal and plantar interosseous muscles, which are innervated by the medial and lateral plantar nerves. The foot is inverted by the tibialis anterior and posterior, triceps surae, and extensor hallucis longus, which are innervated by the tibial nerve.

16. **The answer is E.** An embolus from the deep veins of the lower limb would travel through the femoral vein, the iliac veins, the inferior vena cava, the right atrium, the right ventricle, and the pulmonary trunk and into the pulmonary arteries, where it could obstruct and occlude these vessels. If not obstructed, blood from the pulmonary artery passes to the lungs, pulmonary veins, left atrium, left ventricle, ascending aorta, and coronary arteries; to the body tissues; and then to the venous system, including the renal veins and sinusoids of the liver.

17. **The answer is A.** Flat foot is characterized by disappearance of the medial portion of the longitudinal arch, which appears completely flattened. The plantar calcaneonavicular (spring)

ligament supports the head of the talus and the medial side of the longitudinal arch. The planar calcaneocuboid (short plantar) ligament supports the lateral portion of the longitudinal arch. The other ligaments support the ankle joint.

18. **The answer is D.** The posterior cruciate ligament prevents forward displacement of the femur on the tibia when the knee is flexed. The anterior cruciate ligament prevents backward dislocation of the femur on the tibia when the knee is extended. The medial meniscus acts as a cushion, or shock absorber, and forms a more stable base for the articulation of the femoral condyle. The tibial and fibular collateral ligaments prevent medial and lateral displacement, respectively, of the two long bones.

19. **The answer is E.** The lateral longitudinal arch is formed by the calcaneus, cuboid bone, and lateral two metatarsal bones, whereas the medial longitudinal arch of the foot is formed by the talus, calcaneus, navicular bone, cuneiform bones, and medial three metatarsal bones.

20. **The answer is E.** The deep iliac circumflex artery does not supply the hip joint. However, this joint receives blood from branches of the medial and lateral femoral circumflex, superior and inferior gluteal, and obturator arteries.

21. **The answer is D.** The lateral meniscus, like the medial meniscus, lies outside the synovial cavity but within the joint cavity. However, the lateral meniscus is nearly circular, whereas the medial meniscus is C-shaped or forms a semicircle. The lateral meniscus is smaller than the medial meniscus and less frequently torn in injuries than the medial meniscus. In addition, the lateral meniscus is separated from the fibular collateral ligament by the tendon of the popliteal muscle, whereas the medial meniscus attaches to the tibial collateral ligament.

22. **The answer is C.** The ventral root of a thoracic spinal nerve contains sympathetic preganglionic fibers, which have cell bodies located in the lateral horn of the gray matter of the spinal cord, and general somatic efferent fibers, which have cell bodies located in the anterior horn of the gray matter of the spinal cord. The dorsal root ganglion contains cell bodies of GSA and general visceral afferent (GVA) fibers, and the sympathetic chain ganglion contains cell bodies of postganglionic sympathetic nerve fibers.

23. **The answer is B.** The azygos vein receives the hemiazygos and accessory hemiazygos veins and drains into the superior vena cava. The internal thoracic vein drains into the subclavian vein. The right superior intercostal vein drains into the azygos vein, and the left superior intercostal vein drains into the left brachiocephalic vein.

24. **The answer is C.** The great cardiac vein is accompanied by the anterior interventricular artery, which is a branch of the left coronary artery. The circumflex branch of the left coronary artery runs along with the coronary sinus. The right marginal artery is accompanied by the small cardiac vein, and the posterior interventricular artery is accompanied by the middle cardiac vein.

25. **The answer is B.** The right and left coronary arteries arise from the ascending aorta, and reduced blood flow in the ascending aorta causes decreased blood flow in the coronary arteries. Blockage of the pulmonary trunk or coronary sinus minimally affects blood flow in the coronary arteries. Blockage of the origin of the aortic arch or the descending aorta increases blood flow in the coronary arteries.

26. **The answer is B.** The right lymphatic duct drains the right sides of the thorax, upper limb, head, and neck, and the thoracic duct drains the rest of the body.

27. **The answer is D.** The third rib articulates with the body of the sternum rather than the manubrium. The manubrium of the sternum articulates with the body of the sternum, the first and second ribs, and the clavicle.

28. **The answer is D.** Gray rami communicantes contain postganglionic sympathetic nerve fibers but contain no other nerve fibers.

29. **The answer is B.** The dorsal root contains both GSA and GVA fibers. The sympathetic trunk contains preganglionic sympathetic fibers. The greater splanchnic nerve and white rami

communicantes contain GVA and preganglionic sympathetic fibers. The gray rami communicantes contain sympathetic postganglionic (GVE) fibers.

30. **The answer is C.** Because the anterior cardiac vein drains directly into the right atrium, its diameter is unchanged. However, all other cardiac veins drain into the coronary sinus, and they are dilated.

31. **The answer is D.** The mediastinum does not contain the lungs; it contains the thymus, esophagus, trachea, and heart.

32. **The answer is B.** The genioglossus protrudes the tongue. The hyoglossus and styloglossus muscles retract the tongue. The palatoglossus elevates the tongue. The geniohyoid elevates the hyoid bone and the floor of the mouth.

33. **The answer is D.** The pulmonary veins carry oxygenated blood, and the pulmonary artery carries deoxygenated blood. The right atrium (which contains the crista terminalis and pectinate muscle) and the right ventricle (which contains the septomarginal trabecula) carry deoxygenated blood.

34. **The answer is C.** The ulnar nerve arises from the lower trunk of the brachial plexus, which is formed by ventral primary rami of C8 and T1. Abduction of the index finger is done by the palmar interosseous muscle, which is innervated by the ulnar nerve. Lateral rotation of the arm is performed by the deltoid and teres minor muscles, which are innervated by the axillary nerve. The ring finger is extended by the extensor digitorum, which is innervated by the radial nerve. The forearm is flexed by the biceps brachii and brachialis muscles, which are innervated by the musculocutaneous nerve. Pronator teres and pronator quadratus muscles, which pronate the forearm, are innervated by the median nerve.

35. **The answer is C.** The cardinal ligament provides the major support for the uterus. Therefore, the weakness of the cardinal ligament may result in uterine prolapse. The transversalis fascia, ovarian ligament, arcuate pubic ligament, and piriformis muscles do not support the uterus.

36. **The answer is A.** An indirect inguinal hernia occurs lateral to the inferior epigastric vessels, whereas a direct inguinal hernia arises medial to these vessels. The other statements are not related to the indirect inguinal hernia.

37. **The answer is B.** The vagus nerve supplies parasympathetic fibers to the thoracic and abdominal viscera, including the transverse colon. The descending colon, sigmoid colon, prostate, rectum, and other pelvic viscera are innervated by the pelvic splanchnic nerves.

38. **The answer is C.** The bile duct traverses the head of the pancreas; thus, a tumor located there could compress this structure. The duodenojejunal junction comes into contact with the tip of the uncinate process and the interior portion of the body of the pancreas. The other structures are not closely associated with the head of the pancreas.

39. **The answer is C.** The arterial supply to the pancreas is from both the celiac trunk and superior mesenteric artery. Other organs, including the liver, spleen, gallbladder, and stomach, receive blood from the celiac trunk.

40. **The answer is C.** The superior rectal vein is part of the portal venous system. All the other veins belong to the systemic (caval) venous system.

41. **The answer is C.** Hirschsprung disease (congenital megacolon) is abnormal dilatation of the lower colon proximal to the inactive segment and caused by the absence of enteric ganglia (parasympathetic postganglionic neuron cell bodies) in the myenteric plexus in the wall of the colon due to the failure of neural crest cells to migrate into the walls of the hindgut or colon. Abnormal rotation of the hindgut as they return to the abdominal cavity can cause volvulus or strangulation (twisting) of the gut. Abnormal formation of the urorectal septum or deficient (incomplete) separation of the cloaca results in anal agenesis.

42. **The answer is C.** The deep perineal space contains a segment of the dorsal nerve of the penis in males. The deep perineal space is bounded superiorly by the superior fascia and inferiorly

by the inferior fascia (perineal membrane) of the urogenital diaphragm. The superficial transverse perineal muscles and the greater vestibular glands are found in the superficial perineal space. The Colles fascia is the deep membranous layer of the superficial perineal fascia and forms the inferior boundary of the superficial perineal space.

43. **The answer is C.** The ileum is the most common site of Meckel diverticulum, which is located on the antimesenteric border of the ileum. This fingerlike pouch (diverticulum) is the remnant of the proximal portion of the embryonic yolk stalk (vitelline duct), which may be connected to the inner surface of the umbilicus via a fibrous cord or fistula. The other digestive organs are not associated with the development of the Meckel diverticulum.

44. **The answer is B.** The inferior hypogastric (pelvic) plexus contains preganglionic parasympathetic fibers from the pelvic splanchnic nerves. The lumbar and sacral splanchnic nerves and the sacral sympathetic chain ganglia contain preganglionic sympathetic fibers. The vagus nerve does not supply parasympathetic nerve fibers to the pelvic organs.

45. **The answer is B.** The urinary bladder receives parasympathetic fibers from the pelvic splanchnic nerve, not the vagus nerve. The greater, lesser, lumbar, and sacral splanchnic nerves contain sympathetic preganglionic fibers.

46. **The answer is C.** Carcinoma of the uterus can spread directly to the labium majus through the lymphatics that follow the round ligament of the uterus. This ligament extends from the uterus, enters the inguinal canal at the deep inguinal ring, emerges from the superficial inguinal ring, and merges with the subcutaneous tissue of the labium majus. The other ligaments do not reach the labium majus.

47. **The answer is C.** The iliohypogastric nerve does not supply the scrotum. The scrotum is innervated by the anterior scrotal branch of the ilioinguinal nerve, the genital branch of the genitofemoral nerve, the posterior scrotal branch of the perineal branch of the pudendal nerve, and the perineal branch of the posterior femoral cutaneous nerve.

48. **The answer is C.** Although the pubic crest forms a part of the pelvic inlet (pelvic brim), it does not contribute to the formation of the pubic outlet. The pelvic outlet (lower pelvic aperture) is bounded posteriorly by the sacrum and coccyx; laterally by the ischial tuberosities and sacrotuberous ligaments; and anteriorly by the pubic symphysis, the arcuate ligament, and the rami of the pubis and ischium.

49. **The answer is A.** Compared with the male pelvis, the female pelvis is characterized by presence of the oval inlet, larger outlet, larger pubic angle, shorter and wider sacrum, and wider and shallower cavity.

50. **The answer is E.** The cauda equina is formed by dorsal and ventral roots of the lumbar and sacral spinal nerves. Thus, it is crushed at the level of the L5 vertebra, whereas the other structures are not. The vertebral artery, which arises from the subclavian artery, ascends through the transverse foramina of the upper six cervical vertebrae. The spinal cord ends at the level of the L2 vertebra. The filum terminale externus (filum of the dura) extends from the apex of the dura at the level of the S2 vertebra to the dorsum of the coccyx. The denticulate ligament, a lateral extension of the pia between the dorsal and ventral roots of the spinal nerves, consists of 21 pairs of processes, the last one lying between the T12 and L1 spinal nerves.

51. **The answer is C.** The suboccipital nerve supplies the suboccipital muscles, including the rectus capitis posterior major. The dorsal primary rami of the spinal nerves innervate the deep muscles of the back, including the splenius capitis and iliocostalis muscles. The spinal accessory nerve innervates the trapezius muscle, and the dorsal scapular nerve innervates the levator scapulae muscle; these are the superficial muscles of the back.

52. **The answer is C.** To obtain cerebrospinal fluid (CSF) contained in the subarachnoid space, the needle should penetrate the dura mater and arachnoid mater. The denticulate ligament, pia mater, annulus fibrosus, and nucleus pulposus should not be penetrated during a lumbar puncture.

53. **The answer is D.** The levator scapulae are attached to the transverse processes of the upper cervical vertebrae. All of the other muscles are attached to the spinous processes.

54. **The answer is B.** The transverse cervical nerve innervates the skin over the anterior cervical triangle; the great auricular nerve innervates the skin behind the auricle and over the parotid gland. The ansa cervicalis innervates the infrahyoid muscles, including the sternohyoid, sternothyroid, and omohyoid muscles. The superior laryngeal nerve divides into the internal laryngeal nerve, which supplies sensory fibers to the larynx above the vocal cord, and the external laryngeal nerve, which supplies the cricothyroid and inferior pharyngeal constrictor muscles.

55. **The answer is D.** The common carotid artery normally bifurcates into the external and internal carotid arteries at the level of the superior border of the thyroid cartilage. The thyroid isthmus crosses the second and third tracheal rings. The cricoid cartilage is at the level of CV6, and its lower border marks the end of the pharynx and larynx. The sternal angle is at the level of the intervertebral disk between TV4 and TV5, where the aortic arch begins and ends. The jugular notch is at the level of TV3.

56. **The answer is D.** The lateral pterygoid muscle is paralyzed because it inserts on the articular disk and capsule of the temporomandibular joint. The temporalis muscle inserts on the coronoid process, and the medial pterygoid and masseter muscles insert on the medial and lateral surfaces of the ramus and angle of the mandible, respectively. The buccinator muscle inserts into the orbicularis oris at the angle of the mouth.

57. **The answer is C.** Damage to the oculomotor nerve results in ptosis (drooping) of the eyelid because the levator palpebrae superioris is innervated by the oculomotor nerve. The trochlear nerve innervates the superior oblique, and the abducens nerve innervates the lateral rectus. The oculomotor nerve innervates the remaining ocular muscles. The facial nerve innervates the orbicularis oculi, which functions to close the eyelids.

58. **The answer is A.** The superior petrosal sinus lies in the margin of the tentorium cerebelli. The falx cerebri contains the inferior and superior sagittal sinuses, and the falx cerebelli encloses the occipital sinus. The diaphragma sellae forms the dural roof of the sella turcica. The straight sinus runs along the line of attachment of the falx cerebri and tentorium cerebelli.

59. **The answer is A.** Arachnoid granulations are tuftlike collections of highly folded arachnoid that project into the superior sagittal sinus and the lateral lacunae, which are lateral extensions of the superior sagittal sinus. They absorb the CSF into dural sinuses and often produce erosion or pitting of the inner surface of the calvaria. The CSF is produced in the ventricles of the brain.

60. **The answer is E.** The great cerebral vein of Galen and the inferior sagittal sinus unite to form the straight sinus.

61. **The answer is B.** The tendon of the tensor veli palatini curves around the pterygoid hamulus to insert on the soft palate. The tensor tympani inserts on the handle of the malleus, the levator veli palatini inserts on the soft palate, the superior pharyngeal constrictor inserts on the median raphe and the pharyngeal tubercle, and the stylohyoid inserts on the body of the hyoid.

62. **The answer is C.** The pterygomandibular raphe serves as a common origin for the superior pharyngeal constrictor and buccinator muscles. None of the other choices are involved with the pterygomandibular raphe.

63. **The answer is D.** The tensor veli palatini is innervated by the trigeminal nerve, the levator veli palatini and palatoglossus are innervated by the vagus nerve, the cricothyroid is innervated by the external laryngeal branch of the superior laryngeal nerve, and the geniohyoid muscle is innervated by the first cervical nerve through the hypoglossal nerve.

64. **The answer is E.** The mylohyoid muscle indents the submandibular gland and divides it into superficial and deep parts. The deep portion of the gland is located between the mylohyoid muscle laterally and the hyoglossus and styloglossus muscles medially. Posteriorly, the gland lies against the posterior digastric and stylohyoid muscles.

65. **The answer is B.** The auditory (eustachian) tube connects the nasopharynx with the middle ear cavity. The vestibule and semicircular canals are parts of the inner ear. The external ear and inner ear communicate with the nasopharynx.

66. **The answer is D.** The action of the lateral pterygoid muscles opens the jaws. The medial pterygoid, masseter, and temporalis muscles are involved in closing the jaws. The buccinator presses the cheek to keep it taut.

67. **The answer is C.** Parasympathetic preganglionic fibers in the lesser petrosal nerve enter the otic ganglion where they synapse, and postganglionic parasympathetic fibers join the auriculotemporal nerve to supply the parotid gland for secretion of saliva. The other conditions are not caused by a lesion of the lesser petrosal nerve.

68. **The answer is D.** The musculus uvulae are innervated by the vagus nerve. A lesion of the vagus nerve results in deviation of the uvula toward the opposite side of the injury. An injury of the right vagus nerve causes paralysis of the right uvular muscle, which means that the uvula deviates toward the left. A lesion of the hypoglossal nerve causes deviation of the tongue toward the injured side on protrusion. A lesion of the trigeminal nerve (mandibular division) causes paralysis of the mastication muscles.

69. **The answer is D.** The superior thyroid artery does not supply the palatine tonsil. The palatine tonsil receives blood from the lesser palatine branch of the maxillary artery, the ascending palatine branch of the facial artery, the dorsal lingual branches of the lingual artery, and the ascending pharyngeal artery.

70. **The answer is D.** The parasympathetic secretomotor fibers for mucous glands in the nasal cavity run in the facial nerve, the greater petrosal nerve, the nerve of the pterygoid canal, and the pterygopalatine ganglion. The lesser petrosal nerve contains parasympathetic preganglionic fibers for the parotid gland. The facial nerve in the facial canal contains parasympathetic fibers for submandibular and sublingual salivary glands but not for nasal mucosal glands. The superior cervical ganglion and the deep petrosal nerve contain sympathetic postganglionic nerve cell bodies and/or fibers, which supply blood vessels in the lacrimal gland and the nasal and palate mucosa.

71. **The answer is C.** Tethered cord syndrome is frequently associated with meningomyelocele or intraspinal lipomatous growth. Meningomyelocele is a protrusion of the spinal cord and the meninges through the unfused arch of the vertebra. Spinal bifida occulta is a condition caused by failure of the vertebral arch to fuse, with no protrusion of the spinal cord and the meninges. Kyphosis is an abnormal accentuation of lumbar curvature. Herniated disk represents a protrusion of the nucleus pulposus through the annulus fibrosus of the intervertebral disk into the intervertebral foramen or into the vertebral canal, compressing the spinal nerve roots. Scoliosis is a lateral deviation of the spine resulting from unequal growth of the vertebral column.

72. **The answer is D.** The quadratus femoris muscles—the flexors of the thigh—are innervated by the femoral nerve, which originates from the spinal cord at L2 to L4. In contrast, the hamstring muscles—the extensors of the thigh—are innervated by the sciatic nerve, which originates from L4 to S3. Therefore, the lesion occurs at the level of L5 (between L4 and S3).

73. **The answer is B.** The median nerve enters the palm of the hand through the carpal tunnel deep to the flexor retinaculum, giving off a muscular branch (recurrent branch) to the thenar muscles, including the abductor pollicis brevis, flexor pollicis brevis, and opponens pollicis. The ulnar nerve enters the hand superficial to the flexor retinaculum and lateral to the pisiform bone, supplying the hypothenar muscles and adductor pollicis. The patient can adduct his thumb but not oppose it. Therefore, the median nerve is injured. The radial nerve and the anterior and posterior interosseous nerves do not supply the muscle that opposes the thumb.

74. **The answer is B.** The tibial nerve innervates the triceps surae, plantaris, and posterior tibialis, which plantar flex; innervates the flexor digitorum longus and brevis, flexor hallucis longus and brevis, and flexor digiti minimi brevis, which flex toes; and supplies sensory innervation on the sole of the foot. The common peroneal nerve divides into the deep peroneal nerve, which

innervates muscles of the anterior compartment that dorsiflex the foot, and the superficial peroneal nerve, which innervates the peroneus longus and brevis that dorsiflex the foot. The saphenous nerve is a cutaneous nerve and does not supply the muscles.

75. **The answer is C.** Lung cancer in the apex of the lung compresses the cervical sympathetic trunk and stellate ganglion, causing ptosis, miosis, enophthalmos, and anhidrosis, which are symptoms of Horner syndrome. Injury of the other nerves does not cause ptosis, miosis, enophthalmos, or anhidrosis.

76. **The answer is D.** The ulnar nerve supplies sensation to the fourth and fifth digits and innervates the hypothenar muscles, the dorsal interosseous muscles that abduct the fingers, and the medial half of the flexor digitorum profundus (to the ring and little fingers or fourth and fifth digits) that flexes the distal interphalangeal joints. Claw hand is a condition in which the ring and little fingers are hyperextended at the metacarpophalangeal joints and flexed at the interphalangeal joints. The axillary and anterior interosseous nerves do not supply the hand. Injury to the radial nerve results in wrist drop. Injury to the median nerve causes an ape hand (flattening of the thenar eminence).

77. **The answer is D.** The long thoracic nerve innervates the serratus anterior muscle. Paralysis of this muscle causes a "winged scapula," in which the vertebral or medial border and inferior angle of the scapula protrude away from the thorax. Other nerves do not supply the serratus anterior muscle.

78. **The answer is C.** The medial brachial cutaneous nerve supplies the skin on the medial aspect of the arm. The axillary nerve supplies the skin of the lateral side of the arm. The musculocutaneous nerve supplies the lateral side of the forearm as the lateral antebrachial cutaneous nerve. The medial antebrachial cutaneous nerve supplies the medial aspect of the forearm. The radial nerve gives off the posterior brachial and posterior antebrachial cutaneous nerves.

79. **The answer is D.** The internal thoracic or internal mammary artery arises from the subclavian artery. Other arteries do not give rise to the internal thoracic artery. The superior epigastric artery is a branch of the internal thoracic artery.

80. **The answer is C.** The recurrent laryngeal nerve runs behind the thyroid gland in a groove between the trachea and esophagus and is vulnerable to injury during thyroidectomy. This nerve innervates all of the laryngeal muscles, except the cricothyroid muscle, which is innervated by the external laryngeal nerve. The internal laryngeal nerve is sensory to the larynx above the vocal cord. The hypoglossal and glossopharyngeal nerves do not supply the larynx and are not closely associated with the thyroid gland.

81. **The answer is C.** Thyroglossal duct cyst results from the incomplete obliteration of the duct through which the thyroid gland migrates to the root of the neck. Inferior parathyroid glands and the thymus migrate in the neck lateral to the thyroglossal duct. The tongue and submandibular glands form and remain in the floor of the primitive mouth.

82. **The answer is B.** The middle ear cavity develops from pharyngeal pouch 1. Pharyngeal groove 1 forms the external auditory canal; auricular hillocks form the auricle; pharyngeal membrane 1 forms the tympanic membrane; and pharyngeal pouch 2 forms the crypts of the palatine tonsil.

83. **The answer is B.** The lunate bone articulates with the radius and triquetrum.

84. **The answer is C.** The hook of the hamate provides attachment for the flexor digiti minimi brevis and opponens digiti minimi muscles. Therefore, its fracture may cause paralysis of these muscles.

85. **The answer is E.** The base of the proximal phalanx of the thumb is the site of attachment for the flexor pollicis brevis, which, along with the opponens pollicis, forms the thenar eminence. It is also the site of attachment for the adductor pollicis brevis.

86. **The answer is D.** The middle phalanx of the ring finger is the site of attachment for the flexor digitorum superficialis.

87. **The answer is A.** The scaphoid bone forms the floor of the anatomic snuffbox, and its fracture may cause a deep tenderness. When fractured, the proximal fragment may undergo avascular necrosis because the blood supply is interrupted.

88. **The answer is D.** The left renal vein receives the left testicular vein.

89. **The answer is A.** The gallbladder receives bile and concentrates and stores it.

90. **The answer is E.** The superior mesenteric artery gives off the middle colic artery.

91. **The answer is C.** The kidney produces and excretes urine.

92. **The answer is B.** The right suprarenal vein drains into the inferior vena cava. However, the left renal vein receives the left suprarenal vein.

93. **The answer is D.** The uterine cervix is the common site of uterine cancer.

94. **The answer is B.** The ureter descends retroperitoneally on the psoas muscle in the abdomen and runs under the uterine artery in the pelvis.

95. **The answer is C.** The rectum returns its venous blood to the portal vein via the superior rectal vein and to the inferior vena cava (caval or systemic venous system) via the middle and inferior rectal veins.

96. **The answer is A.** The detrusor muscle in the wall of the bladder is innervated by sympathetic nerves.

97. **The answer is E.** The iliacus muscle, together with the psoas major muscle, inserts on the lesser trochanter.

98. **The answer is E.** The margin of the rectus abdominis forms the medial boundary of the inguinal triangle.

99. **The answer is C.** The prostate gland secretes a fluid that produces the characteristic odor of semen.

100. **The answer is B.** The seminal colliculus or verumontanum of the prostatic urethra receives the ejaculatory duct.

101. **The answer is A.** The frontal sinus opens into the hiatus semilunaris of the middle nasal meatus by way of the frontonasal duct or infundibulum.

102. **The answer is E.** The superior orbital fissure transmits the ophthalmic vein, trochlear nerve, and other structures.

Index

Note: Page locators followed by "f" and "t" indicate figures and tables, respectively.

A

B

D

F

J

K

L

M

N

Q

T

U

V

W

X

Z